Audiologists' Desk Reference

VOLUME 1

Diagnostic Audiology Principles, Procedures, and Protocols

A Singular Audiology Text
Jeffrey L. Danhauer, Ph.D.
Audiology Editor

Audiologists' Desk Reference

VOLUME 1

Diagnostic Audiology Principles, Procedures, and Protocols

James W. Hall, III, Ph.D.
Division of Hearing and Speech Sciences
and
Department of Otolaryngology
School of Medicine
Vanderbilt University
Nashville, Tennessee

H. Gustav Mueller, III, Ph.D.
University of Northern Colorado
Greeley, Colorado
and
Division of Hearing and Speech Sciences
School of Medicine
Vanderbilt University
Nashville, Tennessee

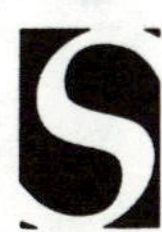

Singular Publishing Group, Inc.
San Diego · London

Singular Publishing Group, Inc.
401 West "A" Street, Suite 325
San Diego, California 92101-7904

19 Compton Terrace
London N1 2UN, U.K.

Typeset in 10/12 Times by So Cal Graphics
Printed in the United States of America by McNaughton and Gunn

Library of Congress Cataloging-in-Publication Data

Hall, James W. (James Wilbur), 1948–
Audiologists' desk reference : diagnostic audiology principles and procedures / James W. Hall III and H. Gustav Mueller III.
p. cm.
Includes index.
"A Singular audiology text."
ISBN 1-56593-269-2 (v. 1)
1. Audiometry—Handbooks, manuals, etc. 2. Hearing disorders—Diagnosis—Handbooks, manuals, etc. 3. Hearing disorders in children—Diagnosis—Handbooks, manuals, etc. I. Mueller, H. Gustav. II. Title.
[DNLM: 1. Audiometry—handbooks. 2. Hearing Disorder—handbooks.
WV 39 H177a 1996]
RF294.H32 1996
617.8—dc20
DNLM/DLC
for Library of Congress

96-28454
CIP

Contents

How To Use *The ADR* Volume I

"That book is good
Which puts me in a working mood.
Unless to Thought is added Will, Apollo is an imbecile."

Fragments on the Poetic Gift
Ralph Waldo Emerson (1803–1882)

Rare is the person who will pick the *Audiologist's Desk Reference* (ADR) up and read it from cover to cover. The ADR is, as the title clearly implies, a *reference*, that is, a repository of information which one will consult, hopefully often. What kind of information you might ask? The audiologically-important facts and details you vaguely recall learning in graduate school, or reading sometime in a journal article, but can't quite remember precisely when you need them most. The facts and details you will find in this book are practical and useful, because the ADR is a clinical book, written by we clinicians for you clinicians.

"Life being short, and the quiet hours of it few,
we ought to waste none of them in reading valueless books".

Sesame and Lilies (1865)
John Ruskin (1819–1900)

What you're looking for in the ADR should be easy to find. Just consult the topical summary of contents at the beginning of each chapter. Or look up the topic in the index. You might even flip through any of the many chapters covering the broad scope of clinical audiology from diagnostic test procedures and protocols, including ECochG, ABR, OAE, CAPD, and vestibular assessment. And there's the always hard-to-find normative test data for neonates, children, and adults. Setting up a newborn hearing screening program and looking for a review of the educational and economic rationale for early identification of hearing impairment in young children? It's in the ADR. No need to worry about making a trip to the library or borrowing your friendly physician's books, as we incorporated in the ADR essential medical information from syndromes to CT scans to clinical pharmacology.

"In science, read, by preference, the newest works; in literature, the
oldest. The classic literature is always modern".

Caxtonia. Hints on Mental Culture
Edward Bulwer-Lytton, Baron Lytton (1803–1873)

Hungry for some audiologic inspiration after a long day in the clinic, or just plain curious to know whether Georg von Bekesy ever got married, and if not why not? Read any of the numerous biographical sketches, and examine the photographs, of important personages in audiology and hearing science, from Hallowell Davis to Marion Downs.

But wait . . . . There's more!

ADR Volume II will be also consulted every day by the practicing audiologist. In it, we summarize everything you need to know about hearing aids and current hearing aid fitting strategies. From hearing conservation to auditory rehabilitation, all the important facts and concepts are here in a handy and fun-to-read format. Volume II concludes with an comprehensive glossary of audiologic and medical terminology.

> "Affect not as some do that bookish ambition to be stored with books and have well-furnished libraries, yet keep their heads empty of knowledge; to desire to have many books, and never use them, is like a child that will have a candle burning by him all the while he is sleeping"
>
> *The Compleat Gentleman* (1622)
> **Henry Peacham (c. 1576–c.1643)**

Become aquainted with all the friendly features of the ADR—Clinical Concepts, Technical Tips, Lists, Protocols, Tables, Historic Reverberations, and the occasional Audioid. We hope that you keep the ADR handy and use it regularly!

James W. Hall III dedicates the ADR Volume I to:

James F. Jerger
Mentor, Teacher, Colleague, and Friend
and to
Missy Hall
who 25 years ago didn't realize she was also marrying audiology.

To all the interns, residents, graduate students, and rookie audiologists who, for the past 25 years, have continually asked "Can you tell me where I can find __________ ? Thanks for your persistence, I finally have a simple answer: It's in *The Book!* **HGM**

CHAPTER 1

Principles of Auditory Science

In This ADR Chapter

Perspective

"Whoever, in the pursuit of science, seeks after immediate practical utility, may generally rest assured that he will seek in vain. All that science can achieve is a perfect knowledge and a perfect understanding of the action of natural and moral forces."

Hermann Ludwig Ferdinand von Helmholtz (1821–1894)
Academic Discourse, Heidelberg

Audiology is built on a foundation of physical, biologic, and social sciences. Everyday audiologic practice taps knowledge from a variety of academic disciplines, among them mathematics, physics, psychology (and psychophysics), general and neurobiology, chemistry, and computer science. The fund of scientific knowledge necessary for a career in clinical audiology should be acquired during years of formal study before the first patient is seen. This ADR chapter barely scrapes the surface of this essential information. What follows herein are simply some of the facts, figures, and principles of auditory science which are important in clinical audiology, yet may occasionally elude the recollection of audiologists.

FOUNDATIONS OF AUDITORY SCIENCE

Classic Quote

ALBERT EINSTEIN on science

"The whole of science is nothing more than a refinement of everyday thinking."

Albert Einstein
Physics and Reality, 1936.

Anatomic Directions and Terms for Description of the Orientation of Structures

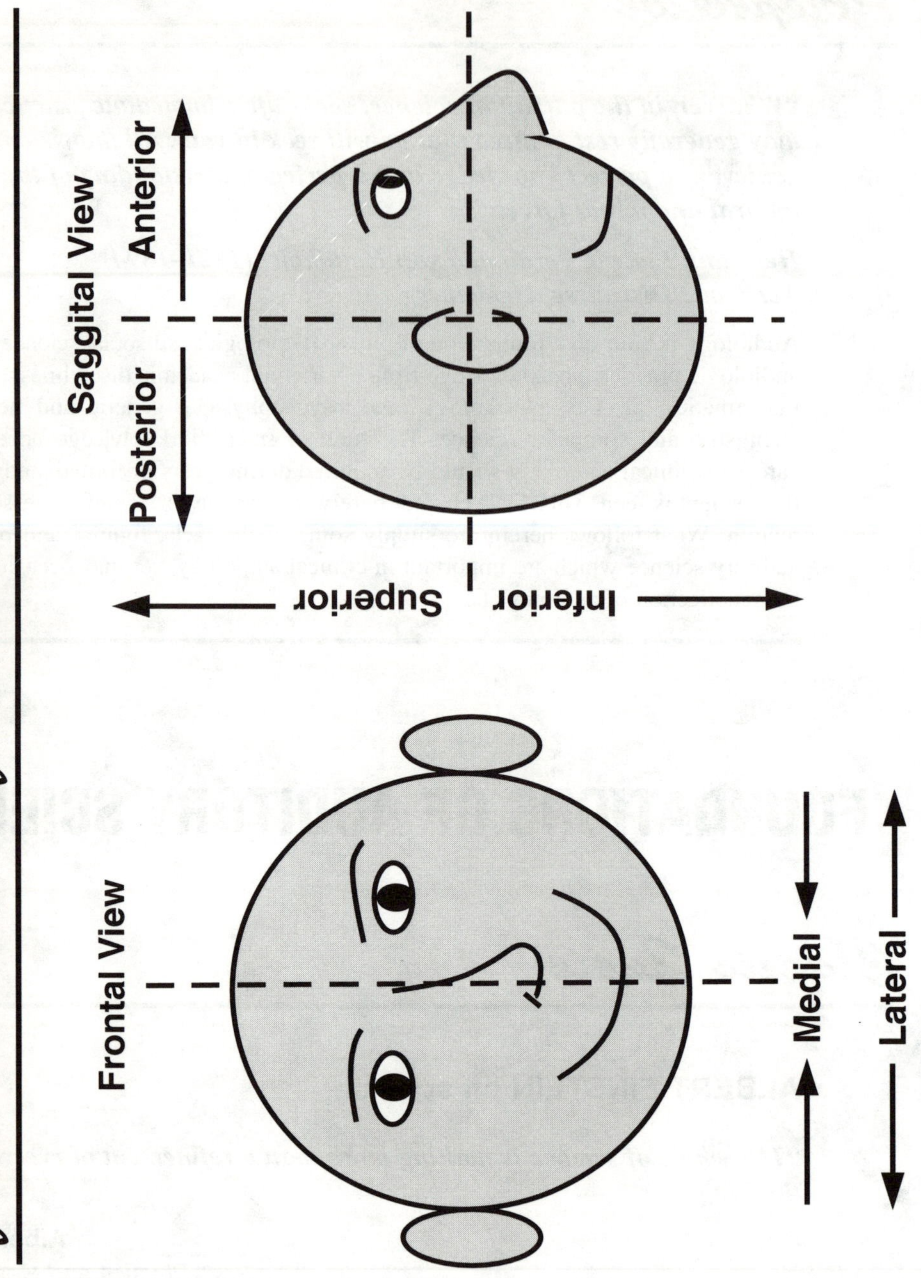

Systems in the Body

A system consists of two or more organs that are functionally related. The 11 systems in the body (with the corresponding medical specialties) are:

- **skeletal:** bones and related cartilages (orthopedics or osteology)
- **articular:** joints and ligaments (rheumatology)
- **muscular:** tissues that work on systems 1 and 2 (sports medicine)
- **digestive:** digestive tract (stomach, intestines, and related structures including glands [gastroenterology]
- **vascular:** heart and blood vessels and lymphatic system (cardiology)
- **nervous:** peripheral and central nervous system, with associated nerves, ganglia, and sense organs (neurology, neurosurgery, audiology, otolaryngology, ophthalmology)
- **respiratory:** lungs and air passageways (pulmonary medicine)
- **urinary:** kidneys and urinary passages (nephrology and urology)
- **reproductive:** organs of reproduction (gynecology and urology)
- **endocrine:** ductless (endocrine) glands in the body (e.g., pituitary, thyroid, parathyroid, adrenal) which produce internal secretions (e.g., hormones) into blood or lymph (endocrinology)
- **integumentary:** skin, nails, hair (dermatology)

Classic Quote

Georg von Bekesy on Hearing Research

"One of the most important features of scientific research is the detection of errors. The writer believes that positive results and failures ought to be discussed together. Only by such complete reporting can we get a true conception of a piece of work, of the manner of its development, and of the limitations of its principles.

"One way of discovering errors is to repeat the same measurements by different methods . . . A way of avoiding errors is to work as a team. The several members of a team can supplement one another's skills and check the procedures. In team research, however, it often happens that the dull, routine work is left to the younger members and not checked by the more experienced."

"Another way of dealing with errors is to have friends who are willing to spend the time necessary to carry out a critical examination of the experimental design beforehand and the results after the experiments have been completed. An even better way is to have an enemy. An enemy is willing to devote a vast amount of time and brain power to ferreting out errors both large and small, and this without compensation. The trouble is that really capable enemies are scarce; most of them are only ordinary. Another trouble with enemies is that they sometimes develop into friends and lose a good deal of their zeal. It was in this way that the writer lost his three best enemies."

Source: Georg von Bekesy. *Experiments in Hearing.* New York: McGraw-Hill Book Company, 1960, pp. 7–9.

Historical Reverberation

Georg von Bekesy (1899–1972)

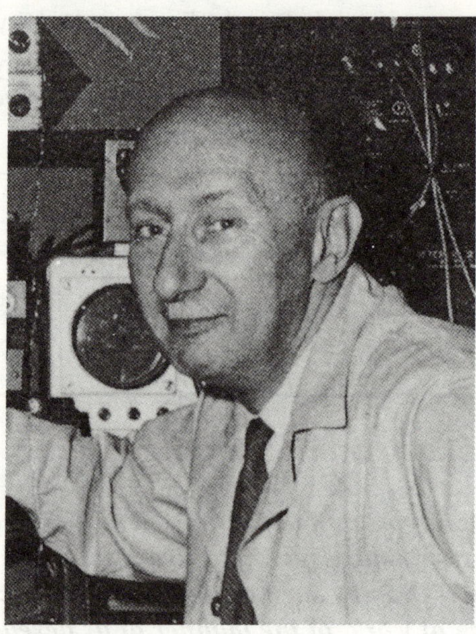

Georg von Bekesy

Georg von Bekesy is dead at the age of 73—the community of auditory scientists has lost its most distinguished member. Those of us who were close to his work feel an emptiness, as if a personal friend had departed. So much contemporary research depends on his contributions that his absence appears almost inconceivable. Yet, it is true, and we are left to pursue our efforts without the help of his continued discoveries.

Von Bekesy began his life in Budapest on 3 June 1899, the son of an Hungarian diplomat. His early years took him to Munich, Constantinople, and Zurich where he finished his secondary education, and to Bern where he studied chemistry. Returning to Hungary, he obtained a Ph.D. in Physics from the University of Budapest in 1923. He remained in Budapest until 1946, except for a short interlude at Siemens and Halske in Berlin—then a center of communication technology. During this whole period, he worked at the Royal Hungarian Institute for Research in Telegraphy and, during part of it, held the chair of Experimental Physics at the University of Budapest. It was then that he made his most important contributions to our knowledge of hearing and of the auditory system and received his first awards—the Denker Prize in Otology, the Leibnitz Medal of the "Akademie der Wissenschaften" in Berlin, the Guyol Prize for Speech and Otology from Groningen University, and the Academic Award of the Hungarian Academy of Science.

Von Bekesy was the first man able to see how the minuscule cochlea, the seat of the auditory sense cells, responded to sound. First on models of the cochlea, later on preparations of temporal bones and even in the ears of live animals, he observed an unexpected pattern of traveling waves. It is almost unbelievable that, after all the theorizing in the 19th century and the beginning of the 20th, a pattern was left that had not been described previously. But von Bekesy discovered it, and it was explained only ex post facto with the help of physical constants he determined.

A feature of the pattern did confirm an earlier prediction. It was von Helmholtz's hypothesis that every tone produced a local vibration maximum along the cochlear spiral, and that the location of this maximum moved from the apex of the spiral to its base when the sound frequency was increased from low to high. Von Bekesy also found that the location of the maximum and the subjective pitch obeyed nearly the same function of sound frequency, strengthening another hypothesis of von Helmholtz.

The continuity of thought between von Helmholtz and von Bekesy is highly significant, and one might say that von Bekesy began where von Helmholtz had left off. As von Helmholtz's work dominated auditory research during the last half of the 19th century and somewhat beyond, Bekesy's investigations did the same for at least 50 years of the century. However, their approach to science differed radically. Whereas von Helmholtz's forte had lain in theoretical inference, his successor excelled in ingenious experimentation. When von Bekesy took over, an era of dominant speculation ended and gave way to empiricism.

Having uncovered the mode of sound propagation in the cochlea and clarified the mechanisms of sound transmission to the cochlea, von Bekesy began to investigate how mechanical vibration was transduced into nerve impulses. However, this happened later, after he had left Hungary because of events that developed in middle Europe after World War II. He first stopped in Stockholm at the invitation of the Caroline Institute and worked in the Department of Telegraphy and Telephony of the Royal Institute of Technology. Here he invented a new psychophysical method and devised an automatic audiometer to go with it. Both are widely used in clinical hearing testing and auditory research.

After a year in Stockholm, von Bekesy moved on to the Psycho-acoustic Laboratory at Harvard University, where he held the special title of a Senior Research Fellow in Psychophysics. He remained in this position until 1966, when he moved to Honolulu to become Professor of Sensory Sciences at the University of Hawaii. At Harvard, the emphasis of his work gradually shifted from mechanics of the ear to electrophysiology and, later, to other sense modalities, especially the sense of touch. It was during this time that the recognition of his work reached its peak. He received doctoral degrees honoris causa from several countries, and many scientific awards, among them the Gold Medal of the Acoustical Society.

Perhaps von Bekesy's biophysical experiments on the cochlea are his most important contribution to science—they won him the 1961 Nobel Prize for Physiology or Medicine. But the greatness of his work is reflected equally in its vast scope and its systematic organization around key problems. His experiments range from acoustics through anatomy and physiology to psychophysics. Although most of them deal with hearing, they also invade the senses of touch, sight, smell, and taste. But it is was not diversity that von Bekesy sought. On the contrary, he was after unity. He discovered great similarities between the senses of touch and hearing and thought that the enhancement of contrasts in sensory stimuli was a general sensory property produced by fundamentally the same physiological process of neural inhibition.

To accomplish as much as he did, von Bekesy had to devote almost his entire life to science. He arrived at the laboratory early in the morning and returned after dinner. He remained a bachelor, feeling that marriage would distract him too much from his work. But he was not a recluse. On the contrary, he liked the company of people with whom he could talk about subjects other than science, especially art. Art was von Bekesy's second love. He collected paintings, sculpture, china, and beautiful old books. They came from various countries and various periods. The diversity of his collections matched the diversity of his scientific interests. But he did not collect superficially. To him, every object of art seemed to be associated with its history and the technique that produced it. It also seemed to evoke a specific sensory effect that linked a purely aesthetic enjoyment to scientific curiosity.

Von Bekesy died of a long and painful ailment that led to one of his last articles, entitled: "Localization of Visceral Pain and other Sensations before and after Anesthesia."

He shall never be forgotten!

Source: Obituary written by J. J. Zwislocki, Laboratory of Sensory Communication, Syracuse University and published in *Journal of the Acoustical Society of America*, 1972.

ANATOMY AND PHYSIOLOGY OF THE AUDITORY SYSTEM

The Temporal Bone

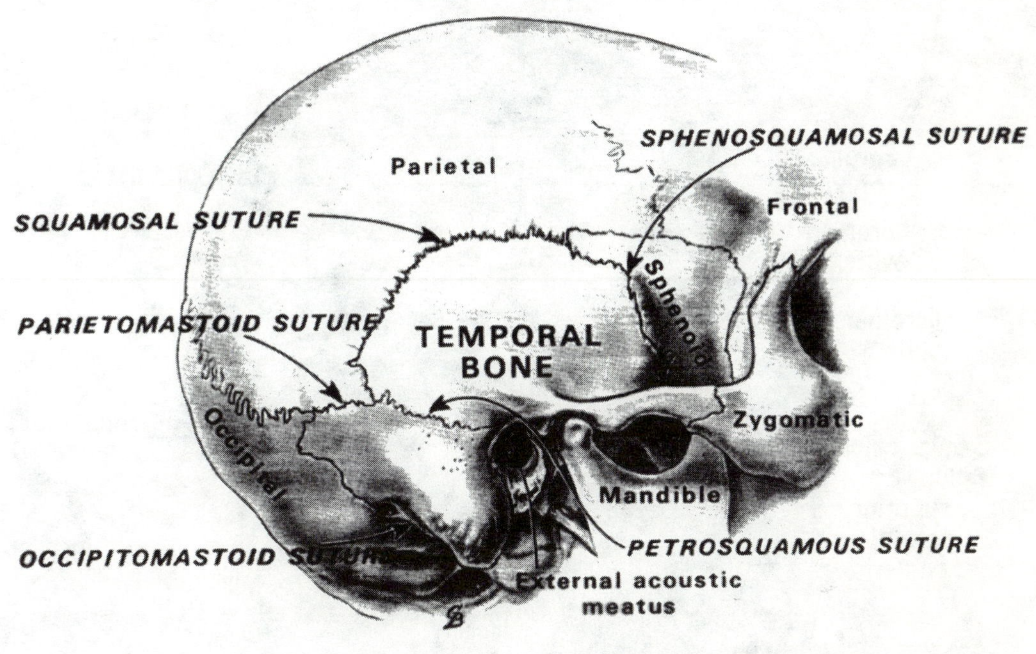

The Skull Base

View from above showing foramen (openings through the skull), the anterior, middle, and posterior fossa (depressions), and the exit/entrance sites of some cranial nerves

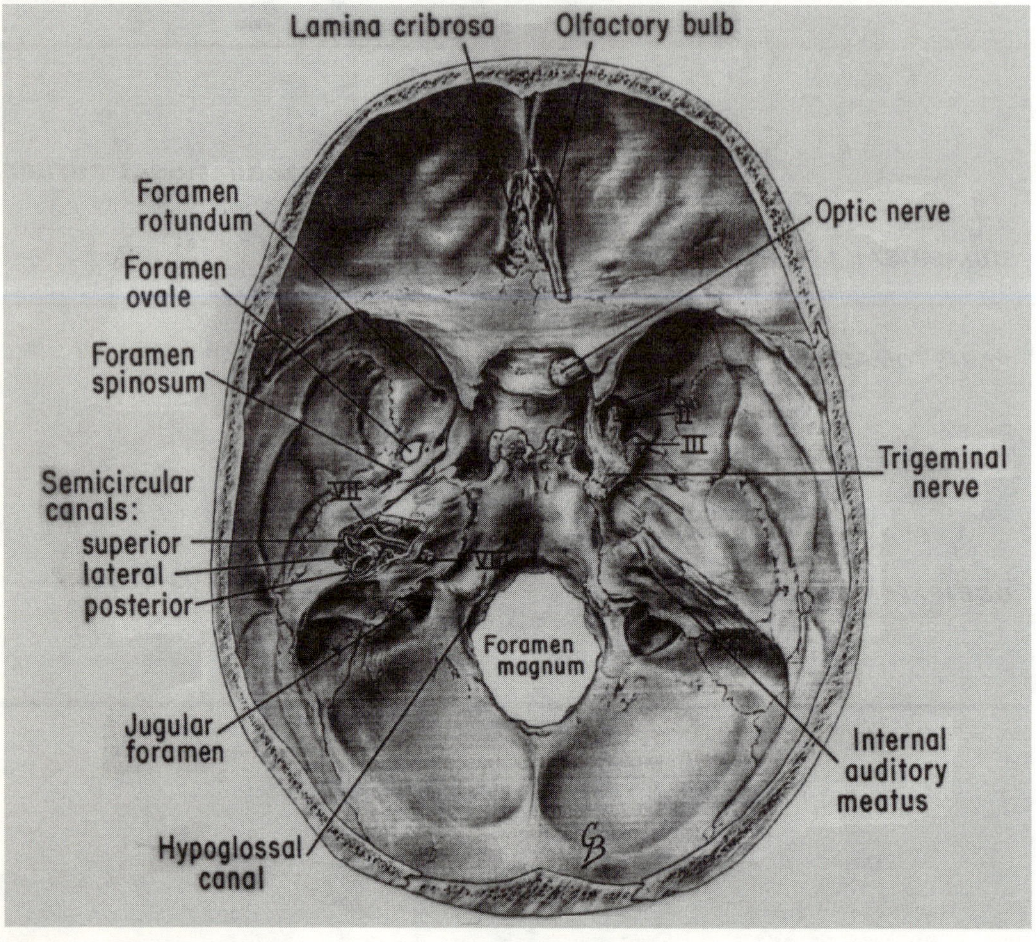

Anatomic Features of the External Ear

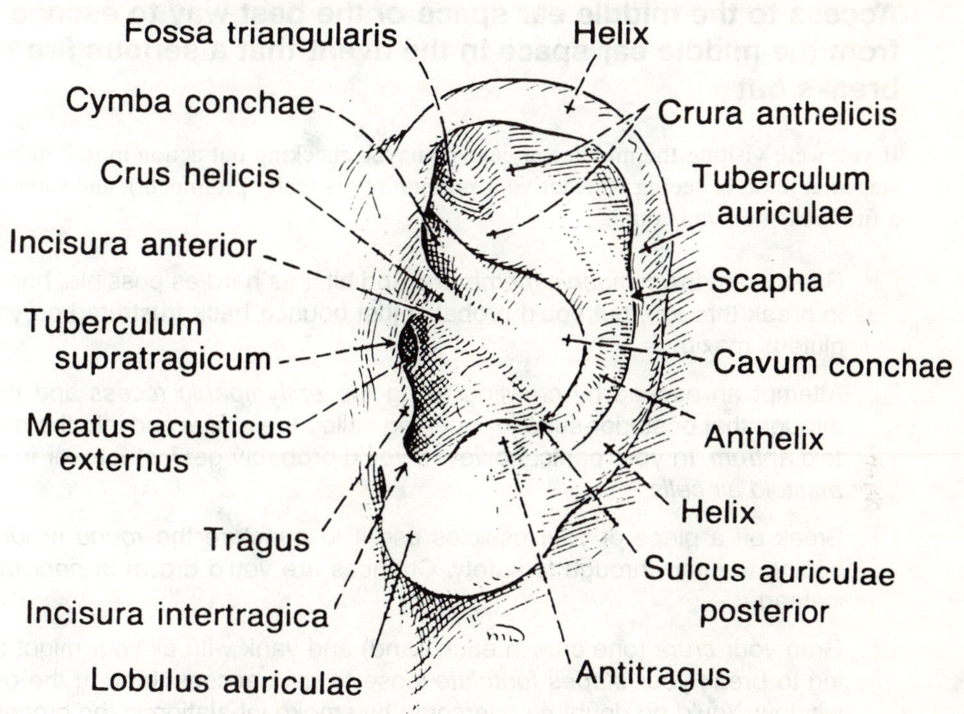

Clinical Concept

Access to the middle ear space *or* the best way to escape from the middle ear space in the event that a serious fire breaks out

If you were visiting the middle ear cavity (maybe checking out action in that incudostapedial joint, or seeing whether your promontory is really prominent), and suddenly a fire broke out, you could:

- ☐ Run toward the *tympanic membrane* and hit it as hard as possible, hoping to break through, but you'd probably just bounce back frustrated on your gluteus maximus.
- ☐ Attempt an escape by crawling along the *epitympanic recess* and then through that posterior-superior opening called the *aditus* and into the *mastoid antrum*. In your panic, however, you'd probably get lost forever in the *mastoid air cells*.
- ☐ Break off a piece of your ossicles use it to puncture the *round window*, hoping to jump through to safety. Chances are you'd drown in *perilymph* instead.
- ☐ Grab your *crura* (one crus in each hand) and yank with all your might trying to break your *stapes footplate* loose to gain access through the oval window. You'd no doubt be overcome by smoke inhalation in the process.
- ☐ Or, if you'd been a serious student of middle ear anatomy, you let out a hearty "Geronimo" and dive feet or head first into the *eustachian tube*, and slide to probable salvation. Just hope that a poorly timed swallow doesn't propel you down the esophagus.

Source: The first author vaguely recalls hearing a story like this in his Introduction to Audiology course at Northwestern University in 1972, taught by Earl "Happy" Harford, Ph.D.

Anatomy of Middle Ear Ossicles

Malleus, incus, and stapes with an emphasis on stapedial structure and dimensions. The manubrium of the malleus is connected to the medial side of the tympanic membrane, whereas the stapes footplate is set within the oval window.

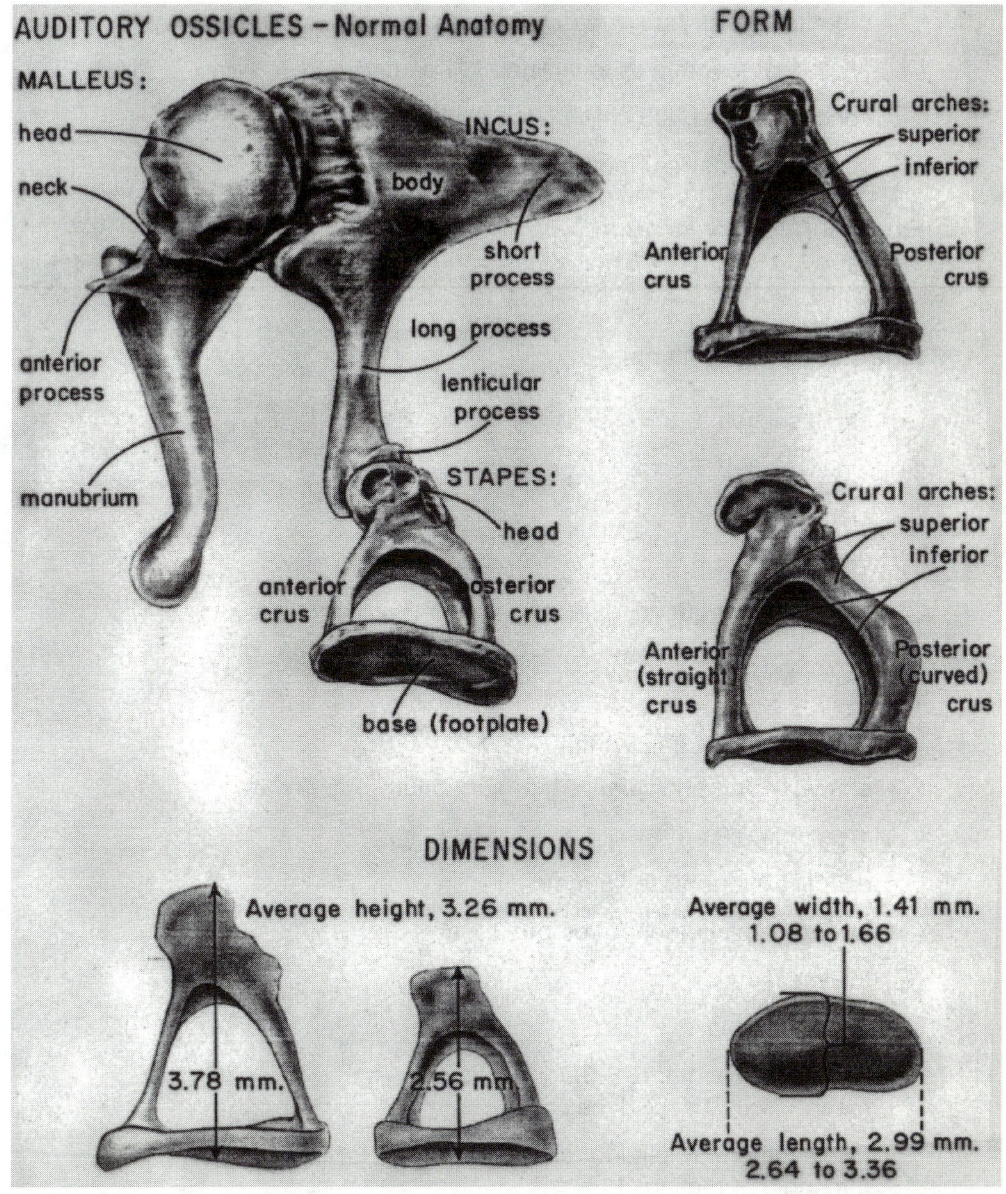

Source: From H. R. Schuknecht, 1993. *Pathology of the Ear* (2nd ed.). Baltimore: Williams & Wilkins. Reprinted with permission.

Dimensions of Outer and Middle Ear Structures

Pinna (male)

- ☐ length: 60–75 mm, mean = 67 mm
- ☐ breadth: 30–39 mm, mean = 34.5 mm
- ☐ angle that length axis is inclined to head: 15°
- ☐ concha volume: 2.5 cm^3
- ☐ concha resonance frequency: 4.5 kHz

External Auditory Meatus

- ☐ cross section: 0.3 = 0.5 cm^2

External Auditory Canal

- ☐ cross section: 0.3 = 0.5 cm^2
- ☐ length: 2.3–2.97 cm
- ☐ diameter: 0.7 cm
- ☐ volume: 1.0 cm^3
- ☐ resonance frequency: 2.6 kHz

Tympanic Membrane

- ☐ diameter along the manubrium: 7.5–9 mm
- ☐ diameter perpendicular to the manubrium: 7.5–9 mm
- ☐ area: 0.5–0.9 cm^2
- ☐ effective area: 42.9–55 mm^2
- ☐ inward displacement of umbo: 2 mm
- ☐ thickness: 0.1 mm
- ☐ weight: 14 mg
- ☐ breaking strength: 0.4–3.0 $\times$ 10^6 dynes/cm^2, mean = 1.61 $\times$ 10^6 dynes/cm^2
- ☐ displacement amplitude for low-frequency tones at threshold of feeling: 10^{-2} cm
- ☐ displacement amplitude for a 250 Hz tone:

- 12.5 A at 75 dB SPL, 7.5 A at 70 dB SPL,
- 5 A at 65 dB SPL (1 A = 10^{-10} m, thus 1 mm = 10,000 A)

Middle Ear Cavity

- ☐ total volume: 2.0 cm^3
- ☐ volume of ossicles: 0.5–0.8 cm^3

Malleus

- ☐ weight: 23–32 mg
- ☐ length from end of manubrium to end of lateral process: 5.8 mm
- ☐ total length: 7.6–9.1 mm

Incus

- ☐ weight: 25–32 mg
- ☐ length of long process: 7.0 mm
- ☐ length of short process: 5.0 mm

Stapes

- ☐ weight: 2.05–4.34 mg, mean = 2.86 mg
- ☐ height: 2.50–3.78 mm, mean = 3.26 mm
- ☐ length of footplate: 1.08–1.66 mm, mean = 1.41 mm
- ☐ area of footplate: 2.65–3.75 mm^2, mean = 3.2 mm^2
- ☐ width of elastic ligament: 0.015–0.1 mm
- ☐ amplitude of displacement for a constant eardrum pressure of 1 dynes/cm^2:
  - 125 Hz: 75×10^{-8} cm
  - 200 Hz: 28×10^{-8} cm
  - 400 Hz: 20×10^{-8} cm
  - 750 Hz: 18×10^{-8} cm
  - 500 Hz: 10×10^{-8} cm
  - 2000 Hz: 6×10^{-8} cm
  - 2500 Hz: 2×10^{-8} cm
- ☐ maximum displacement: 0.1 mm

Oval Window

- ☐ dimensions: 1.2 × 3 mm to 2.0 × 3.7 mm *human*
- ☐ area: 1.12–1.27 mm^2, mean = 1.20 mm^2 *(cat)*
- ☐ mean: 1.4 mm^2 *(guinea pig)*

Round Window

- ☐ dimensions: 2.25 × 1.0 mm
- ☐ area: 2 mm^2

Cochlea

- ☐ number of turns: $2^{5/8}$
- ☐ volume: 98.1 mm^3 (including the vestibule proper)
- ☐ length of cochlear channels: 35 mm

Helicotrema

- ☐ area: 0.8–0.04 mm^2

Basilar Membrane

- ☐ length: 25.3–35.5 mm, mean = 34 mm
- ☐ width, basal end: 0.08–0.16 mm
- ☐ width, apical end: 0.423–0.651 mm, mean = 0.5

Organ of Corti

- ☐ cross–sectional area, basal end: 0.00053 mm^2
- ☐ cross–sectional area, apical end: 0.0223 mm^2

Outer Hair Cells

- ☐ number: 12,000
- ☐ cell body length: 20 mm (basal end), 50 mm (apical end)
- ☐ cell body width: 5 mm
- ☐ cilium width: 0.05 mm at its base to 0.2 mm at tip
- ☐ arrangement: 100–150 stereocilia per outer hair cell
  - ✓ cilia 6–7 rows in W or V pattern per outer haircell
  - ✓ cilia in outermost row have tips embedded in the tectorial membrane
  - ✓ angle in V-shape 120° in the basal turn and 60° in the apical turn

Inner Hair Cells

☐ number: 3,500

☐ arrangement:

- 40–60 cilia per cell arranged, in a shallow U shape
- 204 rows of cilia per cell
- length of cilia longer in apical turn than in basal turn
- lengths and diameters vary among individual coils of the cochlea, and within a single cell

Spiral Ligament

☐ cross-sectional area:

- 0.543 mm^2 near basal end
- 0.042 mm^2 at the apex

Scala Vestibuli

☐ volume: 54 mm^3

Scala Tympani

☐ volume: 37.4 mm^3

Cochlear Duct

☐ volume: 6.7 mm^3

☐ length: 35 mm

Perilymph

☐ volume: scala vestibuli, 10–15 ml
scala tympani, 6–8 ml
total, 16–23 ml

☐ K^+ concentration: 4 meq/liter* (scala vestibuli)

☐ Na^+ concentration: 139 meq/liter (scala vestibuli)

☐ pH: 7.4–7.8

☐ viscosity: 1.030–1.050, in relation to H_2O at 27°C

☐ protein: 70–100 mg/10 ml

Endolymph

- ☐ volume: scala media, 2.7 ml
- ☐ K^+ concentration: 144 meq/liter*
- ☐ Na^+ concentration: 13 meq/liter
- ☐ pH: 7.5
- ☐ viscosity: saccule, 1.030–1.050, in relation to H_2O at 27°C
- ☐ surface tension: 52 dynes/cm^3 *guinea pig* (at 23°C)
- ☐ protein: 20–30 mg/1000 ml

* *meq/liter: milliequivalent per liter*

Source: Yost, W. A. (1994). *Fundamentals of Hearing: An Introduction.* (3rd ed, p.180). Copyright 1994 Academic Press.San Diego: Academic Press. Reprinted with permission.

Anatomy of the Labyrinth

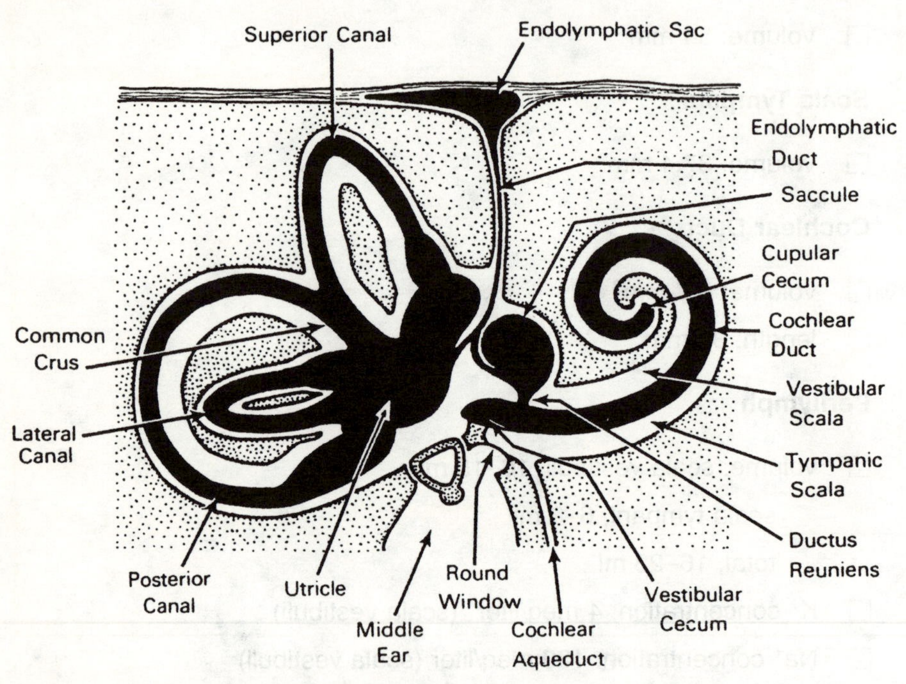

Cross Section Through the Cochlea

Classic view of the cochlea showing scalae (compartments) and important anatomic features.

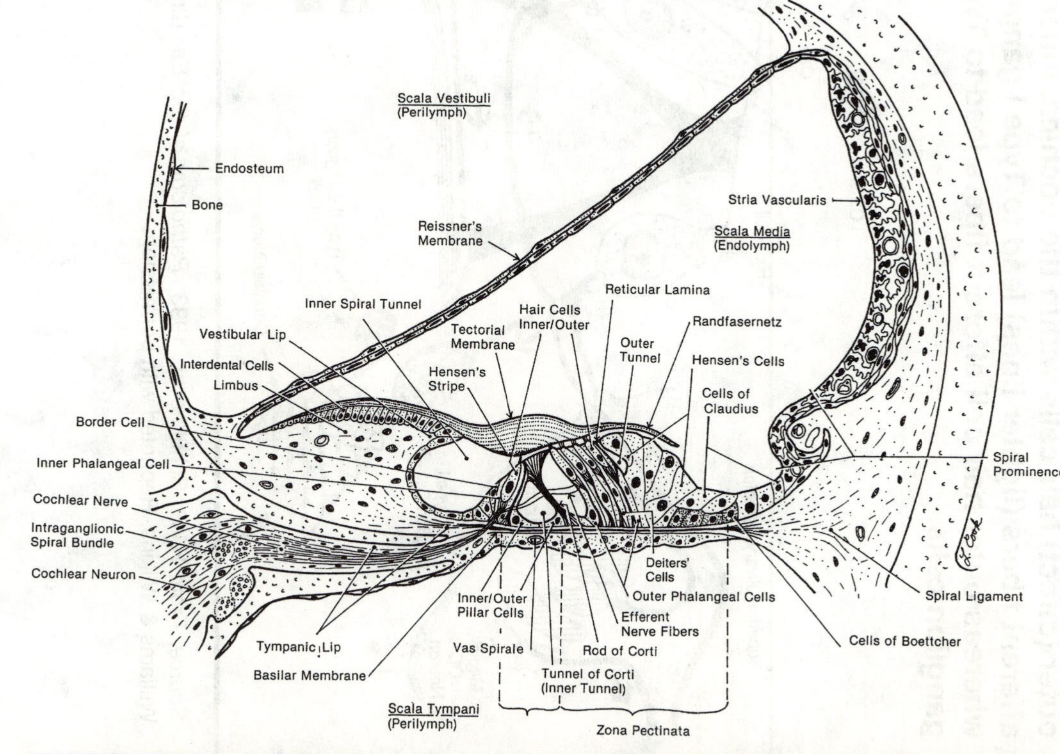

Source: From H. R. Schuknecht, 1993, *Pathology of the Ear* (2nd ed.). Baltimore: Williams & Wilkins. Reprinted with permission.

Distribution of Afferent vs. Efferent Innervation of Outer vs. Inner Hair Cells

Efferent innervation (dark lines) of the inner (indirect) and outer (direct) hair cells within the cochlea. Inner hair cell afferent fibers (lighter lines) lead to Type I ganglion cells, whereas outer hair cell afferent fibers lead to Type II ganglion cells.

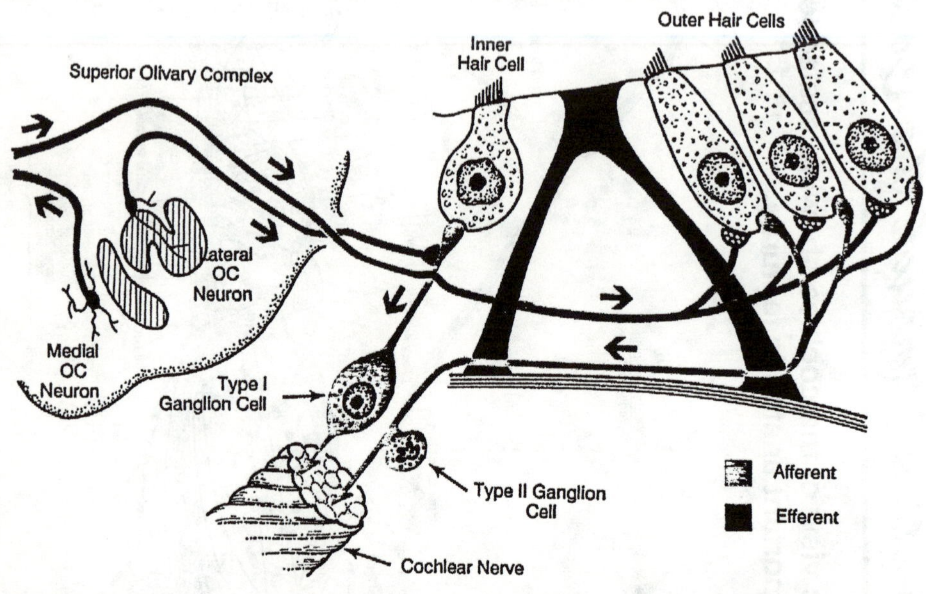

Source: From H. R. Schuknecht, 1993. *Pathology of the Ear* (2nd ed.) Baltimore: Williams & Wilkins. Reprinted with permission.

Relation of Type I and Type III Afferent Fiber Innervation to Inner and Outer Hair Cells

Many afferent fibers innervate a single inner hair cell, whereas one afferent fiber innervates many outer hair cells. About 95% of all afferent fibers synapse on inner hair cells, even though outer hair cells outnumber inner hair cells by a

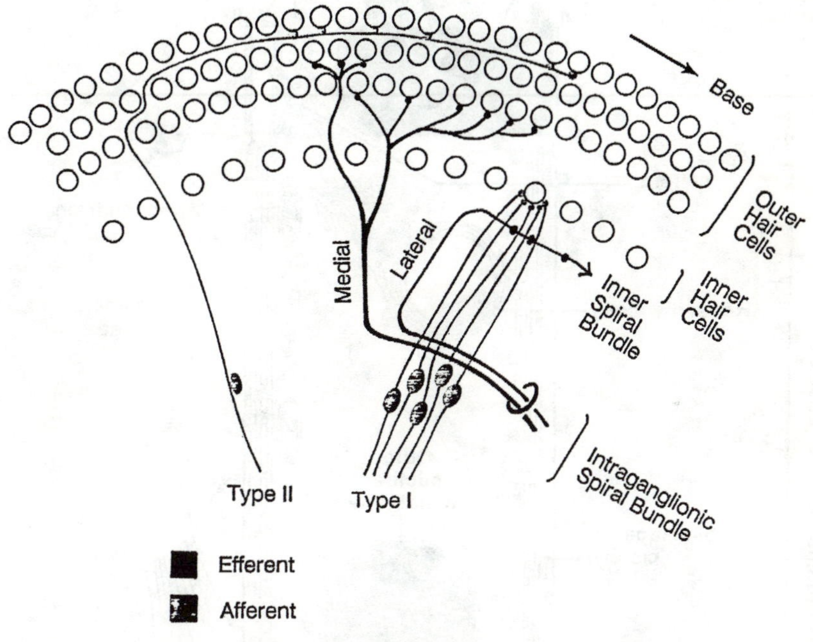

Source: From H. R. Schuknecht, 1993. *Pathology of the Ear* (2nd ed.). Baltimore: Williams & Wilkins. Reprinted with permission.

Outer Hair Cell Anatomy

Note the unique construction of the wall including subsurface cistern, with adjacent mitochondrion. Efferent nerve endings make direct contact (synapse) with the base of the outer hair cells.

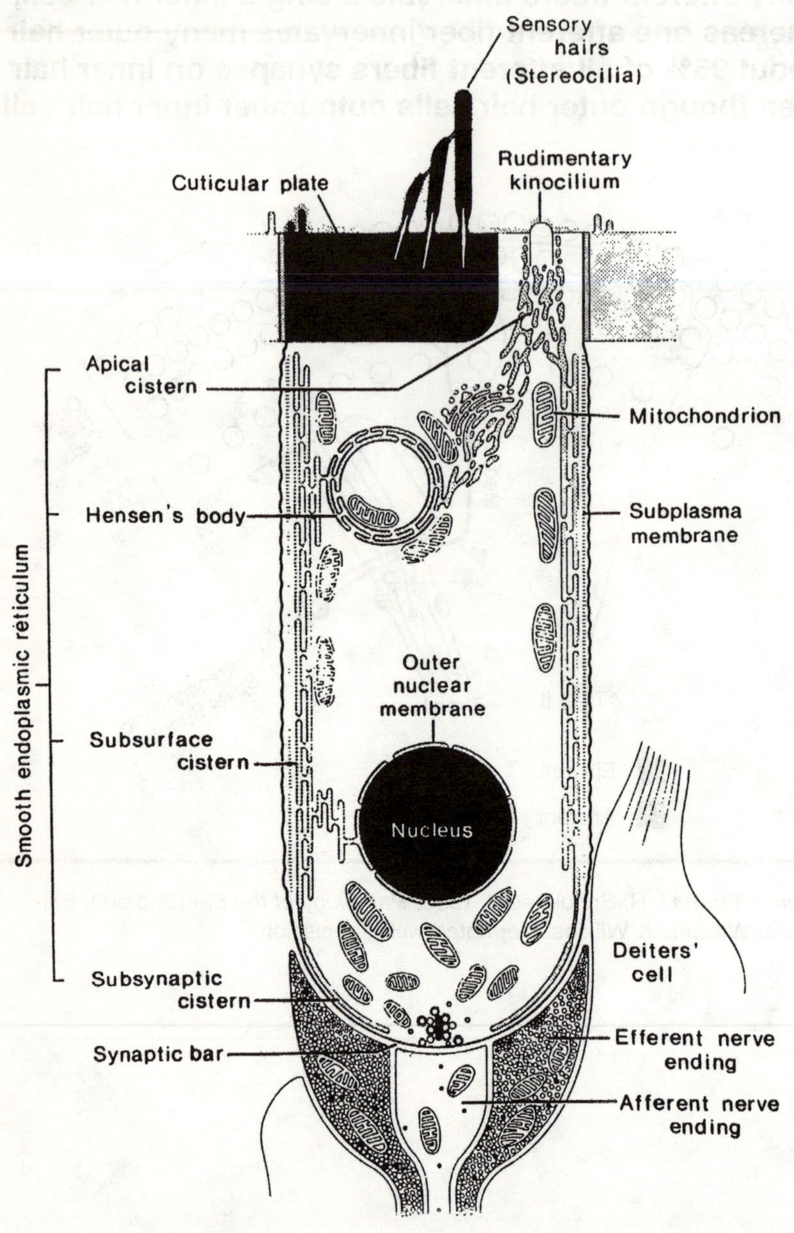

Source: From H. R. Schuknecht, 1993. *Pathology of the Ear* (2nd ed.). Baltimore: Williams & Wilkins. Reprinted with permission.

Inner Hair Cell Anatomy

Afferent nerve endings make direct contact (synapse) with the base of the outer hair cells, whereas efferent nerve endings only make contact with the afferent fibers.

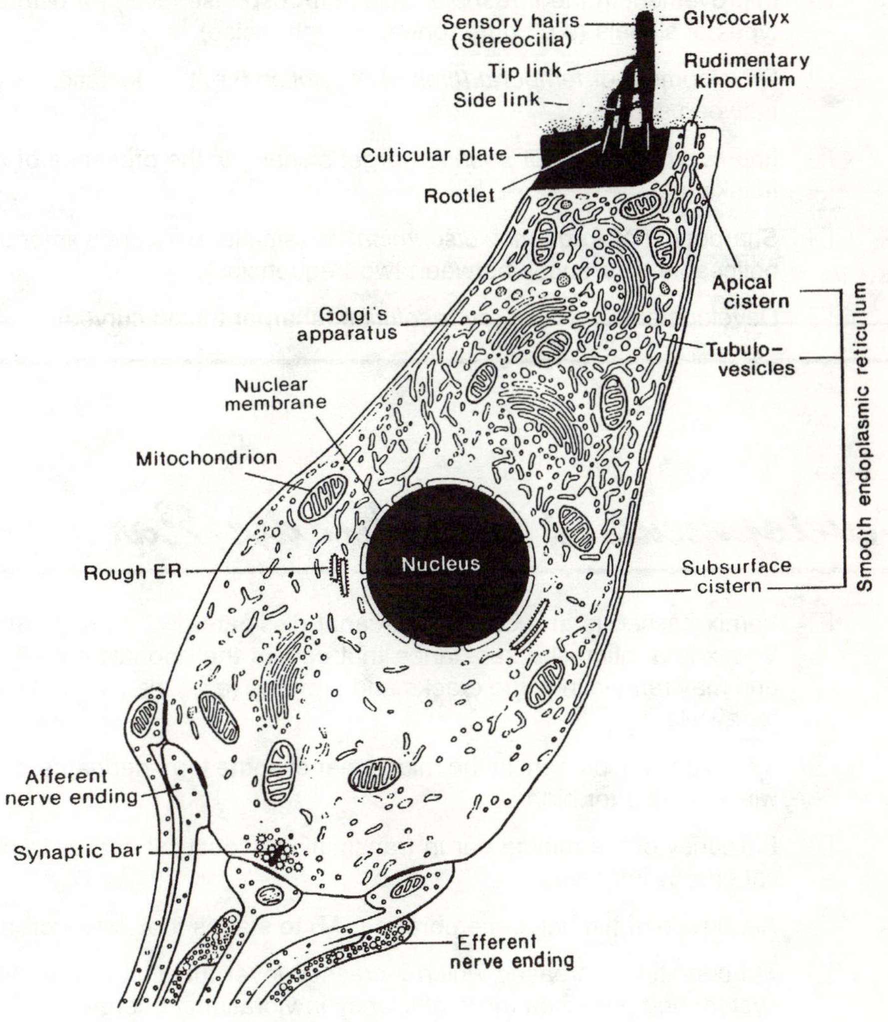

Source: From H. R. Schuknecht, 1993. *Pathology of the Ear* (2nd ed.). Baltimore: Williams & Wilkins. Reprinted with permission.

DEVELOPMENT OF THE AUDITORY SYSTEM

Features of Auditory System Development

- ☐ Improvement in the *threshold* (minimum response level) for different types of signals (e.g., pure tones, speech, noise).
- ☐ Development of *temporal (timing) resolution* (i.e. the detection of gaps between sounds).
- ☐ Improved detection of *sounds* (target signals) *in* the presence of *noise* or masking.
- ☐ Sharpening of *frequency discrimination* (smaller difference limens or just-noticeable differences between two frequencies).
- ☐ Development of *frequency resolution* (sharper tuning curves).

Development of the Middle Ear

- ☐ Vernix casseous in external ear canal dissipates within days after birth. Vernix is a lotion-like substance that covers the neonate's body at birth, and may remain in some cracks and crevices (e.g., the external ear canal) for awhile
- ☐ Mesenchyme, present in the middle ear of some term neonates, dissipates within days after birth
- ☐ Efficiency of the middle ear in transmitting acoustical energy to mechanical energy improves
- ☐ Areal ratio of tympanic membrane (TM) to stapes footplate increases
- ☐ TM curvature increases which increases lever function of the middle ear system and produces more efficiency in vibrational energy
- ☐ TM thickness decreases
- ☐ Lever function of the ossicles improves

Classic Quote

Development of the cochlea by three Frenchpersons

" Information . . . concerning the maturation of structures involved in the cochlear mechanism could help towards understanding the enhanced effects of noise and ototoxic drugs during cochlear development "

M. Lenoir, J-L. Puel, and R. Pujol
Stereocilia and tectorial development in the rat cochlea: A SEM study.
Anatomic Embryology, 175, 477–487, 1987.

Important Principles of Cochlear and Eighth Nerve Maturation (before and soon after term birth)

General

- ☐ There are three general developmental factors to consider, including maturation of:
  - structure
  - physiology
  - biochemistry
- ☐ Afferent innervation (hair cell to auditory nerve) precedes Efferent innervation.
- ☐ The basal region (high-frequency region in the mature cochlea) of the cochlea matures earlier than the apical region (low-frequency region in the mature cochlea) by 1 to 2 weeks.

Stria vascularis

- ☐ Stria vascularis increases in volume.
- ☐ Three cell types of the stria differentiate:
  - marginal cells (they face the endolymph)
  - intermediate cells (a layer between marginal cells)
  - basal cells (dividing stria from spiral ligament)

- ☐ Stria matures from the base to the apex.
- ☐ Melanin in the stria vascularis increases with development. Melanin may play a role in:
  - ✔ energy conversion
  - ✔ energy storage
  - ✔ energy release which probably generates the endocochlear potential

Endocochlear potential (EP)

- ☐ Adult mammals have a positive electrical polarization of 80 to 90 mV versus the perilymph (in the scala vestibuli and scala tympani). See Cochlear Potentials on page 30.
- ☐ Endolymph ionic composition is similar to intracellular fluids in K^+ (potassium) and Na^+ (sodium) concentration.
- ☐ Perilymph ionic composition resembes extracellular fluids.
- ☐ Maintenance of EP is dependent on stria vascularis activity.
- ☐ EP development is most rapid in the first 2 weeks after birth.
- ☐ EP development is dependent on the maturation of the stria.

Eighth Nerve

- ☐ There are two types of eighth nerve fibers (afferent and efferent).
- ☐ Afferent fibers lead proximally (centrally) to the spiral ganglion.
  - ✔ Type I: innervate inner hair cells (IHC)
  - ✔ Type II: innervate outer hair cells (OHC)
- ☐ Efferent fibers project distally (peripherally) from the brainstem down to the cochlea.
  - ✔ Lateral system: runs from the lateral olivary nuclei to innervate IHCs via synapses on afferent auditory dendrites
  - ✔ Medial system: runs from the ventro-medial nuclei of the trapezoid body to direct synapses with OHCs
  - ✔ Lateral efferent maturation precedes the medial efferents

Summary of Cochlear Development

Developmental Event	Time of Emergence in Weeks After Conception
☐ hair cell differentiation	?
☐ afferent eighth nerve fibers in cochlear epithelium	10
☐ inner hair cells histologically distinguished	10–12
☐ outer hair cells histologically distinguished	12+
☐ synapses between hair cells and afferent eighth nerve fibers	11–12
☐ development of stereocilia on inner hair cells	12
☐ development of stereocilia on outer hair cells	12+
☐ efferent eighth nerve fiber endings below inner hair cells	14
☐ maturation of inner hair cell—eighth nerve synapse	15
☐ onset of hearing function by structural criteria	20
☐ efferent synapses with outer hair cells	22
☐ maturation of outer hair cell—eighth nerve synapse	22
☐ stereocilia maturation (inner and outer hair cells)	22
☐ outer hair cells and related structures appear mature	30
☐ normal (mature) auditory sensitivity and frequency resolution	??

Source: Adapted from: Pujol, R., & Lavigne-Rebillard M. (1992). Development of neurosensory structures in the human cochlea. *Acta Otolaryngologica (Stockh) 112:* 259–264.

Audioid

How important is the impedance matching function of the middle ear?

Air has a characteristic acoustic impedance of about 40 dyne sec/cm^3, whereas cochlear fluids (which are similar to sea water) have a characteristic acoustic impedance of 161,000 dyne sec/cm^3. The ratio of characteristic impedances of the air and the fluid is approximately 4000. Only 0.1% of the energy in a sound wave traveling through the air will be transmitted into water. Most of the energy (99.9%) will be reflected back from the water into the air. This impedance mismatch corresponds to a 30 dB loss in hearing sensitivity.

Source: Adapted, Green DM. *An Introduction to Hearing*. Hillsdale, NJ: Lawrence Erlbaum Associates, 1976, pp. 61, 62.

Key References

Early development of the auditory system

Altschuler RA, Bobbin RP, Hoffman DW. (eds). *Neurobiolology of Hearing: The Cochlea.* New York: Raven Press, 1986.

Arnold WJ. The spiral ganglion of the newborn baby. *Amer Otol 3:* 266–269, 1982.

Dallos P, Geisler CD, Matthews JW, Ruggero MA, Steele CR. (eds). *The Mechanics and Biophysics of Hearing.* New York: Springer-Verlag, 1990.

Eimas PD, Siqueland PD, Juscyzk PW, Vigorito J. Speech perception in infants. *Science* 171: 303–306, 1971.

Gray L, Rubel EW. Development of absolute thresholds in chickens. *J Acoust Soc Amer* 77: 1162–1172, 1985.

Gray L. Development of a frequency dimension in chicken *(Gallus gallus). J Comp Psychol* 105: 85–88, 1991.

Krmpotic-Nemanic J, Kostovic I, Bogdanovic N, Fucic A, Judas M. Cytoarchitectonic parameters of developmental capacity of the human associative auditory cortex during postnatal life. *Acta Otolaryngologica (Stockh)* 105: 463–466, 1988.

Lavigne-Rebillard M., Pujol R. Auditory hair cells in human fetuses: Synaptogenesis and ciliogenesis. *J Electron Microscopy Technique* 15: 115–122, 1990.

Morrongiello BA, Gotowiec A. Recent advances in the behavioral study of infant audition: The development of sound localization skills. *J Speech Lang Pathol Audiol* 14: 51–63, 1990.

Peck JE. Development of hearing. Part III. Postnatal development. *J Amer Acad Audiol* 6: 113–123, 1995.

Pujol R, Lavigne-Rebillard, M. Development of neurosensory structures in the human cochlea. *Acta Otolaryngologica (Stockh)* 112: 259–264, 1992.

Romand R. (ed). *Development of Auditory and Vestibular Systems II.* Amsterdam: Elsevier, 1991.

Rubel EW. Auditory system development. In Gottlieb G, Krasnegor NA. (eds). *Measurement of Audition and Vision in the First Year of Postnatal Life: A Methodological Overview.* Norwood NJ: Ablex, pp. 53–90, 1985.

Ruah CB, Schachern PA, Zelterman D, Paparella MM, Yoon TH. Age-related morphologic changes in the human tympanic membrane. *Arch Otolaryngol Head Neck Surg* 117: 627–634, 1991.

Sanes DH, Constantine-Paton M. Altered activity patterns during development reduce neural tuning. *Science* 221: 1184–1185, 1983.

Trehub SE, Schneider BS. (eds). *Auditory Development in Infancy.* New York: Plenum, 1985.

Werner LA, Gillenwater JM. Pure-tone sensitivity of 2- and 5-week-old infants. *Inf Behav Dev* 13: 355–375, 1990.

FUNCTION OF THE AUDITORY SYSTEM

Audioid

What is the relationship between middle ear mass, stiffness, and resonant frequency?

The resonant or natural vibration frequency of the middle ear is found when mass and stiffness components are equal. As mass of the middle ear system *increases*, the resonant frequency *decreases*; as stiffness of the middle ear system *increases*, the resonant frequency *increases*. The resonant frequency of the middle ear is in the 1000 to 2000 Hz region.

Audioid

Why and how is hearing sensitivity decreased in ossicular chain abnormalities?

With total absence of the tympanic membrane and the ossicles, there is a hearing loss of about 39 dB. This is caused by the loss of the areal ratio and lever action (27 dB) plus the loss of 12 dB due to round-window related cancellation of energy.

With disarticulation of the ossicular chain, there is a loss of the areal ratio and lever action contribution of the middle ear system (tympanic membrane and ossicles) of 27 dB. An additional 12 dB is lost due to round window cancellation of energy. Finally, the disarticulated tympanic membrane and ossicles in combination dampen and constrain energy transmission by an addtional 12 dB. As a result, the sum total hearing loss is about 54 dB.

Source: Marleen Ochs, personal communication, Vanderbilt University

Amplification Produced by the Middle Ear System

Mechanical advantages offered by the middle ear, including the area ratio between the tympanic membrane and the oval window, and the lever ratio of the ossicular chain.

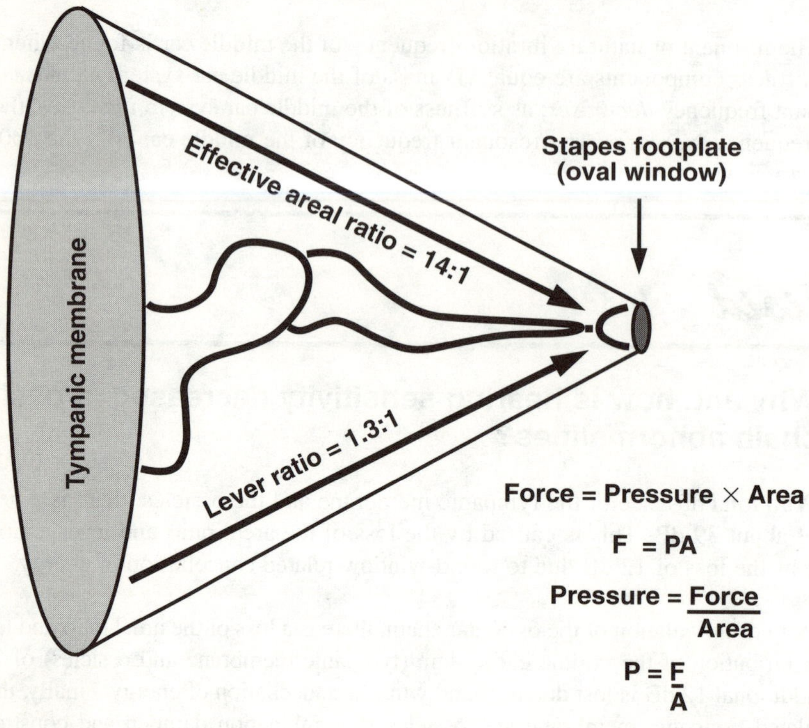

Force = Pressure × Area

$$F = PA$$

$$\text{Pressure} = \frac{\text{Force}}{\text{Area}}$$

$$P = \frac{F}{A}$$

Cochlear Potentials

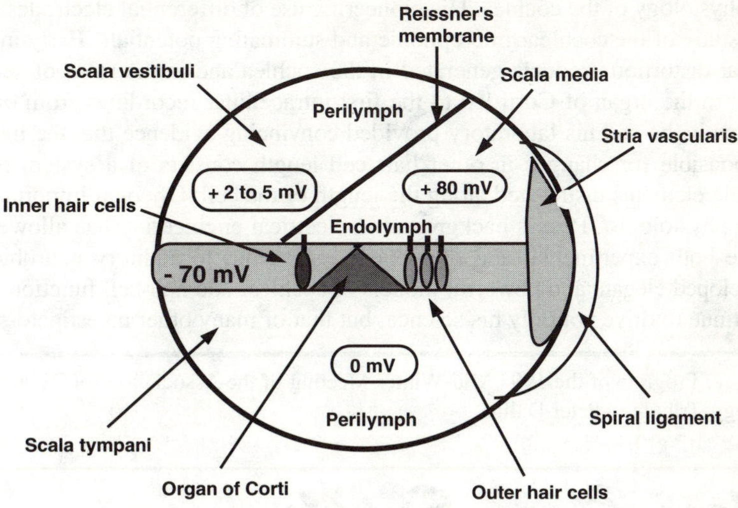

Endolymph potential of + 80 mV = endocochlear potential

Potential difference across hair cells at stereocilia = 150 mV

Mover and Oscillator

Cochlear Biophysics: Peter Dallos, Ph.D.

Peter was born in Budapest, Hungary. While he was attending the Technological University of Budapest, Hungary's liberal government was overthrown by Soviet troops, and he decided to emigrate to the West. He came to the United States in 1956, and completed his undergraduate degree at the Illinois Institute of Technology. Peter then received his master's and doctoral degrees in electrical engineering from Northwestern University where he studied ocular fixation. While still in graduate school, he came to the attention of Ray Carhart, then Chairman of the Division of Audiology at Northwestern. Upon the completion of Peter's doctorate in 1962, Carhart asked him to join the division. There Peter founded the Auditory Physiology Laboratory, and immersed himself in cochlear electrophysiology. He rapidly rose to a position of preeminence in the field, and by 1969 he was a full Professor. Peter was the driving force behind a new Department of Neurobiology and Physiology at Northwestern, and from 1981-1984 he served as its first chairman. Since 1986, he has been the John Evans Professor of Neuroscience. Peter has served on many committees and boards of the National Institutes of Health and of several professional societies. He has received numerous national and international awards, including Guggenheim and Fogarty Fellowships and a Jacob Javits Award. He served as President of the ARO in 1992–1993.

Peter's scientific contributions to our understanding of the biophysics and elecrophysiology of the peripheral auditory system are too numerous to allow more than a brief summary of highlights. His research has always focused upon the biophysics and electrophysiology of the cochlea. His pioneering use of differential electrodes revolutionized the study of the cochlear microphonic and summating potentials. Early interests in nonlinear distortion products generated in the cochlea and in the roles of sensory receptor cells in the organ of Corti led to the first intracellular recordings from outer hair cells. Recently, he and his laboratory provided convincing evidence that the molecular motor responsible for changes in outer hair cell length consists of a system of independent motile elements distributed along the length of the cell. Of equal importance to his skill as a physiologist, Peter's background in electrical engineering has allowed him to integrate both experimental and theoretical approaches to auditory neurobiology. He has developed elegant and powerful models of cochlear and hair cell function. These models continue to drive not only his science, but that of many other investigators in the field.

Source: Program of the 1994 Mid-Winter Meeting of the Association for Research in Otolaryngology. Tribute to Peter Dallos.

Cochlear Blood Supply

Circulation of the cochlea including arteries supplying blood to the cochlea and veins draining blood from the cochlea. Arterial blood supply to the cochlea travels from the vertebral-basilar system.

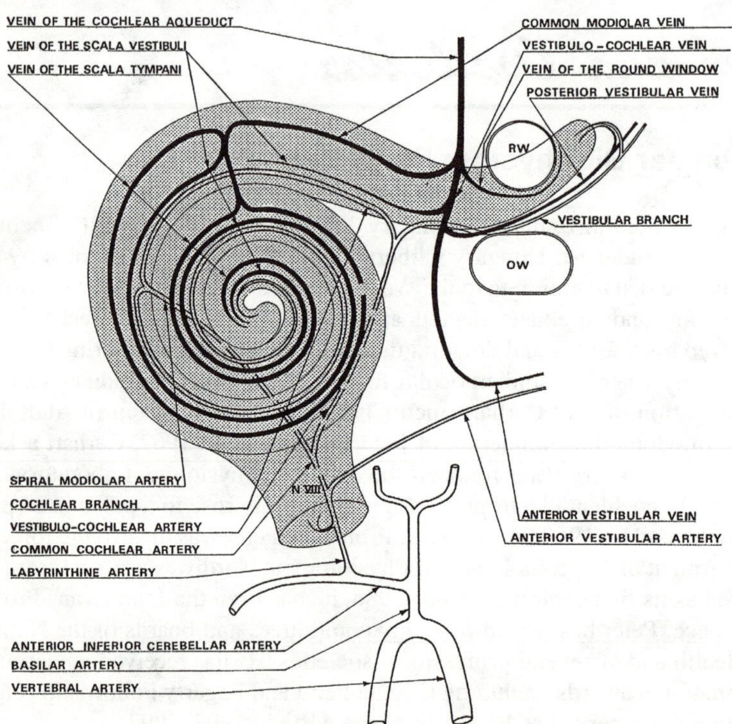

Tuning Curves

Schematic of tuning curves illustrating several characteristic frequencies and the concept of the Q10 value.

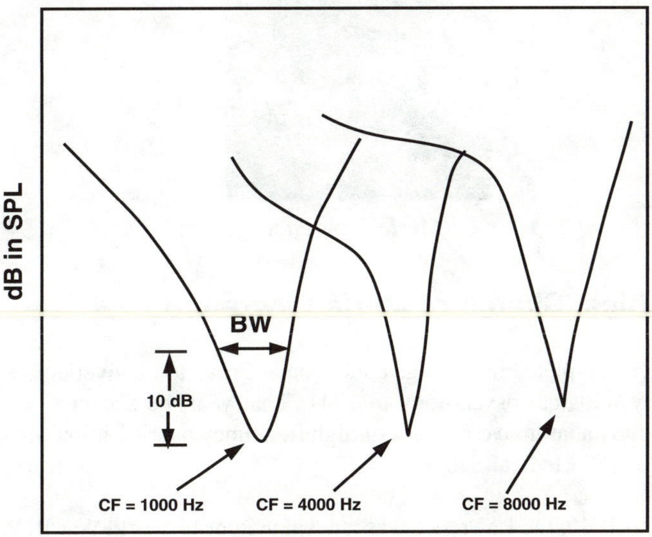

CF = charcteristic frequency (best threshold)
Q10 = CF/bandwidth (BW) of tuning curve = quality factor
High Q10 = narrow bandwidth = more frequency
Low Q10 = broad bandwidth = less frequency resolution

Historical Reverberation

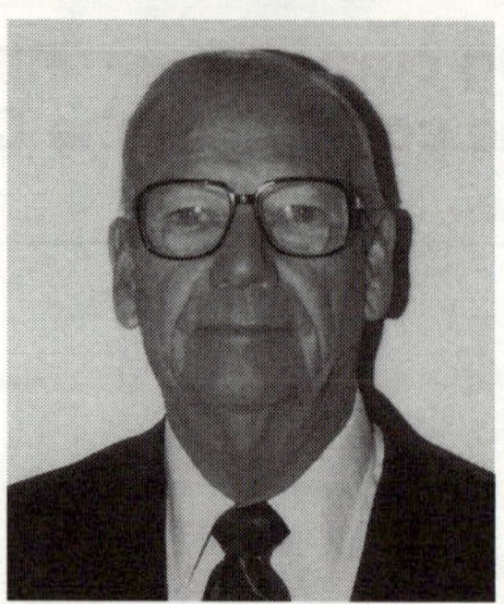

Merle Lawrence

Biographical Sketch of Merle Lawrence

Dr. Lawrence completed his college education at Princeton University, receiving his doctorate in physiological psychology in 1941. That year, he accepted a postdoctoral fellowship to study anatomic correlates of high freqeuncy hearing impairment at Johns Hopkins Hospital and Medical School.

From 1941 to 1946, Dr. Lawrence was a naval aviator in World War II. When discharged from active duty in the U.S. Navy, with the rank of Lt. Commander, Dr. Lawrence had flown 78 combat missions and received the Purple Heart medal. Toward the end of the War, he was a research test pilot and participated in tests of the acoustic properties of microphones in oxygen masks.

After the War, Dr. Lawrence joined the Department of Psychology at Princeton and then, in 1952, assumed a joint-appointment as Professor of Otolaryngology and Psychology at the University of Michigan. From 1961 to his retirement in 1985 he also served as Director of the Kresge Hearing Research Institute at Michigan. During these years, Dr. Lawrence published 5 books and over 200 journal articles. Among these many publications were classic papers on cochlear physiology. Selected publications include the textbook "Physiological Acoustics" (1954) co-authored with Ernst G. Wever, and the journal articles (arranged chronologically) "The locus of distortion in the ear" (1940), "The nature of cochlear activity after death" (1941) with co-authors E. G.Wever and C. W. Bray, "A note on recent developments in auditory theory" (1954) co-authored with E.G. Wever and G. von Bekesy, "Onset and growth of aural harmonics in the overloaded ear" (1956), "Dynamic range of the cochlear transducer" (1965), "Middle ear muscle influence on binaural hearing" (1965), "Control mechanisms of inner ear microcirculation" (1980), and "Attachment of the tectorial membrane revealed by scanning electron microscope" (1980).

Source: Program for American Academy of Audiology's 4th Annual Convention, Nashville, Tennessee, April 1992.

NEUROSCIENCE CONCEPTS AND FACTS

Anatomy of Neuron

Shows presynaptic cell (upper portion) and postsynaptic cells (lowermost portion). Axons may extend to lengths of greater than 1 meter, but they are thin (between 0.2 to 20 mm). The action potential is initiated in the region of the axon hillock.

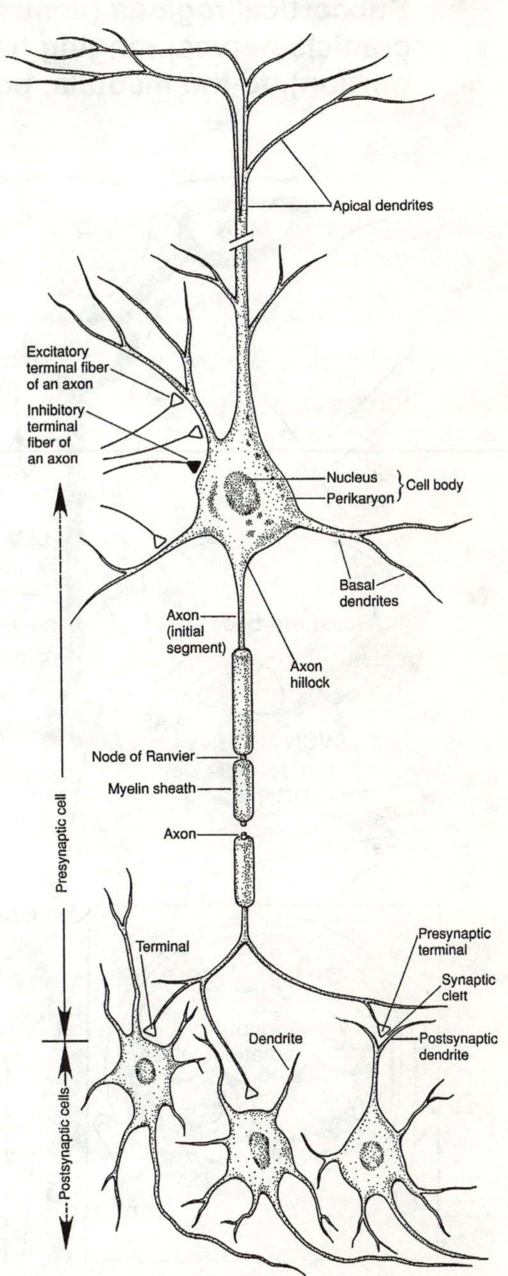

Source: Kandel ER, Schwartz JH, Jessell, TM (Eds). (1991). *Principles of Neural Science* (3rd ed.). Norwalk, CT: Appleton & Lange. Reprinted with permission.

Brainstem with Cranial Nerve Origins

Subcortical regions (ventral view) showing origins of the cranials nerves, ranging from the spinal cord (lowest portion), to the medulla, pons, and midbrain (upper region)

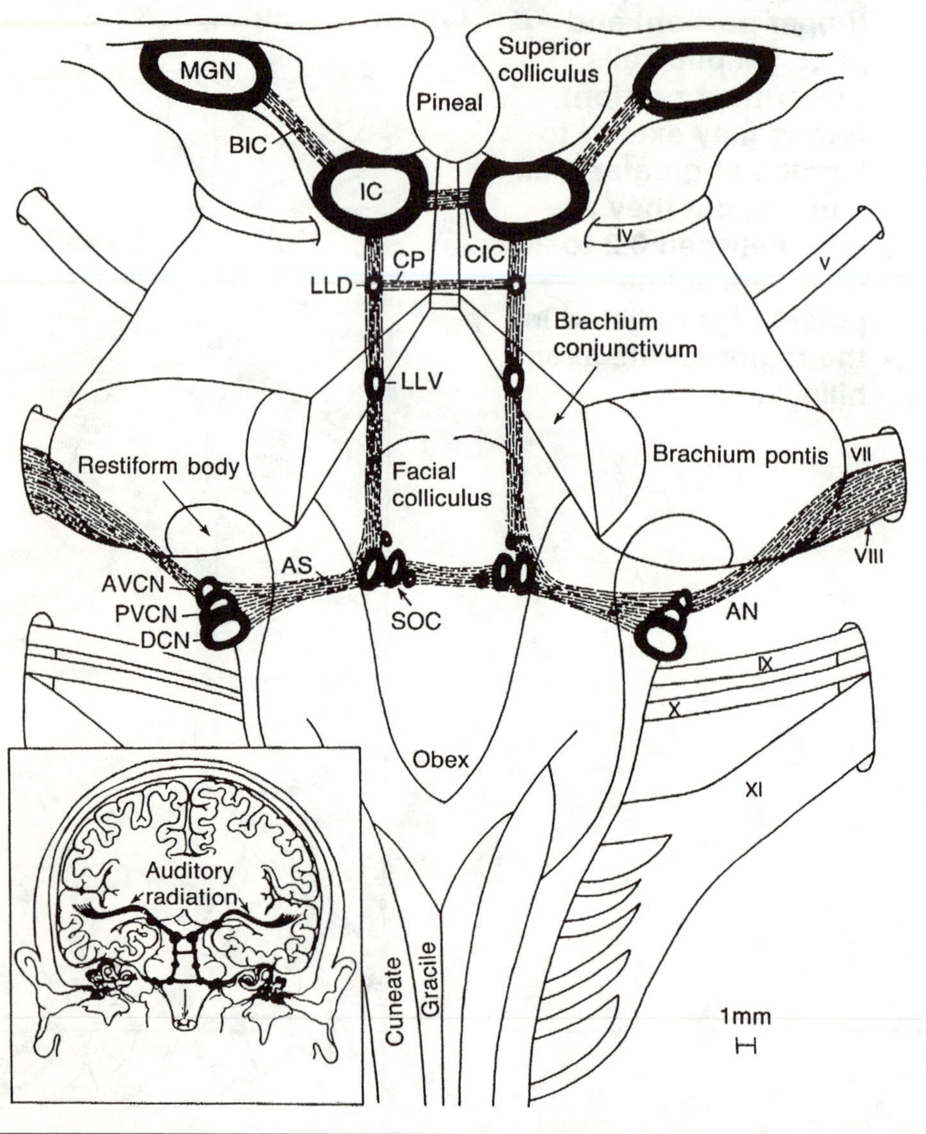

Technical Tip

How to Remember the 12 Cranial Nerves (an international beer drinkers' guide)

On:	**olfactory** (sensory for smell)
Old:	**optic** (sensory for vision)
Olympus:	**oculomotor** (motor for visual convergence and accommodation)
Towering:	**trochlear** (motor for rotating eyes down and out)
Tops:	**trigeminal** (sensory for face and motor for muscles of mastication and tongue)
A:	**abducent** (motor for lateral eye muscles)
Finn:	**facial** (motor for face muscles and sensory for tongue and soft palate)
and	**acoustic** (sensory for hearing and balance)
German:	**glossopharyngeal** (sensory for tonsils, pharynx, and soft palate; motor for muscles of pharynx and stylopharyngeus)
Viewed:	**vagus** (sensory for ear, pharynx, larynx, viscera; motor for muscles of pharynx, larynx, tongue, smooth muscles of viscera)
Some:	**spinal accessory** (motor for muscles of pharynx, larynx, soft palate, and neck)
Hops:	**hypoglossal** (motor for strap muscles of neck and muscles of tongue)

Cranial Nerves, Functions, and Dysfunctions

Cranial Nerve	Function	Disorders Associated with Lesions
I Olfactory	Smell	Anosmia
II Optic	Vision	Vision loss

(continued)

Cranial Nerve		Function	Disorders Associated with Lesions
III	Oculomotor	Eye movements, pupillary constriction, and accommodation	Ptosis, diplopia, loss of accommodation, mydriasis
IV	Trochlear	Eye movement	Diplopia
V	Trigeminal	Facial sensation, mastication, and proprioception	Facial numbness and weakness
VI	Abducens	Eye movement	Diplopia
VII	Facial	Facial expression; taste; sensation of tonsils, soft palate, external and middle ear; salivation	Upper and lower facial weakness, loss of taste for anterior two-thirds of tongue, dry mouth, dysarthria
VIII	Vestibulocochlear	Equilibrium and hearing	Vertigo, nystagmus, disequilibrium, hearing impairment, deafness
IX	Glossopharyngeal	Pharyngeal elevation; taste; sensation of the base of the tongue, epiglottis, uvula, pharynx, auditory tube; parotid secretion	Dysphagia; dysarthria; loss of taste, posterior one-third of tongue; anesthesia of pharynx; dry mouth
X	Vagus	Taste; sensation of epiglottis, larynx, trachea, stomach, small intestine, transverse colon; muscles of deglutition and phonation; cardiac suppression; visceral movement and secretions	Dysphagia, hoarseness, palatal weakness, cardiac dysfunction, dysfunctions of the viscera
XI	Spinal Accessory	Phonation, head and shoulder movement	Hoarseness, weakness of head and shoulder muscles
XII	Hypoglossal	Tongue movements	Dysarthria, weakness or wasting of tongue muscles

Source: Compiled from Golper LA (1992) as adapted from Gilroy J. (1990). *Basic Neurology.* New York: Pergamon.

Summary of Cranial Nerve Functions

Classification	Functions	Structures Innervated	Cranial Nerves
☐ **Afferent fibers**			
General somatic	Touch, pain, temperature, and proprioception	Skin, skeletal muscles of head and neck, mucus membrane of mouth, and teeth	V, VII, IX, X
Special somatic	*Hearing, vision, balance*	*Cochlea, vestibular organ*	*II, VIII*
General visceral	Mechanical, pain, temperature, and proprioception	Pharynx, larynx, gut	V, VII, IX, X
Special visceral	Olfaction, taste	Taste buds, olfactory epithelium	I, VII, IX, X
☐ **Motor fibers**			
General somatic	Control of skeletal muscle (somatic)	Extraocular and tongue muscles	III, IV, XVI, XII
General visceral	Control of autonomic effectors	Tear glands, sweat glands, gut	III, VII, IX, X
Special visceral	Control of skeletal muscles (branchiomeric)	Muscles of facial expression, jaw, neck, larynx, and pharynx	V, VII, IX, X, XI

Source: Kandel ER, Schwartz JH, Jessell TM (Eds). (1991) *Principles of Neural Science* (3rd ed). Norwalk, CT: Appleton Lange.

Clinical Concept

Functions of the Components of the Central Nervous System

☐ **Spinal cord**

The most caudal part of the central nervous system, the spinal cord controls movement of the limbs and the trunk. It receives and processes sensory information from the skin, joints, and muscles of the limbs and trunk. The spinal cord continues rostrally as the *brain stem*.

☐ **Brain stem**

The brain stem receives sensory information from the skin and muscles of the head and provides the motor control for the muscles of the head; it also contains several collections of cell bodies, called *cranial nerve nuclei*. Some of these nuclei receive information from the skin and muscles of the head; others control motor output to muscles of the face, neck, and eyes. Still others are specialized for information from the special senses: for hearing, balance, and taste. In addition, the brain stem conveys information from the spinal cord to the brain and from the brain to the spinal cord; and it regulates levels of arousal and awareness. This is accomplished by the diffusely organized reticular formation. The brain stem consists of three parts, the *medulla, pons*, and *midbrain.*

☐ **Medulla oblongata**

The *medulla oblongata*, which lies directly above the spinal cord, includes several centers responsible for such vital autonomic functions as digestion, breathing, and the control of heart rate.

☐ **Pons**

The *pons*, which lies above the medulla, conveys information about movement form the cerebral hemisphere to the cerebellum.

☐ **Cerebellum**

The *cerebellum* lies behind the pons and is connected to the brain stem by several major fiber tracts called *peduncles.* The cerebellum modulates the force and range of movement and is involved in the learning of motor skills.

☐ **Midbrain**

The *midbrain*, which lies rostral to the pons, controls many sensory and motor functions, including eye and the coordination of visual and auditory reflexes.

☐ **Diencephalon**

The *diencephalon* lies rostral to the midbrain and contains two structures. One, the *thalamus*, processes most of the information reaching the cerebral cortex from the rest of the central nervous system. The other, the *hypothalamus*, regulates autonomic, endocrine, and visceral function.

Cerebral hemispheres

The *cerebral hemispheres* consist of the *cerebral cortex* and three deep-lying structures: the *basal ganglia*, the *hippocampus*, and the *amygdaloid nucleus*. The basal ganglia participate in regulating motor performance; the hippocampus is involved with aspects of memory storage, and the amygdaloid nucleus coordinates autonomic and endocrine responses in conjunction with emotional states.

Brainstem with Cranial Nerve Origins

Subcortical regions (lateral view) showing origins of the cranials nerves, ranging from the spinal cord (lowest portion), to the medulla, pons, and midbrain (upper region)

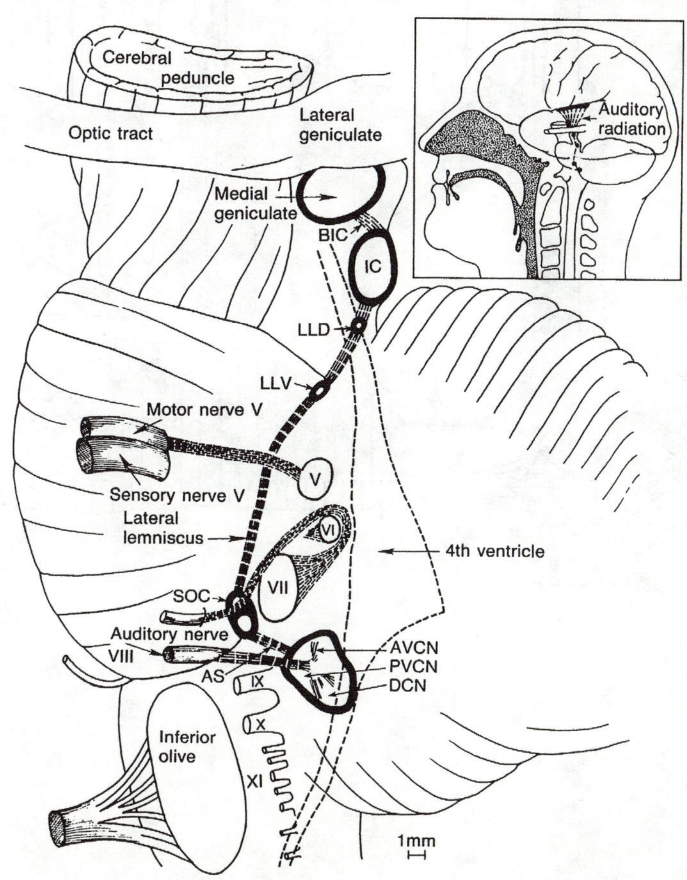

Autonomic Nervous System

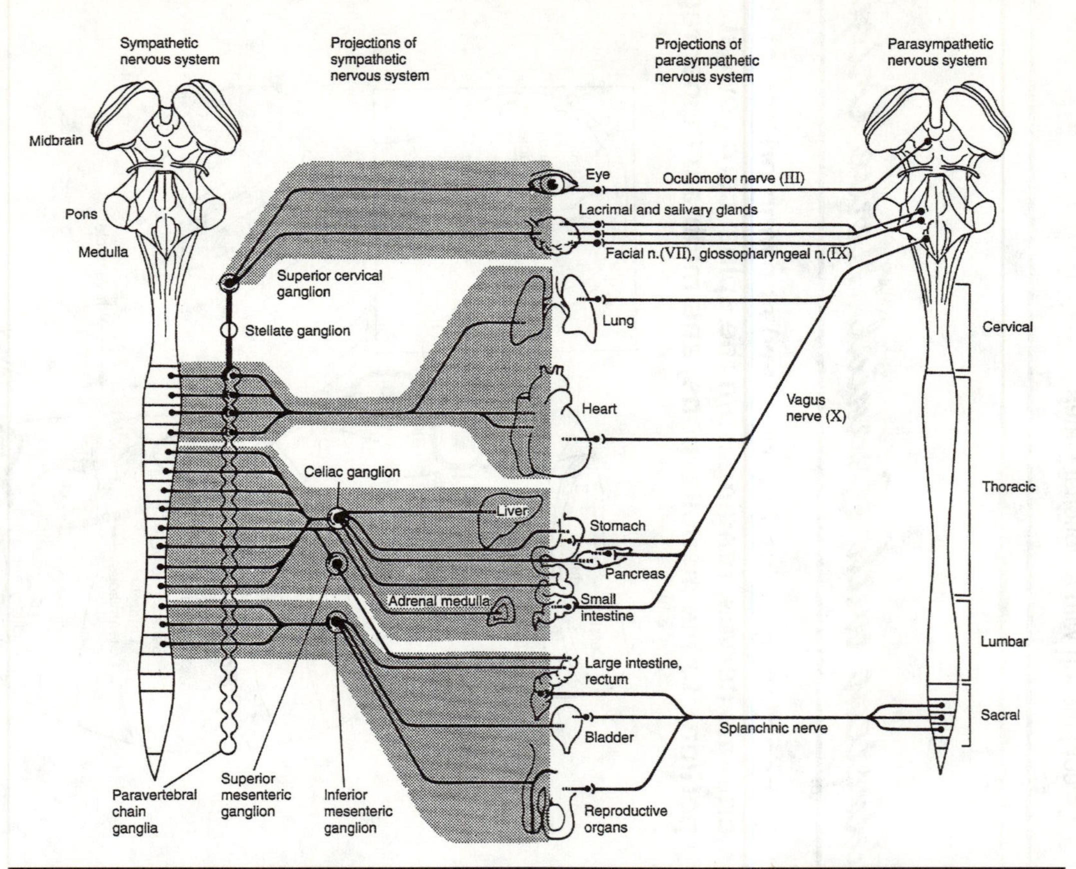

Source: Kandel, ER, Schwartz, JH, Jessell, TM (Eds.)., (1991). *Principles of Neural Science* (3rd ed.). Norwalk, CT: Appleton Lange. Reprinted with permission.1

Estimated Number of Neurons at Various Levels of the Afferent (Ascending) Auditory System

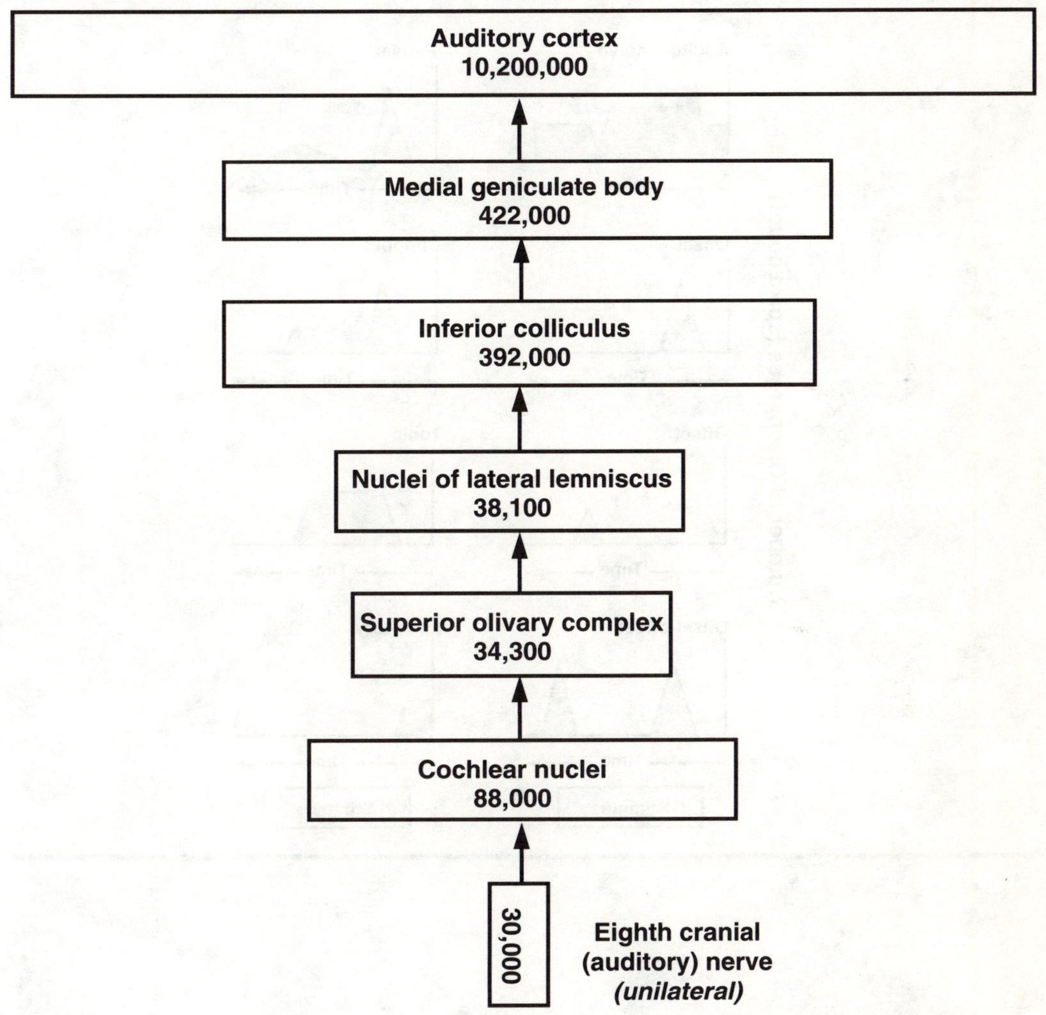

From Chow KL. Numerical estimates of the auditory central nervous system of the rhesus monkey. *J Comp Neurol 95:* 159–175, 1951; and Schuknecht HF. *Pathology of the Ear* (2nd ed.) Philadelphia: Lea & Febiger, 1993, p. 69.

Poststimulus Time Histograms of Auditory CNS Neurons

Illustration of eight different functional types of neurons in the central auditory nervous system.

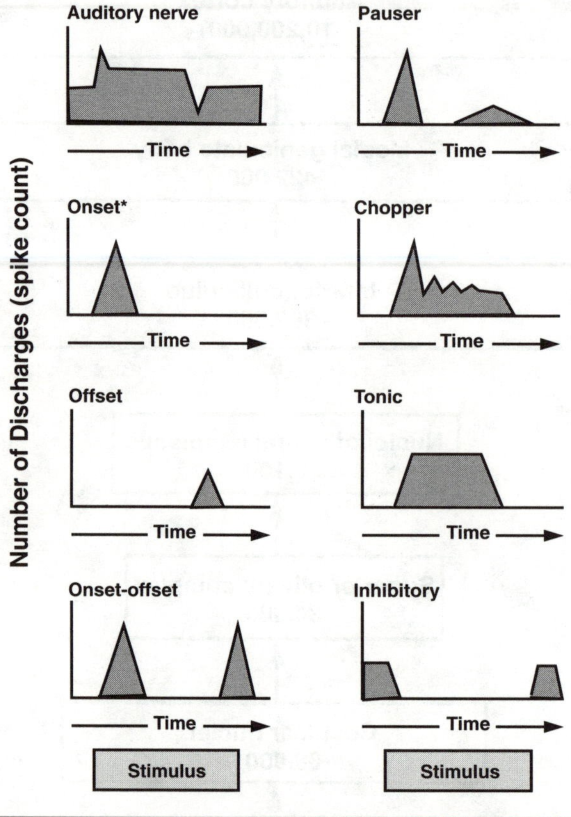

Vertebral-Basilar Vascular System

System gives rise to the anterior inferior cerebellar artery and blood supply to portions of the auditory brainstem, the eighth cranial nerve, and the cochlea.

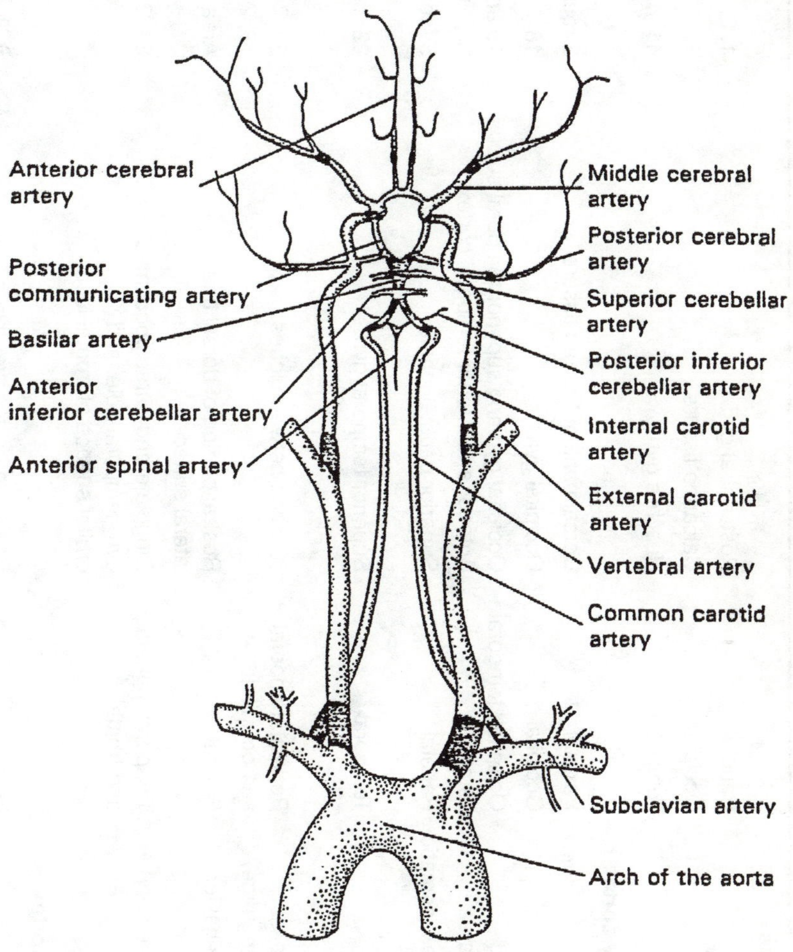

Major Sensory, Association, and Motor Cortices

Functional Designation	Lobe	Location in Lobe	Brodmann's Area
☐ **Primary sensory cortex**			
Somatic sensory	Parietal	Postcentral gyrus	1, 2, 3
Visual	Occipital	Calcarine fissure	17
Auditory	Temporal	Heschl's gyrus	41, 42
☐ **Higher order sensory cortex**			
Somatic sensory II	Parietal	Dorsal bank of Sylvian fissure	2 (opercular portion)
Visual II	Occipital	Occipital gyri	18
Visual III, IIIa, IV, V	Occipital, temporal	Occipital gyri and superior temporal sulcus	19 and area rostral to 19
Visual inferotemporal area	Temporal	Anterior and inferior temporal cortex	21, 20
Posterior parietal cortex (somatic sensation, vision)	Parietal	Superior parietal lobule	5 (somatic), 7 (visual)
Auditory	Temporal	Superior temporal gyrus	22
☐ **Association cortex**			
Parietal-temporal-occipital (polymodal sensory, language)	Parietal, temporal, and occipital	Junction between lobes	39, 40, and portions of 19, 21, 22, 37
Prefrontal (cognitive behavior and motor planning)	Frontal	Rostral portion of dorsal and lateral surface	Area rostral to 6
Limbic (emotion and memory)	Temporal, parietal, and frontal	Cingulate and parahippocampal gyri, temporal pole, and orbital surface of frontal lobe	23, 24, 38, 28, 11
☐ **Higher-order motor cortex**			
Premotor (including supplementary motor area)	Frontal	Rostral to postcentral gyrus	6, 8
Primary motor cortex	Frontal	Precentral gyrus	4

Source: Kandel ER, Schwartz JH, Jessell TM (Eds). (1991) *Principles of Neural Science* (3rd ed). Norwalk, CT: Appleton Lange.

Movers and Oscillators

Neuroanatomists and Neurophysiologists

Paul Broca (1824–1880)

A French neurosurgeon who demonstrated in a case study that the third convolution in the frontal lobe on the left side of the brain is important in speech production. Broca also introduced other theories on the localization of brain functions.

John Hughlings Jackson (1834–1911)

An English neurologist who, with careful postmortem studies, localized and defined the functions of certain cerebral cortex areas of the brain, including those involved in motor activities, sensory perception, and language. He also described how the presence of some abnormal neurologic findings are related to lower central nervous system centers that lack control because of pathology in higher central nervous system regions.

Santiago Ramon y Cajal (1852–1934)

A Spanish neuroanatomist, one of the most famous, who made significant contributions to current understanding of the anatomy and histology of neurons, neuroglial cells, synapses, and a variety of regions of the peripheral and central nervous system. Ramon y Cajal and Camillo Golgi (an Italian anatomist, 1844–1926) shared the 1906 Nobel Prize for Physiology and Medicine.

Louis Antoine Ranvier (1835–1922)

A French histologist who described in 1878 details of the myelin covering some peripheral nerves, including interruptions in myelin sheaths.

Theodore Schwann (1810–1882)

A German physician who described the cellular composition of animal and vegetable tissues, along with the gross anatomy of nerves and, specifically and for the first time, the neurilemma surrounding nerves.

Neurotransmitters

Small-molecule transmitter substances and their key biosynthetic enzymes in the central auditory nervous system

Transmitter		Enzymes
☐	Acetylcholine	Choline acetyltransferase (specific)
☐	Biogenic amines	
	Dopamine	Tyrosine hydroxylase (specific)
	Norepinephrine	Tyrosine hydroxylase and dopamine b-hydroxylase (specific)
	Epinephrine	Tyrosine hydroxylase and dopamine b-hydroxylase (specific)
	Serotonin	Tryptophan hydroxylase (specific)
	Histamine	Histidine decarboxylase (specificity uncertain)
☐	Amino acids	
	g-Aminobutyric acid	Glutamic acid decarboxylase (probably specific)
	Glycine	General metabolism (specific pathway undetermined)
	Glutamate	General metabolism (specific pathway undetermined)

Source: Kandel ER, Schwartz JH, Jessell TM (Eds). (1991). *Principles of Neural Science* (3rd ed). Norwalk, CT: Appleton Lange.

Cerebral Spinal Fluid Pathways

Pathways originate in the choroid plexus and bathe the brain

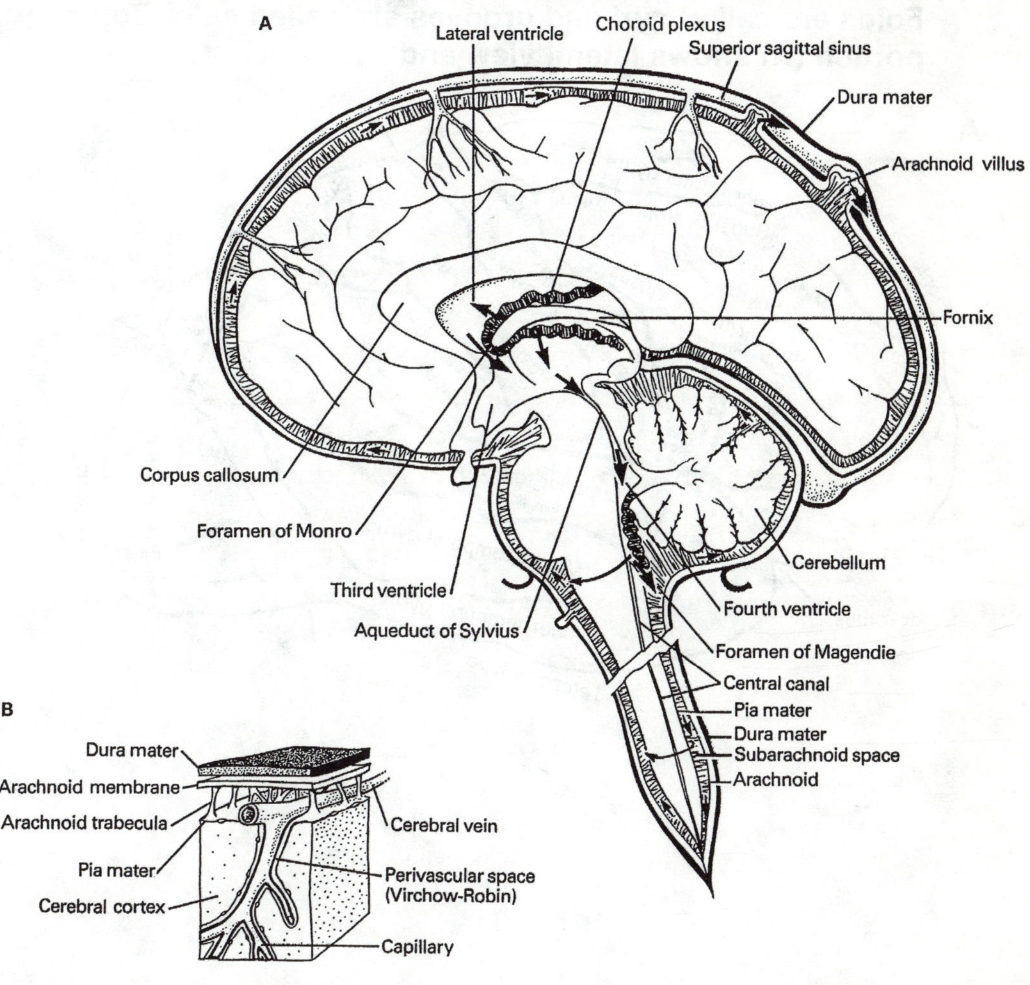

Major Divisions of the Human Cerebral Cortex

Folds are called gyri and grooves are called sulci. Top portion (A) shows lateral view and

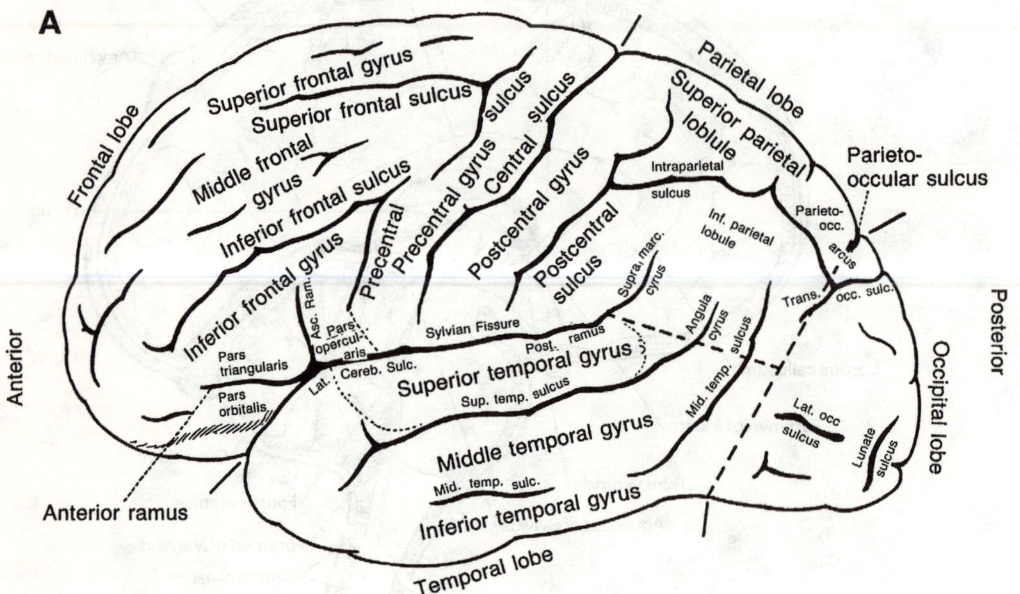

bottom portion (B) shows medial view.

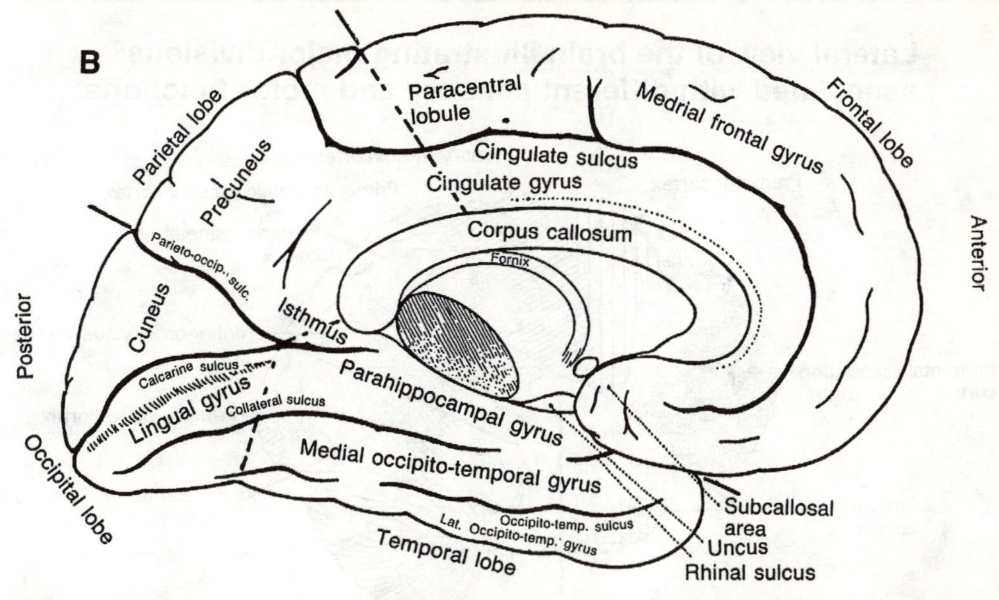

Source: Kandel, ER, Schwartz, JH, & Jessell, TM, (Eds.). (1991). *Principles of Neural Science* Norwalk, CT: Appleton Lange. Reprinted with permission.

Regions of Human Cerebral Cortex

Lateral view of the brain illustrating major divisions associated with different sensory and motor functions.

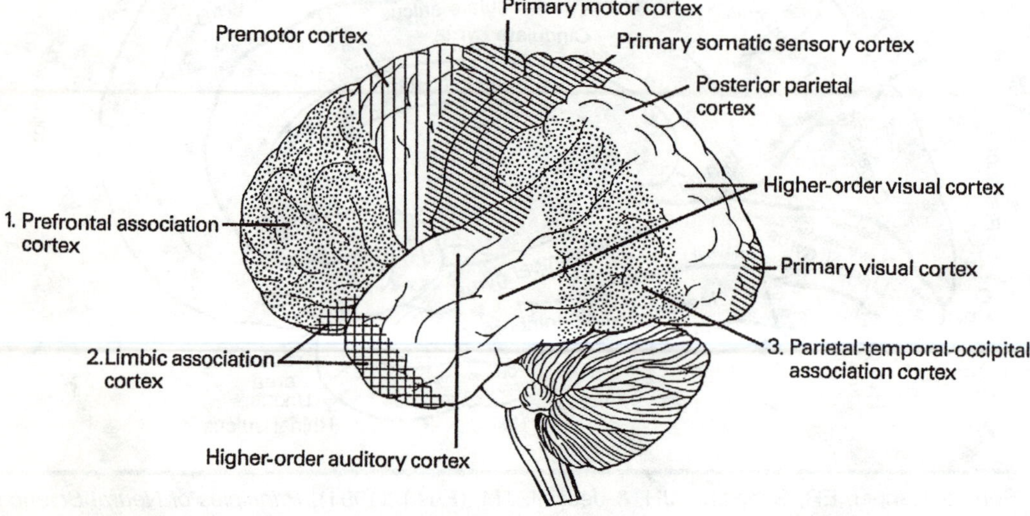

Cytoarchitectonic Areas of the Brain

Areas described by Korbinian Brodmann in the early 1900s. Areas 41 and 42 represent the primary auditory cortex.

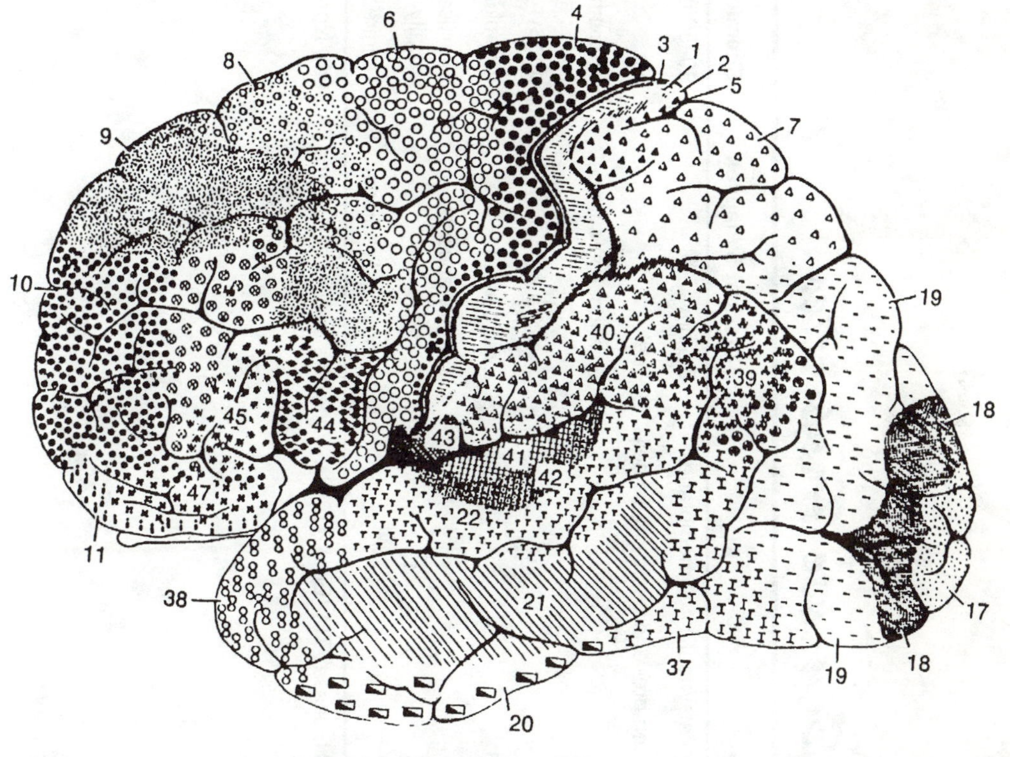

Source: Kandel, ER, Schwartz, JH, & Jessell, TM (Eds.). (1991). *Principles of Neural Science* (3rd ed.). Norwalk, CT: Appleton Lange. Reprinted with permission.

Summary of Synapse Properties

Property	Electrical Synapses	Chemical Synapses
☐ Distance between pre- and postsynaptic cell membranes	3.5 nm	30–50 nm
☐ Cytoplasmic continuity between pre- and postsynaptic cells	Yes	No
☐ Ultrastructural components	Gap junction channels	Presynaptic active zones and vesicles; postsynaptic receptors
☐ Agent of transmission	Ionic current	Chemical transmitter
☐ Synaptic delay	Virtually absent	Significant: at least 0.3 ms, usually 1–5 ms or longer
☐ Direction of transmission	Usually bidirectional	Unidirectional

Source: Kandel ER, Schwartz JH, Jessell TM (Eds). (1991). *Principles of Neural Science* (3rd ed). Norwalk, CT: Appleton Lange.

Connections to and from Thalamic Nuclei

Thalamic portions serving auditory function are in italics

Nuclei	Principal Afferent Inputs	Major Projection Sites	Function
☐ **Relay nuclei**			
Anterior nuclear group	Mammillary body of hypothalamus	Cingulate gyrus	Limbic
Ventral anterior	Globus pallidus	Precortex (area 6)*	Motor
Ventral lateral	Dentate nucleus of cerebellum through brachium conjunctivum (superior cerebellar peduncle)	Motor and premotor	Motor
Ventral posterior			
Lateral portion	Dorsal column-medial lemniscal and spinothalamic pathways	Somatic sensory cortex of parietal lobe	Somatic sensation (body)
Medial portion	Sensory nuclei of trigeminal nerve (V)	Somatic sensory cortex of parietal lobe	Somatic sensation (face)
Medial geniculate	*Inferior colliculus through brachium of inferior colliculus*	*Auditory cortex of temporal lobe*	*Hearing (areas 41 and 42)**
Lateral geniculate	Retinal ganglion cells through optic nerve and optic tract	Visual cortex (area 17)*	Vision
Lateral dorsal	Cingulate gyrus	Cingulate gyrus	Emotional expression
Lateral posterior	Parietal lobe	Parietal lobe	Integration of sensory information
Pulvinar	Superior colliculus, temporal, parietal, and occipital lobes	Temporal, parietal, and occipital lobes	Integration of sensory information
Medial dorsal	Amygdaloid nuclear complex, olfactory, and hypothalamus	Prefrontal cortex	Limbic

(continued)

Nuclei	Principal Afferent Inputs	Major Projection Sites	Function
☐ **Diffuse-projection nuclei**			
Midline nuclei	Reticular formation and hypothalamus	Basal forebrain	Limbic
Intralaminar, centro-median, and centro-lateral nuclei	Reticular formation, spinothalamic tract, globus pallidus, and cortical areas	Basal ganglia and cortex	
Reticular nucleus	Cerebral cortex and thalamic nuclei, brain stem	Thalamic nuclei	Modulation of thalamic activity

Source: Kandel ER, Schwartz JH, Jessell TM (Eds). (1991). *Principles of Neural Science* (3rd ed). Norwalk, CT: Appleton Lange.

Four Important Steps in Synaptic Transmission

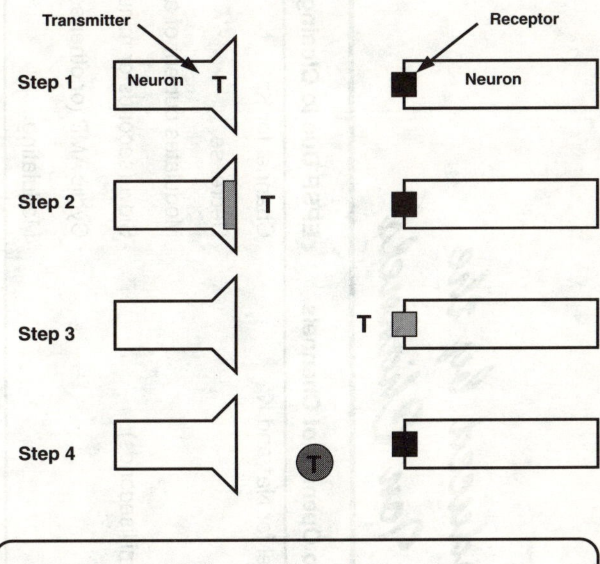

STEP 1: synthesis of neurotransmitter substance

STEP 2: transmitter is released into the synaptic cleft

STEP 3: transmitter binds to the postsynaptic receptor

STEP 4: transmitter substance is removed or destroyed

Source: Kandel, ER, Schwartz, JH, & Jessell, TM (Eds.). (1991). *Principles of Neural Science* (3rd ed.). Norwalk, CT: Appleton Lange.

Synaptic Excitation Produced by the Opening and Closing of Ion Channels

Properties	EPSP* Due to Opening of Channels	EPSP Due to Closing of Channels
Ion channels involved	Cation channel for Na^+ and K^+	Channel for K^+
Effect on total membrane conductance	Increase	Decrease
Contribution to action potential	None	Modulates current of action potential
Time course	Usually fast (milliseconds)	Slow (seconds or minutes)
Intracellular second messenger	None	Cyclic AMP (or other second messenger)
Nature of synaptic action	Mediating	Modulating

*EPSP = excitatory post-synaptic potentials

GENERAL AUDITORY SCIENCE FACTS, FIGURES, AND FINDINGS

Movers and Oscillators

Physical Sciences

Blaise Pascal (1623–1662)

A French scientist and, later in life, religious philosopher who is particularly remembered for his work on fluids and the barometer.

Andre Marie Ampere (1775–1836)

A French mathematician and scientist who also wrote poetry and suffered several personal tragedies (his father was beheaded during the French revolution, and his first wife died). Ampere defined important principles in electricity and made major contributions in the understanding of electromagnetism after he finally married again.

Archimedes (287–212 B.C.)

A Greek philosopher who was the first well-known physicist, often considered the person who founded the study of mechanics. He is especially known for his work on liquids and solving the problem of the lever.

Robert Boyle (1627–1691)

Irish physicist who collaborated with Robert Hooke, in a laboratory he built in his house in Oxford, on experiments that described the compressive properties of air.

Gustav Theodor Fechner (1801–1887)

A German scientist and mathematician known as the father of psychophysics who in 1860 published the classic text *Elemente der Psychophysik*. Fechner derived a law from work done by Weber which defines the relationship between acoustic stimulus intensity and the sensation of hearing. Importantly, this was the pioneering systematic and scientific attempt to relate the physical world with the human sense organs and brain. Psychophysics was later developed further by numerous others, notably SS Stevens.

Herman von Helmholtz (1821–1894)

A German physiologist, physicist, and physician with broad scientific interests and accomplishments ranging from physiological optics to applied physics (hydrodynamics and thermodynamics) to physiological acoustics. Helmholtz developed comprehensive theories of hearing which included the functions of the tympanic membrane, the ossicles, and cochlear biomechanics.

Ernst Heinrich Weber (1795–1878)

A German anatomist and physiologist from Leipzig who studied wave motion with one of his two scientist brothers (Eduard Friedrich Weber, 1806–1871). Weber also studied sensory function, and defined the relation between the sensation of sound (i.e., hearing) as some constant proportion of the stimulus intensity.

Georg Simon Ohm (1787–1854)

A German mathematician and physicist who made important contributions to the study of electricity, although his discoveries were initially unappreciated and he lived most of his life poor and feeling dejected.

Sir Charles Wheatstone (1802–1875)

A British scientist who popularized a device invented in 1833 by SH Christie for measuring an unknown resistance by comparing it with a known standard. In a graduate school course, the first author once built a Wheatstone bridge with the help of physics graduate students at Rice University. Principles of the Wheatstone bridge were incorporated into early electromechanical devices for clinical measurement of middle ear impedance.

Normal Statistical Distribution

Distribution illustrates mean and standard deviations in scores above and below the mean, related to standard score equivalents, and stanines.

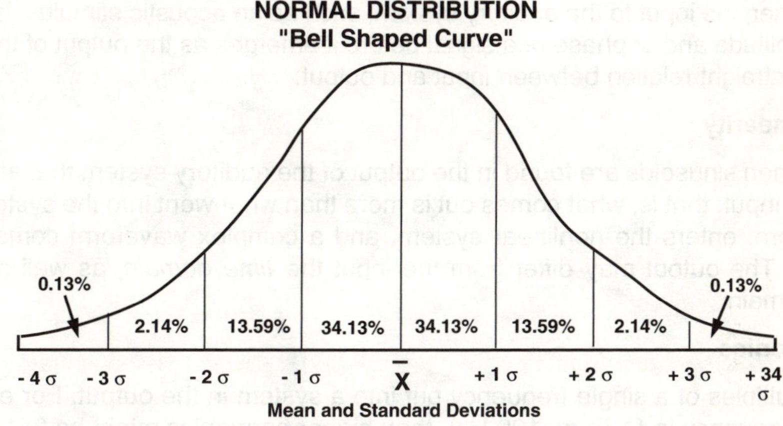

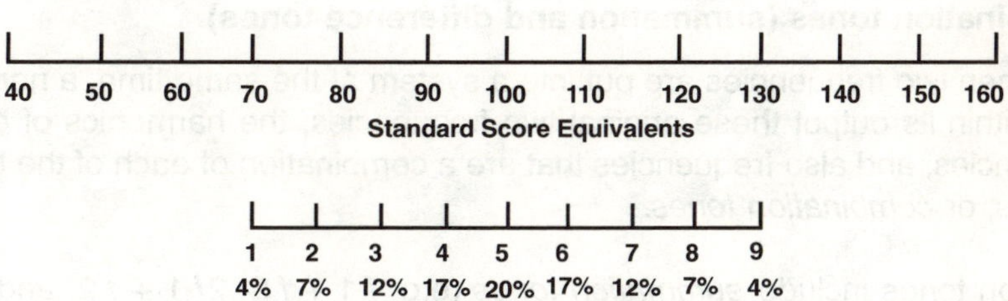

Technical Terminology

Linearity/nonlinearity of the auditory system. See LIST: combination tones in this chapter.

☐ **Linearity**

When the input to the auditory system, such as an acoustic stimulus, is changed only in amplitude and/or phase of a signal before it emerges as the output of the system. There is a straight relation between input and output.

☐ **Nonlinearity**

When sinusoids are found in the output of the auditory system that are not present in the input; that is, what comes out is more than what went into the system. A simple waveform enters the nonlinear system, and a complex waveform comes out the other end. The output may differ from the input the *time domain*, as well as the frequency domain.

☐ **Harmonics**

Multiples of a single frequency put into a system in the output. For example, if the input frequency is $f1$ (e.g., 100 Hz), then higher harmonics might be $2f1$, $3f1$, and so on (or 200 Hz, 300 Hz, etc).

☐ **Combination tones (summation and difference tones)**

When two frequencies are put into a system at the same time, a nonlinear system has within its output these original two frequencies, the harmonics of each of the two frequencies, and also frequencies that are a combination of each of the two original frequencies, or *combination tones.*

Combination tones include *summation tones* (e.g. $f1 + f2$, $2f1 + f2$, and *difference tones* (e.g., $2f1 - f2$, $2f2 - f1$). Combination tones are mathematically predictable.

Musical Scales and Audiometric Frequencies

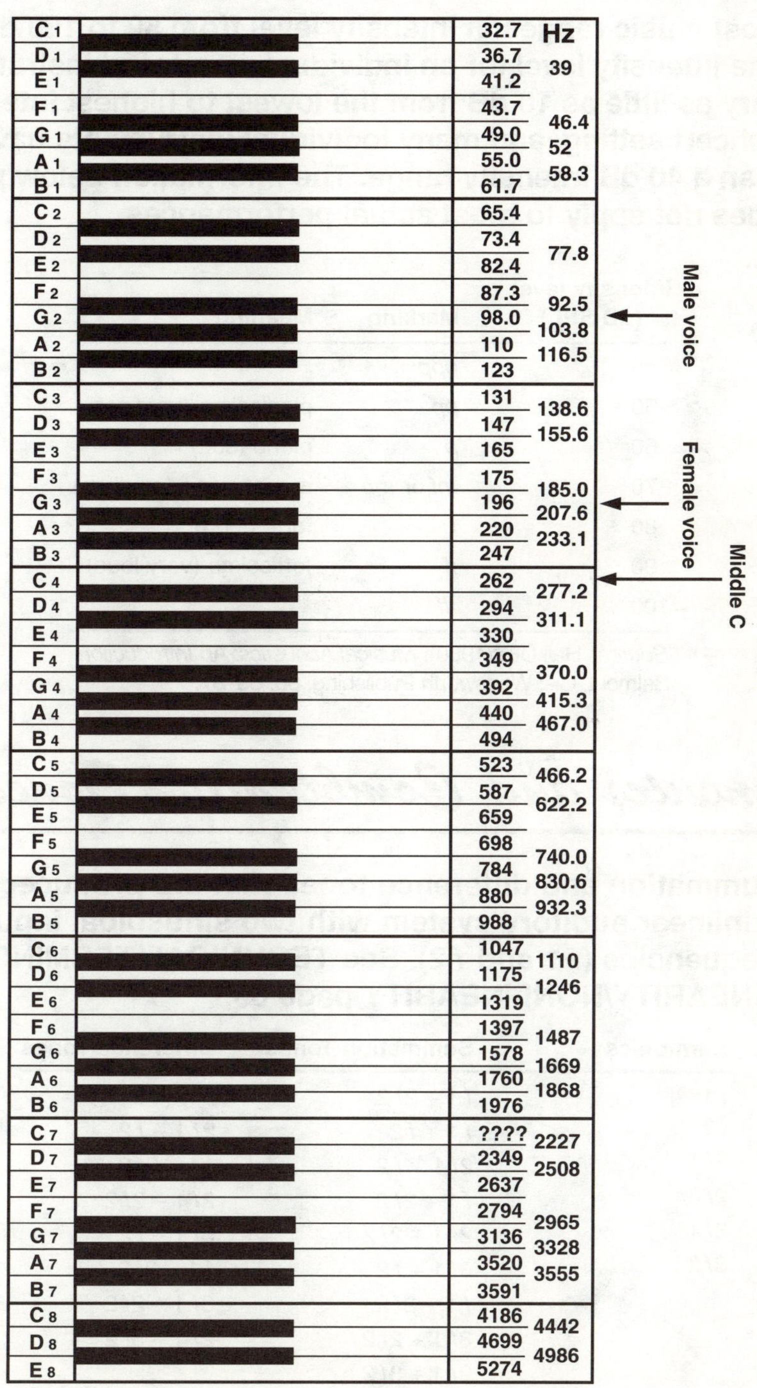
C1 32.7
Hz
D1 36.7
39
E1 41.2
F1 43.7
46.4
G1 49.0
52
A1 55.0
58.3
B1 61.7
C2 65.4
D2 73.4
77.8
E2 82.4
F2 87.3
92.5
G2 98.0
103.8
A2 110
116.5
B2 123
Male voice
C3 131
138.6
D3 147
155.6
E3 165
F3 175
185.0
G3 196
207.6
A3 220
233.1
B3 247
Female voice
C4 262
277.2
D4 294
311.1
E4 330
F4 349
370.0
G4 392
415.3
A4 440
467.0
B4 494
Middle C
C5 523
466.2
D5 587
622.2
E5 659
F5 698
740.0
G5 784
830.6
A5 880
932.3
B5 988
C6 1047
1110
D6 1175
1246
E6 1319
F6 1397
1487
G6 1578
1669
A6 1760
1868
B6 1976
C7 ????
2227
D7 2349
2508
E7 2637
F7 2794
2965
G7 3136
3328
A7 3520
3555
B7 3591
C8 4186
4442
D8 4699
4986
E8 5274

Music Sound Levels with Dynamic Markings

Most music ranges in intensity level from 50 to 100 dB SPL. The intensity level for an individual woodwind instrument may vary as little as 10 dB from the lowest to highest intensity in a concert setting, and many individual instruments have less than a 40 dB intensity range. The information below probably does not apply to most actual performances.

Intensity level (dB SPL)	Marking	Meaning
40	*ppp*	
50	*pp*	pianissimo (very soft)
60	*p*	piano (soft)
70	*mf* or *mp*	mezzopiano (medium)
80	*f*	forte (loud)
90	*ff*	fortissimo (very loud)
100	*fff*	

Source: Hall DE. (1980). *Musical Acoustics: An Introduction.* Belmont, CA: Wadsworth Publishing, pp. 86–87.

Harmonics and Combination Tones

Summation and difference tones that are produced by the nonlinear auditory system with two sinusoidal input frequencies (*f* 1 and *f* 2). See TECHNICAL TERMINOLOGY: LINEARITY/NONLINEARITY page 63.

Harmonics	Summation Tones	Difference Tones
$f1$	$f1 + 2f2$	$f1 - f2$
$f2$	$f1 + f2$	$2f1 - f2$
$2f1$	$2f1 + f2$	$f1 - 2f2$
$2f2$	$f1 + 2f2$	$2f1 - 2f2$
$3f1$	$2f1 + 2f2$	$3f1 - f2$
$3f2$	$3f1 + f2$	$f1 - 3f2$
	$f1 + 3f2$	$3f1 - 2f2$
	$3f1 + 2f2$	$2f1 - 3f2$
	$2f1 + 3f2$	

Technical Terminology

Masking Level Difference (MLD), or the binaural masking phenomenon. See MLD, page 67.

- ☐ **Monotic:** stimuli are presented to only one ear
- ☐ **Diotic:** stimuli are presented to both ears
- ☐ **Dichotic:** different stimuli are presented to each of two ears.
- ☐ **S_m:** signal is presented in the monaural condition (i.e., to one ear).
- ☐ **M_m:** masker is presented in the monaural condition (i.e., to one ear).
- ☐ **M_mS_m:** a monotic condition in which the signal and masker are presented to one ear.
- ☐ **M_o:** masker is presented in diotic condition (i.e., binaural presentation with no interaural phase differences).
- ☐ **S_o:** signal is presented in diotic condition (i.e., binaural presentation with no interaural differences).
- ☐ **M_oS_o:** the signal and the masker are presented binaurally to each ear in the diotic condition (i.e., with no interaural phase differences).
- ☐ **M_oS_π, M_oS_m, $M_\pi S_\pi$, M_oS_π, $M_\pi S_o$:** various dichotic presentations of the signal and masker. That is, the signal and/or maskers are out of phase between ears.
- ☐ **S_π:** signal is presented to both ears, but the signal for one ear is 180° out of phase with the signal to the other ear.
- ☐ **M_π:** masker is presented to both ears, but the masker for one ear is 180° out of phase with the masker to the other ear.
- ☐ **MLD:** Masking level difference (i.e., the difference in the intensity level of a signal required for detection with a masking noise in a binaural diotic or dichotic listening condition versus a monotic listening condition). Also sometimes referred to as BMLD (binaural masking level difference).

Clinical Concept

Masking Level Difference (MLD), or the binaural masking phenomenon. See MLD (below) and TECHNICAL TERMINOLOGY: MLD, page 65.

- ☐ The MLD is the improvement in the detection of a signal, such as a pure tone or spondee words, when presented within a masker (e.g., white noise) that is not in (out of) phase with the signal (e.g., M_oS_π) in comparison to when the signal and masker are presented to one ear or to both ears in phase (e.g., M_mS_m or M_oS_o).
- ☐ The signal is always easier to hear in dichotic out-of-phase conditions than in diotic conditions (same signal or masker phase to each ear).
- ☐ The size of the MLD (the improvement in detection or the threshold of the signal when out of phase with the masker) is greatest for low frequency (<1000 Hz) pure tones, especially those below 500 Hz with relatively long durations (>100 msec) than for higher frequency and/or shorter pure tone signals.
- ☐ The use of interaural differences in the timing of the signal versus masker by the listener probably is a major factor contributing to the MLD.
- ☐ The MLD phenomen presumably reflects functions of neurons in the brainstem (e.g., the superior olivary complex) which are especially sensitive to timing differences in the information arriving from the two ears.

Masking Level Difference (MLD)

The binaural masking phenomenon. The maximum MLD is displayed for different stimulus (masker and signal) conditions. The masker is a broad band white (Gaussian) noise. The signal is a pulsed, low frequency (below 1000 Hz), long duration (more than 100 msec) pure tone. See TECHNICAL TERMINOLOGY: MLD (page 65) *and* CLINICAL CONCEPT: MLD above.

Interaural Condition	MLD in dB Compared to the Monaural (M_mS_m) Condition
M_mS_m, M_oS_o, $M_\pi S_\pi$	0
$M_\pi S_m$	6
M_oS_m	9
$M_\pi S_o$	13
M_oS_π	15

Source: Adapted from Yost WA. (1994). *Fundamentals of Hearing: An Introduction* (3rd ed). San Diego: Academic Press, p. 180. Copyright 1994 Academic Press. Reprinted with permission.

Everyday Sound Levels

Intensity Level (dB SPL)	Sound Source or Condition
0	threshold of 3000 Hz pure tone in free field
10	falling pin and normal breathing
15	rustling leaves (in a breeze)
20	whisper at 3 to 4 ft
30	empty auditorium
40	quiet living room or library or quiet town
50	quiet interior of automobile or department store
50–60	average conversational speech at 5 ft from talker
65	typical newborn intensive care unit
70	average city traffic or inside moving (cheap) car
80	shouting at 5 ft from shouter or heavy traffic
90	platform at subway station as train arrives or Niagara Falls (shout those sweet nothings in his ear)
100	a riveter 35 ft away or machine shop
110	rock 'n roll concert in front row (not unplugged!) or loud thunder (Rolling Thunder Review)
120	boiler factory
130	machine gun fire at close range (keep low while making sound level measurements)
140–150	50 to 100 ft behind jet airplane engine
140	threshold of pain
180	space rocket at blastoff (outside)

Volume-dependent Changes in SPL in a Closed Cavity

Relationship of sound intensity in dB sound pressure level (SPL) within a hard-walled cavity as a function of the volume of the cavity.

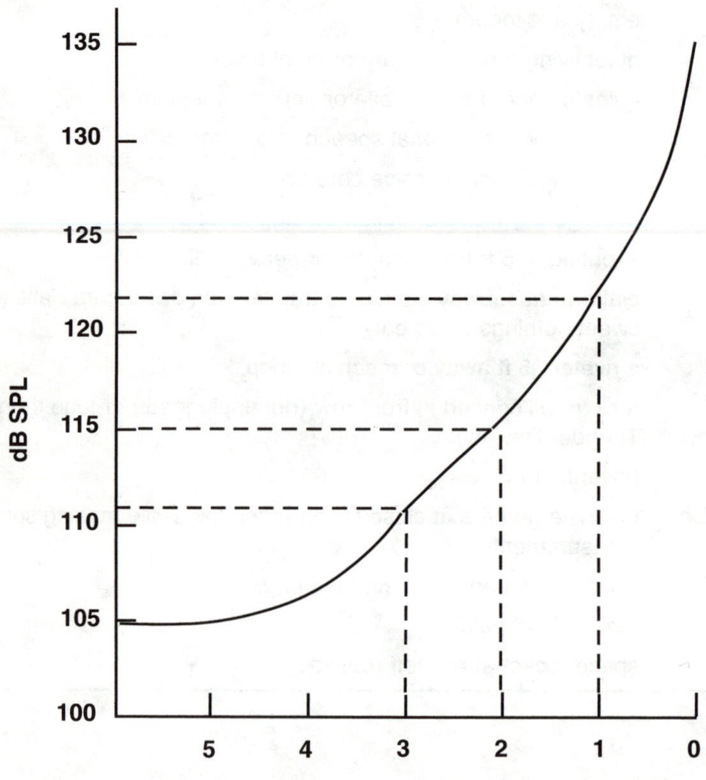

Classic Quote

Georg von Bekesy on Hearing Research design and development

"When in a field of science a great deal of progress has been made and most of the pertinent variables are known, a new problem may most readily be handled by trying to fit it into the existing framework. When, however, the framework is uncertain and the number of variables is large the mosaic approach is much the easier.

Of great importance in any field of research is the selection of problems to be investigated and a determination of the particular variables to be given attention. No doubt the verdict of history will be that the able scientists were those who picked out the significant problems and pursued them in the proper ways, and yet these scientists themselves would probably agree that in this phase of their work fortune played a highly important role. When a field is in its early stage of development the selection of good problems is a more hazardous matter than later on, when some general principles have begun to be developed. Still later, when the broad framework of the science has been well established, a problem will often consist of a series of minor issues."

Source: Georg von Bekesy, *Experiments in Hearing*. New York: McGraw-Hill Book Company, 1960, pp. 7–9.

Velocity of Sound in Different Media

Medium	Velocity m/sec	Velocity ft/sec
air (0°C)	331	1087
oxygen	317	1041
hydrogen (0°C)	1270	4165
water (20°C)	1461	4794
iron	5130	16,820
glass	5500	18,033

Source: Compiled from Rusk RD. (1960) *Introduction to College Physics (2nd ed).* New York, NY: Appleton-Century-Crofts, Inc., p. 374. Yes, the first author has kept his college physics text all those years.

The Speed of Sound

Item	Speed
☐ flow of glacier	0.00001 in/sec
☐ worm crawling	0.015 ft/sec
☐ person walking briskly	4 mi/hr
☐ automobile on autobahn	110 mi/hr
☐ *sound wave in air*	*760 mi/hr = 331.36 m/sec = 1087.13 ft/sec*
☐ jet airplane	1500 mi/hr
☐ Rusty Wallace in #2 Miller Genuine Draft NASCAR	200 mi/hr
☐ rifle bullet	0.5 mi/sec
☐ electron in radio tube	2000 mi/sec
☐ light wave	186,300 mi/sec

Laws in Auditory Science

(and some related definitions too)

Ampere: Common unit of current.

Archimedes Principle: A body that is partially or wholly submerged in a liquid is buoyed up to a force equal to the weight of the displaced liquid. That is, a floating body always displaces its own weight.

Bernoullis' Principle: Pressure of a fluid or air is least where its velocity is greatest.

Boyle's Law: The volume of a given mass of gas varies inversely as the pressure assuming that the temperature is held constant, or $P_1/P_2 = V_2/V_1$. That is, if pressure on a volume of air is tripled, the volume decreases to one third the original volume.

Density: The density of any substance is defined as the mass per unit volume of the substance.

Energy: The capacity of anything (or any body) to do work.

Fechner's Law: The magnitude of sensations vary as the logarithm of the physical stimulus, or $\psi = k \log (I/I_o)$.

Hooke's Law: When an elastic body is deformed, the strain produced is proportional to the acting stress, as long as the elastic limit is not exceeded.

Inverse Square Law: The amount of power (e.g., sound intensity at a microphone) at various distances from a sound source will vary inversely with the square of the distance.

Newton's First Law: When forces acting on a body in any direction are balanced by opposing forces, the body is in equilibrium. If a body is at rest, it will remain at rest, whereas if it is in motion, it will remain in motion in the same direction and at the same speed.

Newton's Second Law: The acceleration (time-rate of change of velocity) of any body is directly proportional to the force acting on the body, and inversely proportional to the mass of the body. That is, $F=ma$, or $a=F/m$.

Newton's Third Law: Whenever one body exerts a force on a second body, the second body exerts a force on the first body that is equal in magnitude but opposite in direction. The terms *action* and *reaction* are used in explaining this law.

Ohm's Electrical Law: The amount of dc current in amperes in any circuit is equal to the net effective electromotive force (or emf) in volts acting in the circuit divided by the total resistance of the circuit in ohms, *or 1 (amp) = emf (volts)/R (total ohms).*

Ohm's Acoustical Law: The ability of the ear to analyze and distinguish between two tones that have frequencies that are different and not harmonically related.

Pascal's Principle: An increase in pressure on any portion of the surface of a confined liquid (or any fluid, such as inner ear fluids) is transmitted undiminished to every other portion of the liquid (or fluid). Pressure is independent of the size and shape of the container.

Power Law: Loudness is proportional to the 0.3 power of the intensity, as defined by Stevens, 1957. Or, equal stimulus ratios produce equal sensation ratios. The relation between loudness *(L)* and sound pressure *(p)* is defined by the equation: $L = k(p-p_o)^{0.6}$, where k is a constant and p_o is the threshold value.

Resonance: Relatively large vibrations (increased energy) whenever the frequency of the driving force matches a natural oscillation frequency of the system on which it is acting.

Simple Harmonic Vibration (motion): Vibratory motion in which the restoring force is proportional to the displacement.

Specific Gravity: The specific gravity of a substance is defined as the ratio of the density of the substance to the density of water.

Speed: The rate at which a body travels in any direction.

Velocity: The rate at which a body travels in a definite direction.

Vector Quantity: A quantity will possesses both magnitude and direction (e.g., velocity, acceleration, displacement). As opposed to a *scalar quantity*, which is completely described by a number and a unit, without the directional quantity (e.g., a volume that is described in cubic centimeters, gallons, or some other appropriate measure).

Power: The time rate of doing work.

Relation between Auditory Threshold and Duration of Tonal Stimulus

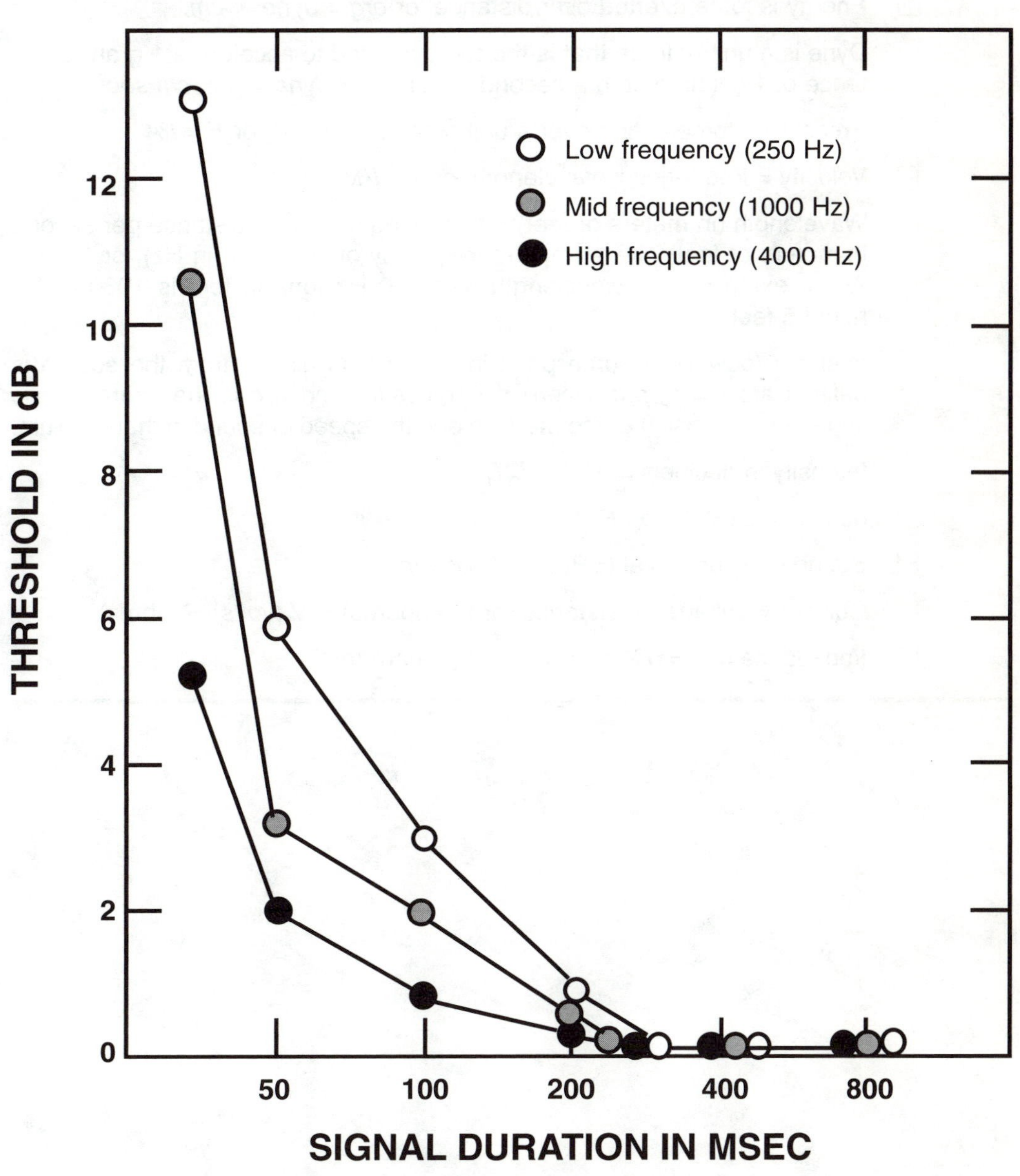

Formulae, Equations, and Expressions in Hearing Science

- ☐ Energy is force exerted over distance, or *erg = dyne × cm.*
- ☐ Dyne is a unit of force that is the force needed to accelerate 1 gram a distance of 1 centimeter in a second squared, or $dyne = g \times cm/sec^2$
- ☐ Pressure = force acting over a unit area, or $P = F/A$, or $F = PA$
- ☐ Velocity = frequency x wavelength, or $v = f/\lambda$
- ☐ Wavelength (in meters or feet) = the speed of sound (distance per second in meters or feet) divided by the frequency of vibration (in Hz), or $\lambda = c/f$. As an example, the wavelength of a 220 Hz tone in feet is 1080/220 = about 5 feet.
- ☐ Intensity (power) at some point in a free field distant from the source is defined as: $I = p^2/p_oc$, where p is pressure and p_oc is the characteristic impedance (density) of the medium and the speed of sound in that medium.
- ☐ Intensity in decibels = $10 \log I_2/I_1$
- ☐ decibel (dB) = $10 \log P_1/P_2$
- ☐ Sound pressure level (SPL) = $20 \log p/p_{ref}$
- ☐ Current = Voltage / resistance, or I (amperes) = *V (volts)/R* (ohms)
- ☐ Impedance = $Z = R^2 + (Xm - Xs)^2$ [square root]

Clinical Concept

Duration and Frequency of Acoustic Stimuli

For relatively brief, transitory (not continuous) sounds, there is an inevitable trade-off between the duration of the sound and its frequency content. The relationship is inverse. That is, as the duration of the sound is decreased, the bandwidth of its spectrum (the range of frequencies that compose the sound) increases.

Critical Bandwidths for 11 Audiometric Test Frequencies

Center Frequency in Hz	Critical Bandwidth Hz	Critical Bandwidth 10log
125	70.8	18.5
250	50	17
500	50	17
750	64	18
1500	79.4	19
2000	100	20
3000	158	22
4000	200	23
6000	376	25.75
8000	501	27

Selected Units and Conversions

- ☐ 1 kilogram (kg) = 1000 grams (gm) = 2.204622 pounds (lb), or 1 lb = 1/2.204622 km

  Note: the criterion for low birth weight of 1500 gm = 3.3 lb
- ☐ 1 meter = 100 centimeters (cm)
- ☐ 1 kilometer (km) = 1000 meters (m)

  Note: *a 10 K race = 6.2 miles*

  Note: if you are driving 100 km/hour your speed is 60 mph
- ☐ 1 slug = 32.174 lb
- ☐ 1 pound (lb) = 16 ounces (oz) = 453.59 gm
- ☐ 1 ounce (oz) = 28.349 gm
- ☐ 1 foot (ft) = 12 inches (in)

  Note: in days gone by the unit of one foot was roughly the actual length of the King's foot
- ☐ 1 inch (in) = 2.54 cm
- ☐ 1 mile = 5280 feet (ft)
- ☐ circumference of a circle = $2\pi r$
- ☐ deci = 1/10
- ☐ deka = 10
- ☐ centi = 1/100
- ☐ hecto = 100
- ☐ milli = 1/1000
- ☐ kilo = 1000
- ☐ micro = 1/1,000,000
- ☐ mega = 1,000,000
- ☐ air density = 0.080 lb/ft^3 = 1.293 kg/m^3 = 0.001293 gm/cm^3
- ☐ Temperature in Fahrenheit (F) degrees = 9/5 (Celsius degrees) +32
- ☐ Temperature in Celsius (C) degrees = 5/9 (Fahrenheit degrees) –32

CHAPTER 2

Pure Tone Audiometry

In This ADR Chapter

Perspective

In the beginning of audiology, there was pure tone audiometry.

From the early systematic descriptions of pure tone hearing thresholds in the 1930s by C. C. Bunch, to the massive "normative" studies at state fairs around the Midwest, to the refinement of techniques for clinical measurement by Hughson and Westlake, and later Raymond Carhart and James Jerger, to ANSI and ISO standards for equipment and threshold levels, pure tone audiometry has traditionally been the mainstay of clinical audiometry. Nowadays, of course, we don't (or at least we shouldn't!) rely as much on pure tone audiometry to describe auditory function clinically.

The current test battery includes a variety of procedures, in addition to pure tone audiometry, that are far more sensitive to peripheral and central auditory system dysfunction, and more accurately measure or predict hearing handicap. These other procedures are described elsewhere in the ADR. The role of pure tone audiometry in the overall audiologic test battery is addressed, specifically, in Chapter 13, Diagnostic Audiometry. What you'll find in this ADR chapter are tips, technical data, and other odds and ends which you may want to seek out from time to time as you go about your daily clinical duties.

FOUNDATIONS OF PURE TONE AUDIOMETRY

Historical Reverberation

Raymond Carhart, the "Father of Audiology"

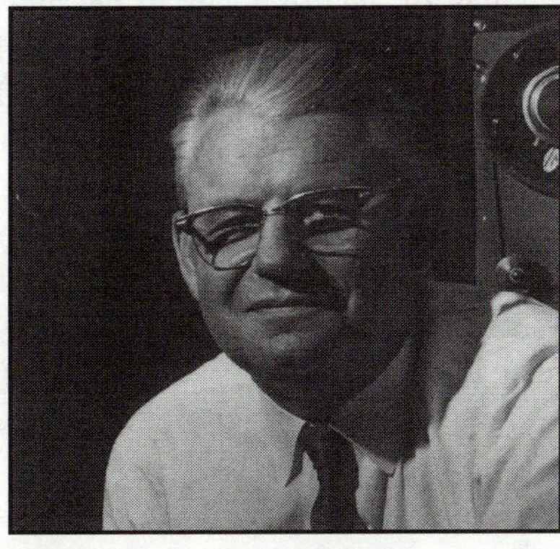

Raymond Carhart, Ph.D.

Raymond Carhart, Professor of Audiology at Northwestern University, died suddenly on October 2, 1975 at the age of 63.

Carhart was born on March 28, 1912 in Mexico City. He attained his bachelor's degree in Speech and Psychology at Dakota Wesleyan in 1932. His graduate work in Speech Pathology, Experimental Phonetics, and Psychology at Northwestern University led to a master's degree in 1934 and a doctoral degree in 1936. He remained at Northwestern University throughout his career except for the years from 1944 to 1946, when he served in the U.S. Army Medical Corps as Director of the Acoustic Clinic at Deshon General Hospital in Butler, Pennsylvania. He established an academic program in Audiology, the first in the United States, in 1947 and was appointed Professor of Otolaryngology at Northwestern's Medical School in 1952. He headed the program in Audiology from 1947 to 1975, and directed Northwestern's Hearing Clinics from 1947 to 1959. He headed the Auditory Research Laboratories there until his death.

Carhart exerted a significant influence on the development of his field. He held chairmanships, trusteeships, and consultantships in literally dozens of organizations at the local, state, and national levels. He was accorded many honors. Among those that he cherished most were his Associate Fellowship in the American Laryngological, Rhinological and Otological Society and his Fellowships in the Acoustical Society of America and the American Speech and Hearing Association. He served the latter organization as President in 1957 and was awarded the Honors of the Association in 1960.

Carhart served the National Institutes of Health in a variety of roles, including membership on both the Communicative Sciences Study Section and the National Advisory Council. In 1963 he was granted a Research Career Award by NIH. The seriousness with which he accepted that award is reflected by the fact that almost half of his publications appeared during the 11½ years he held it.

Carhart's contributions to acoustics were wide-ranging. His very early work was concerned with the acoustics of the vocal tract. Throughout his career he was concerned with basic problems of psychoacoustics including such issues as forward and backward masking, masking level differences, binaural fusion and lateralization, and both threshold and supra-threshold power integration. Nevertheless, his major contributions to his field resulted from the attention he gave to problems relating to clinical audiology. His contributions to the evolution and refinement of speech audiometry and the application of this tool to the assessment of the efficiency of hearing aid performance in the individual patient are widely recognized. If any aspect of Carhart's research efforts can be singled out as representative of his most significant contribution, it is his work relating to the refinements in techniques of interpreting the pure tone audiogram. Over the years he maintained close contact with the most fundamental level of clinical audiology. Through the routine inspection of audiometric test data, he was able to detect individual deviations from expected patterns of response. Consideration of the mechanisms underlying such behavioral deviations often led him to systematic explorations of the phenomena, and the results of those investigations frequently yielded refinements in audiometric techniques that aided in differentiating among various disorders of the hearing mechanism.

Although Carhart's influence touched countless individuals and organizations, those who knew him as a teacher will probably remember him best. He was a superb teacher and part of his success undoubtedly resulted from his abiding respect for his students as individuals. He personally led 45 of them to the successful completion of doctoral or postdoctoral study. In 1972 when the Communicative Disorders Department at Northwestern moved into new quarters, Carhart's former students searched for a way to honor their teacher. They finally decided to commission a portrait of him to be presented to the department for display in the new building. The inscription on that portrait is an accurate characterization of the man. It reads simply "Raymond Carhart, Teacher, Scholar, and Friend. From his students."

Information graciously provided courtesy of Laszlo Stein, Ph.D., and Tom Tillman, Ph.D.

Classic Quote

Raymond Carhart and James Jerger on the preferred method for clinical determination of pure-tone thresholds

"The Hughson-Westlake ascending method for establishing pure-tone auditory threshold is recommended for general use when audiometry is performed with a five-decibel intensity interval. The procedure, which presents stimuli for a second or two so as to elicit on-effect responses from the subject, encourages stability of reactions and yields measurement of the unadapted level of acuity. According to the theory of on-effect, the Hughson-Westlake method should yield thresholds which are clinically equivalent to those obtained by similar short tonal presentations patterned in descending or 'threshold crossing' sequences. Experimental exploration with 36 normal hearing subjects confirmed this expectation. Adoption of the Hughson-Westlake method is recommended over the other methods which also elicit on-effect for the purpose of gaining uniformity of procedure throughout the field of clinical audiometry."

Source: Carhart R, & Jerger J. Preferred method of clinical determination of pure-tone thresholds. *J Speech Hearing Dis, 24*:330–345, 1959.

Measurement of Pure Tone Hearing Thresholds

Step by Step

Preferred method for pure tone audiometry (technique based on the Carhart-Jerger modified Hughson-Westlake method)

☐ Use pure tone signals of 1 to 2 seconds duration

☐ Seat the patient comfortably in a sound-treated booth with his or her profile toward you (viewing the patient from the side) but facing slightly away from you. This arrangement reduces the chance that the patient will detect any inadvertent cues from you, but still permits you to observe his or her facial expressions.

☐ Position a talk-back microphone close enough to the patient for you to hear him speak at a low conversational level. Let the patient know that you'll be talking with him, and that you can hear him. This information is usually comforting to the patient, and lessens the chance that he'll grumble or cuss aloud about you or your audiometric technique. On the other hand, some teeny boppers take this information as a cue to grab the microphone and show off their best Bon Jovi or Guns 'N Roses impression.

☐ Instruct the patient to respond when he just barely hears the stimulus (e.g., beeping sounds or, for children, little birdies). Tell the patient he should respond even if he thinks that he heard the sound.

☐ Response modes include (in order of preference):

- ✔ pressing a button (one button for both ears or separate buttons for the right versus left ear). In the South, patients don't press the button—they mash it.
- ✔ raising a finger or hand.
- ✔ giving a verbal response to when the stimulus is heard (e.g., "Yes"). This is least preferable because jaw movements may alter ear canal acoustics or, in rare cases, temporarily close off ear canal and influence threshold measurements.

☐ Briefly inspect each ear for any evidence of abnormality and to estimate the likelihood of ear canal collapse. Be sure to otoscopically inspect the ear canal before inserting anything into it.

- ☐ For air conduction assessment, carefully place the right and left earphones over the correct ears, or insert ER-3A plugs into ear canals. Use loudspeakers for sound-field audiometry, not traditional earphones.
- ☐ For bone conduction measurement, place the bone oscillator on the mastoid, not touching the ear and not over hair. Verify a stable placement of the oscillator after the earphones for masking are in place.
- ☐ Close both doors of your double-walled sound booth on the way to your audiometer. You paid good money for that booth; take full advantage of your investment.
- ☐ Present a pure tone signal (e.g., 1000 Hz) to the better ear at an intensity level comfortably above the patient's presumed threshold
  - ✔ about 30 to 40 dB HL for normal hearing sensitivity
  - ✔ about 70 dB HL for hearing loss
- ☐ If the patient does not respond, increase the stimulus intensity by 15 dB increments until the patient does respond.
- ☐ Decrease the intensity level of stimulus presentations in 10 to 15 dB increments until the patient responds.
- ☐ Begin the search for threshold when the patient doesn't respond to two presentations at an intensity level.
- ☐ Increase the intensity level in 5 dB increments and continue ascending until the patient responds.
- ☐ Go back down another 10 dB, and present the stimulus once more.
- ☐ Increase the intensity level again in 5 dB increments, seeking a response.
- ☐ Don't forget to consider the need for masking the nontest ear, if indicated. Guide-lines for masking for air- and bone-conduction pure tone audiometry are summarized later in this chapter.
- ☐ The patient's threshold for the stimulus frequency is found when he or she responds three times at an intensity level.
- ☐ Go on to the next audiometric frequency, or to the other ear if a threshold for all audiometric frequencies for one ear has been found.
- ☐ When pure tone audiometry is completed, leave the audiometer in the "neutral position." That is, with:
  - ✔ the earphone (versus bone conduction or speaker) output selected

- ✓ a pure tone signal (usually 1000 Hz) selection, versus microphone or tape output
- ✓ the attenuator (hearing loss dial) at or near 0 dB HL. Never leave the audiometer with a very high intensity level selected. The next patient might get blasted inadvertently.

Sources: Carhart R, Jerger JF. Preferred method for clinical determination of pure-tone thresholds. *J Speech Hear Dis 24:* 330–345, 1959; Hughson W, Westlake H. Manual for program outline for rehabilitation of aural casualties both military and civilian. *Trans Am Acad Ophthalmol Otolaryngol 48 (Suppl.):* 1–15, 1944; and first author's clinical experience.

Classic Quotes

Stanley Smith (S.S.) Stevens and Hallowell Davis in 1938 on tonal lacunae

"Tonal lacunae are commonly understood to be isolated regions of frequencies to which the ear is not sensitive. The sensitive regions between tonal lacunae are called tonal islands. In most cases of supposed insensitivity to certain frequencies, it is found that, by increasing the intensity of the stimulating tone, a value is found which results in a sensation of hearing. In other words, tonal lacunae turn out to be regions of relative rather than absolute insensitivity."

Source: Stevens SS, Davis H. *Hearing: Its Psychology and Physiology.* New York: John Wiley & Sons, Inc., 1938: p. 63.

ADR NOTE: Lacunae are empty or missing spaces. Latin *lacuna* = pool

Audiogram of Familiar Sounds

This graphic display of intensity levels and frequencies can be helpful in counseling patients about their audiometric findings.

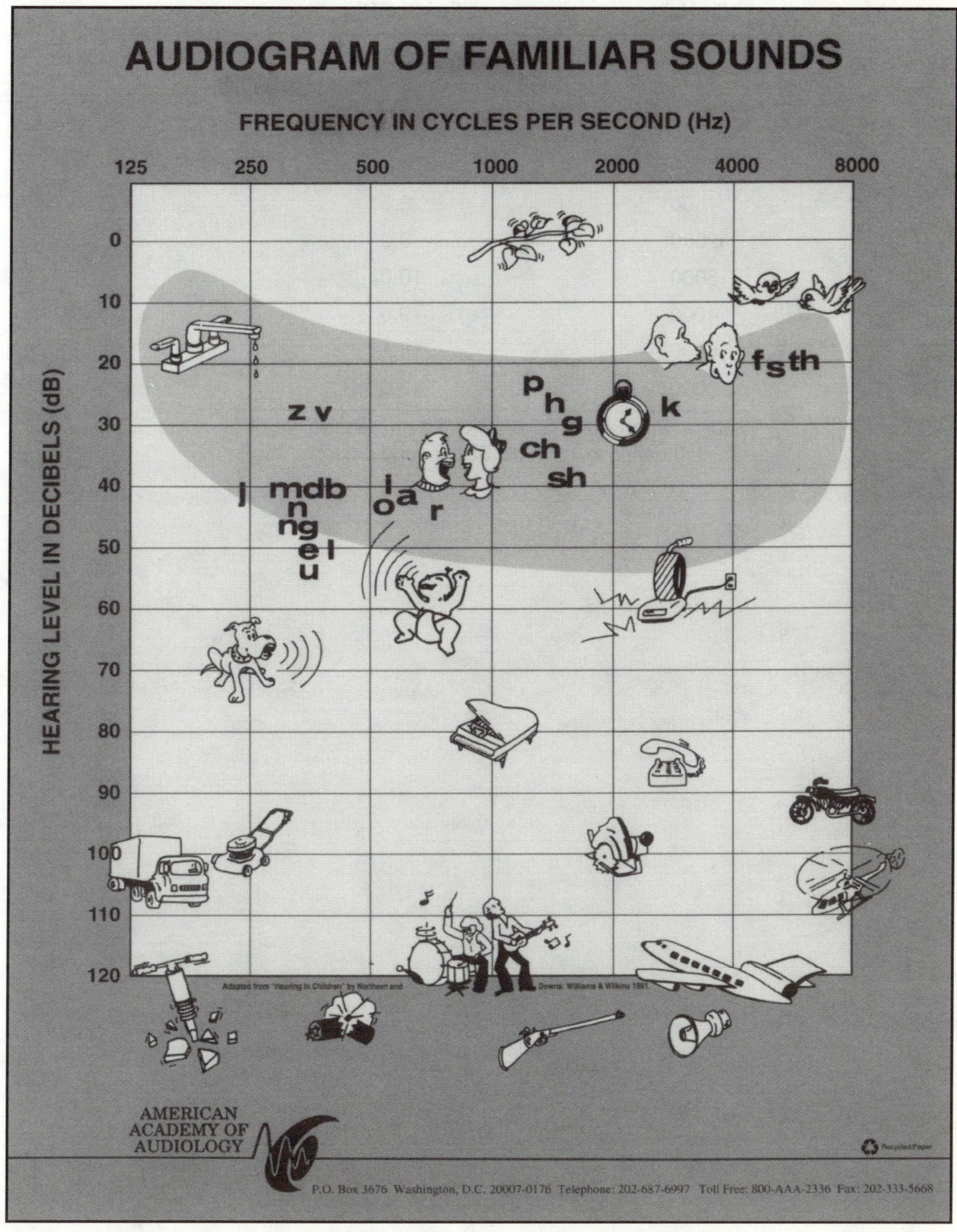

Source: Courtesy of the American Academy of Audiology and Dr. Jerry Northern

ANSI Standard Reference Threshold Sound Pressure Levels

Frequency (in Hz)	Normal Hearing Threshold Level (in dB SPL)
125	45.5
250	25.5
500	11.5
1000	7.0
1500	6.5
2000	9.0
3000	10.0
4000	9.5
6000	15.5
8000	13.0

Source: From ANSI S3.6-1969, i.e. the equivalent of 0 dB HL (hearing level) in dB SPL (sound pressure level)

Acceptable Noise Levels in dB SPL in Audiometric Test Rooms

Table assumes normal hearing threshold level is 0 dB HL Re ANSI (1969).

	Frequency (Hz) Octave Band Level Measurements									
Test Condition	**125**	**250**	**500**	**1000**	**1500**	**2000**	**3000**	**4000**	**6000**	**8000**
Supra-aural earphones (dB SPL)	34.5	23.0	21.5	22.5	29.0	34.5	39.0	42.0	41.0	45.0
Sound field or bone conduction (dB SPL)	28.0	18.5	14.5	12.5	14.0	8.5	8.5	9.0	14.0	20.5

Source: From the ANSI Criteria for Permissible Ambient Noise During Audiometric Testing (ANSI, 1977) and Wilber LA. Pure tone audiometry: air and bone conduction. In Rintelmann W. (ed), *Hearing Assessment* (2nd ed.). Austin, TX: Pro-Ed, 1991: p. 19.

Classic Quote

Jay W. Sanders on Masking in Audiology

"Of all the clinical procedures used in auditory assessment, masking is probably the most often misused and the least understood. For many clinicians, the approach to masking is a haphazard, hit-or-miss bit of guess work with no basis in any set of principles."

Source: Sanders JW. In J Katz (ed), *Handbook of Clinical Audiology*. Baltimore: Williams & Wilkins, 1972, p. 111.

Hood Plateau Method for Determining Adequate Masking in the Measurement of Bone-conduction Pure Tone Thresholds

Hypothetical results are shown for a 500 Hz signal with a normal hearing ear (open circles) and an ear with mild conductive hearing loss (filled circles).

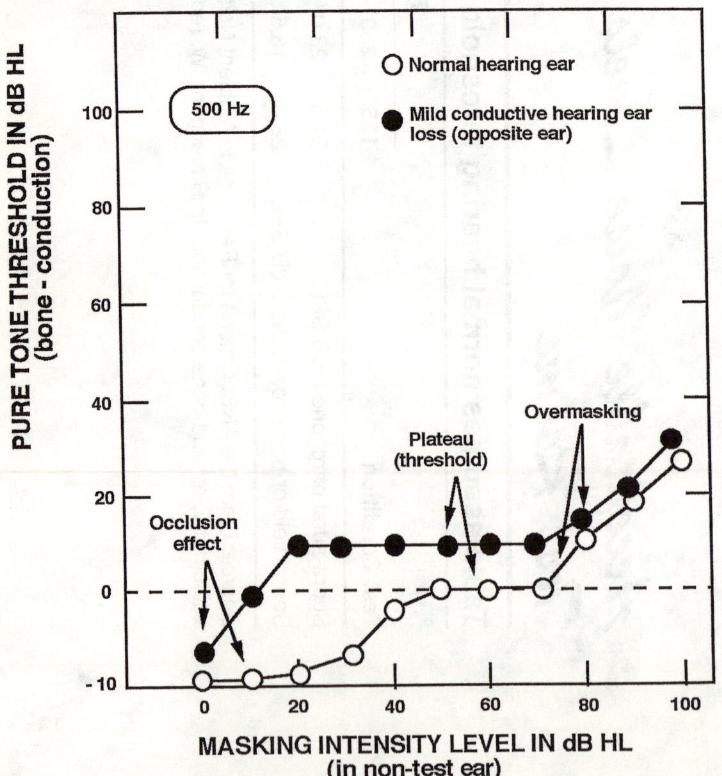

Technical Tip

Masking made simple

ASSUMPTIONS

- ☐ **Assumption #1: Clinical application of aural immittance measurement.** Routine use of tympanometry and acoustic reflex measurement is the most efficient and effective approach for determining whether peripheral auditory dysfunction has a middle ear component. Decisions on the use of masking, e.g. whether the hearing loss is sensorineural versus conductive or mixed, are predicated initially on the results of immittance measures.
- ☐ **Assumption #2: Masking formulae and the plateau method have clinical disadvantages.** The clinical application of formulae (e.g., Goldstein & Newman, 1985; Beedle, 1971; Liden, Nilsson & Anderson, 1959; Martin, 1986) or the plateau method of masking (Hood, 1960) for determining appropriate masking levels for each test frequency for air- and bone-conduction signals can be confusing and/or time consuming. Consistency and simplicity in technique is always desirable in clinical audiology.
- ☐ **Assumption #3: Insert earphones are preferable to supra-aural earphones in pure tone and speech audiometry.** Interaural attenuation is highest, and the likelihood of unwanted crossover of the signal to the nontest ear or of masking from the nontest ear to the test ear is lowest when insert earphones are used. See **Interaural Attention Figure** in this ADR chapter for minimal interaural values for deeply inserted ER-3A earphone plugs.
- ☐ **Assumption #4: It's okay to go for maximum masking.** There is no clinical contraindication to the use of maximum masker intensity levels, as long as overmasking (crossover of the masking signal from the nontest ear to the test ear) is avoided. That is, efforts to calculate the minimum effective masking levels are probably unwarranted and unecessary. "Go for the max."

GUIDELINES

- ☐ Always apply maximum masking (MM) for bone-conduction pure tone audiometry and whenever air-conduction pure tone or speech thresholds (using insert earphones) exceed 50 dB.
- ☐ Follow the simple equation (Silman & Silverman, 1991):

$$MM = Bt - IA - 5\text{ dB}$$

  where MM = maximum masking, Bt = bone conduction threshold of the test ear, and IA = interaural attenuation.
- ☐ Determine IA by reference to minimum values published for ER-3A earphones for audiometric frequencies (summarized on page 96).
- ☐ Ask the patient to lateralize the response (i.e., to give a side-specific—right ear or left ear—response). This can be a verbal response or the use of a separate button for each hand (ear).

Clinical Concept

Liden Formula for Masking

Determining minimum and maximum effective masking levels:

☐ Air conduction

M_{min} = At – 40 + (Am – Bm)
M_{max} = Bt + 40, provided M_{max} is less than D

☐ Bone Conduction

M_{min} = Bt + (Am – Bm)
M_{max} = Bt + 40, provided M_{max} is less than D

where,

A = air conduction threshold
B = bone conduction threshold
t = test ear
m = masked ear
D = discomfort level

Source: Adapted from Liden G., Nilsson G., Anderson H. (1959). Narrow band masking with white noise. *Acta Otolaryngologica 50:* 116–124.

Clinical Concepts

Clinical Tests of Bone Conduction

GENERAL PRINCIPLES

☐ There are three mechanisms underlying bone conduction hearing:

- the inertial response of the middle ear ossicles and the inner ear fluids
- the distortional response of the cochlear bony labyrinth
- radiation of sound energy into external ear canal

☐ When a signal is presented to the head via bone conduction, the apparent direction or image of the bone-conducted sound will shift toward the ear which receives the signal at a higher sound intensity or with a leading phase.

☐ In patients with mixed hearing impairments, or sensory hearing impairments of varying configurations, there may be interactions among the degree of sensory (bone conduction) hearing impairment and the outcome of clinical bone conduction tests.

TESTS

☐ Bing

One ear canal is occluded. If both ears are normal, low frequency (1000 Hz and below) sounds lateralize to occluded ear. Lateralization does not occur if there is middle ear dysfunction. Occlusion presumably eliminates the escape of low frequency sounds from the ear canal, producing an apparent increase in sound intensity.

☐ Weber

Bone-conducted signals presented to a midline site (e.g., the forehead) lateralize to an ear with middle ear dysfunction (conductive hearing loss). The middle ear dysfunction (e.g., fluid or purulence) increases the mass and friction properties of the impedance of the ossicular chain which, in turn, increase the inertial bone conduction component and increase intensity of the bone-conducted signal.

☐ Runge

One ear canal is filled with water. If that ear is normal, low frequency bone-conducted signals are lateralized to that ear. Lack of lateralization is consistent with middle ear dysfunction (conductive hearing loss) on the test (filled ear canal) ear. Filling the ear canal with water presumably loads the tympanic membrane which increases the inertia of the ossicular chain and, as as result, increases the perceived intensity level in the test ear.

☐ Gelle

Air pressure in the ear canal is increased or, in modified versions of the Gelle test, also decreased. Patients with normal hearing note a decrease in hearing sensitivity for air- and bone-conducted signals. Patients with conductive hearing loss due to ossicular abnormalities (fixation or disarticulation) note a decrease in hearing sensitivity for air- but not bone-conducted signals, especially for lower frequencies. This latter outcome is described as a negative Gelle test.

Source: Adapted from Schuknecht HF. *Pathology of the Ear* (2nd ed). Philadelphia: Williams & Wilkins. 1993, p. 82.

Reference Levels for Bone Conduction

Reference RMS equivalent threshold force levels (dB re 1 N) for B-71 bone oscillator (vibrator) used with a P-3333 Headband (ANSI S3.26-1981).

Frequency (in H_z)	Threshold Force Level (dB re 1 n)
250	61.0
500	59.0
1000	39.0
2000	32.5
3000	28.0
4000	31.0

Source: From Melnick W. Instrument calibration. In Rintelmann W (ed.). *Hearing Assessment* (2nd ed). Austin, TX: Pro-Ed, 1991, p. 827.

Volume Unit (VU) Meter

The VU meter permits precise presentation of auditory signals in deciBels (dB).

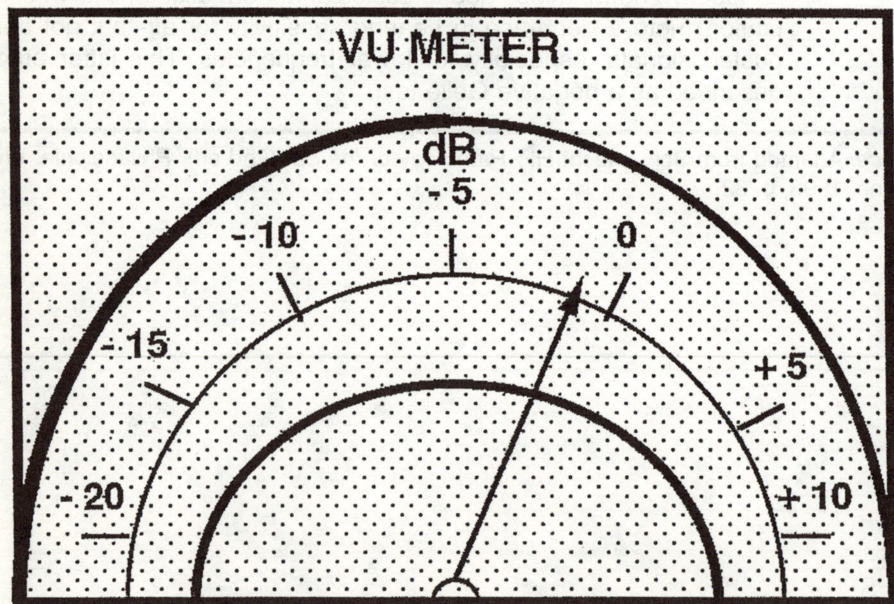

NOTE: At Vanderbilt University, these devices are referred to as VU2 meters.

Air Conduction Pure Tone Threshold as a Function of Age

For otologically normal persons (according to ISO 1999 standard (1990).

	Frequency in Hertz							
Age (years)	**250**	**500**	**1000**	**2000**	**3000**	**4000**	**6000**	**8000**
Men								
25	0	0	0	0	1	1	1	1
30	0	1	1	1	2	2	3	3
35	1	1	1	2	3	5	5	6
40	1	2	2	3	6	8	9	1
45	2	3	3	5	8	12	13	16
50	3	4	4	7	12	16	18	23
55	4	5	5	10	16	22	25	30
60	5	6	7	12	20	28	32	39
65	7	8	9	15	25	35	40	49
70	8	9	11	19	31	43	49	59
75	10	11	13	23	37	52	59	71
Women								
25	0	0	0	0	0	0	1	1
30	0	1	1	1	1	1	2	2
35	1	1	1	2	2	3	3	4
40	1	2	2	3	4	4	6	7
45	2	3	3	4	5	7	9	11
50	3	4	4	6	8	9	12	15
55	4	5	5	8	10	12	16	21
60	5	6	7	1	13	16	21	26
65	7	8	9	13	17	20	27	33
70	8	9	1	16	20	24	32	41

Source: From Rosler G. Progression of hearing loss caused by occupational noise. *Scand Audiol 23:* 13–37, 1994.

Earphones and Other Transducers

Comparison of Reference Threshold Levels Among Different Earphones (for 0 dB HL)

	Reference Threshold Levels re 20mPA (0.0002 dynes/cm^2)			
Frequency (in Hz)	**Western Electric 705A**	**Telephonics TDH-3**	**Telephonics(b) TDH-49 and 50**	**Telex 1470 (c)**
125	45.5	45.0	47.5	47.0
250	24.5	25.5	26.5	27.5
500	11.0	11.5	13.5	13.0
1000	6.5	7.0	7.5	6.5
1500	6.5	6.5	7.5	5.0
2000	8.5	9.0	11.0	8.0
3000	7.5	10.0	9.5	7.5
4000	9.0	9.5	10.5	8.5
6000	8.0	15.5	13.5	17.5
8000	9.5	13.0	13.0	17.5

Sources: Michael PL, Bienvenue GR. Real-ear threshold level comparisons between the Telephonics TDH-39 earphone with a metal outer shell and the TDH-39, TDH-49, and TDH-50 earphones with plastic outer shells. *Journal of the Acoustical Society of America 61:* 1640–1642, 1977; Michael PL, Bienvenue GR. Calibration data for the Telex 1470-A audiometric earphones. *Journal of the Acoustical Society of America 67:* 1812–1815, 1980.

Technical Tips

Insert Earphones

- ☐ Be careful to leave the small plastic coupler in the tube when removing the foam plug after testing a patient. The plastic coupler may come out of the tube with the disposable foam plug. Consider securing the coupler in the tube with a very small dab of cement.
- ☐ Have bags of adult- and pediatric-size foam plugs within arm's reach of your ER-3A insert transducers in the sound booth, or wherever you use them.
- ☐ Make sure that the red tube is connected to the right transducer (box) and the blue tube is connected to the left transducer. Reversing the tubes might result in inadvertant reversal of the earphones when assessing a patient.
- ☐ Periodically inspect the tubing for occlusion with debris, cracks, or kinking (compression). Always suspect such problems if a patient shows an unexpected apparent mild conductive hearing loss.
- ☐ Do the same for the actual ear plugs whenever a patient shows an unexpected apparent mild conductive hearing loss.
- ☐ Always discard the disposable foam plugs immediately after use. In this day of necessary concern about universal precautions, disposable foam plugs are a major advantage of insert earphones.
- ☐ *NOTICE TO ALL CLINICAL AUDIOLOGISTS:* With any earphone, always verify that phone plugs are pushed all the way into the audiometer and sound booth wall panel jacks. If the earphone plugs appear to be secure, but are really not plugged all the way in, the result may be a 20 to 30 dB reduction in signal intensity. This may lead to a spurious unilateral (or bilateral) mild conductive hearing loss. When you have doubts, push on the plug as hard as you can. If you hear a clicking sound, the plug wasn't in the jack all the way.

Advantages Cited for Insert (ER-3A) Earphones

- ☐ General
  - ✓ increased interaural attenuation
  - ✓ increased ambient noise attenuation
  - ✓ elimination of ear canal collapse
  - ✓ increased patient comfort
- ☐ Auditory evoked response stimulation
  - ✓ reduced transducer ringing
  - ✓ reduced electrical (stimulus) artifact with separation of transducer and inverting electrode

Interaural Attenuation Values for Supra-aural Versus Insert Earphones

Auditory signals are less likely to cross over from the test ear to the nontest ear for insert earphones, especially in the lower frequency region.

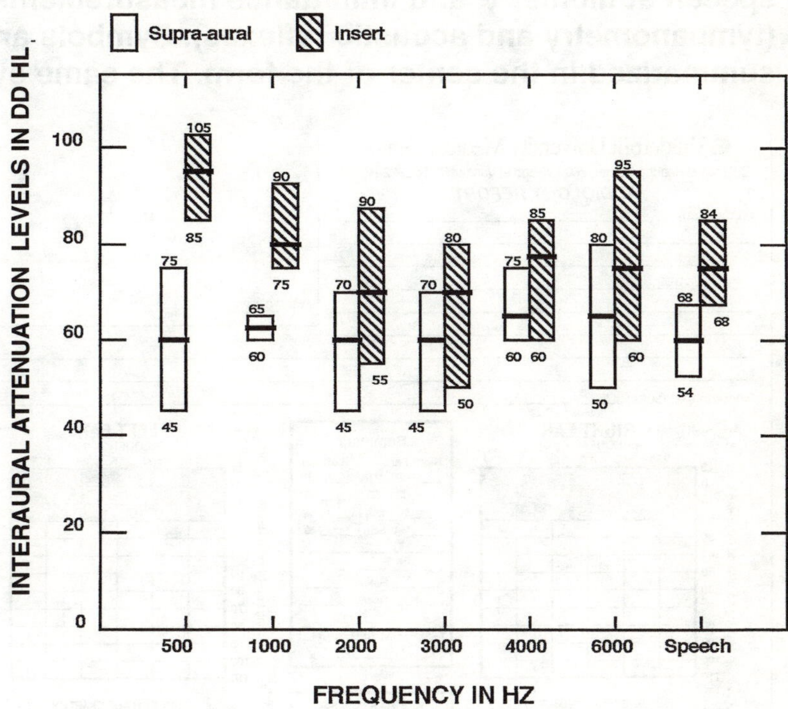

Audiograms and Audiometric Patterns

Example of a "Separate Ear" Audiogram Form

Audiogram form including findings for pure tone and speech audiometry, and immittance measurements (tympanometry and acoustic reflexes). Symbols are summarized in the center of the form. The same symbols

Vanderbilt University Medical Center
Balance & Hearing Center, 2600 Village at Vanderbilt, Tel. 322-HEAR
AUDIOLOGY REPORT

Impressions: ____

Recommendations: ____

RIGHT EAR
FREQUENCY (Hz)
250 500 1K 2K 4K
Hearing Level in dB (ANSI-69)
-10 0 10 20 30 40 50 60 70 80 90 100 110

Summary

Right Ear		Left Ear
____ dB	PTA	____ dB
____ dB	ST	____ dB
____ %	PB_M	____ %
____ %	SSI_M	____ %
____	Reflex	____
____	Decay	____

WEBER
____ Hz

LEFT EAR
FREQUENCY (Hz)
250 500 1K 2K 4K
Hearing Level in dB (ANSI-69)
-10 0 10 20 30 40 50 60 70 80 90 100 110

SPEECH AUDIOMETRY
% Correct: 0 20 40 60 80 100
dB HL: 20 40 60 80 100

KEY TO SYMBOLS

	unmasked	masked
AC	○	●
BC	△	▲
SAL	◇	
No Response ↘		
ACOUSTIC REFLEX	uncrossed □	crossed ☒
SSI	□	■
PB	○	●

IMPEDANCE AUDIOMETRY
Compliance in cm^3: 0 0.3 0.6 0.9 1.2 1.5
mmH$_2$O: -400 -300 -200 -100 0 100 200

Crossed
REFLEX PATTERN
Uncrossed
□ Normal ■ Abnormal

Referred by: ____ Audiologist: ____

WHITE COPY — Medical Records / YELLOW COPY — Otolaryngology / PINK COPY — Audiology MC 0905 (4/92)

Example of a Sound Field Audiogram Form

Note findings for pure tone and speech audiometry and immittance measurements (tympanometry and acoustic

Vanderbilt University Medical Center
Balance & Hearing Center, 2600 Village at Vanderbilt, Tel. 322-HEAR
AUDIOLOGY REPORT

Impressions: ______

Recommendations: ______

SOUND FIELD AUDIOGRAM

FREQUENCY (Hz): 250, 500, 1K, 2K, 4K

Hearing Level in dB (ANSI-69): -10, 0, 10, 20, 30, 40, 50, 60, 70, 80, 90, 100, 110

SOUND FIELD AUDIOMETRY

Test Method:

VRA Play Audiometry

BOA Other ______

Speech Results:

Sound Field

SAT ____ SRT ____

Headphone

Right SAT ____ SRT ____

Left SAT ____ SRT ____

Reliability: ______

ELM Results: ______

HEARING AID EVALUATION

Hearing Aids:

A: ______ #1

B: ______ #2

Speech Results:

	SRT	WDS Q	WDS N	LEVEL (HL)
S				
A				
B				

Word List: ______

Tape Live Voice

S/N Ratio: ______

Tolerance: ______

RIGHT EAR
IMPEDANCE AUDIOMETRY

Compliance in cm³: 0, 0.3, 0.6, 0.9, 1.2, 1.5
mmH₂O: -400, -300, -200, -100, 0, 100, 200

KEY TO SYMBOLS

S = Sound Field (unaided)
A = Hearing Aid #1
B = Hearing Aid #2
Δ = Bone

LEFT EAR
IMPEDANCE AUDIOMETRY

Compliance in cm³: 0, 0.3, 0.6, 0.9, 1.2, 1.5
mmH₂O: -400, -300, -200, -100, 0, 100, 200

Referred by: ______ Audiologist: ______

WHITE COPY — Medical Records / YELLOW COPY — Otolaryngology / PINK COPY — Audiology

MC 3536 (3/92)

Four Common Air-conduction Audiogram Configurations

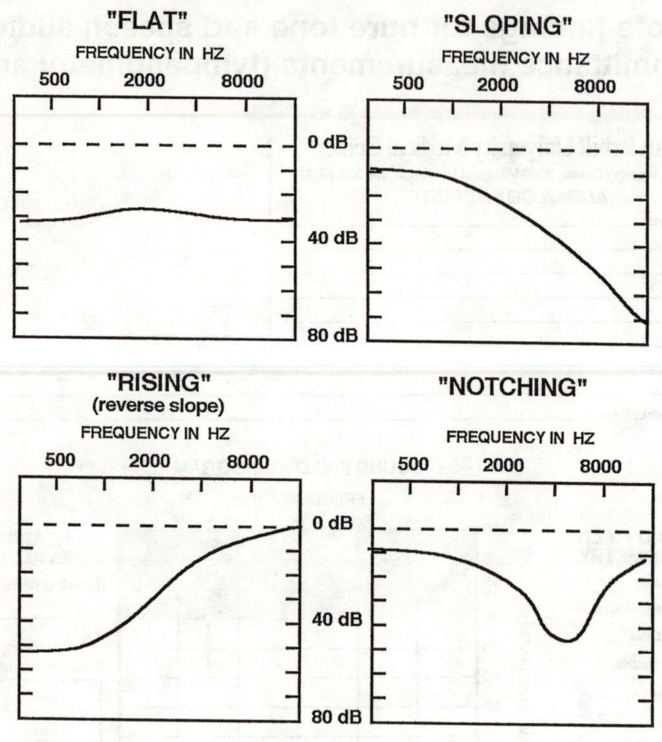

Audioid:

What name did James Jerger give to his newest boat?

"AUDacious"

Audiogram Configurations Encountered Most Often in Clinical Hearing Assessment

Different configurations are often associated with different causes of hearing loss or etiologies.

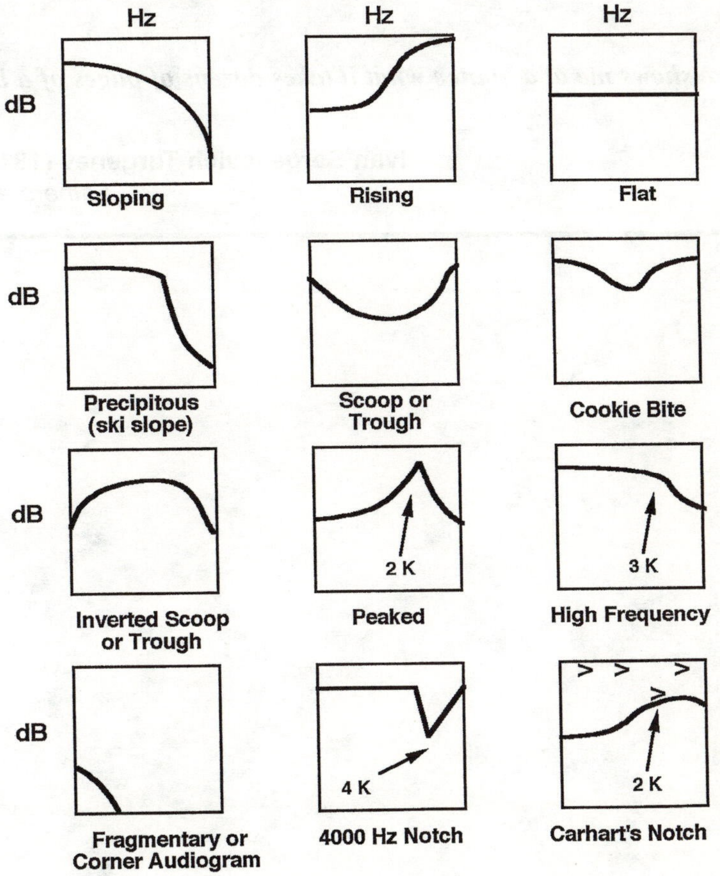

Classic Quote

An anonymous ancient Chinese audiologist, and a more recent Russian, probably on the value of graphing hearing findings with an audiogram

"One picture is worth more than a thousand words."

—Chinese proverb

"A picture shows me at a glance what it takes dozens of pages of a book to expound."

Ivan Sergeyevich Turgenev (1818–1883)
Fathers and Sons

Schematic Illustration of Insert Earphone and TIPtrode

Components of the Etymotics Research (ER) 3A "insert" earphone. Advantages of insert earphones are summarized in Tables and Lists in this ADR chapter. The insert earphone can also be adapted as an electrode (known as the TIPtrode) for auditory evoked response measurement (*lower portion of figure*).

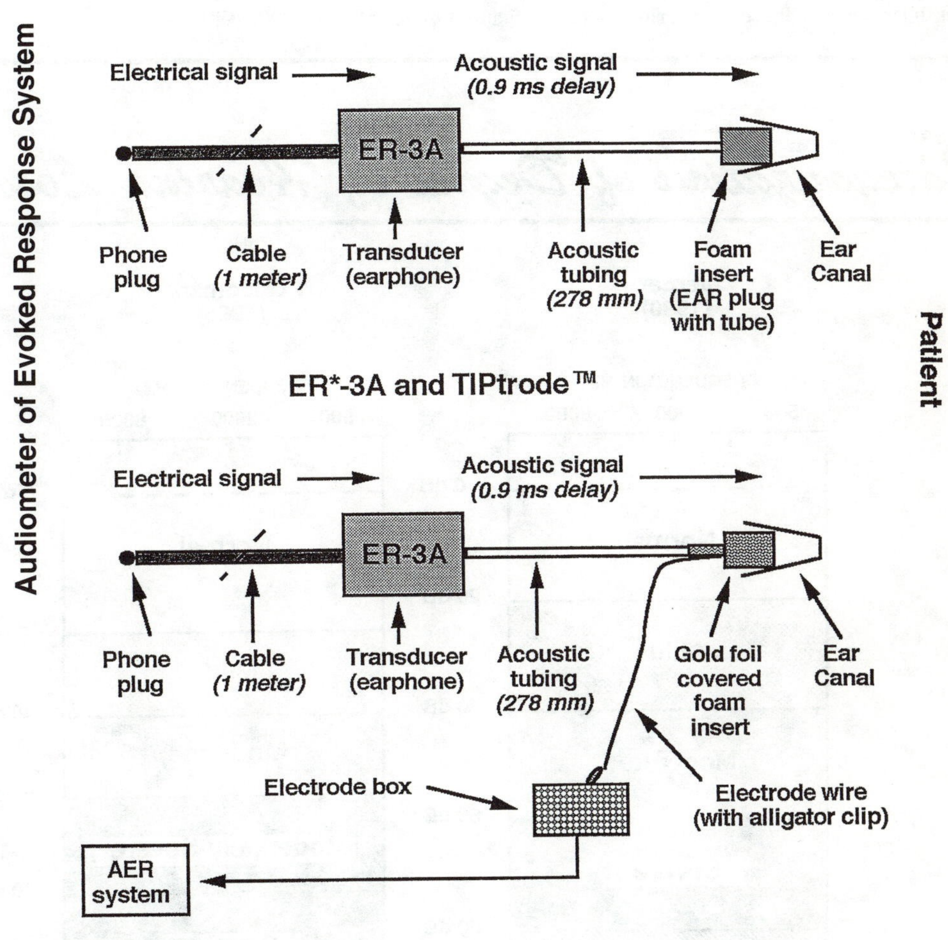

Key References

Classification of degree of hearing loss (ordered chronologically). See ADR Volume II (Chapter 19) for AMA guidelines for evaluation of hearing handicap.

Fletcher H. *Speech and Hearing*. New York: Van Nostrand, 1929.

Goodman A. Reference zero levels for pure-tone audiometer. *Asha 7*: 262–263, 1965.

American Academy of Otolaryngology and American Council of Otolaryngology. Guide for evaluation of hearing handicap. *JAMA 241*: 2055-2059, 1979.

Jerger J, Jerger S. Measurement of hearing in adults. In MM Paparella, DA Shumrick (eds). *Otolaryngology* (2nd ed). Philadelphia: WB Saunders, 1980, p. 1226.

Clark JG. Uses and abuses of hearing loss classification. *Asha 23*: 493–500, 1981.

Categorization of Degree of Hearing Loss

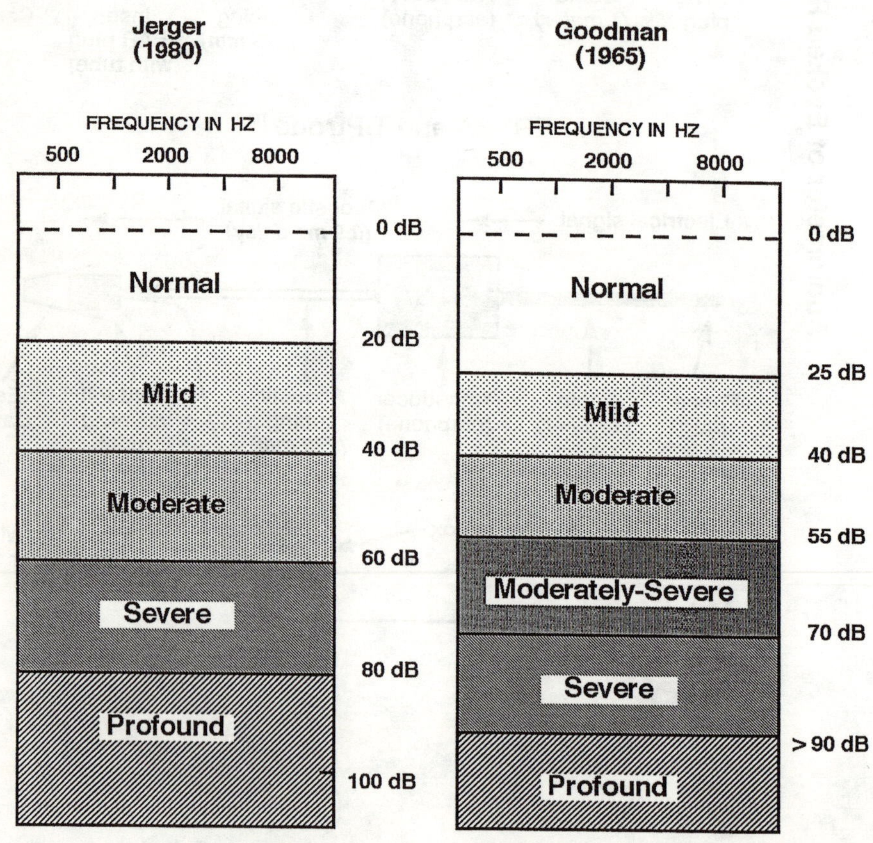

General "Separate Ear" Audiogram Form

The key to symbols is located in the center of the figure. Top portion is for plotting results of pure tone audiometry. The darker horizontal line at 20 dB HL is the limit of the clinical normal region for adults. Results of speech audiometry including performance intensity (PI) functions are plotted on the graphs in the middle section of the figure. Tympanograms, and the acoustic reflex pattern for ipsilateral and contralateral conditions, are plotted in the lower section of the figure. A normal tympanogram peak falls within the rectangle in the tympanometry graph. The small hatched rectangular box next to each ear represents the transducer (earphone) for each condition. The outcome of reflex measurement for each condition (normal, abnormal, or absent) is indicated by the box.

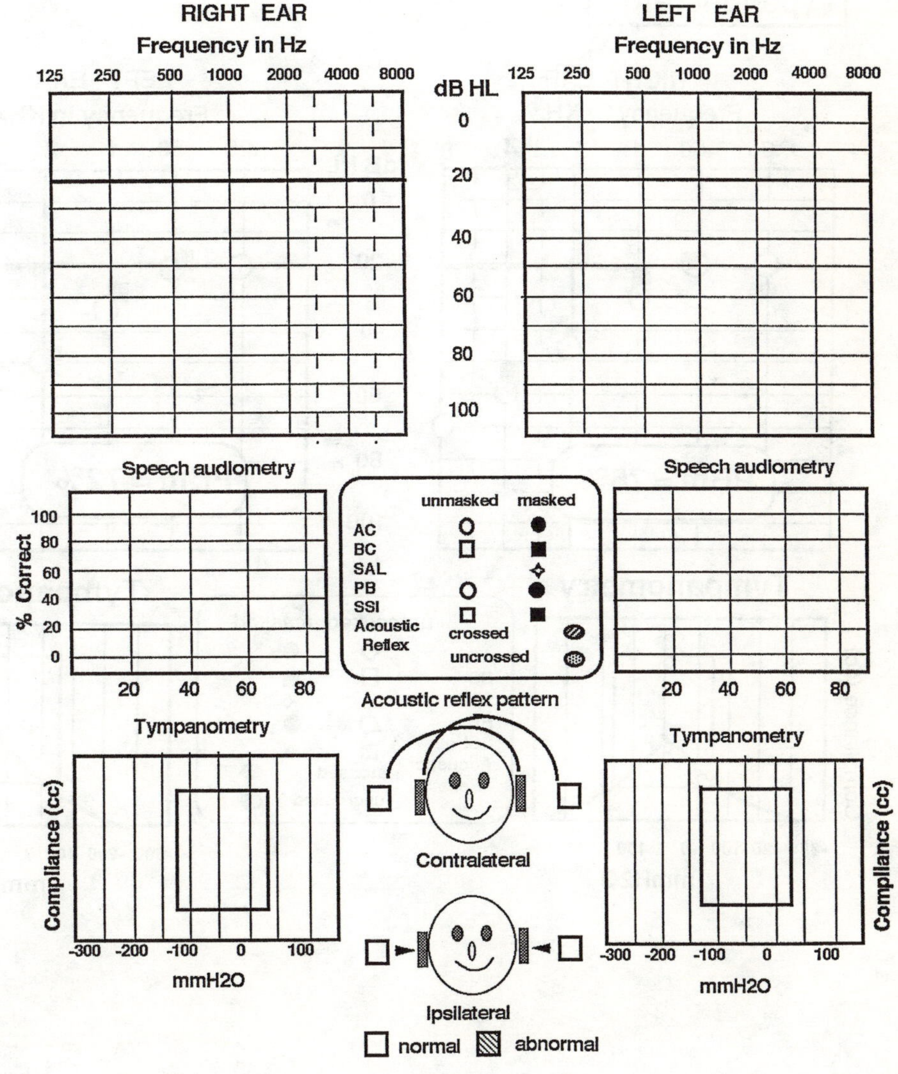

Audiometric Findings Characteristic of Peripheral Presbycusis

Circles indicate pure tone thresholds for air-conduction signals, where as black squares indicate masked bone-conduction thresholds. Pb_m refers to maximum score on phonetically balanced word recognition test. Tympanogram peaks are within the normal range (box within tympanometry graph).

Presbycusis (peripheral)

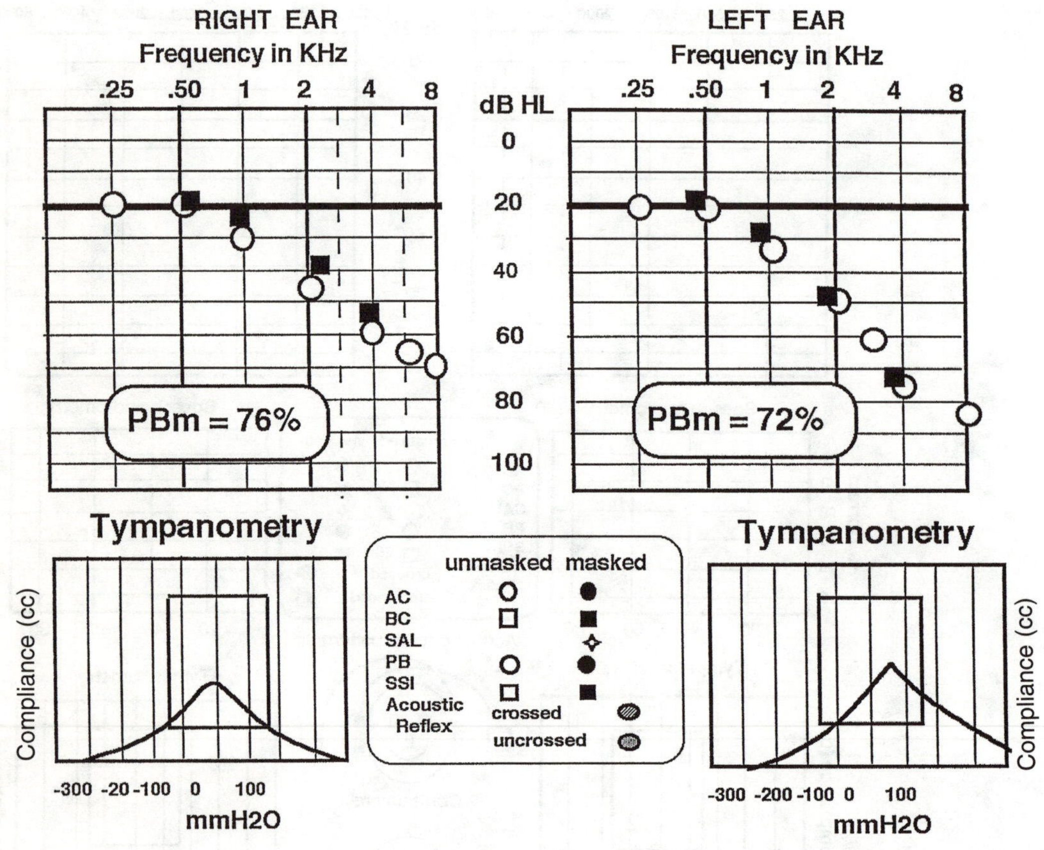

Audiometric Findings Characteristic of Noise Exposure

Circles indicate pure tone thresholds for air-conduction signals, where as black squares indicate masked bone-conduction thresholds. Pb_m refers to maximum score on phonetically balanced word recognition test. Tympanogram peaks are within the normal range (box within tympanometry graph).

Noise exposure

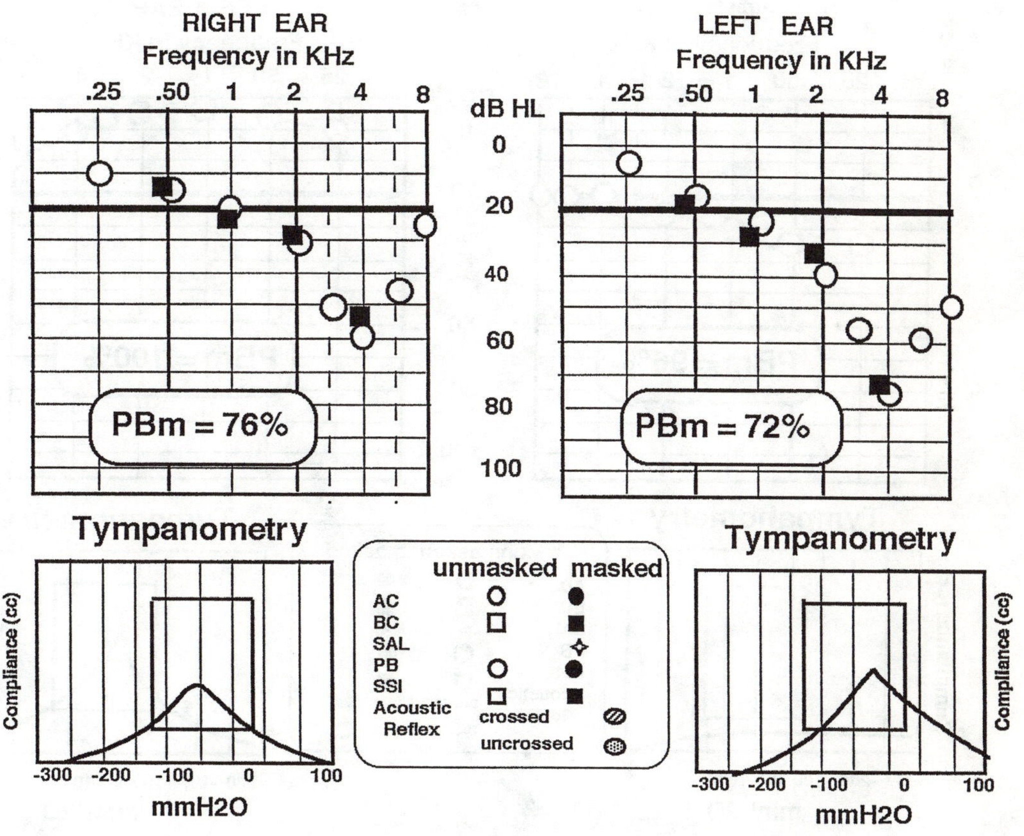

Audiometric Findings Characteristic of Otitis Media with Effusion

Circles indicate pure tone thresholds for air-conduction signals, where as black squares indicate masked bone-conduction thresholds. Pb_m refers to maximum score on phonetically balanced word recognition test. The right ear tympanogram is type B (no peak) and is outside of the normal range (box within tympanometry graph).

Otitis media with effusion
(right ear)

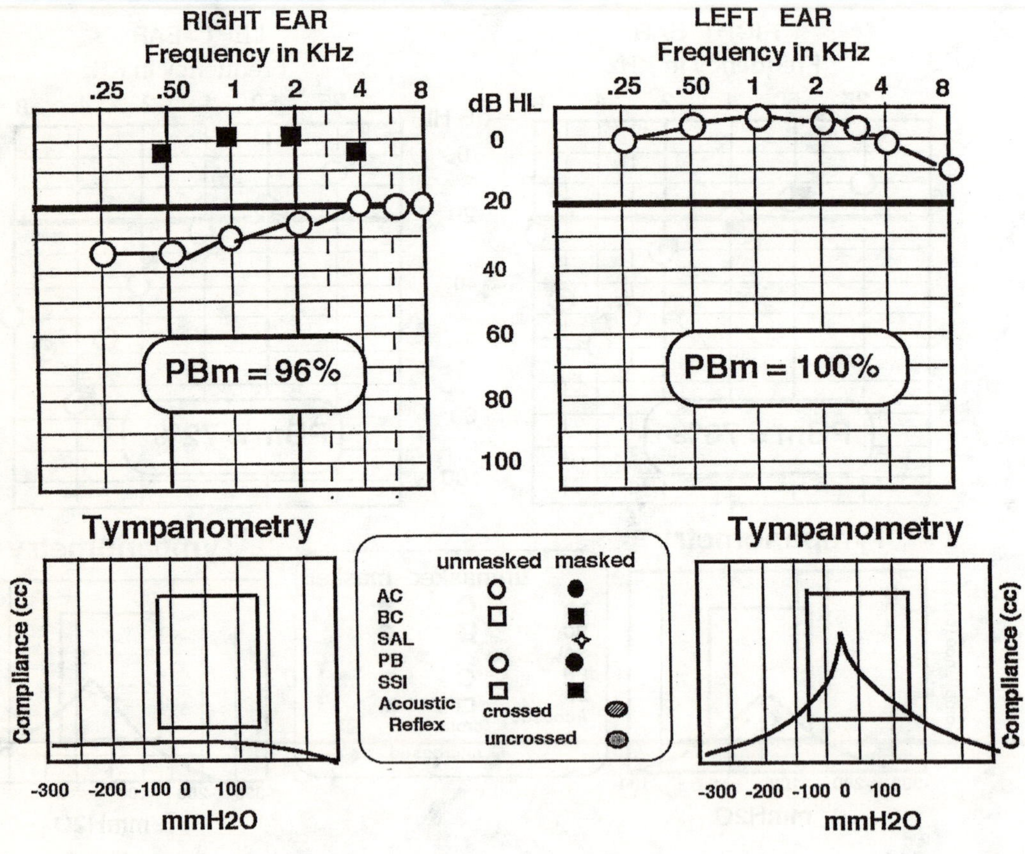

ETC.

Schematic Description of Four Tuning Fork Tests

The square in the region of the ear represents the middle ear, whereas the adjacent oval represents the cochlea. Open symbols indicate normal status, whereas filled symbols indicate abnormal status.

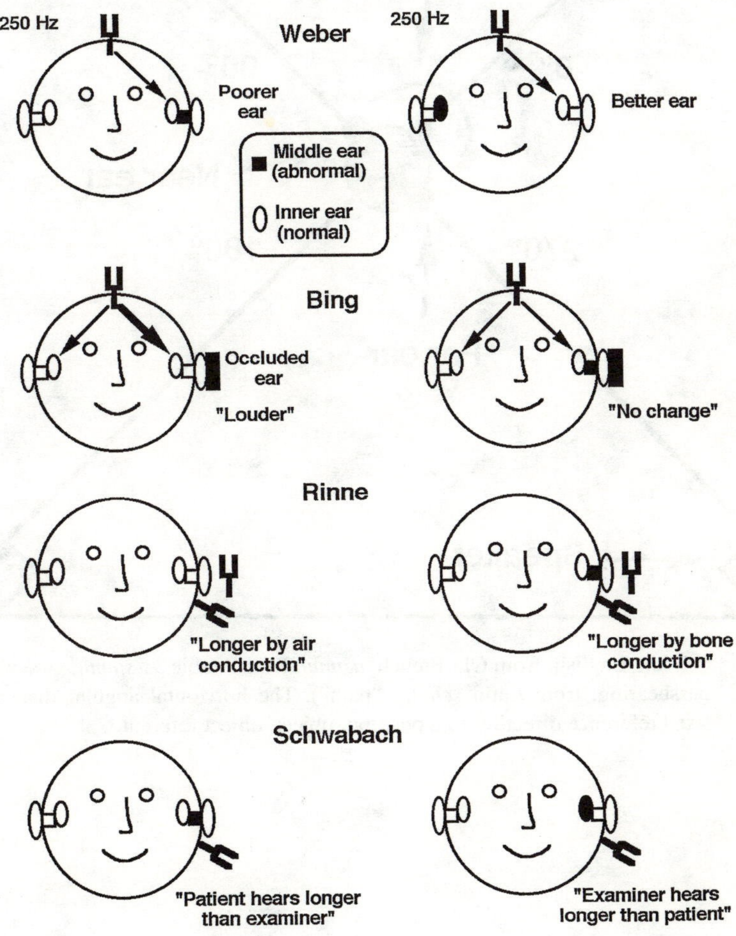

Concept of Azimuth* in Sound Field Measurement of Auditory Function

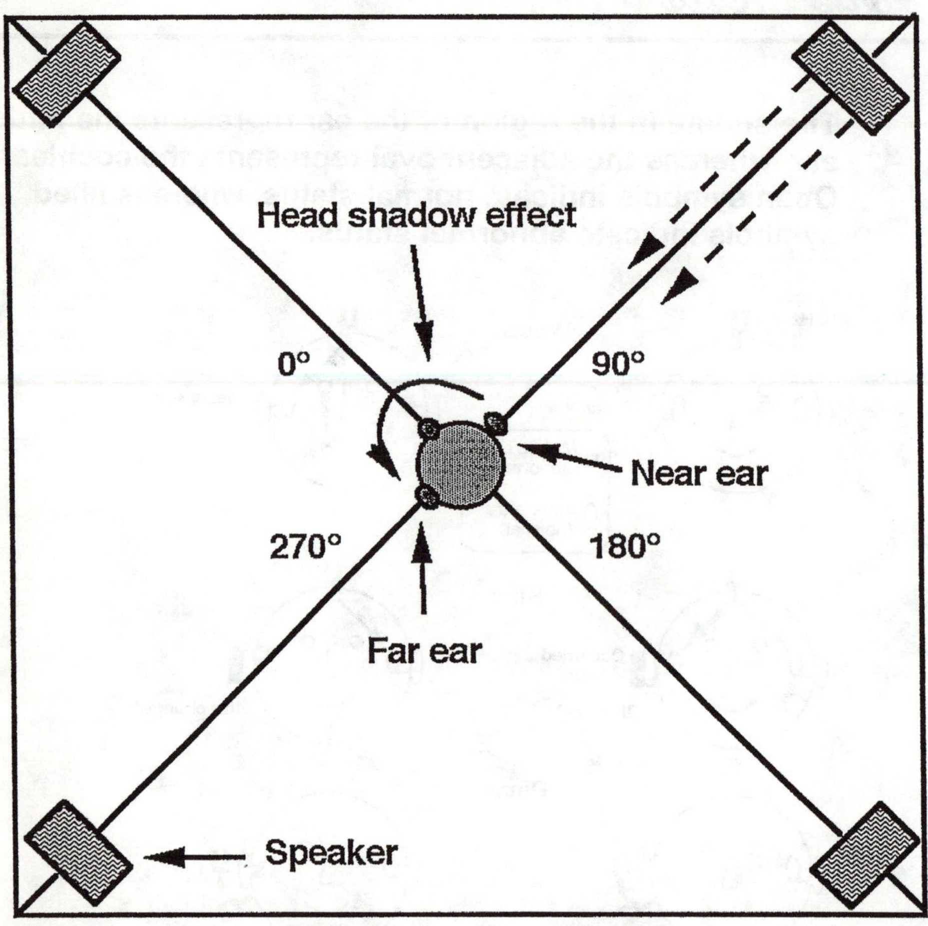

**Definition:* (Middle English, from Old French *azimut*, from Arabic *as-sumut*, "the way", compassbearing, from Latin *semita*, "path"). The horizontal angular distance from a fixed reference direction to a position, object, object referent.

Technical Tip

Assessment of suspected pseudohypacusis *or* how to outfool the malingerer

- ☐ Advance warning signals that a patient might feign a hearing loss include:
  - refer by a lawyer
  - refer by U.S. Department of Labor (USDL)
  - compensation for an injury, accident, or noise exposure may hinge on the outcome of the hearing evaluation
  - the patient's history and complaints are inconsistent with your clinical impressions of the patient's hearing ability
  - previous audiometry yielded highly inconsistent results
  - the patient frequently asks how the results are coming out, or how he's doing
- ☐ Perform acoustic reflex measurement first, and estimate hearing loss with Sensitivity Prediction by the Acoustic Reflex (SPAR) or, minimally, by analyzing acoustic reflex threshold for a broad band noise (BBN) signal. A BBN acoustic reflex threshold of 85 dB or better strongly suggests hearing sensitivity within normal limits. See Chapter 4 for details.
- ☐ If possible, assess otoacoustic emissions (OAE) before or immediately after pure tone audiometry and analyze patient findings according to normative data. See Chapter 5 for details. Feel free to let patients watch the testing, preferrably after you've given them an inservice on what a normal response looks like on the computer monitor. Their nervousness and sweating at this point may provide further confirmation of malingering.
- ☐ Perform spondee threshold assessment first, give the patient plenty of opportunity to respond, yet don't give the patient much of a reference for intensity. For example,
  - Use tape or CD recorded speech materials (minimizes visual cues!)
  - Begin at 0 dB HL
  - Ascend in 5 dB steps
  - Present three or more words at each intensity level
  - Document any half-word responses (e.g., The word is "hotdog" but the patient says, "Uh, uh, I think I heard dog").
- ☐ Use the same general technique for pure tone audiometry:
  - Sneak up on them and don't give them anything to hang their response on.

- ✔ Consider asking the patient to tell you how many beeps he hears, then present either one, two, or three in quick succession
- ✔ Ask the patient to say "yes" when he hears the tones, and "no" when he doesn't. Don't be discouraged, however, if most patients don't fall for this ploy. It seems like some patients have visited the library and studied the Pseudohypacusis chapter of an introductory audiology textbook.

☐ Begin word recognition testing at 40 dB HL and keep presenting the words even though the patient assures you that he or she can't hear them. How do they always know that they aren't hearing them anyhow? Sometimes, patients will lose patience and begin to occasionally repeat the words, even though they volunteered no pure tone thresholds anywhere near 40 dB.

☐ Document any increase in the vocal intensity of the patient's response to words when masking noise is presented to the nontest "hearing impaired" ear.

☐ Take the time to inspect the pattern of audiometric findings for:

- ✔ a pure tone average that is > 7 dB worse than the speech threshold
- ✔ unusually good acoustic reflex threshold for BBN signal
- ✔ normal OAEs and some or all test frequencies
- ✔ discrepancy between pure tone audiogram and the patient's word recognition performance

☐ Consider frequency-specific auditory evoked response assessment to better define hearing status. A good choice is the auditory middle latency response to tone burst stimuli of, for example, 500 Hz, 1000 Hz, 2000 Hz, and 4000 Hz. See Chapter 8 for details.

☐ Consider confronting patients with your objective, electrophysiologic evidence that their hearing is actually quite good. Maybe they didn't quite understand the task. Do they want to give it one more try?

CHAPTER 3

Speech Audiometry

In This ADR Chapter

Perspective

If you had to select a single audiologic procedure to measure "hearing," it would have to be some speech audiometry measure. Our ability to perceive and understand speech is, by far, our most important hearing function. Theoretically, speech audiometry is an attempt at "communicometry"—measurement of our communication ability. Given the importance of speech audiometry in the measurement of communication abilities and disorders, it's not surprising that intensive investigation of speech audiometry materials and procedures has continued essentially unabated for over 50 years. Publications, and advances, in some other early audiologic frontiers, such as pure tone audiometry, have generally run their course and become few and far between. Speech audiometry research, on the other hand, remains vibrant, highly productive, and on the cutting edge of technological advances.

From the beginning, speech audiometry research has been a multidisciplinary effort uniting basic scientists (e.g., psychoacousticians, speech scientists), industrial research and development types (especially those employed by telephone companies), military investigators (pilots must hear well under adverse listening conditions), and clinical audiology researchers. Indeed, a listing of those who have dabbled in, or seriously investigated, speech audiometry questions would be very long and would, really, be a "who's who" roster of audiologists. It's hard to find a doctoral-level audiologist in his or her 40s, 50s, or 60s who didn't present or publish at least one or two speech audiometry papers at some point in his or her career.

With the development of the CD medium for recorded speech materials, CD-ROM options for personal computers, and other technological advances, it would appear that we have not yet seen the "golden era" of speech audiometry. What seems to be needed most now is for clinical audiologists to catch up with this rapidly advancing technology. In approaching speech audiometry, audiologists might well ponder the following quotation:

"A foolish consistency is the hobgoblin of little minds, adored by little statesmen and philosophers and divines. With consistency a great soul has simply nothing to do . . . . Speak what you think today in hard words and tomorrow speak what tomorrow thinks in hard words again, though it contradict everything you said today."

Ralph Waldo Emerson (1803–1882)
Self-Reliance

FOUNDATIONS OF SPEECH AUDIOMETRY

Dream Team for Speech Audiometry

Psycho-Acoustics Laboratories at Harvard University in the late 1940s and early 1950s

☐ **Captain**

- Stanley Smith "Smitty" Stevens

☐ **Team Members**

- Hallowell Davis
- James Egan
- Ira Hirsh *
- Clarence Hudgins
- Clifford Morgan
- Gordon Peterson
- Douglas Ross **

* Rookie

** The ADR first author had the pleasure of meeting Dr. Ross unexpectedly in the Vanderbilt Audiology Clinic. A retired physician living in Nashville, Dr. Ross underwent a basic audiologic assessment, performed by Dr. Hall, in 1990. Emerging from the sound booth, Dr. Ross proclaimed "I haven't heard those words [PAL PB words] in over 40 years." He then went on to relate some of his fascinating experiences as a medical student research assistant at the Harvard PAL in the late 1940s.

Mover and Oscillator

Ira Hirsh

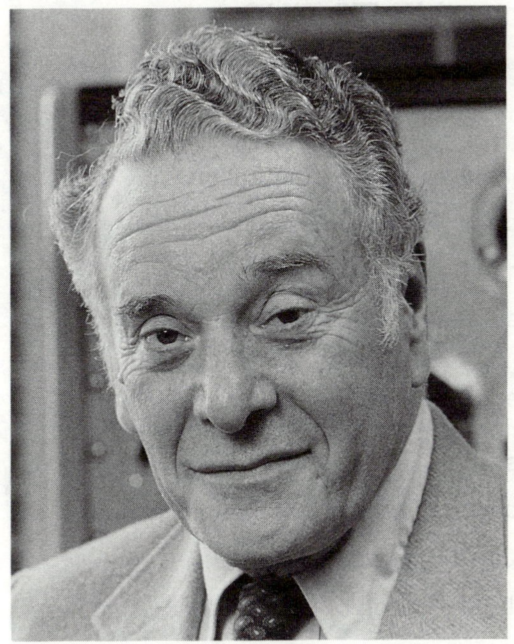

Ira Hirsh

Dr. Hirsh's first graduate studies were in audiology with Raymond Carhart at Northwestern University. He continued his graduate studies at Harvard University, completing his dissertation under S. S. Stevens in 1948.

In addition to his classic book, *The Measurement of Hearing* (1952), Hirsh has published 130 articles in professional journals, among them such important contributions to the literature as "Development of Materials in Speech Audiometry" (*J Speech Hear Dis* 17: 1952) with co-authors and CID colleagues Hallowell Davis, S. Richard Silverman, and others. His research interests encompass binaural hearing, speech perception, the effects of noise, and the temporal aspects of auditory perception.

Dr. Hirsh is a member of numerous professional societies and has received a variety of professional honors including the Gold Medal of the Acoustical Society of America.

Ira Hirsh is currently the Mallinckrodt Distinguished University Professor Emeritus in Psychology and Audiology at Washington University in St. Louis, Missouri. He is also Senior Scientist at the Central Institute for the Deaf (CID) in St. Louis, having served previously as Director of CID.

Historical Reverberation

EVERYTHING (except audiology's advancement beyond exclusive reliance on standardized word recognition assessment) IN ITS TIME

How long it took . . .

	How long it took	
☐	Lincoln to travel to inaurguration	12 days
☐	Europe to hear Lincoln died	2 weeks
☐	Spain to hear of Columbus' voyage	5 months
☐	Drake to travel around the world	34 months
☐	Immittance measurements to be regularly applied clinically after the introduction of commercially available instrumentation in late 1960s	3 years
☐	Application of ABR in infants and children after discovery in 1970–1971	3 years
☐	For all Declaration of Independence signatures	6 years
☐	Regular clinical application of OAE after discovery in 1978	16 years
☐	Audiologists to dispense more than 50% of all hearing aids in the United States	50 years
☐	Universal use of standardized, recorded (taped or CD) speech materials for word recognition assessment, after development of materials at PAL in late 1940s	> 55 years and still waiting

Spectra for Different Categories of Speech Sounds

Frequency composition (spectra) and approximate intensity ranges, within conversational speech, for different categories of speech sounds.

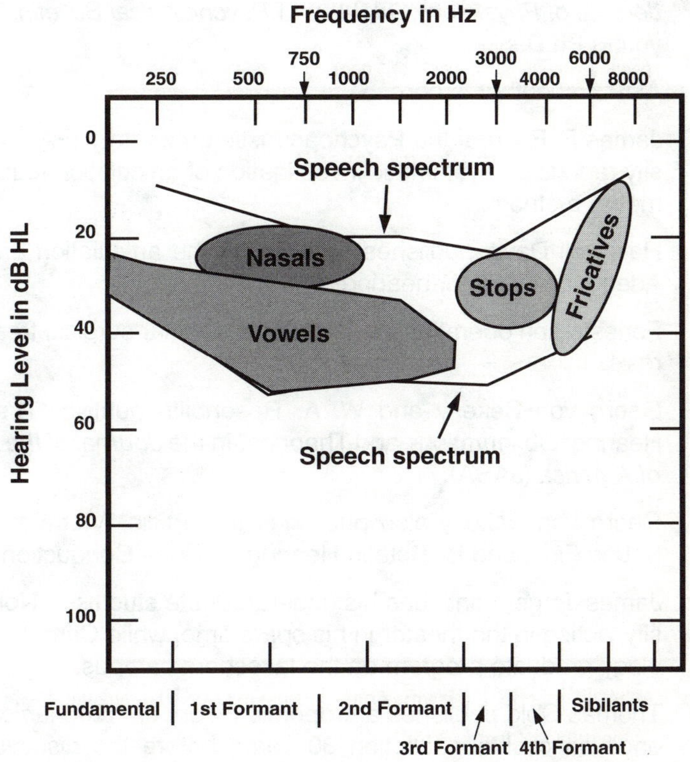

Sources: Tyler R. Measuring hearing loss in the future. *Brit J Audiol, (Suppl. 2):* 29–40, 1979; Liden G. Speech audiometry, an experimental and clinical study with Swedish language material. *Acta Otolaryngologica (Suppl. 114),* 1954; as in Olsen WO, Matkin ND. Speech audiometry. In *Hearing Assessment*, 2nd ed (WF Rintelmann, ed). Austin, TX:Pro-Ed, 1991, p. 64.

Historical Reverberation

1948—One of Our Favorite Years

- ☐ Ira Hirsh completes his doctoral dissertation at Harvard University under the direction of S. S. Stevens.
- ☐ The young and prolific Dr. Hirsch publishes a series of three papers on binaural summation and interaural summation and inhibition in the *American Journal of Physiology, JASA*, and *Psychological Bulletin*. Take notice all you young Ph.D.s.
- ☐ ADR first author is born.
- ☐ James P. Egan of the Psychoacoustic Laboratory (PAL) at Harvard University reports on systematic investigation of articulation testing (speech audiometry) methods.
- ☐ Hallowell Davis publishes a paper on the articulation area and the Social Adequacy Index for hearing.
- ☐ Fenestration operations emerge as a popular surgical treatment for otosclerosis.
- ☐ Georg von Bekesy and W. A. Rosenblith publish "The Early History of Hearing: Observations and Theories" in the *Journal of the Acoustical Society of America* (JASA).
- ☐ Georg von Bekesy also publishes the article "Vibration of the Head in a Sound Field and Its Role in Hearing by Bone Conduction" in JASA.
- ☐ James Jerger continues his undergraduate studies at Northwestern University, acting in the theater in his spare time, while Carhart develops the audiology graduate program on the lakeshore campus.
- ☐ Thomas Gold publishes a prophetic theory on "mechanical resonator" influence on cochlear function 30 years before the discovery of otoacoustic emissions.
- ☐ Dix, Hallpike, and Hood publish observations on loudness recruitment (the ABLB) in one of the first attempts at differential diagnosis of cochlear versus eighth cranial nerve dysfunction with audiometric procedures.
- ☐ Along this line, H. C. Huizing publishes a study on "The Symptom of Recruitment and Intelligibility of Speech" in *Acta Otolaryngologica* (Stockholm).
- ☐ Research on recruitment is also reported by two other early big names in auditory science—Luscher and Zwislocki.
- ☐ Leo Doerfler publishes a paper entitled "Neurophysiological Clues to Auditory Acuity" in the *Journal of Speech and Hearing Disorders*.

- ☐ Baseball's legendary "Sultan of Swing" Herman "Babe" Ruth dies of laryngeal cancer on August 16 at the age of 53 years. A hitting pitcher (or really a pitching hitter), Babe held the home run title for three consecutive years (1919, 1920, and 1921). He also would have held his own at AAA Conventions in the party category, as he was known for his ability to drink beer all night long and then play baseball better than his teammates the next (actually later the same) day. Audiology's own Roger A. Ruth proudly claims the Babe as a relative, although the authors are still awaiting some evidence in support of this bold assertion.
- ☐ The Bekesy audiometer, reported 1 year earlier by its namesake, is developed for clinical use by Rufus Grason, the co-founder of Grason Stadler, Inc., in the Boston area.
- ☐ A couple of vans (van Dischoeck and van Gool) publish a paper entitled "The Detailed Audiogram" in the *Archives of Otolaryngology.*
- ☐ P. M. Morse publishes the textbook *Vibration and Sound* (McGraw-Hill).
- ☐ Dawson's rudimentary signal averager, reported 1 year earlier, is used in recording sensory (somatosensory) evoked responses.
- ☐ E. H. Johnson reports in *American Annals of Deaf* on the effectiveness of different methods of communication of pupils in a school for the deaf.
- ☐ William G. "Bill" Hardy of Johns Hopkins publishes a paper on "Special Techniques for the Diagnosis and Treatment of Psychogenic Deafness" in the *Annals of Otology, Rhinology, and Laryngology.*
- ☐ Edwin G. Boring co-authors the textbook *Foundations of Psychology* which includes several chapters on hearing-related topics. Professor Boring was a mentor of S. S. Stevens and Hallowell Davis in the 1930s.
- ☐ The Olympics were held in London.
- ☐ The well-respected psychoacoustician J. Donald Harris of the Naval Medical Research Laboratory in New London, Connecticut publishes "Discrimination of Pitch: Suggestions Toward Method and Procedure" in the *American Journal of Physiology.*
- ☐ Two years after his classic publication on acoustic impedance measurements in normal and pathologic ears, Otto Metz continues his studies on clinical applications of impedance measures, including research on stapedius reflex contractions and loudness recruitment.
- ☐ Among others publishing articles on various auditory topics include J. E. Bordley, M. R. Breakley, H. de Vries, P. W. Johnson, H. G. Kobrak, J. C. R. Licklider, I. Pollak, and H. W. Rudmose.

SPEECH THRESHOLDS

Audioid

The reason why audiologists speak in spondees at Annual AAA Convention parties.

Spondee: *n. Prosody*. A metrical foot consisting of two long or stressed syllables. (Middle English *sponde*, from Old French *spondee*, from Latin *spondeum*, from Greek *spondeious* [*pous*]. "[meter] used at libation," from *sponde*, libation.)

Source: From W. Morris (ed). *The American Heritage Dictionary of the English Language.* New York: American Heritage Publishing Co., 1973, p. 1248.

Spondee Words and Familiarization

Words used in measurement of speech reception (or recognition) threshold (SRT). Words are ordered according to the difference in correct responses attributed to familiarization, that is, when the listener was first introduced to the words (familiarized) versus when the listener heard them initially (unfamiliarized).

	Correct responses[a]		
Word	Unfamiliar	Familiar	Familiarization Effect[b]
baseball	22	23	1
airplane	19	21	2
iceberg	18	21	3
sunset	18	18	0
hardware	17	24	7
armchair	16	17	1
playground	16	16	0
stairway	16	16	0
woodwork	16	22	6
workshop	16	21	5
birthday	14	14	0
eardrum	14	18	4

Word	Correct responses[a]		Familiarization Effect[b]
	Unfamiliar	Familiar	
doormat	13	13	0
northwest	13	17	4
railroad	13	17	4
grandson	12	16	4
sidewalk	12	16	4
farewell	11	12	1
mousetrap	11	15	4
mushroom	11	15	4
whitewash	11	19	8
horseshoe	10	9	1
hotdog	10	19	9
oatmeal	10	18	8
pancake	10	15	5
cowboy	9	20	11
daybreak	8	14	6
toothbrush	8	14	6
drawbridge	7	18	11
greyhound	7	14	7
inkwell	7	18	11
schoolboy	7	12	5
padlock	6	14	8
duckpond	3	16	13
headlight	3	11	8
hothouse	1	6	5

Source: Conn M, Dancer J, Ventry IM. A spondee list for determining speech recognition threshold without prior familiarization. *J Speech Hear Disord* 40: 388–396, 1975

[a]Correct responses for each word among 25 listeners. If all listeners had repeated a word correctly, the score would be 25.

[b]Correct responses among 25 listeners when each listener was familiarized minus not familiarized to the words. A larger difference reflects a greater effect of familiarization.

Clinical Concept

Limitations of SPEECH RECEPTION THRESHOLD (SRT) in clinical audiometry. Speech reception threshold is also known as SPEECH RECOGNITION THRESHOLD (SRT) and SPEECH THRESHOLD (ST).

☐ Validity in estimating hearing threshold

- ✔ The recognition of spondee words is not very predictive of communicative function.
- ✔ Spondee words are not representative of the speech used in everyday communication.
- ✔ There is little or no standardization of spondee materials from clinic to clinic.
- ✔ There is little or no standardization in the methods used to measure spondee thresholds from clinic to clinic (e.g., intensity increments, familiarization with words, response criterion).
- ✔ Monitored live-voice (MLV) presentation, a very unstandardized technique, continues to be used by most audiologists.

☐ Cross-check of pure tone thresholds

- ✔ The reliability of pure tone thresholds is not in question for most first-time patients.
- ✔ In follow-up pure tone audiometry, repeatability would be better assessed by comparison of pure tone thresholds for each test session.
- ✔ SRT (ST) is indicated and useful in the audiometric assessment of patients suspected of pseudohypacusis (malingerers).
- ✔ SRT (ST) is indicated and useful in the audiometric assessment of very young and/or difficult-to-test patients for whom pure tone audiometry cannot be successfully completed.

☐ Reference intensity level for other auditory tests (e.g., word recognition tests)

- ✔ Spondees aren't a good reference for determining a level for presentation of word recognition test material, (i.e., sensation level) because the two tests utilize different stimuli.
- ✔ If the idea of a speech-based sensation level for word recognition is applied, it would be more appropriate to use a measure of speech detection threshold, rather than recognition threshold.

- ✓ If you feel compelled to employ a sensation level approach for selecting a single intensity level for a word recognition test, an even more appropriate and legitimate audiometric reference would be pure tone hearing sensitivity.

Source: Adapted from Wilson RH, Margolis RH. Measurements of auditory thresholds for speech stimuli. In *Principles of Speech Audiometry*. (Konkle DF, Rintelmann WF, eds). Baltimore: University Park Press, 1983, p. 101.

General Guidelines for Speech Threshold Testing of Children

Approximate Level of Function *	Type of Measurement	Test Stimuli	Response Task	Type of Reinforcement
≥ 10 years	Conventional SRT	Spondee	Verbal	Verbal (Intermittent)
5 to 10 years	Conventional SRT	Child's spondee list	Verbal	Verbal (Intermittent)
30 months to 6 years	Modified SRT	Selected child's spondees	Picture or object pointing	Social, visual, or tangible
Less than 3 years	SAT	Repetitive speech utterance	Conditioned	Play, visual, or tangible
Limited	SAT	Repetitive speech utterance	Unconditioned response	None

Source: From Olsen W, Matkin N. Speech audiometry. In Rintelmann W. (ed). *Hearing Assessment* (2nd ed). Austin, TX, Pro-Ed, 1991, p. 55. Reprinted with permission.

* Dependent on cognitive, motor, and language development and attending behavior

PURE TONE vs. SPEECH THRESHOLDS

Classic Quote

Ira Hirsh on the relation between speech and pure tone audiometry.

"In spite of the seeming unimportance of measuring the threshold of intelligibility or the Hearing Loss for Speech, the very fact that this Hearing Loss can be predicted so well from the audiogram suggests that we may profitably use a measurement of the Hearing Loss for Speech as a check on the accuracy of the pure-tone audiogram. Inconsistency between the Hearing Loss for Speech and the average Hearing Loss for frequencies of 500, 1000, and 2000 cps should make the clinician suspicious of one or the other of these measurements.

Carhart (1946) has tested the correlation between Hearing Loss for Speech and different estimates of the audiogram. The three-tone average mentioned above seems to correlate best with the Hearing Loss for Speech in a large number of clinical observations. More recently, Fletcher (1950) has suggested an even simpler formula. He reports that Hearing Loss for Speech is best predicted by noting the Hearing Loss for the middle three frequencies and then taking the average of the smallest two. In most cases the average three-tone and this two-tone average are almost the same.

Another favorable result of the close relation between the audiogram and Hearing Loss for Speech has to do with children. The difficulty in obtaining reliable responses to pure tones from most children is well known to most clinicians. Children who have acquired some language can, however, give reliable responses (i.e., can repeat words) when a speech test is used . . . .

So far as the relation between the audiogram and Discrimination Loss is concerned, we can only point out that here lies one of the greatest points of ignorance in contemporary clinical audiology."

Source: From Hirsh I. *The Measurement of Hearing*. New York: McGraw-Hill Book Company, 1952, pp. 148–149. Reprinted with permission.

Historical Reverberation

Old but good papers on speech and pure tone hearing thresholds. Complete citations are listed in the reference list at the end of this chapter.

Important persons in the initial descriptions of the relation between pure tone hearing versus speech thresholds and recognition were, chronologically:

- ☐ Fletcher (1929)
- ☐ Steinberg and Gardner (1940)
- ☐ Hughson and Thompson (1942)
- ☐ Carhart (1946)
- ☐ Fletcher (1950)
- ☐ Carhart (1971)

Technical Tips

Agreement between pure tone and speech thresholds

- ☐ The accuracy of pure tone thresholds is confirmed by close agreement between the conventional pure tone average (PTA) for 500, 1000, 2000 Hz and a speech threshold measure.
- ☐ Agreement between the PTA and speech threshold should agree within ±7 dB.
- ☐ Perform SRTs first so that you don't waste lots of time obtaining invalid pure tone threshold findings.
- ☐ When the hearing threshold value for one of the three convention pure tone frequencies is more than 20 different than the other two, compare the speech threshold to an average of the best two thresholds (Fletcher, 1950).
- ☐ If the speech threshold is >7 dB better than the pure tone average, accuracy of the pure tone thresholds is in doubt. Possible reasons should be explored by trouble-shooting and, if necessary, further audiologic assessment.
- ☐ For additional confirmation of the accuracy of pure tone findings, consider analysis of acoustic reflex thresholds (especially for a broad band noise signal), otoacoustic emissions, and threshold estimations with frequency-specific auditory evoked response recordings.
- ☐ Always calculate your PTA as soon as pure tone audiometry is completed for the test ear. Don't put it off until later. Buy a calculator watch (like the first ADR author has) if that will help you adhere to this simple but important audiologic axiom.
- ☐ If you're under a time crunch, don't bother measuring a speech threshold for patients who volunteer consistent pure tone thresholds of 10 dB or better for all audiometric frequencies.

Normal Data

PB Word Recognition Scores vs. Pure Tone Averages

Disproportionate loss in speech intelligibility with the lower boundary of PB_{max} score (PAL PB word lists) shown as a function of PTA_2 (1000, 2000, and 4000 Hz). For any given value of PTA_2, any score below the tables values of PB_{max} must be considered disproportionately poor (e.g., an abnormal audiologic finding).

PTA_2	PB_{max} (%)	PTA_2 (dB)	PB_{max} (%)	PTA_2 (dB)	Pb_{max} (%)
0	89	31	57	61	26
1	88	32	56	62	25
2	87	33	55	63	24
3	86	34	54	64	23
4	85	35	53	65	22
5	84	36	52	66	21
6	83	37	51	67	20
7	82	38	50	68	19
8	81	39	49	69	18
9	80	40	48	70	17
10	79	41	47	71	16
11	78	42	46	72	15
12	77	43	45	73	14
13	76	44	44	74	13
14	75	45	43	75	12
15	74	46	42	76	11
16	73	47	41	77	10
17	72	48	40	78	9
18	71	49	39	79	8
19	70	50	38	80	7
20	69	51	37	81	6
21	68	52	36	82	5
22	67	53	35	83	4
23	65	54	34	84	3
24	64	55	32	85	2
25	63	56	31	86	1
26	62	57	30		
27	61	58	29		
28	60	59	28		
29	59	60	27		
30	58				

Source: From Yellin, MW, Jerger J, Fifer RC. Norms for disproportionate loss in speech intelligibility. *Ear and Hearing 10:231–234,* 1989.

ADR NOTE: See Kamm (1995) for similar information with NU-6 words.

Normal Data

SSI Scores vs. Pure Tone Averages

Lower boundary of SSI_{max} score as a function of PTA_1. For any given value of PTA_1, any score below the tables values of SSI_{max} must be considered disproportionately poor (e.g. an abnormal audiologic finding).

PTA_2	PB_{max} (%)	PTA_2 (dB)	PB_{max} (%)	PTA_2 (dB)	PB_{max} (%)
0	86	31	55	61	25
1	85	32	54	62	24
2	84	33	53	63	23
3	83	34	52	64	22
4	82	35	51	65	21
5	81	36	50	66	20
6	80	37	49	67	19
7	79	38	48	68	18
8	78	39	47	69	17
9	77	40	46	70	16
10	76	41	45	71	15
11	75	42	44	72	14
12	74	43	43	73	13
13	73	44	42	74	12
14	72	45	41	75	11
15	71	46	40	76	10
16	70	47	39	77	9
17	69	48	38	78	8
18	68	49	37	79	7
19	67	50	36	80	6
20	66	51	35	81	5
21	65	52	34	82	4
22	64	53	33	83	3
23	63	54	32	84	2
24	62	55	31	85	1
25	61	56	30		
26	60	57	29		
27	59	58	28		
28	58	59	27		
29	57	60	26		
30	56				

Source: From Yellin MW, Jerger J, Fifer RC. Norms for Disproportionate Loss in Speech Intelligibility. *Ear and Hearing 10:231–234,* 1989.

CLINICAL FACTS AND FACTORS

Factors Influencing Speech Audiometry Outcome

Factor		Influence
✔ familiarity with material	+	increased response accuracy with familiarity
✔ tape-recorded vs. live voice	+	increased standardization for tape-recorded materials
✔ test materials	++	considerable differences in scores among different test materials
✔ response scoring method	+	aural monitoring and interpretation can lead to errors in scores. Have patient write response down, or use a picture pointing task or the synthetic sentence identification speech material.
✔ carrier phrase for speech threshold	–	
✔ carrier phrase in word recognition	–	
✔ length of word lists for recognition	?	
✔ presentation level in dB	+	determination of maximum performance may require more than one presentation level

Note: ++ = very important, + = important, ± = sometimes important, ? = questionable importance, – = not important.

ADR NOTE: See speech audiometry references at the end of the chapter.

Technical Tip

Seven (7) reasons why you shouldn't routinely use the monitored-live-voice (MLV) method for presentation of word recognition materials

- Word recognition scores obtained for different talkers are not equivalent.
- Word recogntion scores for the same talker at different times are not equivalent.
- "Each speaker of word recognition materials constitutes a different test that may produce different psychometric articulation functions (percent correct performance as a function of presentation level)" (Wiley et al., 1994, p. 29).
- With MLV presentation, the acoustic characteristics of the signal are highly variable, just as Jennifer's voice is distinctly different from Jay's, and Gus has totally different vocal characteristics than both of them (e.g., pitch, articulation, rate of speech, dialect).
- With MLV presentation, the difficulty of the items (single words) is dependent, in part, on who's talking.
- Most testers today are not sitting in a sound-treated control room. Background sounds reaching the patient through the open microphone may confuse the patient and influence test results.
- With current CD recorded speech audiometry materials, and progressive presentation techniques (e.g., patient control of the rate of words), you need not sacrifice quality, reliability, and validity to obtain speed.
- A variety of word recognition test materials are commercially available in compact disc (CD), digital audio tape (DAT), and, of course, cassette tape recording formats. Sources for these materials are listed elsewhere in this ADR chapter. You spend your hard-earned cash on CDs of your favorite bands and music because the quality is superior. Don't your patients deserve the same audio quality?

Technical Tips

What do you do when the patient can't provide an adequate oral response or when the tester can't aurally monitor the patient's response?

☐ **Indications**

- Patient is apraxic or dysarthric
- Patient is a laryngectomee or severely hoarse
- Tester has hearing loss that affects aural monitoring of patient response

☐ **What to do**

- Use the SSI (synthetic sentence identification) test in the 0 dB MCR (message-to-competition ratio) condition because the patient can respond by pointing to the sentence heard
- Use a picture pointing test, such as the WIPI (*Word Intelligibility by Picture Identification*)
- Use a written response mode, that is, the patient writes down each word heard

Technical Tips

How to minimize test time and maximize information gained

- ☐ Don't measure speech reception (recognition) thresholds if they aren't likely to contribute to your understanding of the patient's auditory status. For example, the SRT is of little value:
  - ✔ if pure tone thresholds are entirely normal within the speech frequency region, especially for a cooperative adult or older child
  - ✔ if the patient is returning for a follow-up assessment and all other findings are unchanged
  - ✔ for the majority of patients
- ☐ Use recorded word recognition materials that include the 10 most-difficult words first, and stop for the test ear if the patient scores 90% or 100% on these words.
- ☐ With relatively young adult or "with it" older patients, use recorded word recognition materials that have a brief interval between each word, or let the patient control the rate of word presentation.
- ☐ Don't use word materials that include a carrier phrase.
- ☐ Present this word list initially at 80 dB HL to the better hearing ear.
- ☐ If you're lucky, the patient will score 90 or 100% at 80 dB HL, and you will have obtained the maximum score *and* ruled out rollover simultaneously. Then, do the same on the poorer hearing ear.
- ☐ Keep score as the test proceeds; don't wait until the end of the test for both ears.

Technical Tips

Indicators for central auditory assessment with speech audiometry *or* when you should consider central auditory assessment with speech audiometry

- Patient complains of difficulty understanding speech despite a normal audiogram and good word recognition scores
- Other audiometric findings suggest retrocochlear or central auditory dysfunction
- Patient has a history of neurologic disease or dysfunction, such as stroke, multiple sclerosis, head injury, or brain tumor
- For school-age children, patient has poor academic performance, learning disability, language disorder, or attention deficit disorder, or presents with a history of chronic middle ear disease
- For any child who had one or more risk indicators associated with central nervous system dysfunction as a neonate, such as asphyxia, hyperbilirubinemia, meningitis, or intraventricular hemorrhage

Technical Tips

What do you do when the patient doesn't speak English or is not a native English speaker?

- If possible, use an appropriate tape-recorded or compact disc speech audiometry material in the patient's native language, for example the Spanish language version of the SSI (synthetic sentence identification) test.
- If no commerically available materials are handy, ask a bilingual family member or friend to write down 10 to 20 common words in the patient's native language.
- Then, give this "assistant" a very short course in the monitored live voice technique. Explain that you may be lowering the intensity of the words so that their loved one may not clearly hear each word (otherwise the assistant will keep repeating the missed words at increasing intensity levels in an attempt to get a correct response!).
- Ask the "assistant" to nod his or her head up and down to indicate a correct (yes) response, and side to side for an incorrect (no response).
- Measure the patient's speech reception threshold or, as indicated, their speech detection (awareness) threshold, and/or roughly estimate word recognition performance at a suprathreshold level.
- Be sure to keep the list of words in the patient's native language in the clinical record so it will be available if he or she returns to your clinic.

PB vs. SSI Speech Audiometry Findings Characteristic of Peripheral High Frequency Sensory (Cochlear) Hearing Loss (Presbycusis)

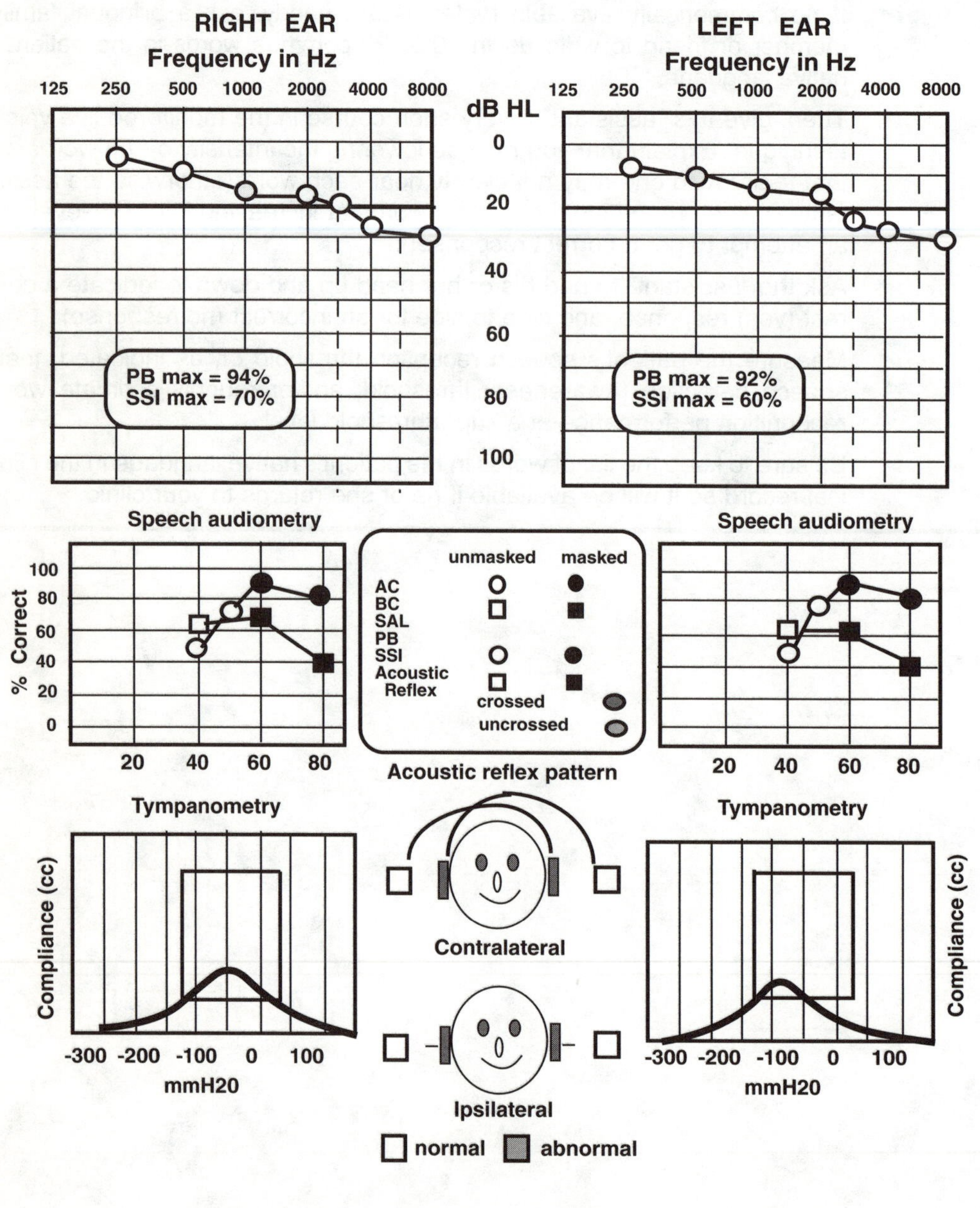

PB vs. SSI Speech Audiometry Findings Characteristic of Central Auditory Nervous System Dysfunction

Pattern shown for post-stroke patient.

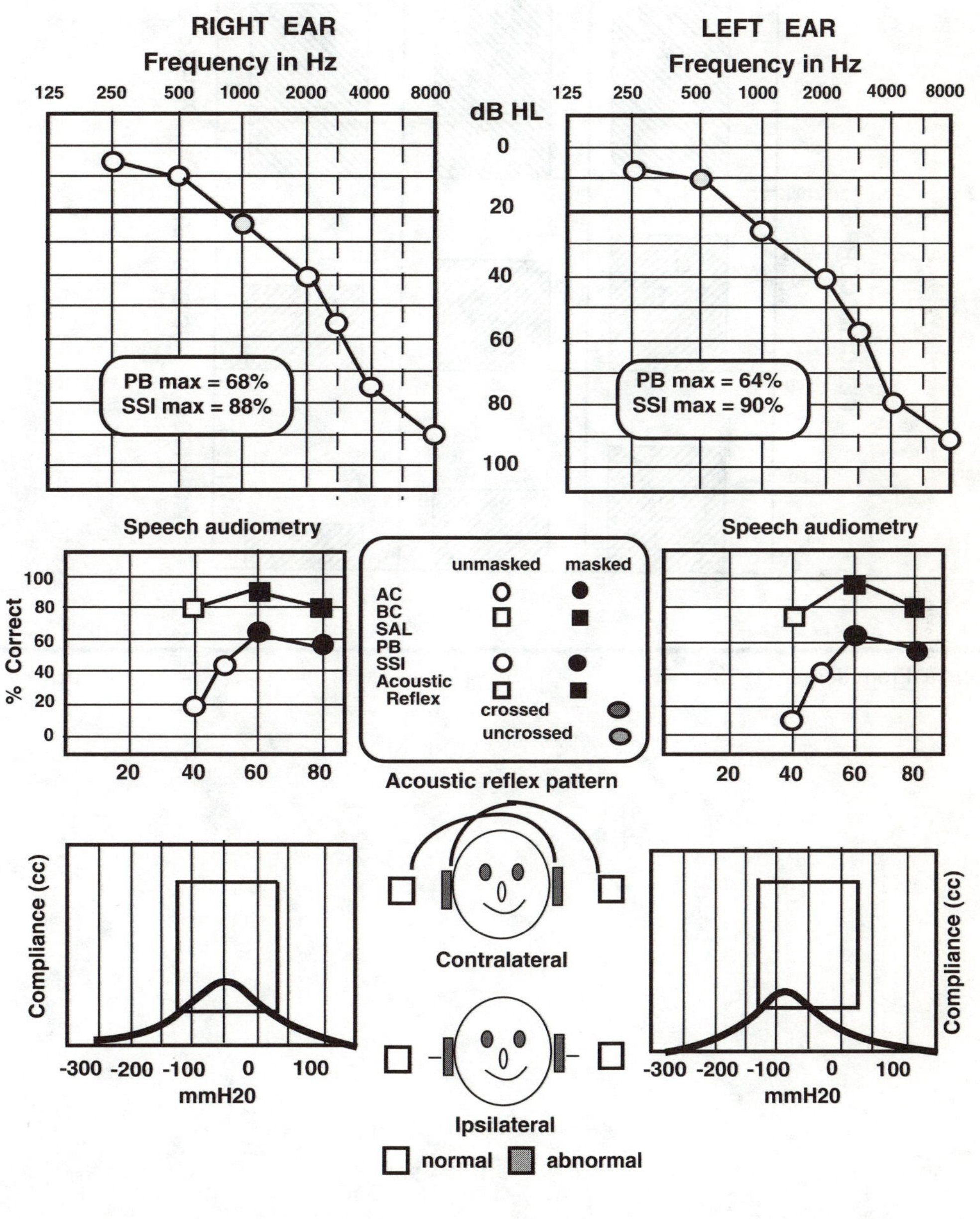

Speech Audiometry Findings in Presbycusis

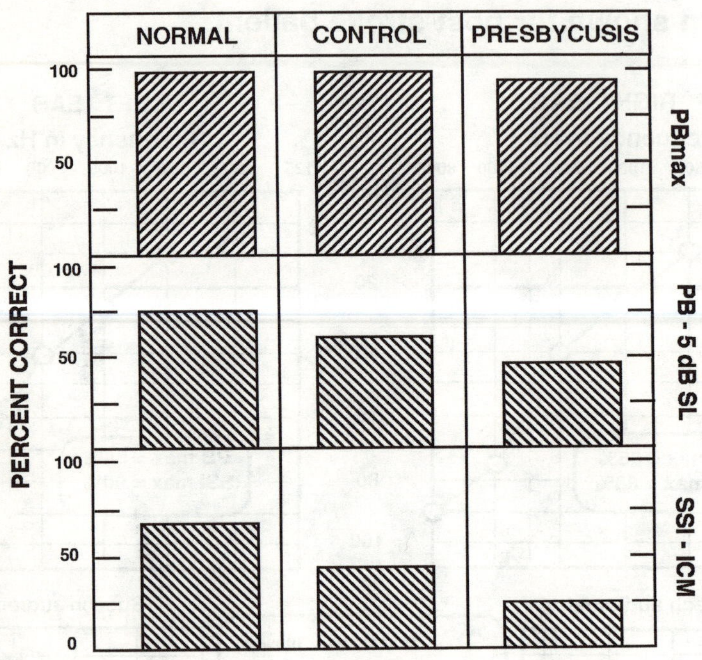

Source: From Jerger (1973).

Key References

Speech Audiometry

Beattie RC, Edgerton BJ, Svihovec DV. An investigation of Auditec of St. Louis recordings of Central Institute for the Deaf Spondees. *J Amer Audiology Soc* 1: 97–101, 1975.

Berger K. A speech discrimination task using multiple-choice key words in sentences. *J Auditory Res* 3: 247–262, 1969.

Boothroyd A. Developments in speech audiometry. *Sound* 2: 3–10, 1968.

Carhart R. Monitored live voice as a test of auditory acuity. *J Acoust Soc Amer* 17: 339–349, 1946.

Carhart R. Observations on the relations between thresholds for pure tones and for speech. *J Speech Hear Disord* 36: 476–483, 1971.

Carhart R, Porter LS. Audiometric configurations and prediction of threshold for spondees. *J Speech Hear Res* 14: 486–495, 1971.

Conn MJ, Dancer J, Ventry IM. A spondee list for determining speech reception threshold without prior familiarization. *J Speech Hear Dis* 40: 388–396, 1975.

Dubno JR, Dirks DD, Morgan DE. Effects of age and mild hearing loss on speech recognition in noise. *J Acoust Soc Amer* 76: 87–96, 1984.

Egan JP. Articulation testing methods. *Laryngoscope* 58: 955–991, 1948.

Erber NP. Use of the auditory numbers test to evaluate speech perception abilities of hearing-impaired children. *J Speech Hear Disord* 45: 527–532, 1980.

Erber NP, Witt LH. Effects of stimulus intensity on speech perception by deaf children. *J Speech Hear Disord* 42: 271–278, 1978.

Fairbanks G. Test of phonemic differentiation: The rhyme test. *J Acoust Soc Amer* 30: 596–600, 1958.

Feeney MP, Franks JR. Test-retest reliability of a distinctive feature difference test for hearing aid evaluation. *Ear and Hearing* 3: 59–65, 1982.

Fifer R, Jerger J, Berlin C, Tobey E, Campbell J. Development of a dichotic sentence identification test for hearing impaired adults. *Ear and Hearing* 4: 300–305, 1983.

Finitzo-Hieber, T, Gerling IJ, Matkin ND, Chaerow-Skalka E. A sound effects recognition test for the pediatric evaluation. *Ear and Hearing* 1: 271–276, 1980.

Fletcher H. *Speech and Hearing*. Princeton, NJ: Von Nostrand Reinhold, 1929.

Fletcher H. A method of calculating hearing loss for speech from an audiogram. *Acta Otolaryngol* (Suppl 90), 26–37, 1950.

Fry DB. Word and sentence tests for use in speech audiometry. *Lancet* 2: 197–199, 1961.

Fry DB, Kerridge PMT. Tests for the hearing of speech by deaf people. *Lancet* 1: 106–109, 1939.

Gardner H. Application of high-frequency consonant discrimination word list in hearing-aid evaluation. *J Speech Hear Dis* 36: 354–355, 1971.

Gaeth J. A scale for testing speech discrimination. Final Report No. RD-2277-S, Society of Rehabilitation Services, Department of Health, Education and Welfare, 1970.

Griffiths J. Rhyming minimal contrasts: A simplified diagnostic articulation test. *J Acoust Soc Amer* 42: 236–241, 1967.

Haskins H. *A phonetically balanced test of speech discrimination for children*. Unpublished master's thesis. Northwestern University, 1949.

Hirsh I, Davis H, Silverman S, Reynolds E, Eldert E, Benson R. Development of materials for speech audiometry. *J Speech Hear Disord* 17: 321–337, 1952.

House A, Williams C, Hecker M, Kryter K. Articulation testing methods: Consonantal differentiation with closed-response set. *J Acoust Soc Amer* 37: 158–168, 1965.

Hughson W, Thompson EA. Correlation of hearing acuity for speech with discrete frequency audiograms. *Arch Otolaryngol* 36: 526–540, 1942.

Jerger S, Lewis S, Hawkins J, Jerger J. Pediatric speech intelligibility test. I. Generation of test materials. *Int J Pedi Otorhinolaryngol* 2: 217–230, 1980.

Kalikow D, Stevens K, Elliott L. Development of a test of speech intelligibility in noise using sentence materials with controlled word predictability. *J Acoust Soc Amer* 61: 1337–1351, 1977.

Katz DR, Elliott LL. *Development of a new children's speech discrimination test.* Paper presented at the convention of the American Speech-Language-Hearing Association, Chicago, November 18–21, 1978.

Lehiste I, Peterson G. Linguistic considerations in the study of speech intelligibility. *J Acoust Soc Amer* 31: 280–286, 1959.

Ling D. Auditory coding and reading—an analysis of training procedures for hearing-impaired children. In M Ross, TG Giolas (eds). *Auditory Management of Hearing-Impaired Children.* Baltimore: University Park Press, pp. 181–218, 1985.

Olsen WO, Van Tassell DJ, Speaks CE. *Preparation of isophonemic word list and sentence test materials.* Paper presented at the Annual Convention of the American Speech-Language-Hearing Association, Toronto, Ontario, Canada, November 1982.

Olsen WO, Van Tassell DJ, Speaks CE. *Further evaluation of isophonemic word list and sentence test materials.* Paper presented at the Annual Convention of the American Speech-Language-Hearing Association, Cincinnati, Ohio, November 1983.

Olsen WO, Van Tassell DJ, Speaks CE. *List equivalence of isophonemic word lists.* Paper presented at the Annual Convention of the American Speech-Language-Hearing Association, Detroit, November 1986.

Owens E, Schubert E. Development of the California consonant test. *J Speech Hear Res* 20: 463–474, 1977.

McPherson D, Pang-Ching G. Development of a distinctive feature discrimination test. *J Auditory Res* 19: 235–246, 1979.

Pederson O, Studebaker G. A new minimal-contrasts closed-response-set speech test. *J Auditory Res* 12: 187–195, 1972.

Raffin M, Thornton AR. Confidence levels for differences between speech discrimination scores: A research note. *J Speech Hear Res* 23: 5–18, 1980.

Resnick S, Dubno J, Hoffnung S, Levitt H. Phoneme errors on a nonsense syllable test. *J Acoust Soc Amer* 58(Suppl): 114, 1975.

Ross M, Lerman J. A picture identification test for hearing impaired children. *J Speech Hear Res* 13: 44–53, 1970.

Schultz M, Schubert E. A multiple choice discrimination test (MCDT). *Laryngoscope* 79: 382–399, 1969.

Sergeant L, Atkinson JE, Lacroix PG. The NSMRL tri-word test of intelligibility. *J Acoust Soc Amer* 65: 218–222, 1979.

Siegenthaler B, Haspiel G. Development of two standard measures of hearing for speech by children. Department of Health, Education and Welfare Project No. 2372, Contract OE5 10–003, 1966.

Silverman SR, Hirsh I. Problems related to the use of speech in clinical audiometry. *Ann Otol Rhinol Laryngol* 64: 1234–1244, 1955.

Speaks C, Jerger J. Method for measurement of speech indentification. *J Speech Hear Res* 8: 185–194, 1965.

Thornton AR, Raffin MJM. Speech-discrimination scores modeled as a binomial variable. *J Speech Hear Res* 21: 507–518, 1978.

Tillman T, Carhart R. An expanded test for speech discrimination utilizing CNC monosyllabic words. Northwestern University Auditory Test No. 6. USAF School of Aerospace Medicine Technical Report, Brooks Air Force Base, Texas, 1966.

Wilson RH, Antablin JK. A picture identification task as an estimate of word-recognition performance on nonverbal adults. *J Speech Hear Disord* 45: 223–238, 1980.

WORD RECOGNITION

Classic Quote

Tom Tillman and Wayne Olsen in 1973 on word recognition assessment, particularly the problems inherent in monitored-live-voice (MLV) presentation of word recognition materials.

"In general it is the slope of the articulation function for a given test that determines the precision with which it will separate the performance of individuals or the performance of a single individual under different listening conditions . . . . it is obvious than no standarized test is possible unless recorded tests are employed, that is, because of talker differences tests administered via monitored-live-voice defy standardization."

Source: Tillman TW, Olsen WO. Speech audiometry. In Jerger J (ed). *Modern Developments in Audiology* (2nd ed). New York: Academic Press, 1973, pp. 52–53.

Clinical Concept

Word recognition presentation level *or* reasons why a single intensity level is usually the wrong intensity level.

- ☐ PB_{max} for patients will not be consistently obtained when word lists are presented only at a single intensity level.
- ☐ Reliance on the most comfortable listening (loudness) level will not result in measurement of the PB_{max}. For most patients, the intensity level for the PB_{max} will be higher than the most comfortable listening (loudness) level.
- ☐ Adding a fixed sensation level value to the SRT also will not result in a reliable PB_{max} score.
- ☐ The intensity level at which the PB_{max} score is found varies considerably from one patient to the next.
- ☐ Variability in the intensity level at which the PB_{max} score is found is greatest among patients with sensorineural hearing loss.
- ☐ The inherent and unavoidable errors in estimating PB_{max} from the score at a single intensity level may result patient misdiagnosis and mismanagement.

ADR NOTE: A good reference:

Wiley TL, Stoppenbach DT, Feldhake LJ, Moss KA, Thordardottir ET. Audiologic practices: What is popular versus what is supported by evidence. *American Journal of Audiology 4*: 26–34, 1994.

Sensitivity of Word Recognition Test Materials

Ability to discriminate real differences in hearing abilities among patients. Ironically, there appears to be an inverse relation between the popularity of these word recognition materials and their ability to sort out differences in hearing function.

- ☐ Most sensitive to differences in hearing loss among patients
  - ✓ Harvard (PAL) PB-50 words lists
  - ✓ Nonsense Syllable Test
  - ✓ California Consonant Test
- ☐ Least sensitive to differences in hearing loss among patients
  - ✓ CID W-22
  - ✓ NU #6

ADR NOTE: A good reference:

Wiley TL, Stoppenbach DT, Feldhake LJ, Moss KA, Thordardottir ET. Audiologic practices: What is popular versus what is supported by evidence. *American Journal of Audiology 4*: 26–34, 1994.

Syllable Identification as a Function of Speech Frequency

Importance of different frequencies for the identification (in percent correct) of a speech signal (syllables) as determined by progressively more high pass or low pass filtering of the signal.

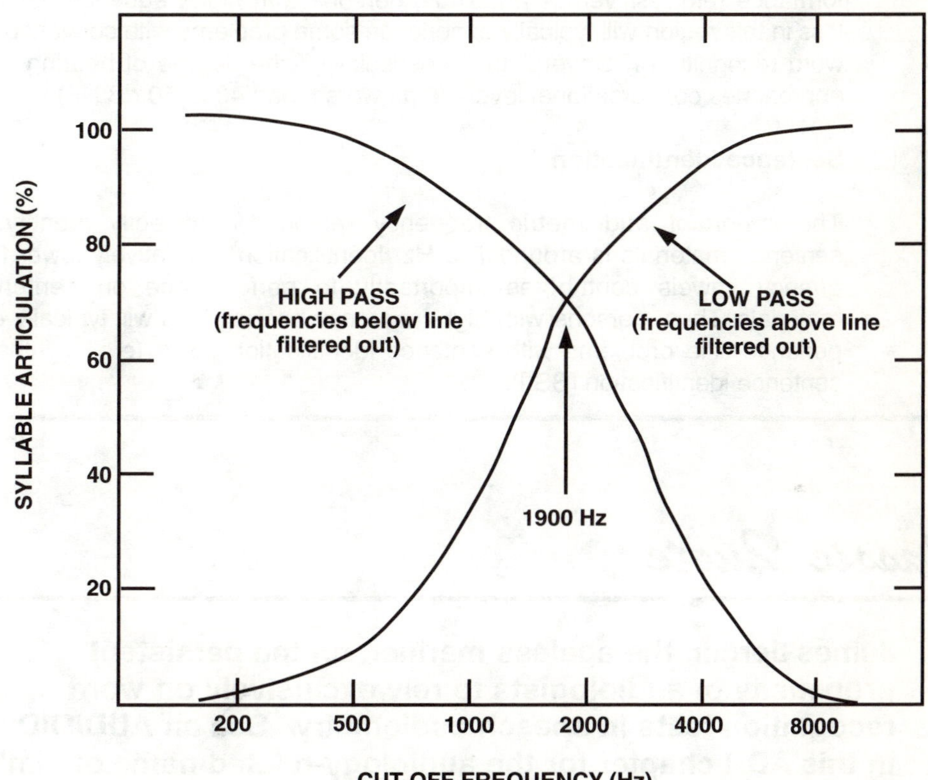

Main points:

1. **Frequencies above about 500 Hz and below about 4000 Hz are important for 100% correct syllable identification.**
2. **The frequency of about 1900 Hz is most important for syllable identification.**

From French NR, Steinberg JC. Factors governing intelligibility of speech sounds. *J Acoust Soc Amer* 19:90–119, 1947, p. 102; Green DH, *An Introduction to Hearing*. Hillsdale, NY: Lawrence Erlbaum Associates, 1976, p. 310.

Technical Tip

Frequency regions most important for performance on word recognition versus sentence identification.

☐ **Word recognition**

The important audiometric frequency region for correctly repeating single-syllable word recognition materials is around 1900 Hz. Identification of high frequency consonants is a critical component in word recognition performance (e.g., /s/ versus /f/). Thus, persons with high-frequency hearing loss in this region will typically experience some problems with conventional word recognition (PB word) tests, especially if the degree of hearing loss approaches conversational levels (e.g., worse than 40 to 50 dB HL).

☐ **Sentence identification**

The important audiometric frequency region for correctly identifying sentence materials is around 750 Hz. Identification of relatively lower frequency vowels contributes importantly to performance on sentence materials. Thus, persons with high-frequency hearing loss will typically experience little problems with sentence identification tasks (e.g., synthetic sentence identification [SSI]).

Classic Quote

James Jerger, the ageless mariner, on the persistent propensity of audiologists to rely exclusively on word recognition tests in speech audiometry. See an AUDIOID in this ADR chapter for the audiology-related name of Jim's current boat.

"We are, at the moment, becalmed in a windless sea of monosyllables. We can sail further only on the fresh winds of imagination."

Source: From Jerger JF. Research priorities in auditory science—The audiologist's view. *Ann Otol Rhinol Laryngol 89 (Suppl 74):* 134–135, 1980, p. 135.

Performance-Intensity (PI) Functions and Corresponding Rollover Indices (RI)

Representative of persons with normal, cochlear, and retrocochlear auditory dysfunction. A rollover index of more than 0.40 is associated with retrocochlear auditory dysfunction.

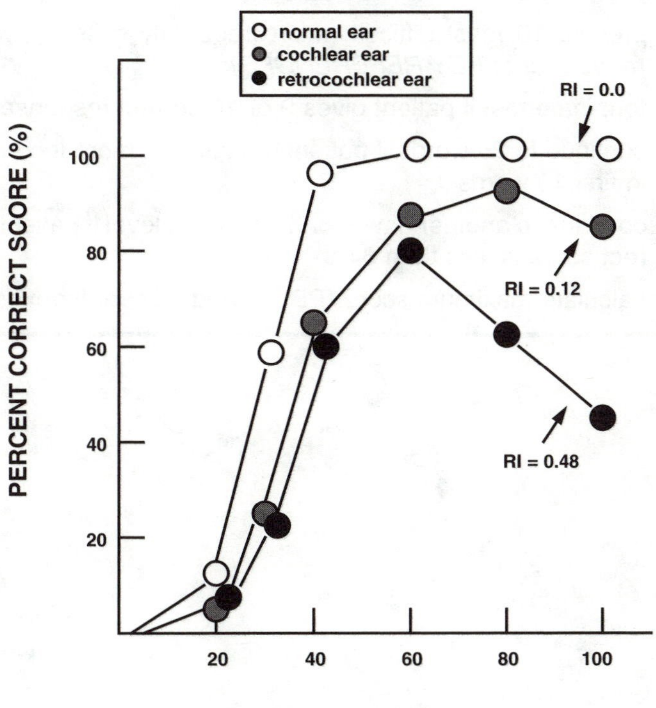

Technical Tip

Clinical Word Recognition Measurement

☐ **Objectives**

- find maximum word recognition score (e.g., PB_{max})
- rule out rollover in test performance
- minimize test time
- minimize factors contributing to inter- and intra-subject variability
- maximize inter-clinic and inter-tester agreement in findings

☐ **Strategy**

- use commercially-available tape-recorded or compact disc materials
- present words at 75 to 80 dB HL (95 to 100 dB SPL) initially
- present 10 most difficult (most frequently missed) words first *(see related list of KEY REFERENCES)*
- terminate test if patient gives 9 or 10 correct responses
- continue to 25 words if patient makes 2 or more incorrect responses in first 10 words
- continue to another (lower or higher) test level if patient's percent correct score is less than 84%
- calculate maximum score (PB_{max}) and rollover index for each ear

Rollover Index (RI) in the Differentation of Cochlear vs. Retrocochlear Dysfunction

Values shown for patients with confirmed eighth nerve lesions versus Ménieře's disease. In the study cited, a rollover index of 0.25 generally differentiated cochlear versus retrocochlear groups.

Factors Potentially Influencing the

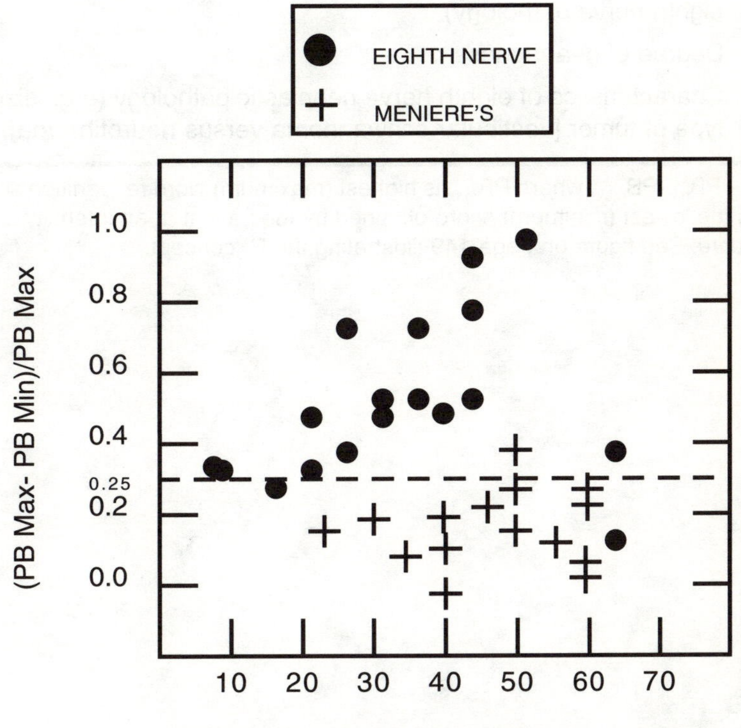

$$\text{Rollover Index} = \frac{(\text{PBmax} - \text{PBmin})}{(\text{PBmin})}$$

From Bess FJ, Josey AF. Humes, LE. Performance intensity functions in cochlear and eighth nerve disorders. *Am J. Otol* 1:27–31, 1979. Reprinted with permission.

Rollover Index (RI) Measure*

- Speech material (e.g., NU-6, PAL PB-50, W-22 word lists)
- Accuracy of PB_{max} measure, e.g. size of intensity increment used in performance intensity (PI) function
- Reliability of PI-PB functions
- Intersubject variability of PI-PB functions
- Subject age in hearing impaired subjects (e.g., neural presbycusis)
- PB_{max}, (e.g., RI) cannot be calculated accurately for very low PB_{max} values (less than 30%)
- Highest intensity level used for determination of the PB_{min}, (e.g., 80 versus 90 versus 100 dB HL).
- Auditory status (e.g., normal hearing versus cochlear pathology versus eighth nerve pathology)
- Degree of hearing loss
- Characteristics of eighth nerve neoplastic pathology (e.g., size of tumor or type of tumor [vestibular schwannoma versus neurofibroma])

*RI = $PB_{max} - PB_{min}/PB_{max}$, where PB_{max} is highest (maximum) word recognition score for an ear and PB_{min} is the lowest (minimum) score obtained by the patient at an intensity level above the maximum score. See figure on page 149 illustrating the RI concept.

Summary of Published Rollover Index (RI) Values

For phonetically balanced (PB) word recognition tests that most effectively differentiated cochlear versus eighth nerve auditory dysfunction.*

Study	Speech Material	RI Value
Jerger and Jerger (1971)	PAL PB-50s	0.40 to 0.45
Dirks, Kamm, Bower, and Betsworth (1977)	PAL PB-50s	0.45
Bess, Josey and Humes (1979)	NU-6	0.25
Meyer and Mishler (1984)	NU-6	0.35

*RI = $PB_{max} - PB_{min}/PB_{max}$, where PB_{max} is highest (maximum) word recognition score for an ear and PB_{min} is the lowest (minimum) score obtained by the patient at an intensity level above the maximum score. See nearby figure illustrating the RI concept.

Audioid

PB_{max}

What candy bar is a hit with audiologists nationwide, and is especially preferred during long speech audiometry sessions?

The PB_{max} of course.

Word Recognition Scores

Thornton and Raffin data on lower and upper limits of the 95% critical differences for word recognition percentage scores. That is, the scores with any given range are really not different from the corresponding (same row) percentage scores, according to how many words were in the list.

Score %	N = 50	N = 25	N = 10	Score %	N = 100
0	0–4	0–8	0–20	50	37–63
2	0–10			51	38–64
4	0–14	0–20		52	39–65
6	2–18			53	40–66
8	2–22	0–28		54	41–67
10	2–24		0–50	55	42–68
12	4–26	4–32		56	43–69
14	4–30			57	44–70
16	6–32	4–40		58	45–71
18	6–34			59	46–72
20	8–36	4–44	0–60	60	47–73
22	8–40			61	48–74
24	10–42	8–48		62	49–74
26	12–44			63	50–75
28	14–46	8–52		64	51–76
30	14–48		10–70	65	52–77
32	16–50	12–56		66	53–78
34	18–52			67	54–79
36	20–54	16–60		68	55–80
38	22–56			69	56–81
40	22–58	16–64	10–80	70	57–81
42	24–60			71	58–82
44	26–62	20–68		72	59–83
46	28–64			73	60–84
48	30–66	24–72		74	61–85
50	32–68		10–90	75	63–86
52	34–70	28–76		76	64–86
54	36–72			77	65–87
56	38–74	32–80		78	66–88

Score %	N = 50	N = 25	N = 10	Score %	N = 100
58	40–76			79	67–89
60	42–78	35–84	20–90	80	68–89
62	44–78			81	69–90
64	46–80	40–84		82	71–91
66	48–82			83	72–92
68	50–84	44–88		84	73–92
70	52–86		30–90	85	74–93
72	54–86	48–92		86	75–94
74	56–88			87	77–94
76	58–90	52–92		88	78–95
78	60–92			89	79–96
80	64–92	56–96	40–100	90	81–96
82	66–94			91	82–97
84	68–94	60–96		92	83–98
86	70–96			93	85–98
88	74–96	68–96		94	86–99
90	76–98		50–100	95	88–99
92	78–98	72–100		96	89–99
94	82–98			97	91–100
96	86–100		80–100	99	94–100
100	96–100	92–100	80–100	100	97–100

Source: Thornton AR, Raffin MJM. Speech-discrimination scores modeled as a binomial variable. *J Speech Hearing Res 21:* 507–518, 1978. Reprinted with permission.

Confidence Levels Associated with Word Recognition Scores

Differences between percent correct scores for 25 word lists.

Put another way, if the second score for a patient (e.g., at another intensity level or for the other ear) is different from the first score at a confidence level of less than 0.05, then there is a very good chance that the scores are really different.

Second Score (in % Correct)	First Score in % Correct										
	0.00	4.00	8.00	12.00	16.00	20.00	24.00	28.00	32.00	36.00	40.00
	1.0000	0.3077	0.1188	0.0455	0.0178	0.0069	0.0014	0.0014	0.0003	0.0001	0.0001
4.00	0.3077	1.0000	0.5961	0.3320	0.1707	0.0873	0.0404	0.0178	0.0093	0.0037	0.0014
8.00	0.1188	0.5961	1.0000	0.6599	0.4065	0.2340	0.1285	0.0673	0.0332	0.0160	0.0069
12.00	0.0455	0.3320	0.6599	1.0000	0.7039	0.4593	0.2801	0.1645	0.0910	0.0477	0.0238
16.00	0.0178	0.1707	0.4065	0.7039	1.0000	0.7188	0.4965	0.3173	0.1936	0.1141	0.0601
20.00	0.0069	0.0873	0.2340	0.4593	0.7188	1.0000	0.7339	0.5222	0.3421	0.2187	0.1285
24.00	0.0014	0.0404	0.1285	0.2801	0.4965	0.7339	1.0000	0.7490	0.5419	0.3628	0.2340
28.00	0.0014	0.0178	0.0673	0.1645	0.3173	0.5222	0.7490	1.0000	0.7642	0.5552	0.3843
32.00	0.0003	0.0093	0.0332	0.0910	0.1936	0.3421	0.5419	0.7642	1.0000	0.7718	0.5687
36.00	0.0001	0.0037	0.0160	0.0477	0.1141	0.2187	0.3628	0.5552	0.7718	1.0000	0.7718
40.00	0.0001	0.0014	0.0069	0.0238	0.0601	0.1285	0.2340	0.3843	0.5687	0.7718	1.0000
44.00	—	0.0003	0.0037	0.0111	0.0316	0.0703	0.1416	0.2501	0.3953	0.5687	0.7718
48.00	—	0.0003	0.0014	0.0037	0.0151	0.0366	0.0801	0.1527	0.2543	0.3953	0.5823

Second Score (in % Correct)	First Score in % Correct										
	0.00	4.0	8.00	12.00	16.00	20.00	24.00	28.00	32.00	36.00	40.00
52.00	—	0.0001	0.0003	0.0014	0.0069	0.0188	0.0424	0.0873	0.1585	0.2627	0.4065
56.00	—	0.0001	0.0001	0.0014	0.0037	0.0093	0.0214	0.0455	0.0910	0.1585	0.2627
60.00	—	—	0.0001	0.0003	0.0014	0.0037	0.0099	0.0226	0.0477	0.0910	0.1645
64.00	—	—	0.0001	0.0001	0.0003	0.0014	0.0037	0.0105	0.0238	0.0500	0.0910
68.00	—	—	—	0.0001	0.0001	0.0003	0.0014	0.0037	0.0105	0.0238	0.0477
72.00	—	—	—	—	0.0001	0.0003	0.0003	0.0014	0.0037	0.0105	0.0226
76.00	—	—	—	—	0.0001	0.0001	0.0003	0.0003	0.0014	0.0037	0.0099
80.00	—	—	—	—	—	0.0001	0.0001	0.0003	0.0003	0.0014	0.0037
84.00	—	—	—	—	—	—	0.0001	0.0001	0.0001	0.0003	0.0014
88.00	—	—	—	—	—	—	—	—	0.0001	0.0001	0.0003
92.00	—	—	—	—	—	—	—	—	—	0.0001	0.0001
96.00	—	—	—	—	—	—	—	—	—	—	—

Source: Adapted from Thornton AR, Raffin MJM. Speech-discrimination scores modeled as a binomial variable. *J Speech Hearing Res* 21: 507–518, 1978.

SPEECH AUDIOMETRY MATERIALS

Summary of Speech Audiometry Test Materials

Test	Number of Items/List	Number of Lists	Response	Sample of Stimulus	Sample of Alternatives
Monosyllables: Open Set					
PB-50	50	20	Repeat word	ache, toil, vow (vc, cvc, cv)	N/A
W-22	50	4	Repeat word	ace, could, toe (vc, cvc, cv)	N/A
CNC	50	10	Repeat word	pack, mop, net (cvc)	N/A
NU-6	50	4	Repeat word	bean, fall, which (cvc)	N/A
HFCDT	25	2	Repeat word	picked, its, tip	N/A
SDS	5 subtests 8 items each	1	Repeat word	digits, easy/hard letters, easy/hard words	N/A
ABL	10	15	Repeat word	ship, rug, fan (cvc)	N/A
PBK-50	50	3	Repeat word	ox, pants, low (vc, cvc, cv)	N/A
Monosyllables: Closed Set					
RT	50	5	Supply initial consonant	got	__ot
MRT	50	6	Mark word	book	book, took, shook, cook hook, look
RMC	50	5	Mark word	thin	thin tin chin shin gin
MCTD	50	4	Mark word	leave	leash league leech weave
OUCRT	224 3 subtests	1	Mark word	pot	pop pock pa pot
CCT	100	1	Mark word	tin	pin thin tin kin
DFDT	50	4	Mark word	fast	fast vast cast mast

Test	Number of Items/List	Number of Lists	Response	Sample of Stimulus	Sample of Alternatives
NST	102 11 subtests	1	Mark syllable	/ti/	pee chee kee fee tee she he thee see
DIP	48	1	Point to picture	peas	peas bees (pictures)
WIPI	25	4	Point to picture	school	shoe boot school broom moon spoon (pictures)
Sentences: Open Set					
CID	50 key words 10 sentences	10	Repeat sentence	Hard *work* is *good* for *everyone.*	N/A
SPIN	50 key words	8	Repeat final word	A spoiled child is a *brat.* She has known about the *drug.*	N/A
BKB	50 key words 16 sentences	21	Repeat sentence	He *dropped* his *money.*	N/A
Sentences: Closed Set					
KSUDT	13 key words 13 sentences	8	Mark word	He painted the porch red.	He painted the STORE PORCH GOURD DOOR BOARD red.
SSI	10	1	Identify sentence	Go change your car color is red.	Entire list of sentences
PSI*	5 nouns 5 sentences-I 5 sentences-II	4 2 2	Point to picture	bear Show me horse 5 pictures eating an apple. A horse is eating	

Source: From Brewer C, Resnick D. Speech discrimination tests. *Seminars in Hearing* 4: 205–220 1983. Reprinted with permission.
*Closed set monosyllable and sentence tests.

Clinical Speech Audiometry Procedures

See Central Auditory Processing Disorders, Chapter X, for additional speech audiometry procedures. Full citations for publications are listed at the end of this chapter.

Type of Procedure	Test	Publication
Word Recognition: Monosyllables Open Set		
Word Tests for Deaf People		Fry and Kerridge (1939)
PB-50	phonetically balance (PB) word lists	Egan (1948)
PBK-50	PB kindergarden lists	Haskins (1949)
W-22	CV, VC, and CVC words*	Hirsh et al. (1952)
CNC	consonant nucleus consonant	Lehiste and Peterson (1959)
NU-6	Northwestern University lists	Tillman et al. (1963)
ABL		Boothroyd (1967)
SDS	speech discrimination scale	Gaeth (1970)
HFCDT	high frequency consonant discrimination	Gardner (1971)
Five Sound Test		Ling (1978)
Word Recognition: Monosyllables Closed Set		
RT	rhyme test	Fairbanks (1958)
Fry Lists		Fry (1961)
MRT	modified rhyme test	House et al. (1965)
DIP	discrimination by identification of pictures	Siegenthaler and Haspiel (1966)
RMC	rhyming minimal contrasts	Griffiths (1967)
MCDT	mulitple choice discrimination test	Schultz and Schubert (1969)
WIPI	word intelligibility by picture identification	Ross and Lerman (1970)
OUCRT	Oklahoma University Closed Response test	Pederson and Studebaker (1972)
NST	nonsense syllable test	Resnick et al. (1975)
CCT	California consonant test	Owens and Schubert (1977)
Perception of Words and Word Patterns		Erber and Witt (1977)
CHIPS	Children's Perception of Speech	Katz and Elliott (1978)
DFDT	distinctive features discrimination test	McPherson and Pang-Ching (1979)
Picture Identification Task		Wilson and Antablin (1980)
ANT	Auditory Numbers Test	Erber (1980)
SERT	sound effects recognition test	Finitzo-Hieber et al. (1980)
DFD	Distinctive Feature Difference test	Feeney and Franks (1982)

Type of Procedure	Test	Publication
Sentences: Open Set		
Sentence Tests for Deaf People		Fry and Kerridge (1939)
CID	Central Institute for the Deaf	Silverman and Hirsh (1955)
Fry Revised Sentences		Fry (1961)
SPIN	speech perception in noise	Kalikow et al. (1977)
BKB		Bench-Kowal-Bamford
Sentences: Closed Set		
KSUDT	Kent State University discrimination test	Berger (1969)
SSI	synthetic sentence identification	Speaks and Jerger (1965)
PSI	pediatric speech intelligibility	Jerger et al. (1980)
Naval Submarine Medical Research Laboratory Tri-Test of Intelligibility		Sergeant et al. (1981)
DSI	dichotic sentence identification	Fifer et al. (1983)

Technical Tips

Advantages of recorded speech audiometry materials (compact disc or tape recording)

- ☐ Tester is not a variable in presentation (even students do O.K.)
- ☐ Patient can't read your lips even if you're looking right at him/her
- ☐ You can take a sip of your favorite beverage while performing the test
- ☐ Since your eyes don't need to be glued to the VU meter, you can:
  - ✔ calculate your patient's PTA
  - ✔ connect your pure tone threshold symbols
  - ✔ rest your eyes
  - ✔ check out the Atlanta Braves or Colorado Rockies score in the daily newspaper
- ☐ Even on the best of days, it's very difficult to speak each sentence in the SSI material at the same time that you recite the story about Davy Crockett, or simultaneously speak the two competing words on the SSW or the four digits on the dichotic digits test.

Compact Disc (CD) Speech Materials

Also see VA Medical Center CD Speech Materials and BYU CD Speech Materials, pages 162–165.

AUDiTEC of St. Louis Compact Discs

CD 101R

- ☐ Spondee word list
- ☐ Children's spondee word list
- ☐ W-22 word lists
- ☐ NU #6 word lists
- ☐ PBK-50 word lists
- ☐ *Word Intelligibility by Picture Identification* (WIPI) pediatric test
- ☐ Multitalker noise
- ☐ Paired comparison sentences
- ☐ Connected discourse

CD 102

- ☐ Speech in Noise (SIN) test

Source: AUDiTEC of St. Louis, 2515 S. Big Bend Blvd., St. Louis, MO 63143
TEL: (800) 669-9065

CD Speech Materials

"Speech and Tonal materials for Auditory Perceptual Assessment" on the Long Beach VA Medical Center compact disc (CD) 1.0.

Track	Channel	Content
1	L	1000 Hz calibration tone
	R	1000 Hz calibration tone
2	L	Spondees, S_π N0 masking-level difference (MLD)
	R	Spondees, S_π N0 masking-level difference (MLD)
3	L	Dichotic synthetic musical chords
	R	Dichotic synthetic musical chords

Track	Channel	Content
4	L	Dichotic chords with 90 msec onset lag
	R	dichotic synthetic musical chords
5	L	Dichotic nonsense syllables (CVs)
	R	Dichotic nonsense syllables (Cvs)
6	L	Dichotic syllables with 90 msec onset lag
	R	Dichotic nonsense syllables
7	L	Dichotic monosyllabic digits (single digit)
	R	Dichotic monosyllabic digits (single digit)
8	L	Dichotic synthetic sentences
	R	Dichotic synthetic sentences
9	L	VIOECITO-consonant segments (CNCs), list 5A *
	R	VIOECITO-vowel segments (CNCs), list 5A
10	L	VIOECITO-consonant segments (CNCs), list 5B *
	R	VIOECITO-vowel segments (CNCs), list 5B
11	L	NU #6, high-pass filtered, list 3C
	R	NU #6, low-pass filtered, list 3C
12	L	NU #6, high-pass filtered, list 4C
	R	NU #6, low-pass filtered, list 4C
13	L	Frequency tonal patterns
	R	Duration tonal patterns
14	L	NU #6, 45% compressed, 0.3 sec reverberation, list 5
	R	NU #6, 45% compressed, list 5
15	L	NU #6, 45% compressed, 0.3 sec reverberation, list 6
	R	NU #6, 45% compressed, list 6
16	L	NU #6, 65% compressed, 0.3 sec reverberation, list 7
	R	NU #6, 65% compressed, list 7
17	L	NU #6, 65% compressed, 0.3 sec reverberation, list 8
	R	NU #6, 65% compressed, list 8
18	L	100 Hz, pulsed phase calibration tone
	R	100 Hz, pulsed phase calibration tone

Source: Noffsinger D, Wilson RH, Musiek FE. Department of Veterans Affairs compact disc recording for auditory perceptual assessment: Background and introduction. *Audiology* 5: 231–235, 1994.

*VIOECITO = vowels in one ear, consonants in the other

For more information contact: Richard H. Wilson, Ph.D., Audiology - 126, VA Medical Center, Mountain Home, TN 37684 or Douglas Noffsinger, Ph.D., Audiology and Speech Pathology (126), VA Medical Center West Los Angeles, Los Angeles, CA 90073

CD Speech Materials

"Speech Recognition and Identification Materials" on the Long Beach VA Medical Center compact disc (CD) 1.1.

Track	Channel	Content
1	L	1000 Hz calibration tone
	R	1000 Hz calibration tone
2	L	CIDs spondaic words (N = 72, 4 sec ISI*), female voice
	R	CID spondaic words (N = 144, 2 sec ISI), female voice
3	L	Maryland CNC, List 1 (1–25), 4.2 sec ISI, male voice
	R	CID W–22, List 1A (1–25), 4.2 sec ISI, male voice
4	L	Maryland CNC, List 1 (26–50), 4.2 sec ISI, male voice
	R	CID W–22, List 1A (26–50), 4.2 sec ISI, male voice
5	L	Maryland CNC, List 3 (1–25), 4.2 sec ISI, male voice
	R	CID W–22, List 2A (1–25), 4.2 sec ISI, male voice
6	L	Maryland CNC, List 3 (26–50), 4.2 sec ISI, male voice
	R	CID W–22, List 2A (26–50), 4.2 sec ISI, male voice
7	L	Maryland CNC, List 6 (1–25), 4.2 sec ISI, male voice
	R	CID W–22, List 3A (1–25), 4.2 sec ISI, male voice
8	L	Maryland CNC, List 6 (26–50), 4.2 sec ISI, male voice
	R	CID W–22, List 3A (26–50), 4.2 sec ISI, male voice
9	L	Maryland CNC, List 7 (1–25), 4.2 sec ISI, male voice
	R	CID W–22, List 4A (1–25), 4.2 sec ISI, male voice
10	L	Maryland CNC, List 7 (26–50), 4.2 sec ISI, male voice
	R	CID W–22, List 4A (26–50), 4.2 sec ISI, male voice
11	L	Maryland CNC, List 9 (1–25), 4.2 sec ISI, male voice
	R	Rush Hughes PB–50 List 8B (1–25), 4.2 sec ISI
12	L	Maryland CNC, List 9 (26–50), 4.2 sec ISI, male voice
	R	Rush Hughes PB–50 List 8B (26–50), 4.2 sec ISI
13	L	Maryland CNC, List 10 (1–25), 4.2 sec ISI, male voice
	R	Rush Hughes PB–50 List 9B (1–25), 4.2 sec ISI
14	L	Maryland CNC, List 10 (26–50), 4.2 sec ISI, male voice
	R	Rush Hughes PB–50 List 9B (26–50), 4.2 sec ISI
15	L	Picture ID Task, List 1A, (1–25), 6 sec ISI
	R	Rush Hughes PB–50 List 10B (1–25), 4.2 sec ISI
16	L	Picture ID Task, List 1A, (26–50), 6 sec ISI
	R	Rush Hughes PB–50 List 10B (26–50), 4.2 sec ISI
17	L	Picture ID Task, List 2A, (1–25), 6 sec ISI
	R	Rush Hughes PB–50 List 11B (1–25), 4.2 sec ISI
18	L	Picture ID Task, List 2A, (26–50), 6 sec ISI
	R	Rush Hughes PB–50 List 11B (26–50), 4.2 sec ISI

Track	Channel	Content
19	L	NU #6 CNC, List 1A (1–25), 4.6 sec ISI, female voice
	R	Competing sentences, male voice
20	L	NU #6 CNC, List 1A (26–50), 4.6 sec ISI, female voice
	R	Competing sentences, male voice
21	L	NU #6 CNC, List 2A (1–25), 4.6 sec ISI, female voice
	R	Competing sentences, male voice
22	L	NU #6 CNC, List 2A (26–50), 4.6 sec ISI, female voice
	R	Competing sentences, male voice
23	L	NU #6 CNC, List 3A (1–25), 4.6 sec ISI, female voice
	R	Competing sentences, male voice
24	L	NU #6 CNC, List 3A (26–50), 4.6 sec ISI, female voice
	R	Competing sentences, male voice
25	L	NU #6 CNC, List 4A (1–25), 4.6 sec ISI, female voice
	R	Competing sentences, male voice
26	L	NU #6 CNC, List 4A (26–50), 4.6 sec ISI, female voice
	R	Competing sentences, male voice
27	L	Synthetic sentence Identification, List #1, 6.5 sec ISI
	R	Davy Crockett competing message story
28	L	Synthetic sentence Identification, List #2, 6.5 sec ISI
	R	Davy Crockett competing message story
29	L	Synthetic sentence Identification, List #3, 6.5 sec ISI
	R	Davy Crockett competing message story
30	L	Synthetic sentence Identification, List #4, 6.5 sec ISI
	R	Davy Crockett competing message story
31	L	Synthetic sentence Identification, List #5, 6.5 sec ISI
	R	Davy Crockett competing message story
32	L	Synthetic sentence Identification, List #6, 6.5 sec ISI
	R	Davy Crockett competing message story
33	L	Synthetic sentence Identification, List #7, 6.5 sec ISI
	R	Davy Crockett competing message story
34	L	Synthetic sentence Identification, List #8, 6.5 sec ISI
	R	Davy Crockett competing message story
35	L	Synthetic sentence Identification, List #9, 6.5 sec ISI
	R	Davy Crockett competing message story

*ISI = interstimulus interval

For more information contact: Richard H. Wilson, Ph.D., Audiology - 126, VA Medical Center, Mountain Home, TN 37684 or Douglas Noffsinger, Ph.D., Audiology and Speech Pathology (126), VA Medical Center West Los Angeles, Los Angeles, CA 90073

Brigham Young University CD Speech Materials

Also, see VA CD Speech Materials, pages 162–163.

- ☐ Track 1: 1000 Hz calibration tone (6 dB down from peaks of words on CD).
- ☐ Track 2: 15 sets each of 300 ms, 270 ms, and 330 ms tone bursts.
- ☐ Track 3: Four randomizations of 13 CID W-1 spondee words (Hirsch et al., 1952) that were reported as homogeneous in numerous published investigations (see KEY REFS in this ADR chapter) with 0.7 sec silent intervals.
- ☐ Track 4: Four randomizations of 13 CID W-1 spondee words (Hirsch et al., 1952) that were reported as homogeneous in numerous published investigations (see KEY REFS in this ADR chapter) with 2.7 sec silent intervals between words.
- ☐ Track 5: Two different randomizations of 36 CID W-1 spondee words with 0.7 second intervals between words
- ☐ Track 6: Two different randomizations of 36 CID W-1 spondee words with 2.7 second intervals between words.
- ☐ Tracks 7–16: Ten isophonemic word lists developed by Olsen, Van Tasell, and Speaks (1982, 1983, 1986) containing 10 words and the same 30 phonemes with 3.5 sec silent intervals between words.
- ☐ Tracks 17–24: CID W-22 word lists 1 through 4. The odd numbered Tracks (17, 19, 21, and 23) contain the 25 most difficult words with the *most difficult* words appearing first. The even-numbered Tracks (19, 20, 22, and 24) contain the 25 easiest words. Ordering of the words in these lists is from data of Thornton and Raffin (1978). The lists use a 3.5 sec interval between words.
- ☐ Tracks 25 and 26: 25 most difficult and the 25 least difficult words respectively selected from among the 200 words in CID W-22 lists Thornton and Raffin (1978). The lists use a 3.5 sec interval between words.
- ☐ Tracks 27–32: Six word lists developed by Harvey Gardner. First two lists were published by Gardner (1971) and the other four lists (A - D) were developed by Gardner for female or male talkers. The lists use a 3.5 sec interval between words.

- ☐ Tracks 33–40: First and second half-lists for PBK-50 Lists 1 through 4 developed Haskins (1949). The lists use a 3.5 sec interval between words.
- ☐ Tracks 41–42: Word Intelligibility by Picture Identification (WIPI) lists 1 and 2 developed by Ross and Lerman (1970). The lists use a 3.5 sec interval between words.

Note: For all speech materials, the left channel stimulus items are spoken by a male talker and the right channel items are spoken by a female talker.

Audiology Overachievement Award

Book Chapter Division, Speech Audiometry Category

Author: Fred H. Bess

Insitutional Affiliation: Vanderbilt University

Reference: Bess FH.
Clinical assessment of speech recognition.
Chapter 6 in DF Konkle, WF Rintelmann (eds).
Principles of Speech Audiometry.
Baltimore: University Park Press, 1983.

Statistics:

- Page length = 74
- Estimated total manuscript page length = 250
- Number of headings = 7
- Number of subheadings = 18
- Number of tables = 10
- Number of figures = 14
- Number of references cited = 215

Word Recognition

NU-6 half lists arranged with the 10 most difficult (most often incorrect) words first

Form A	Form B	Form C	Form D
1. KNOCK	1. RAISE	1. GIN	1. PAD
2. KITE	2. PAGE	2. PICK	2. MATCH
3. TAKE	3. CHALK	3. PIKE	3. DEEP
4. KEEN	4. LAUD	4. SHACK	4. CHIEF
5. PUFF	5. DEATH	5. DAB	5. GAZE
6. HASH	6. THIRD	6. TURN	6. ROT
7. TIP	7. BEAN	7. KEEP	7. HAZE
8. POOL	8. SIZE	8. TOOL	8. CALM
9. BURN	9. MET	9. BITE	9. SOUTH
10. SUB	10. JAR	10. JUICE	10. NICE
11. FAT	11. HURL	11. TON	11. CHAIR
12. YES	12. WEEK	12. FAIL	12. SHAWL
13. FALL	13. CHOICE	13. MERGE	13. SAID
14. WHICH	14. GAP	14. HUSH	14. GOAL
15. SELL	15. MODE	15. MILL	15. SOAP
16. KING	16. BOAT	16. BOUGHT	16. WAG
17. LOT	17. TOUGH	17. DEAD	17. KEG
18. RAID	18. DIME	18. FAR	18. WITCH
19. VINE	19. WHIP	19. THOUGHT	19. LOAF
20. JAIL	20. SURE	20. LEARN	20. READ
21. REACH	21. DOOR	21. LIVE	21. HATE
22. RAG	22. SHOUT	22. ROOM	22. RAIN
23. HOME	23. MOON	23. BOOK	23. NUMB
24. GOOSE	24. NAG	24. YOUNG	24. VOICE
25. LOVE	25. LIMB	25. WHITE	25. LORE

Form E	Form F	Form G
1. CHEEK	1. CHAT	1. RIP
2. RING	2. SHEEP	2. FIT
3. SEIZE	3. THIN	3. PERCH
4. DODGE	4. YOUTH	4. BACK
5. MESS	5. BEG	5. CHECK
6. CAUSE	6. DITCH	6. CAME
7. MOUSE	7. TEAM	7. GET
8. BASE	8. POLE	8. MOB
9. SHALL	9. HALF	9. MAKE
10. MOP	10. LIFE	10. SAIL
11. DATE	11. PAIN	11. SHIRT
12. TELL	12. JUG	12. ROSE
13. CAB	13. RAT	13. GAS
14. PEARL	14. SOUP	14. VOTE
15. COOL	15. VOID	15. MOOD
16. FIVE	16. HIT	16. JUDGE
17. LUCK	17. LATE	17. SUCH
18. TALK	18. PHONE	18. KILL
19. NOTE	19. RUSH	19. TIME
20. GERM	20. LID	20. NEAR
21. SEARCH	21. ROAD	21. HALL
22. WALK	22. BAR	22. DOLL
23. GUN	23. HIRE	23. BONE
24. WIRE	24. NAME	24. LONG
25. WHEN	25. GOOD	25. HAVE

Source: Available from AUDiTEC of St. Louis in digital audiotape (DAT) or cassette format

Key References

Word Recognition lists ordered with 10 most difficult words first.

Also, see LISTS about Word Recognition Measurements and LISTS about CD Speech Audiometry Materials in this ADR chapter.

Keating LW. Error frequency in CID W-22 lists. Unpublished data. Rochester, MN: Mayo Clinic, 1974 (cited in Olsen WO, Matkin ND. Speech Audiometry. In WF Rintelmann, ed. *Hearing Assessment*, 2nd ed.). Austin, TX: Pro-Ed, 1991, p. 85.

Rose DE, Schreurs KK, Miller LE. A ten-word speech discrimination screening test. *Audiology and Hearing Education* (Winter): 15-16, 1979

Hosford-Dunn HL, Runge CA, Montgomery PA. A shortened rank-ordered word recognition list. *The Hearing Journal 36*: 15–19, 1983

Runge CA, Hosford-Dunn, HL. Word recognition performance with modified CID W-22 word lists. *J Speech Hear Res 28*: 355–362, 1985

Note: CID-W22 lists and NU-6 lists are commerically available in this format in a CD or in a tape-recorded format from AUDiTEC of Saint Louis. (Just ask Bill Carver about them, and tell him that Jay and Gus sent you.) W-22 word lists in the 10-most-difficult format are also available from Brigham Young University (BYU)

Clinical Concept

Advantages of Pediatric Speech Intelligibility (PSI) Test

- ☐ Clinical advantages of the PSI include:
  - ✔ Tape-recorded speech materials are commercially available.
  - ✔ The PSI measures peripheral and central auditory abilities.
  - ✔ Test reliability is established and is described statistically.
  - ✔ Word list equivalence is defined.
  - ✔ Practice effects are known. Stable measures of performance (e.g. Minimal practice effects) are obtained after three practice trials.
  - ✔ Sequence effects (e.g. How well a child performs based on prior performance within the closed message set of five items) are not a major factor in test performance.
  - ✔ The restricted task domain format for test items, a form of closed message set, offers distinct advantages for audiologic assessment of children.
  - ✔ Language ability, as derived from the Northwestern Syntax Screening Test (NSST) is taken into account in selecting the PSI test format which is appropriate for the each pediatric patient.
  - ✔ Complete normative data are available for interpreting test performance.

Did You Know?

How the Pediatric Speech Intelligibility (PSI) Test Was Developed

Unlike most speech audiometry materials which are developed by some well-paid, highly educated, experienced (e.g., old) Ph.D. in a laboratory, PSI materials were actually generated by normal children ($N = 87$) between the ages of 3 and 6 years. This unique strategy produced word and sentence picture test items that the average child could recognize and read. Also, the strategy yielded words that were concrete (e.g., a banana or an apple), rather than abstract (e.g., food). Finally, animals were used for the pictures targets, rather than people, to reduce "cross-cultural" differences among children. That is, who cares if the bear is black, or white, or a black and white Chinese panda?

Pediatric Speech Intelligibility (PSI) Test Materials

I. The 20 monosyllabic words in the PSI test

1. bear
2. bird
3. boat
4. book
5. car
6. dog
7. duck
8. fish
9. flag
10. fork
11. frog
12. hat
13. house
14. key
15. knife
16. pig
17. spoon
18. sun
19. train
20. tree

II. Examples of some of the 10 sentences in the PSI test

Format I

1. Show me a rabbit painting an egg.
2. Show me a bear brushing his teeth.
3. Show me a horse eating an apple.

Format II

1. A rabbit is painting an egg.
2. A bear is brushing his teeth.
3. A horse is eating an apple.

III. Examples of some of the 20 competing sentence messages in the PSI test

1. The cat is driving a race car.
2. The mouse is cooking some pork chops.
3. A boy pig is making a snowman.
4. The squirrel is cutting out some paper dolls.

Source: Jerger S, Lewis S, Hawkins J, and Jerger J. Pediatric speech intelligibility test. I. Generation of test materials. *International Journal of Pediatric Otorhinolaryngology 2*: 217–230, 1980.
Note: The PSI is available commercially from: AUDiTEC of St. Louis, 2515 S. Big Bend Blvd., St. Louis, MO 63143. TEL: 800-669-9065

Protocol

Pediatric Speech Intelligibility (PSI) Test Administration

☐ Perform basic audiometric assessment

- Immitance measurement
- Pure tone audiometry

☐ Pretest conditions

- Parent or clinician has the child verbally label each picture target
- Child is intructed to point to the picture of what he/she hears

☐ PSI administration

- Peformance for PSI test items is measured in quiet initially at an intensity level of 30 to 40 dB HL.
- Then the intensity decreased in 10 dB steps until the "knee" of the performance intensity (PI) function is reached.
- Intensity level is further decreased in 5 dB steps until performance is on the order of 0 to 20%.
- Finally, a high intensity level (80 dB HL) is employed.
- If performance at the first test level is poor (less than 60%), intensity is increased in 20 dB steps.
- Peformance for PSI test items is measured in the presence of competing message (the "trick man").
- A message-to-competition (MCR) ratio of 0 dB is used for sentences and +4 dB is used for words.
- Masking is presented to the nontest ear whenever crossover is a possibility.

☐ Sound-field versus earphone presentation

- Usually, sound-field presentation for PI functions is used for younger children that qualify for Format I sentences.
- An exception is the child with an asymmetric audiogram or suspected CAPD (use earphones if possible in these cases).
- With sound-field presentation for PI functions, test items and competing message are delivered through the same loudspeaker.
- Earphone presentation is always used for MCR functions with an ipsilateral (ICM) and contralateral (CCM) competing message. A dichotic condition can be obtained only under earphones.

- ☐ Test interpretation

  - Analyze results separately for PI functions and for MCR functions.
  - Consider the child's receptive language level (RLL).
  - Consult formal guidelines for interpretation of PSI results (see source noted below).
  - Children with normal CNS function or nonauditory CNS dysfunction typically show normal maximum intelligibility (e.g., 100%), no rollover of PI functions, and normal ICM and CCM test performance even at the most difficult MCR for both ears (competing has no adverse effect on test performance).
  - Children with auditory CNS dysfunction may show normal maximum intelligibility (e.g., 100%), but evidence of rollover of PI functions and depressed maximum ICM and CCM test performance at the most difficult MCR for one or both ears. An example of this type of performance pattern is illustrated in Pattern of PSI Test Findings on the following page.

Source: Chapter 4 of the *Pediatric Speech Intelligibility Test Manual for Administration* (S Jerger and J Jerger) available from AUDiTEC of St. Louis, 2515 S. Big Bend Blvd., St. Louis, MO 63143. Tel: (800) 669-9065

Patterns of PSI Test Results

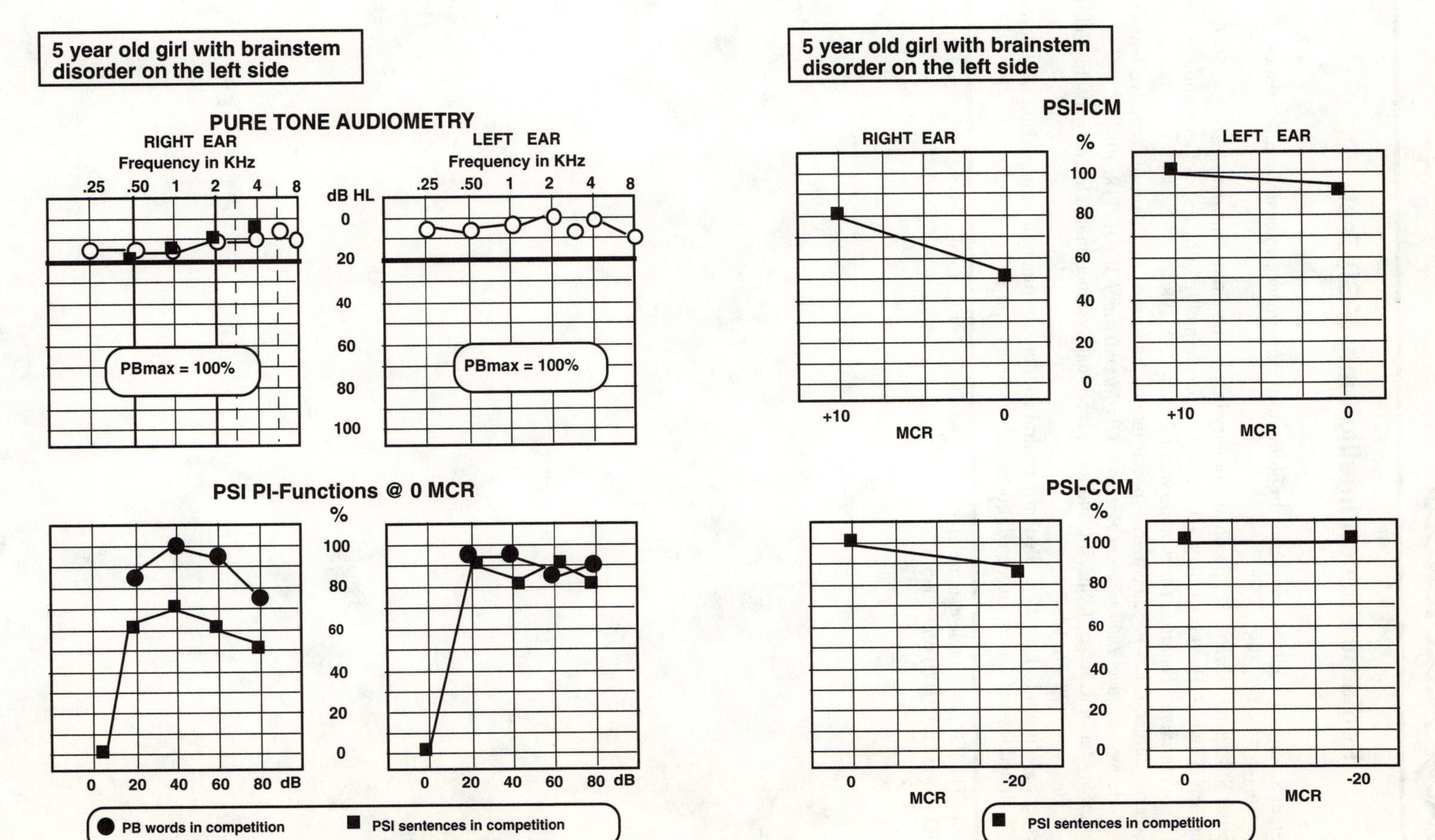

Key References

Pediatric Speech Intelligibility (PSI) Test

Jerger S, Jerger J. Pediatric speech intelligibility test: Performance-intensity characteristics. *Ear and Hearing 3*: 325-333, 1982.

Jerger S, Jerger J, Abrams S. Speech audiometry in a young child. *Ear and Hearing 4*: 56–66, 1983.

Jerger S, Lewis S, Hawkins J, Jerger J. Pediatric speech intelligibility test. I. Generation of test materials. *International Pediatric Otorhinolaryngol 2*: 217–230, 1980.

Jerger S, Jerger J, Lewis S. Pediatric speech intelligibility test. II. Effect of receptive language age and chronologic age. *International Pediatric Otorhinolaryngol 3*: 101–118, 1981.

Jerger S, Martin R, Jerger J. Specific auditory perceptual dysfunction in a learning disabled child. *Ear and Hearing 8*: 78–86, 1987.

Jerger S, Johnson K, Loiselle L. Pediatric central auditory dysfunction: Comparison of children with confirmed lesions versus suspected processing disorders. *Am J Otol 9 (Suppl.)*: 63–71, 1988.

Note: The PSI is available commercially from: AUDiTEC of St. Louis, 2515 S. Big Bend Blvd., St. Louis, MO 63143. Tel: (800) 669-9065

CHAPTER 4

Immittance Measurement

In This ADR Chapter

Perspective

Although the clinical value of measuring middle ear function with aural impedance techniques was clear with the publication in 1946 of a monograph by Otto Metz, the routine incorporation of impedance (immittance) measures in clinical audiology dates back to the early 1970s. The commercial availability of relatively stable and easy-to-operate electroacoustic aural impedance instruments during this time period, combined with the publication of large-scale studies describing and categorizing the patterns of impedance findings characteristic of patients with normal ears, and a variety of otologic pathologies, "impedance audiometry" quickly assumed a pivotal role in clinical audiology.

Before long, most audiologists used impedance measures, or at least tympanometry, on a daily basis in their clinics and offices. Every year many platform sessions at annual conventions were devoted to papers on impedance topics. In less than a decade, the clinical value of impedance measures extended far beyond the use of tympanometry in description of middle ear function. Audiologists were routinely recording acoustic stapedial reflex activity, first for contralateral (crossed) signals, and then for contra- and ipsilateral signals. There were dozens of publications demonstrating the accuracy of hearing loss prediction by the acoustic reflex. Impedance measures also, clearly, could help to differentiate sensory versus neural auditory dysfunction. Analysis of abnormally elevated acoustic reflex thresholds and acoustic reflex decay permitted identification of retrocochlear auditory dyfunctions in approximately 85% of patients with confirmed eighth nerve lesions. And, importantly, this sensitive auditory procedure was "objective" (i.e., electrophysiologic) and took a mere minute or two, a fraction of the test time required to carry out the traditional diagnostic test battery of SISI, tone decay, ABLB, and Bekesy audiometry.

Since the golden days of aural impedance measurement, newer audiologic procedures, such as ABR and OAE, have worked their way into the audiologic test battery. However, there is still no better, quicker, or less expensive single audiologic procedure for assessing the status of the middle ear, cochlea, eighth nerve, and lower auditory brainstem than a performing a complete immittance (*im*pedance or ad*mittance*) test battery.

FOUNDATIONS OF IMMITTANCE MEASUREMENTS

Clinical Concept

Components of Acoustic Immittance (*Im*pedance and Ad*mittance*)

- ☐ Admittance is the reciprocal of impedance. Acoustic admittance a measure of the flow of energy through the middle ear system, whereas impedance is the opposition to this flow.
- ☐ Measured at the tympanic membrane, acoustic impedance = input impedance of the middle ear.
- ☐ The three elements or components of impedance in mechanical (and acoustic) terms are:
  - ✔ mass (a quantity of air moving as a unit)
  - ✔ spring (an enclosed volume of air when compressed)
  - ✔ friction (collisions among air molecules)
- ☐ The ear combines mechanical and acoustic elements.
- ☐ In the middle ear system, the **spring** component includes:
  - ✔ tympanic membrane
  - ✔ air in the ear canal and middle ear
  - ✔ ligaments
  - ✔ tendons
- ☐ In the middle ear system, the **mass** component includes:
  - ✔ the pars flacida of the tympanic membrane
  - ✔ the ossicles
  - ✔ the perilymph within the cochlea
- ☐ In the middle ear system, the **friction** component includes:
  - ✔ viscosity of the perilymph
  - ✔ viscosity of mucous lining of the middle ear cavity
  - ✔ the narrow passages within the middle ear and mastoid cavity
  - ✔ the tympanic membrane
  - ✔ tendons
  - ✔ ligaments

Schematic Diagram of an Electroacoustic Immittance Meter

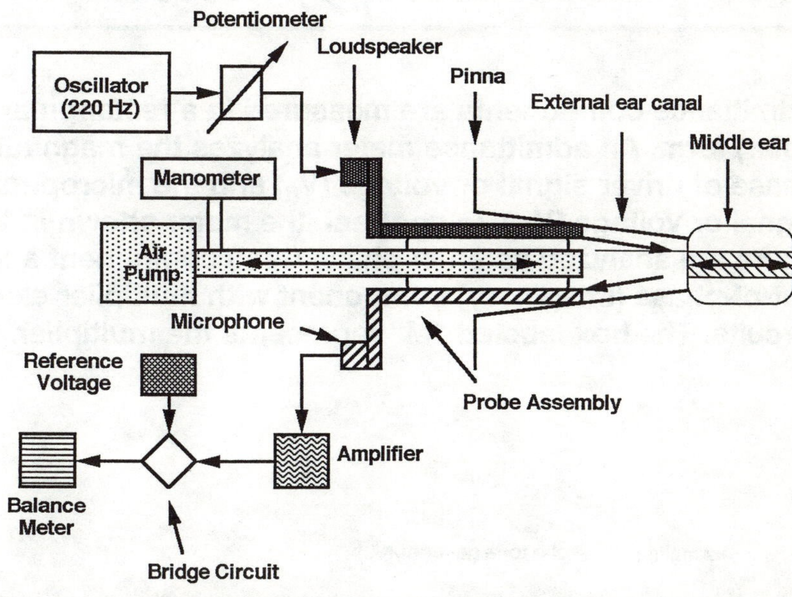

Components of a Conventional Analog (Versus Current Digital) Susceptance (B) and Conductance(G) Meter

Admittance components are measured in a rectangular (vs. polar) form. An admittance meter analyzes the magnitude and phase of driver signal or voltage (V_d) and the microphone signal or voltage (V_m). In contrast, the meter shown in this figure are analyzed as an in-phase (real) component and an out-of-phase (imaginary) component with multiplier electronic circuits. The box labeled "M" represents the multiplier.

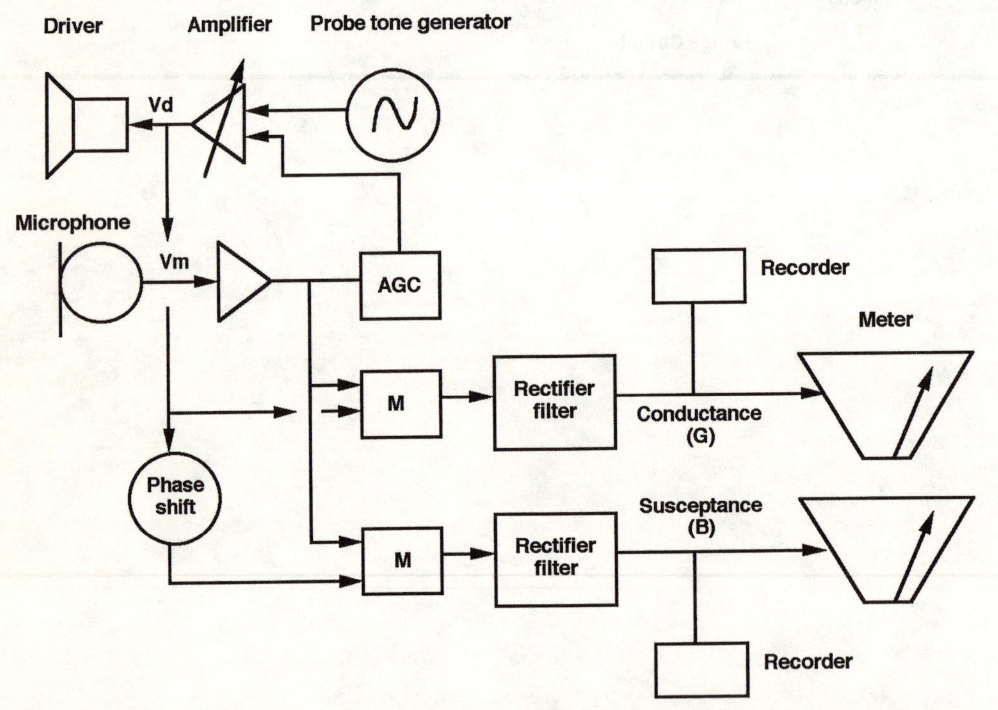

*Summary of Aural Immittance Units**

Quantity	Symbol	SI**	Traditional Units
Acoustic impedance	Z_a		
Acoustic resistance	R_a	$Pa.s/m^3$	Acoustic ohm
Acoustic reactance	X_a		
Impedance phase angle	Φ_z	Radian	Degree
Acoustic admittance	Y_a		
Acoustic conductance	G_a	$m^3/Pa.s$	Acoustic mmho (cgs units implied)
Acoustic susceptance	B_a		
Admittance phase angle	Φ_y	Radian	Degree
Acoustic mass (inertance)	M_a	$Pa.s^2/m^3$	None
Acoustic stiffness	K_a	Pa/m^3	None
Acoustic compliance (capacitance)	C_a	m^3/Pa	None
Acoustic equivalent volume	V_{ea}	m^3	cm^3
Air	P	Pa	mm H_2O

Source: Adapted from: Shanks, J. (1988) Aural acoustic immittance standards. *Seminars in Hearing (Immittance Audiometry), 8*, 307–318.

*The ANSI reference is American National Standards Institute (Draft 1986). Proposed Amercian National Standard Specifications for Instruments to Measure Aural Acoustic Impedance and Admittance (Aural Acoustic Immittance). ANSI S3.6, New York.

**SI = International System of Units used by both the American National Standards Institute (ANSI) and the International Electrotechnical Commission (IEC)

Clinical Concept

Acoustic Impedance Versus Admittance

- ☐ Acoustic *impedance* or $\mathbf{Z_a = R_a + X_a}$, where R = resistance (e.g., the friction component) and X = reactance (e.g., the mass or spring component, also known as the stiffness component), or $X = 2\pi f M/S^2$, where M = mass and S = surface upon which the sound pressure acts.

  Impedance is the opposition to energy flow.

- ☐ Acoustic *admittance* = $\mathbf{Y_a = G_a + B_a}$, where G = conductance (e.g., 1/friction) and B = susceptance (e.g., the mass and spring components).

  Admittance is the flow of energy.

Classic Quote

James Jerger on His Early Studies of the Clinical Value of Impedance Measurements

"In 1960, I was invited to present a paper at the International Congress of Audiology in Bonn, West Germany. This was my first contact with the great names of European audiology, and I was duly impressed. I met Luscher of Switzerland; Langenbeck of Germany; Ewertsen and Bentzen of Denmark; Liden, Klockhoff, and Barr of Sweden; Hood of the United Kingdom; and a host of others. It was a heady experience.

After the Congress I spent a few weeks visiting audiology centers in Denmark and Sweden. In Copenhagen, Professor Ewertsen and his group showed me a new electroacoustic gadget they were trying out in clinic. They called it an "impedancemeter" since it measured impedance characteristics of the middle ear. Another Dane, Otto Metz, had already pioneered the measurement of the acoustic stapedius reflex, by means of a mechanical bridge, during and after World War II. This new device carried the concept a few steps further. In addition to the bridge circuitry necessary to detect stapedius muscle contraction, it had additional circuitry making it possible to measure the absolute static impedance of the middle ear system. In fact, you could measure two dimensions of the static impedance. (1) the vector magnitude, or real component, and (2) the phase angle, or imaginary component. Finally, by means of a calibrated air pump, you could study the way in which the middle-ear impedance changed under conditions of both positive and negative air pressure. A graph of these changes they called a 'tympanogram.' The new system had been designed by Terkildsen and

Scott-Nielsen and fabricated by Madsen Electronics. They called it the model ZO-60.

When I returned to Evanston, I was invited to give a presentation to our department, reporting on what I had seen and heard. In that talk I described the Madsen 'impedancemeter' and predicted that it would probably have a very significant impact on audiometric evaluation. I don't think that anyone took me very seriously on that occasion. They all nodded agreeably but didn't quite see what middle-ear impedance had to do with audiograms. If you wanted to know about the middle ear, after all, you simply tested by bone conduction.

A year later, in 1961, I left Northwestern and moved to Washington, D.C. Here I was associated with both Gallaudet College and the Audiology outpatient clinic of the Veteran's Administration (now the Department of Veteran's Affairs). While at the VA, I ordered a Madsen 'impedancemeter,' now the model ZO-61. It was, I believe, the first Madsen bridge in the USA. But I didn't get to use it very much before I was off again, this time to Houston.

Late in 1962, I joined the Houston Speech and Hearing Center as Director of Research. By this time, Grason-Stadler had come out with the Zwislocki mechanical bridge and, in a colossal demonstration of bad judgment, I bought one of these instead of another Madsen. I still have a photograph of that hardy band of pioneers who traveled to Syracuse in 1963 to take the first course in how to use the new bridge. Alan Feldman was our patient tutor. He told us everything we had to know about the bridge—except that you needed at least three arms and four hands to operate it. I was constantly reminded of Charlie Chaplin on the assembly line in 'Modern Times.'

The Zwislocki bridge was, of course, very good at measuring both the reactive and resistive components of static impedance. It turned out, however, that this middle ear measure was far less interesting than two other measures, the tympanogram and the acoustic reflex, neither of which could easily be assessed with the Zwislocki bridge.

In 1968 I moved again, this time to Baylor College of Medicine as Professor of Audiology. We set up a small audiology clinic in the basement of The Methodist Hospital and began to see patients from the Otolaryngology Service headed by Dr. Bobby Alford. That summer, a very fine gentleman named Jimmy Brown, then the local Madsen representative, came by to show us a new instrument. Madsen Electronics had redesigned the old ZO-61 impedancemeter. The new model, called the ZO-70, eliminated the phase-angle measure and had improved sensitivity for acoustic reflex detection. It was just beginning to appear in the USA. I wanted one desperately but didn't have anything like the money to buy it. Jimmy sensed, however, that I would put it to good use and graciously loaned me an instrument.

We did indeed put it to good use. Throughout 1969, we used it to test every patient coming through our audiology clinic. After seeing the results of what came to be called 'impedance audiometry' (still later, the more politically correct 'immittance audiometry') in a consecutive series of about 400 patients, we thought we had a pretty good grasp of the clinical value of tympanograms, acoustic reflex thresholds, and the static impedance measures. We detailed our experience in a 1970 paper, 'Clinical Experience with Impedance Audiometry,' which was widely read and quoted. The importance of this paper was that it showed how the three components of impedance audiometry, the tympanogram, the static impedance, and the acoustic reflex could be diagnostically effective if used as a total test battery. Previous investigators had studied one or another component and found it unimpressive as a precise diagnostic tool. The 1970 paper reached the same conclusion about the individual components, but showed, paradoxically, that results across the three components fell into distinct categories that could be very useful diagnostically.

As it turned out, this has been a fruitful approach to a number of other test paradigms for diagnostic evaluation. Although some researchers continue to seek one ideal measure of a phenomenon, usually with only limited success, others have exploited the test battery/distinctive pattern approach to better advantage. Some examples are the use of auditory evoked potentials at various latencies rather than the ABR alone, the use of speech audiometric materials sampling a continuum of linguistic complexity rather than intelligibility for monosyllabic (PB) words alone, and the interpretation of evoked otoacoustic emissions within the context of the total audiometric evaluation rather than in relation to audiometric thresholds alone."

Source: Reprinted with permission from Jerger, J. (1993) Introduction to Section IV: Impedance Audiometery. In Alford, B.R., & Jerger, S. (Eds). *Clinical Audiology: The Jerger Perspective* (pp. 282–284). San Diego: Singular Publishing Group.

Audiologic Time Line

Aural immittance meters

Year	Author(s)	Contribution
1833	Wheatstone (Charles)	English physicist popularized SH Christie's electrical bridge circuit for determining an unknown electrical resistance
1926	Stewart	Constructed the first practical acoustic-impedance bridge
1930	Troger	German physicist who systematically studied Impedance at the tympanic membrane
1933	Fay & Hall	Telephone engineers who made aural impedance measurements in human ears (for telephone transducer function)
1934	Schuster	Further refined an acoustic-impedance bridge design which was used by many later investigators
1938	Waetzmann	Used "Schuster type bridge" in acoustic impedance measurement of normal ears
1940	Menzel	Used "Schuster type bridge" in acoustic impedance measurement of three abnormal ears
1946	Metz (Otto)	Dane who published results of a clinical investigation of impedance (static) measures in normal versus pathologic ears that was initiated in 1939 with Schuster-type impedance bridge
1957	Zwislocki	Reliable mechanical-acoustic impedance measurements in human ears with small, portable, calibrated Schuster-type bridge with a variable compensation cavity
1960	Terkildsen & Scott-Nielsen	Electroacoustic impedance device for clincal measurements
1960	Madsen, Inc.	Madsen Electronics manufactured the Terkildsen and Scott-Nielson device for clinical use as Model ZO-60
1962	Grason Stadler	Introduced a clinical version of the Zwislocki mechanical impedance bridge
1970–1973		Commercially available electro-acoustic impedance measuring devices introduced in the U.S.A. by an international variety of manufacturers including Madsen, Grason Stadler, American Electromedics, Amplaid, and Teledyne
1973	Lilly (David)	Comprehensive chapter on impedance meters and measurement in the 2nd edition of Jerger's *Modern Developments in Audiology*

Historical Reverberation

1970—One of Our Favorite Years

- ☐ Jim Jerger publishes the first comprehensive study on clinical applications of impedance measurements in a consecutive series of more than 400 patients appropriately entitled *"Clinical experience with impedance audiometry."*
- ☐ Jewett, Romano, and Williston publish their classic description of the human auditory brainstem response, cautiously entitled "Human auditory evoked potentials: Possible brainstem components detected on the scalp" in the prestigious journal *Science.*
- ☐ Among the hundreds of songs performed in concert by the Grateful Dead over 25 years were the following with lyrics and music, respectively, by the great song-writing team of Robert Hunter and the late great (grate?) Jerry Garcia (with one important exception) and *first* performed live in the year 1970 (site of performance follows each entry).
  - ✓ Brokedown Palace (Fillmore West)
  - ✓ Candyman (Field House, University of Cincinnati)
  - ✓ Friend of the Devil (Family Dog on the Great Highway, San Francisco)
  - ✓ Ripple (Fillmore West)
  - ✓ Till the Morning Comes
  - ✓ To Lay Me Down
  - ✓ Truckin', also written with Weir & Lesh (Fillmore West)
  - ✓ Sugar Magnolia, written by Barlow & Weir (Fillmore West)
- ☐ While we're on the topic, the year 1970 also witnessed an album—*History of the Grateful Dead, Vol. 1 (Bear's Choice)*—recorded live at Bill Graham's Fillmore East on February 13 and 14, plus two other albums (*Workingman's Dead* and the double album *Live Dead*).
- ☐ Herbert Vaughan and Walter Ritter publish a description the scalp topography of the auditory late response, demonstrating that the response receives contribution from the auditory cortex on the superior temporal gyrus. The technique is a precursor of auditory evoked response "brain mapping."
- ☐ A group of Scandinavian researchers (Anderson, Barr, & Wedenberg) show that acoustic reflex measures (thresholds and decay) are valuable in the early detection of acoustic tumors.
- ☐ Another group of Scandinavian investigators (Liden, Peterson, & Björkman) describe methods for analysis, and various clinical applications, for tympanometry.
- ☐ Plomp and Smoorenburg are editors of an oft-cited basic science textbook entitled *Frequency Analysis and Periodicity Detection in Hearing,* which includes contributions from P. Dallos, H. Spoendlin, I. C. Whitfield, and E. Zwicker.
- ☐ Rock star Jimi Hendrix dies in London at the age of 27.

- ☐ Goldman, Fristoe, and Woodcock develop a popular test of auditory discrimination.
- ☐ James Jerger describes the synthetic sentence identification (SSI) test at a symposium in Denmark. Other presenters at the meeting include Raymond Carhart.
- ☐ NFL Monday Night Football first airs. The Cleveland Browns beat the visiting New York Jets by the score of 31 to 21.
- ☐ Mark Ross introduces a picture identification test for hearing impaired children. Naturally, an audiologic test must have an acronym, and this test becomes known as word intelligibility by picture identification, or WIPI.

TYMPANOMETRY AND STATIC IMMITTANCE

Developmental Changes in Neonatal Middle Ear Structure and Function

- ☐ Vernix casseous in external ear canal dissipates within days after birth. Vernix is a lotion-like substance that covers the neonate's body at birth, and may remain in some cracks and crevices (e.g., the external ear canal) for awhile
- ☐ Mesenchyme, present in the middle ear of some term neonates, dissipates within days after birth
- ☐ Efficiency of the middle ear in transmitting acoustical energy to mechanical energy improves
- ☐ Areal ratio of tympanic membrane (TM) to stapes footplate increases
- ☐ TM curvature increases which increases lever function of the middle ear system and produces more efficiency in vibrational energy
- ☐ TM thickness decreases
- ☐ Lever function of the ossicles improves

Did You Know?

Why is a 220 Hz probe tone frequency typically used in immittance measurements?

- ☐ When Terkildsen and Scott-Nielsen (1960) conducted their now-famous experiments, available transducers were nonlinear at higher frequencies.
- ☐ Also, related to early work on this topic, 220 Hz is not an even harmonic of the typical power line frequency used in Europe (50 Hz).
- ☐ A one-component admittance measurement technique can be used with low frequencies as the phase angle is relatively constant in tympanometry.
- ☐ The acoustic stapedial reflex is not apt to be activated with a probe tone frequency in the 220 Hz region, even at high intensity levels.
- ☐ There is a vast accumulated clinical experience with this probe frequency (consider all of the clinical papers published just in the early 1970s).
- ☐ At a low probe frequency, calculations of immittance at the tympanic membrane are more accurate.
- ☐ Standards for immittance devices apply to those that employ a 226 Hz probe tone frequency.

Sources: Van Camp, K. J., Margolis, R. H., Wilson, R. H., Creten, W. L., Shanks, J. E. (1986). *Principles of tympanometry. ASHA Monograph, 24.* Terkildsen, K., & Scott-Nielsen, S. (1960) An electroacoustic impedance measuring bridge for clinical use. *Archives of Otolaryngology 72,* 339–346.

Step-by-Step Protocol

Tympanometry

- ☐ Examine the ear otoscopically for evidence of external ear canal pathology, a perforated tympanic membrane or pressure equalization (PE) or ventilation tube, and general size and shape. Document and consider the interpretation of the results of tympanometry.
- ☐ Instruct patients on what you are about to do, and what you expect of them (e.g., sit quietly without responding to any sounds they might hear). Make sure to tell patients to inform you if they feel any pain. The results of the test are important, but it is okay to discontinue the test anytime if they experience pain or too much discomfort.
- ☐ Select a clean probe-tip that is appropriate for the patient's ear canal and place it on the probe assembly.
- ☐ Keep your clean probe tips organized according to size. Most brands of probe tips are color-coded by size. Two or three sizes typically fit most adult patients. After a quick inspection of the external ear, the experienced clinician is able to select the appropriate-sized probe tip immediately for most patients.
- ☐ Pull gently up and back on the pinna (to straighten the ear canal) and insert a clean probe tip into the external ear canal with a slight twisting motion. Look closely at the fit to verify that the probe tip is well within the ear canal and filling the meatus. If the probe tip slides in real easy, it may be too small.
- ☐ If you can't build up positive pressure, consider troubleshooting (**see TECHNICAL TIP: Seal, page 197**) or select another probe tip (smaller or larger), as appropriate, and insert it into the external ear canal.

  Even experienced clinicians occasionally will experience difficulties obtaining an adquate seal for very young children or elderly patients.
- ☐ For automated tympanometers, simply press the start button to begin tympanometry. Keep in mind, however, that tympanometric technique has important effects on tympanometry findings. You should know the default test parameters used by your equipment manufacturer, including:

  - ✓ positive and negative pressure extremes
  - ✓ direction of pressure change (positive-to-negative or negative-to-positive)
  - ✓ rate of pressure change
  - ✓ probe frequency
  - ✓ immittance component measured (e.g., admittance, impedance, susceptance, conductance, compliance)

- ☐ For manual equipment operation, increase pressure until you have reached +200 mmH_20 (daPa).
- ☐ Plot the tympanogram or save it to a computer. Be sure to mark the patient's name and the test ear on the record form.
- ☐ Note and/or record important tympanometric findings, including:
  - ✓ ear canal volume (see normal values, page 199)
  - ✓ peak amplitude of the tympanogram (see normal values)
  - ✓ pressure point of peak (see normal values, page 199)
- ☐ Interpret the tympanogram as normal or abnormal.
- ☐ Make any necessary changes in tympanometry protocol (e.g., pressure extremes) and repeat test as indicated.
- ☐ If findings are abnormal:
  - ✓ classify the tympanogram and think of possible middle ear pathologies that could be associated with the tympanogram type.
  - ✓ Develop some working hypotheses about which audiometric patterns you will record.
  - ✓ Plan to do bone conduction audiometry, and maybe an audiometric Weber test or the SAL test (see Chapter 2).
  - ✓ Consider an otologic or pediatric referral.
- ☐ Succinctly report the results of tympanometry. Remember, if you are charging for the procedure, the patient's official medical record must show that the test was completed and should include a report of the results. See *ADR* chapter in Volume II on **Billing and Reimbursement** for information on CPT and Diagnosis codes.
- ☐ If after trouble-shooting and probe reinsertion, you still cannot get an adequate seal, it's best to abort the attempt at tympanometry. Don't waste excessive amounts of testing time attempting to obtain an adequate seal, or traumatize or antagonize your patient at the start of the audiologic assessment.
- ☐ Place the probe tip into a container clearly marked for "used" probe tips or into a container with disinfectant.

Tympanometry Types

This system, described by James Jerger, is widely used clinically.

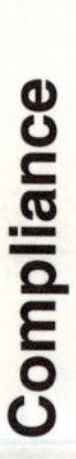
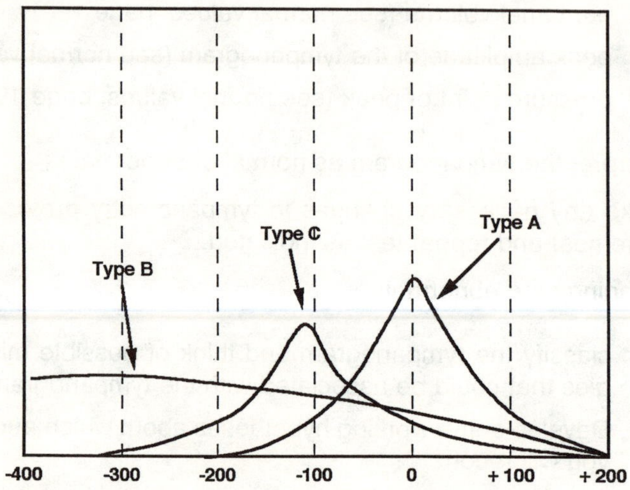

Type A: A relatively sharp maximum at or near 0 mm . . . found in normal and otosclerotic ears.

Type B: Little or no maximum . . . found in ears with serous or adhesive otitis media.

Type C: The maximum is shifted to the left of zero by negative pressure in the middle ear. Slight negative pressure is quite common in many otherwise normal ears, but when the maximum equals or exceeds approximately 100 mm (water) significant negative pressure in the middle ear may be presumed.

Source: From Jerger J. (1970). Clinical experience with impedance audiometry. *Archives of Otolaryngology,* 92, 311–324.

Tympanometry Types

Modified Jerger classification system for tympanometry showing expected normal pressure-compliance region for tympanograms, plus the Ad (d = deep) and As (s = shallow) variations.

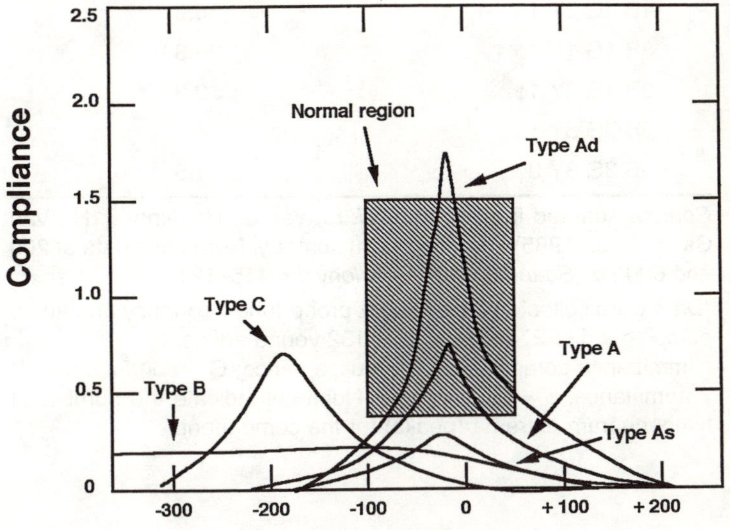

Source: From Jerger J. (1970). Clinical experience with impedance audiometry. *Archives of Otolaryngology, 92*, 311–324. Copyright 1970 American Medical Association. Reprinted with permission.

Normal Data

Proportion of Multi-component Tympanogram Types Found in Adult Subjects with Normal Middle Ear Status*

Tympanogram Type **	Proportion of Normal Subjects (in %)
1B 1G 1Y 1ϕ	56.8
3B 1G 1Y 1ϕ	25.8
3B 1G 3Y 1ϕ	2.3
3B 3G 3Y 1ϕ	4.5
3B 3G 3Y 3ϕ	1.5

Source: Adapted from Creten, W. L., Van de Heyning, P. H., Van Camp, K. J. (1985). Immittance audiometry, Normative data at 200 and 600 Hz. *Scandinavian Audiology 14*, 115–121.

*Data were collected for a 660 Hz probe-tone frequency and an air pump speed of 27 daPa/sec for 132 young adults.

**Immittance components: B = susceptance; G = conductance; Y = admittance; ϕ = phase angle. Numbers indicate the number of tympanogram extrema (peaks) for the component.

Example of a Multicomponent Tympanogram

Example of one of three normal multi-component, i.e., admittance (Y), susceptance (B) and conductance (G), tympanogram types. This type reflects a middle ear system that is massed controlled near ambient ear canal pressure, and is characterized by three peaks (maximum or minimum extremes) for the B component, one for the G component, and one for the Y component. These peaks must occur within a pressure range not exceeding 75 daPa to be classified as normal. The proportion of multipeaked tympanogram patterns recorded in "normal" middle ears is shown in NORMAL DATA, page 194. (from Van Camp et al, 1986).

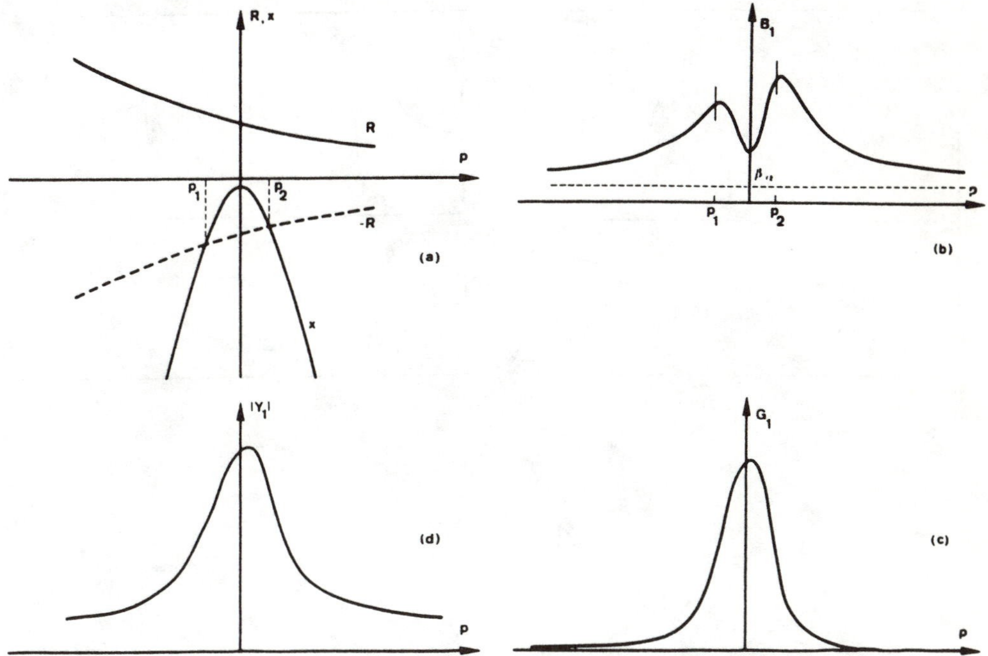

Examples of Normal and Abnormal Multi-component Tympanograms

Normal middle ear (top left). Top right panel represents mild otitis media, bottom left panel represents an ossicular abnormality, or a severe eardrum abnormality, and the bottom right represents another ossicular abnormality, or a severe eardrum abnormality (from Van Camp et al, 1986).

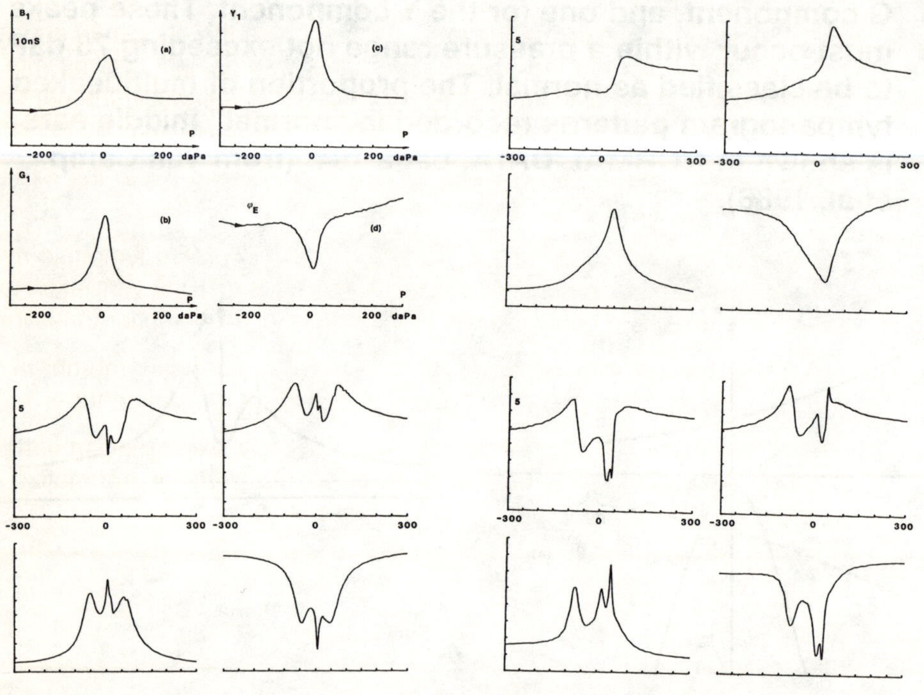

Technical Tip

What to Do When You "Can't Get a Seal"

- ☐ Tightly occlude the end of the probe with your finger and attempt to build up pressure. If pressure doesn't increase, suspect a technical problem with immittance meter (e.g., the manometer) or the probe.
- ☐ Verify that all tubes are completely connected from the immittance meter to the immittance probe, especially the air pressure tube.
- ☐ Verify that the probe tip is snugly fitted to the probe assembly.
- ☐ Pull gently up and back on the pinna (to straighten the ear canal) and reinsert the probe tip into the external ear canal with a slight twisting motion. Look closely at the fit to verify that the probe tip is well within the ear canal and filling the meatus. If the probe tip slides in real easy, it may be too small.
- ☐ Select another probe tip (smaller or larger) and insert it into the external ear canal.
- ☐ Question the patient about the possibility of a perforated tympanic membrane or recent placement of pressure equalization (PE) or ventilation tube, if you are unable to verify visually by otoscopic inspection prior to testing.
- ☐ Examine the ear otoscopically for a perforated tympanic membrane or recent placement of pressure equalization (PE) or ventilation tube.
- ☐ Abort the attempt at tympanometry. Don't waste excessive amounts of testing time attempting to obtain an adequate seal, or traumatize the patient at the start of the audiologic assessment.

Audioid

A_s Versus A_d Tympanograms

What do the "s" and the "d" mean?

A_s refers to a shallow tympanogram, whereas A_d refers to a deep tympanogram.

For clinical purposes, it is sometimes helpful to think of "s" as evidence of stiffness, and "d" as disarticulation, although it's not always quite so simple.

Normal Data

Gradient Values (daPa) for Children and Adults[a]

Subject Group	Normative Gradient
Children[b]	
Mean	133
10th percentile	80
90th percentile	200
Adults[c]	
50th percentile	110
5th percentile	63

Source: Hall J. W. III. Contemporary tympanometry. *Seminars in Hearing 8*: 1988.

[a]Data were collected for a 226 Hz probe frequency at a standard air pump speed of 50 daPa/sec. See text for details on the calculation of GdP.

[b]Data for 88 ears of 46 children between the ages of 3.7 and 5.8 years.

[c]Data for right ears of 83 college students with an average age of 22 years.

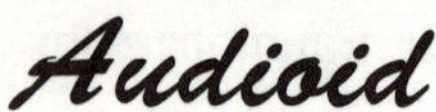

Don't Let the (Middle Ear) Pressure Get to You

1 dekapascal (daPa) of pressure = 1.02 mm H_2O of pressure

Normal Data

Average Values and Ranges for Static Acoustic Admittance (Y), Equivalent Ear Canal Volume (Veq), and Gradient (GR) in Normal Adults and Children[a]

	Children		Adults	
Peak Y (mmhos)	**Mean**	**90% range**	**Mean**	**90% range**
Pump speed = 200 daPa/sec	0.50	0.22–0.81	0.72	0.27–1.38
Pump speed = 400 daPa/sec	0.55	0.22–0.92	0.78	0.32–1.46
Veq (ml)	0.74	0.42–0.97	1.05	0.63–1.46
GR (daPa)	100	59–151	77	51–144

Source: Adapted from Margolis, R. H. & Heller J. W. (1987). Screening tympanometry; criteria for medical referral. *Audiology, 26*, 197–208.

[a]Data were obtained with a screening tympanometer utilizing a 226 Hz probe tone. Static admittance was calculated by subtracting the admittance at 200 daPa from the peak admittance. Equivalent ear canal volume and gradient were equivalent at the two pump speeds (200 and 400 daPa/sec).

Normal Data

Admittance and Impedance Normative Values[a]

Subject Group	Admittance (Y)[b]	Impedance (Z)
Children[c]		
Lower limit	0.35	1100
Median	0.53	1900
Upper limit	0.90	2900
Adults[c]		
Lower limit	0.50	570
Median	0.91	1100

Source: From Hall, J. W. III (1987). Contemporary tympanometry. *Seminars in Hearing, 8*, p. 321.

[a]Data were collected with a 226 Hz probe frequency at a slow air pump (50 daPa/sec for children and 25 daPa/sec for adults).

[b]Under standard barometric conditions, the admittance units are equivalent to volume units (cm^3).

[c]Children were in the age range of 3 to 5 years. Mean age for adults was 25.6 years.

Distribution of Tympanogram Types in Different Pathologies

Group	Number of Subjects	Number of Ears	Tympanogram Type (%) A	B	C
Otosclerosis	60	95	95	1	4
Otitis media	62	118	10	43	47
Cholesteatoma	20	30	4	54	42
Scarred or thickened tympanic membrane	12	20	45	15	40
Discontinuity	18	19	100	—	—

Source: As reported in 172 patients with various middle ear disorders, by Jerger, J., Anthony, L., Jerger, S., Mauldin, L. (1973). Studies in impedance audiometry. III. Middle ear disorders. *Archives Otolaryngology, 97.*

Technical Tip

What's Happening and What You Might Do When You Get a Flat Line (Real Flat) During Tympanometry

Several possible explanations for a very flat apparent tympanogram are:

☐ Probe:

- *Problem:* The probe tip is occluded with debris precluding the immittance device from detecting any changes in admittance as pressure is changed in the external ear canal.
- *Solution:* Disconnect the tubes to the probe tip (one at a time) and follow the manufacturer's recommendations for probe tip cleaning. If that doesn't work, consider the possibility of a defective probe assembly and contact service representative.

☐ Connections between immittance device and probe:

- *Problem:* One of the wires from the immittance meter to the probe is loose or unplugged, precluding the immittance device from delivering a probe tone or from detecting any changes in admittance as pressure is changed in the external ear canal.
- *Solution:* Check and, if necessary, reconnect all wires to the probe and immittance device. Perform a listening check for the probe tone.

☐ Tympanic membrane:

- ✔ *Problem:* The patient has a perforation of the tympanic membrane or a patent ventilation (pressure equalization) tube, plus fluid or other substance in the middle ear space and/or occluded or nonpatent eustachian tube. Attempts to change air pressure in the ear canal are unsuccessful because air escapes into the middle ear space. Tympanometry is the measurement of middle ear immittance as pressure is changed in the ear canal. Therefore, technically, you are not performing tympanometry, and should not plot a tympanogram with this type of patient finding.
- ✔ *Solution:* Note the equivalent ear canal volume. If it is greater than average, and the other ear, the most likely explanation is a hole in the eardrum. Follow up this suspicion with otoscopy and otologic history.

Distribution of Normal Static Compliance Values[a]

Study	No. of Patients	Percentile				
		2.5	**10**	**50**	**90**	**97.5**
Jerger, 1972	825	0.30	0.39	0.67	1.30	1.65
Brooks, 1971	697	0.35	0.42	0.70	1.05	1.40
Rose & Keating (written communication, Nov 8, 1971)	50	0.32	0.43	0.63	1.07	1.35

Source: From Jerger, J., Jerger, S., & Mauldin, L. (1972). Studies in impedance audiometry. I. Normal and sensorineural ears. *Archives of Otolaryngology, 96*, 513–523.

[a]Static compliance as reported in cubic centimeter (cc or cm^3) by various investigators for 220 or 250 Hz probe tone.

Distribution of Maximum Static Compliance Values

Values as Reported in 172 Patients with Various Middle Ear Disorders and in 825 Subjects with No Middle Ear Disorder

Group	Number of Subjects	Number of Ears	Percentiles (in cc)		
			10th	50th	90th
Normal	825	—	0.39	0.67	1.30
Otosclerosis	62	118	0.06	0.29	0.81
Cholesteatoma	20	30	0.04	0.16	0.44
Scarred or thickened tympanic membrane	12	20	0.04	0.37	2.83
Discontinuity	18	19	0.76	1.93	>3.66

Source: From Jerger, J., Anthony, L., Jerger., S., & Mauldin, L. (1973). Studies in impedance audiometry. III. Middle ear disorders. *Archives of Otolaryngology, 97.*

Changes in Tympanograms During the Toynbee and Valsalva Tests of Eustachian Tube Function

See STEP-BY-STEP PROTOCOL: Eustachian tube function tests for a description of these procedures.

R = RESTING PRESSURE
T = PRESSURE AFTER TOYNBEE
T1 = PRESSURE AFTER ONE OPEN-NOSE SWALLOW
T2 = RESIDUAL PRESSURE AFTER MULTIPLE OPEN-NOSE SWALLOWS
V = PRESSURE AFTER VALSALVA
V1 = PRESSURE AFTER ONE SWALLOW
V2 = RESIDUAL PRESSURE AFTER MULTIPLE SWALLOWS

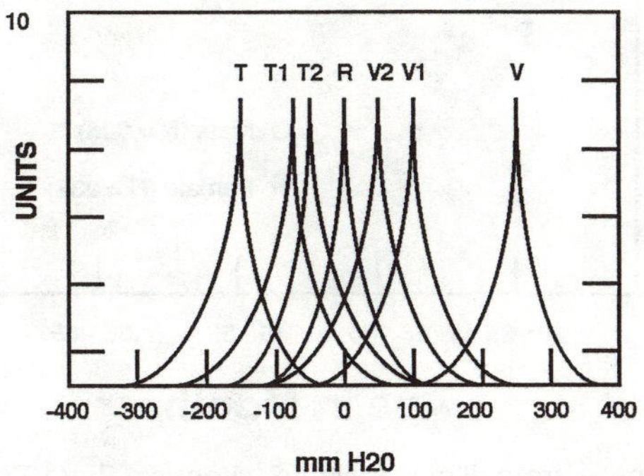

Source: Adapted from Jerger, J. & Northern, J. (1980). *Clinical Impedance Audiometry* (2nd ed.). Acton, MA: American Electromedics.

Static Compliance Changes as a Function of Age and Gender in Children

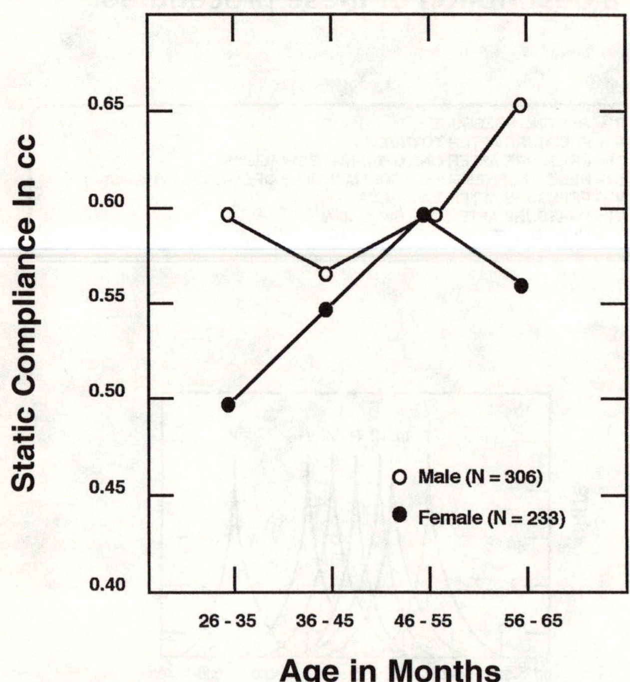

Source: Adapted from Hall, J. W., & Weaver, T. (1979). Impedance audiometry in a young population: The effect of age, sex, and tympanogram abnormalities. *Journal of Otolaryngology, 8*(3), 210–222.

THE ACOUSTIC (STAPEDIAL) REFLEX

Anatomy of the Acoustic Reflex Arc

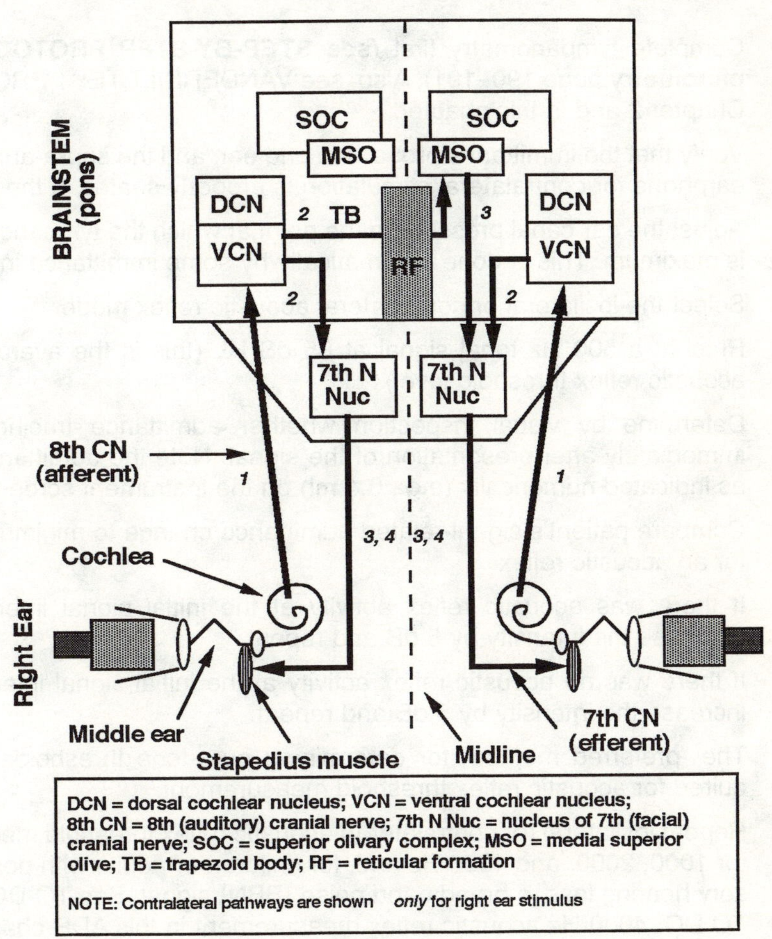

Source: Adapted from work by Erik Borg in rabbits.

STEP-BY-STEP PROTOCOL: Acoustic reflex measurement

Step-by-Step Protocol

Acoustic Reflex Measurement

- ☐ Complete tympanometry first (**see STEP-BY-STEP PROTOCOL: Tympanometry** page 190–191). Also, see VANDERBILT TEST PROTOCOL in Chapter 2 and in this chapter.
- ☐ Verify that the immittance probe is in one ear, and the supra-aural or insert earphone for contralateral stimulation is properly seated in the other ear.
- ☐ Adjust the ear canal pressure to the point at which the tympanogram peak is maximum. This is done automatically by some immittance instruments.
- ☐ Select the ipsilateral or contralateral acoustic reflex mode.
- ☐ Present a 500 Hz tonal signal at 85 dB HL (this is the average normal acoustic reflex threshold level).
- ☐ Determine by visual inspection whether admittance tracing changed immediately after presentation of the signal. Note the admittance change as indicated numerically (e.g., 0.4 ml) on the instrument screen.
- ☐ Compare patient's signal-related admittance change to minimum criterion for an acoustic reflex.
- ☐ If there was acoustic reflex activity at the initial signal intensity level, decrease the intensity by 5 dB and repeat.
- ☐ If there was no acoustic reflex activity at the initial signal intensity level, increase the intensity by 5 dB and repeat.
- ☐ The "preferred method" for determining pure-tone thresholds is not required for acoustic reflex threshold measurement.
- ☐ Repeat ipsilateral (or contralateral) acoustic reflex threshold measurement for 1000, 2000, and 4000 Hz and, for children or adults with possible sensory hearing loss, a broad band noise (BBN) signal. See TO DO OR NOT TO DO: 4000 Hz acoustic reflex measurement in this ADR chapter.
- ☐ Repeat the measurement acoustic reflex thresholds for the other stimulus mode (contralateral or ipsilateral).
- ☐ Plot all acoustic reflex thresholds on an audiogram form (preferably as you measure them).
- ☐ Reverse ears and repeat these procedures.
- ☐ Interpret the acoustic reflex pattern. See pages 215–217 for the clinical significance of different acoustic reflex patterns.
- ☐ Consider measurement of acoustic reflex decay before removing the probe tip from the patient's ear.

Classic Quotes

Stanley Smith (SS) Stevens and Hallowell Davis in 1938 on the Acoustic Reflex

"Contraction of the muscles of the middle ear has been studied directly in animals by attaching mirrors to the tympanic membrane or ossicles or by attaching a delicate myograph directly to the tendons. More recently the electrical activity of the cochlea has been employed in order to observe the effect of contraction upon the transmission of sounds. Luscher has observed directly the movements of the stapedius in a human subject with a defective tympanic membrane . . . . A few individuals are able to contract their intra-aural muscles voluntarily . . . .

From the combined results of human and animal observations, the muscles of the middle ear appear to contract reflexively in response to irritation of the external canal, of the pinna, or of a considerable area of skin surrounding the external ear . . . . One of the present writers (H.D.) finds that the responses of his own intra-aural muscles to light cutaneous stimulation are essentially homolateral. Contraction of the muscles in question seems to occur regularly as part of the act of yawning . . . .

A definite threshold for reflex response of the muscles to sound can be established . . . . The strength of the reflex contraction also varies directly with the intensity of the stimulating sound. Furthermore, the contraction tends to persist as long as the stimulating sound continues . . . .

The acoustic reflex of the middle ear closely resembles the spinal reflexes of skeletal musculature generally, and, in common with them, is abolished by deep anesthesia . . . .

Contraction of the intra-aural muscles causes depression of transmission for low tones . . . . At about 1000 cycles the electrical output of the cochlea is not reduced by the contraction."

Source: From Stevens, S. S., & Davis, H. (1938). *Hearing: Its Psychology and Physiology* (pp. 263–265). New York: John Wiley & Sons, Inc.

Influence of Drugs on the Acoustic Stapedial Reflex

Drug	Effect	Investigator
Chlorpromazine Thioridazine	None	Helfner & Niswander
Phenobarbital	None	Richards et al.
Phenobarbital Phenytoin Primidone Valproic acid Chlorpromazine Ethosuximide	None	Evans
Secobarbital	Minimal increase in threshold	Robinette et al.
Diazepam Meperidine	None	Light et al.
Diazepam Pentymal	None	Liden et al.
Ketamine	Significant increase	Thompson et al.
Curare	Significant increase	Ruth et al.
Ethyl alcohol	Significant increase	Cohill and Greenberg

Source: Reprinted with permission from Hodges A., Ruth, R. (1988). Factors influencing the acoustic reflex. *Seminars in Hearing, 8.*

Types of Acoustic Reflex Deflections

Three distinct patterns for acoustic reflex deflections, including normal (top panel), a normal variant (middle panel), and abnormal (early otosclerosis).

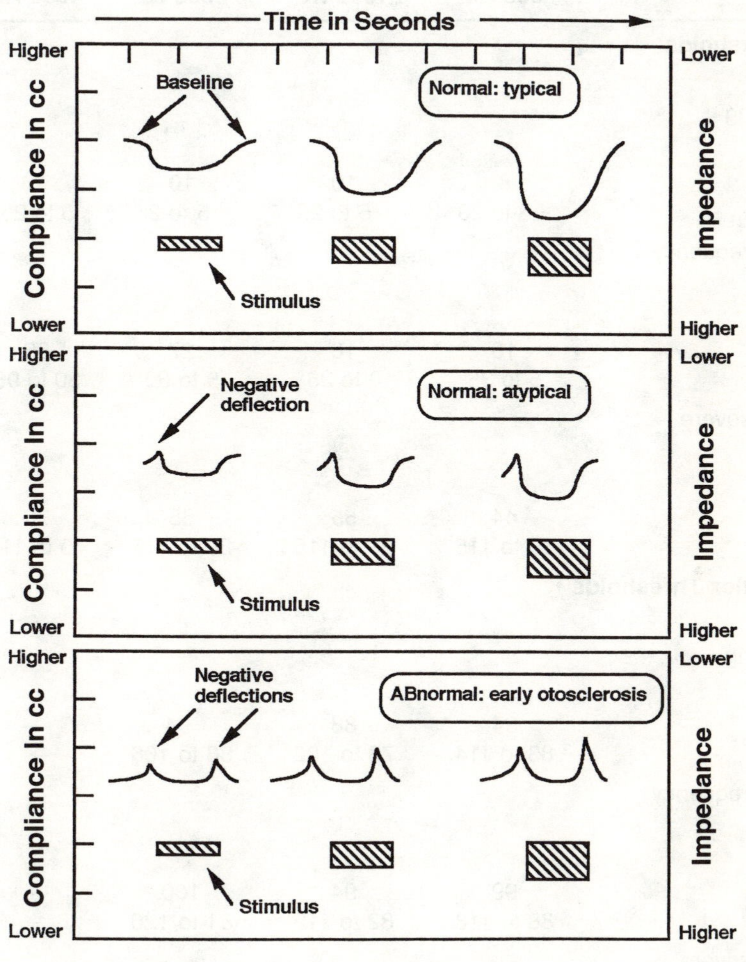

Normal Data

Averages and Ranges for Pure-tone Audiometry Thresholds and Acoustic Reflex Thresholds for Tonal and Broad Band Noise (BBN) Signals.

	Signals				
	500 Hz	**1000 Hz**	**2000 Hz**	**4000 Hz**	**BBN**
Hearing Thresholds (dB HL)					
Normal hearing ($N = 30$)					
mean	8	10	10	13	—
range	−5 to 20	−5 to 25	−5 to 25	5 to 25	
Mild or high frequency hearing loss ($N = 33$)					
mean	16	16	27	55	—
range	5 to 35	0 to 25	5 to 60	30 to 95	
Moderate or severe hearing loss ($N = 63$)					
mean	44	55	65	76	—
range	10 to 115	20 to 115	30 to 115	40 to 115	
Acoustic Reflex Thresholds (dB SPL)					
Normal hearing ($N = 30$)					
mean	94	88	94	—	81
range	83 to 114	78 to 102	86 to 106	—	62 to 95
Mild or high frequency hearing loss ($N = 33$)					
mean	99	94	100	—	89
range	88 to 118	82 to 112	81 to 126	—	76 to 105
Moderate or severe hearing loss ($N = 63$)					
mean	104	102	112	—	100
range	78 to 136	78 to 132	91 to 134	—	85 to 125

Source: Adapted from Silman, S., Gelfand, S. A., & Emmer, M. (1987). Acoustic reflex in hearing loss identification and prediction. *Seminars in Hearing, 8*, 379–390.

Comparison of Crossed Acoustic Reflex Thresholds (dB HL) in Subjects with Normal Tympanograms Versus Minor Tympanogram Abnormalities.

Tympanograms	N	Signal				
		500 Hz	1000 Hz	2000 Hz	4000 Hz	BBN[a]
Normal Tympanogram	539					
Mean		90	89	89	90	82
(Standard Deviation)		(6.4)	(5.3)	(6.1)	(8.5)	(8.8)
Abnormal Tympanogram[b]	212					
Mean		94	93	93	94	88
(Standard Deviation)		(7.4)	(6.8)	(7.4)	(8.9)	(10.2)

Source: From Hall, J. W. III, & Weaver, T. (1979). Impedance audiometry in a young population: The effect of age, sex, and tympanogram abnormalities. *The Journal of Otolaryngology, 8*(3), 210–222.
[a]BBN = broad band noise signal thresholds in dB SPL
[b]Probe A_d = A-deep tympanogram in the probe ear (*N* = 93)
Probe NP = negative pressure of −50 to −100 mm H_2O in the probe ear (*N* = 119)

Acoustic Reflex Thresholds in Subjects with Normal and Abnormal Tympanograms

Percentage of subjects with normal tympanograms and minor tympanogram abnormalities showing no measurable contralateral acoustic reflex for a 4000 Hz signal.

Normal Tympanograms	Minor Tympanogram Abnormality			
	Probe A^d[a]	Probe NP[a]	Bilateral A^d	Bilateral NP
6%	14%	10%	24%	15%
(*N* = 539)	(*N* = 59)	(*N* = 67)	(*N* = 34)	(*N* = 52)

Source: From Hall, J. W. III, & Weaver, T. (1979). Impedance audiometry in a young population: The effect of age, sex, and tympanogram abnormalities. *The Journal of Otolaryngology, 8*(3), 210–222.
[a]Probe A^d = A-deep tympanogram in the probe ear (*N* = 93)
Probe NP = negative pressure of −50 to −100 mm H_2O in the probe ear (*N* = 119)

Acoustic Reflex Presence as a Function of Age in Children

Recorded with a 600 Hz Probe Tone Frequency

Age of Child	Percentage of Subjects with Reflexes
1 month	100
2 months	92
3 months	90
4 months	87
5–11 months	85
1 year	72
2 years	67
3 years	47
4 years	47

Source: From Kankkunen, A., & Liden, G. (1988). Ipsilateral acoustic reflex thresholds in neonates and in normal-hearing and hearing-impaired preschool children. *Scandinavian Audiology, 13*, 139–144, as adapted from Hodges, A., & Ruth, R. A. Subject related factors influencing the acoustic reflex. *Seminars in Hearing, 8, 339–357.*

Acoustic Reflex Findings in Neonates as a Function of Probe Frequency and Presentation Mode

Probe frequency	Stimulus	Presentation	% Reflexes
220 Hz	Broad Band	Ipsilateral	51
660 Hz	Noise		74
220 Hz		Contralateral	49
660 Hz			83
220 Hz	1000 Hz tone	Ipsilateral	43
660 Hz			81
220 Hz		Contralateral	34

Source: From Sprague, B. H., Wiley, T. L., & Goldstein, R. (1983). Tympanometric and acoustic reflex studies in neonates. *Journal of Speech and Hearing Research, 28,* 265–272; and Hodges, A., & Ruth, R. (1988). Factors influencing the acoustic reflex. *Seminars in Hearing*, 8, 339–357.

Acoustic Reflex Decay

Illustration of acoustic reflex normal acoustic reflex time course (*top panel*), and abnormal acoustic reflex decay (*bottom panel*).

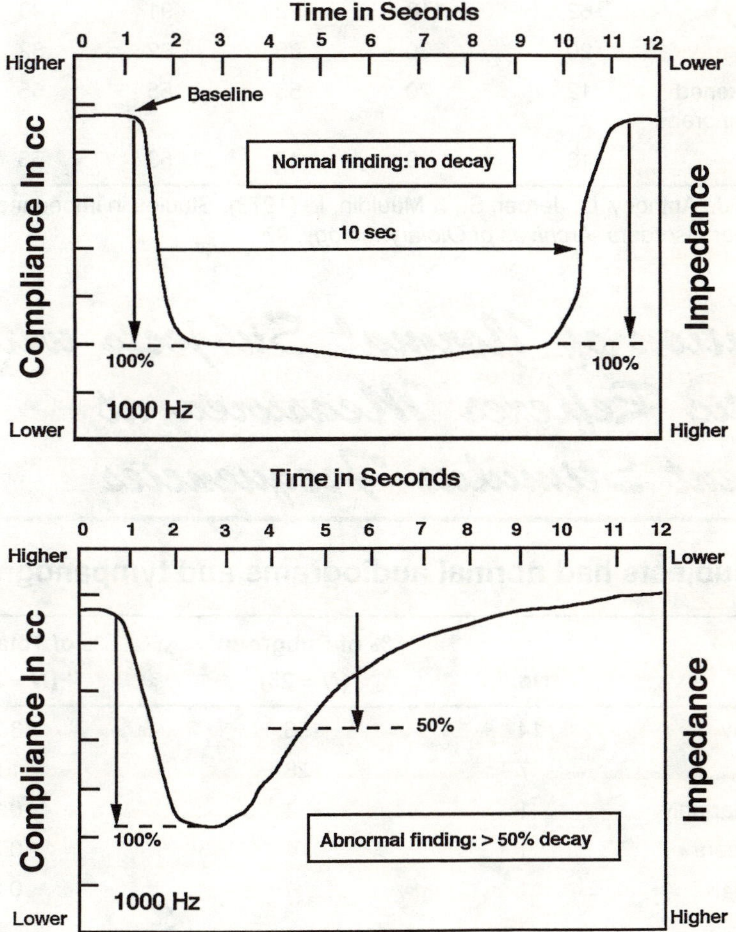

Absence of Stapedius Reflex in 172 Patients with Middle Ear Disorder

Group	Number of Subjects	Number of Ears	Percentage of Subjects at Each Frequency			
			500 Hz	1K Hz	2K Hz	4K Hz
Otosclerosis	60	95	81	77	79	83
Otitis media	62	118	92	91	90	91
Cholesteatoma	20	30	86	82	82	86
Scarred or thickened tympanic membrane	12	20	55	55	55	55
Discontinuity	18	19	47	53	53	58

Source: Jerger, J., Anthony, L., Jerger, S., & Mauldin, L. (1973). Studies in impedance audiometry. III. Middle ear disorders. *Archives of Otolaryngology*, 97.

Proportion of Normal Subjects with Acoustic Reflexes Measured at Different Stimulus Frequencies

All subjects had normal audiograms and tympanograms.

Reflex Absent	No.	% of Subgroup (*N* = 25)	% of Total Group (*N* = 382)
4K, one ear only	14	56	3.7
4K, both ears	7	28	1.8
2K & 4K, one ear only	1	4	0.3
2K & 4K, both ears	1	4	0.3
500, 1K, 2K, & 4K, one ear only	1	4	0.3
500, 1K, 2K, & 4K, both ears	1	4	0.3
Total, subgroup	25	100	6.7

Source: Jerger, J., Jerger, S., & Mauldin, L. (1972). Studies in impedance audiometry. I. Normal and sensorineural ears. *Archives Otolaryngology, 96*, 513–523.
*In subgroup of patients with normal audiograms and tympanograms.

Historical Reverberation

The Origin of the SPAR Acronym. This is a true story, as recollected by an eyewitness (the first author).

The year was 1974, the time was about 5 p.m., and the place was the Audiology Conference room in the bowels of the Methodist Hospital in Houston, Texas. The usual evening Audiology Patient Staffing was under way. Inspired by his recent firsthand observation of the work of Niemeyer and Sesterhenn in Germany, Jim Jerger was conducting a 1000-plus subject study of acoustic reflexes in normal hearing and sensorineurally impaired patients at the Methodist Hospital and other hospitals affiliated with Baylor College of Medicine (Ben Taub County Hospital, the V.A. Hospital). The goal was to describe the use of acoustic reflex data for tone versus noise signals in the estimation of hearing sensitivity. If acoustic reflexes could accurately, and objectively, estimate hearing sensitivity, it would be a very useful tool in pediatric hearing assessment.

The bulk of the research effort was complete. Now came the really important stage of the investigation . . . selecting an appropriate acronym for the procedure. At this time, Jerger had already coined some rather catchy acronyms for other audiologic procedures, such as the SISI, the SAL, the STAT, and the SSI. Chuck Berlin didn't pen the ditty "Acronym Jim" for nothing! Toward the end of the patient staffing on this day, the boss asked for acronym suggestions. After a pregnant pause, someone in the group spoke up. "How about this . . . Predicting Hearing by Acoustic Reflex Thresholds." Jerger tugged at his beard for a moment, and then firmly proclaimed: "No, I don't think so." Over the years, some of us recall him adding "That acronym stinks!" In retrospect, it's likely that Jim had already decided on the acronym before we gathered to meet that day. Being a proud owner of a sizeable sailboat those days (an Eriksen I think), he had a nautical theme in mind. Therefore, the chosen acronym was **S**ensitivity **P**rediction by **A**coustic **R**eflex, or SPAR.*

*__spar__ (*n.*): 1. *Nautical.* A wooden or metal pole, used as a mast, boom, yard, or bowsprit, or in any other way to support rigging.

Technical Tip

How to get some useful information on hearing sensitivity from an uncooperative, difficult-to-test child by recording acoustic reflexes.

Let's say that you're trying to assess a young child audiologically, but you have some doubts about behavioral findings and don't want to (or can't) go on to carry out a sedated ABR. Here's what you might want to do:

☐ *Tympanometry.* If the result is normal, middle ear function is probably normal. Proceed with measurement of acoustic reflex and otoacoustic emissions.

☐ *Acoustic reflexes.* The patient won't cooperate for acoustic reflex measurement with many signals. Ask an assistant or caregiver to amuse your little friend by blowing bubbles. Find acoustic reflex threshold (ART) only for an ipsilateral broad band noise (BBN) signal. If the ART is 85 dB or better, you can probably rule out a communicatively important sensory hearing loss for that ear (see Acoustic Reflex Findings for BBN, page 218). Do the same thing for the other ear.

☐ *Otoacoustic emissions.* Using the same effective bubble-blowing technique to distract your pediatric patient, record OAE bilaterally, at least for the 1000 to 4000 Hz region (see ADR Chapter 5 for details). Some audiologists would begin their audiologic assessment of this child with otoacoustic emissions, and stop the assessment if OAE were within normal limits bilaterally.

The 1974 (original) SPAR Criteria

Used for prediction of hearing loss from acoustic reflex thresholds (ARTs). SPAR = Sensitivity Prediction by Acoustic Reflex.

Noise-Tone Difference (NTD)[a]	Broad Band Noise ART in dB SPL	Prediction[b]
> 20	Anywhere	Normal
15 to 19	≤ 80	Normal
15 to 19	> 80	Normal-Moderate
10 to 14	Anywhere	Mild-Moderate
<10	≤ 90	Mild-Moderate
<10	> 90	Severe
Acoustic reflexes not observed		Profound

Source: From Jerger, J., Burney, P., Mauldin, L., & Crump, B. (1974). Predicting hearing loss from the acoustic reflex. *Journal of Speech and Heaingr Disorders 39*, 11–22.

[a] difference between average ART for signals of 500, 1000, and 2000 Hz and broad band noise ART.

[b] Categories for hearing loss: Normal = pure tone average (PTA) = < 20 dB HL; Mild-Moderate = PTA = 20 to 49 dB HL; Severe = PTA = 50 to 84 dB HL; Profound = PTA = ≥ 85 dB HL

Explanation of Acoustic Reflex Threshold for Broad Band Noise in Sensory Hearing Loss

Illustration of Jerger's explanation for the differentiation in the size of the noise-tone difference in acoustic reflex thresholds for normal vs. sensorineural ears. Critical bands are wider in the impaired ears, resulting in the contribution of fewer bands to hearing over the frequency region.

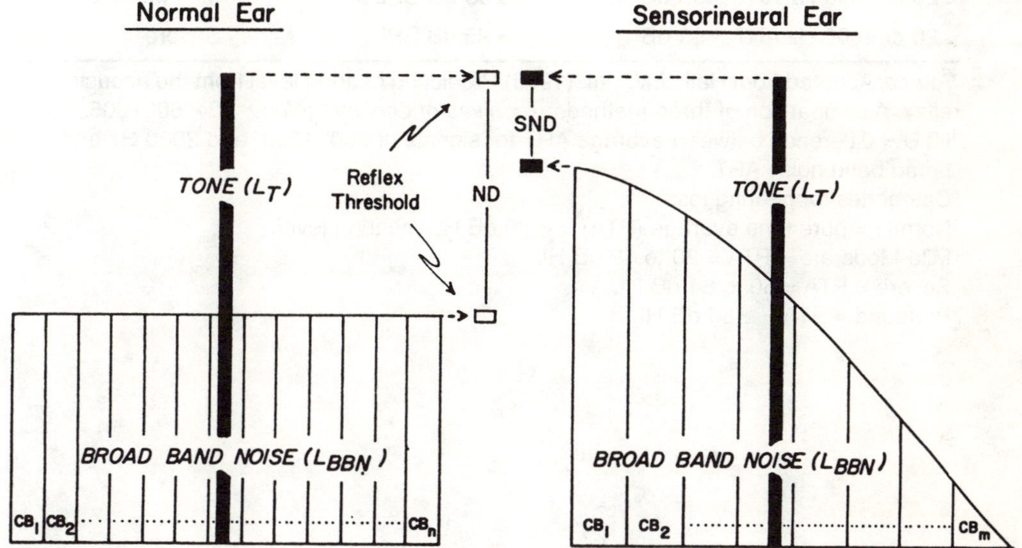

From the original paper on Sensitivity Prediction by Acoustic Reflex (SPAR) by Jerger et al., 1974.

The 1977 (newer and improved) SPAR Criteria for Prediction of Hearing Loss from Acoustic Reflex Thresholds (ARTs)

SPAR = Sensitivity Prediction by Acoustic Reflex

Noise-Tone Difference (NTD)[a]	Broad Band Noise ART in dB SPL	Prediction[b]
≥ 20 *and* 1000 Hz ART ≤ 95 dB HL	Anywhere	Normal
< 20 *or* 1000 Hz ART > 95 dB HL	≤ 95 dB SPL	Mild-Moderate
< 20 or 1000 Hz ART > 95 dB	> 95 dB SPL	Severe

Source: Adapted from Hall, J. W., III. (1978) Predicting hearing level from the acoustic reflex: A comparison of three methods. *Archives of Otolaryngology, 104*, 602–605.

[a]NTD = difference between average ART for signals of 500, 1000, and 2000 Hz and broad band noise ART.

[b]Categories for hearing loss:
Normal = pure tone average (PTA) = < 20 dB HL (hearing level)
Mild-Moderate = PTA = 20 to 49 dB HL
Severe = PTA = 50 to 84 dB HL
Profound = PTA = ≥ 85 dB HL

Effect of Sensory Hearing Loss on Acoustic Reflex Thresholds (ARTs) For Pure Tone Signals vs. a Broad Band Noise (BBN) Signal

Note the nonlinear effect of hearing loss on the pure tone ARTs and the more linear effect on the BBN activated ART. Results are for 539 subjects with sensorineural hearing loss aged 1 to 20 years.

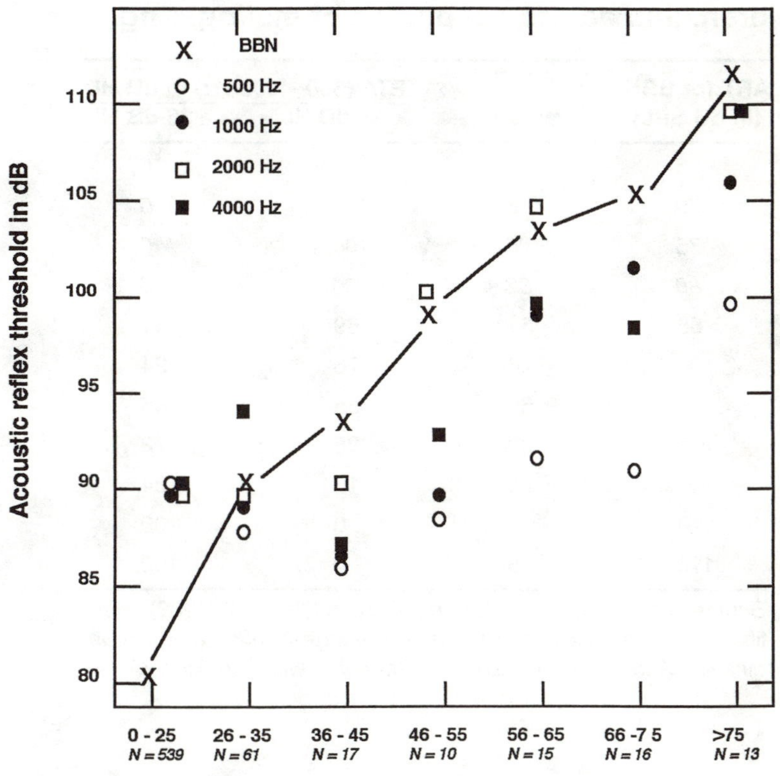

Source: Adapted from Hall, J. W., & Weaver, T. (1979). Impedance audiometry in a young population: the effect of age, sex, and tympanogram abnormalities. *Journal of Otolaryngology, 8*(3), 210–222.

Relation Between Hearing Loss and Acoustic Reflex Thresholds for a Broad Band Noise Signal

The proportion of subjects with no serious hearing loss versus those with serious hearing loss defined by pure tone average (PTA) and shown as function of the level of the acoustic reflex threshold (ART) for a broad band noise (BBN) signal. ART thresholds of 65 through 80 dB are typically associated with communicatively insignificant hearing loss. The ART for a BBN signal is useful in estimation of hearing status of young and difficult to test children, and adults suspected of malingering.

ART for BBN (in dB SPL)	*N*	PTA (500–4000 Hz) in dB HL	
		< 35 dB HL	≥ 35 dB HL
65	*2*	*100%*	*0%*
70	*6*	*100*	*0*
75	*20*	*100*	*0*
80	*32*	*100*	*0*
85	51	69	31
90	76	76	24
95	66	55	45
100	39	28	72
105	25	16	84
110	4	0	100
115	5	0	100

Source: From Hall, J. W., III, Berry, G. A., & Olson, K. (1982). Identification of serious hearing loss with acoustic reflex data. *Scandinavian Audiology, 11*, 251–255. Reprinted with permission.

Clinical Concept

How you can record acoustic reflexes from a patient with a discontinuity of the ossicular chain.

With most patients who have a discontinuity (total break) of the ossicular chain, acoustic reflexes will not be observed when the probe is in the affected ear. The stapedius muscle will be contracting in response to an adequate ipsilateral or contralateral stimulus, but the movement of the stapes and the usual decrease in middle ear admittance will not be transmitted outward to the tympanic membrane where it can be detected by the immittance device.

If, however, the break in the ossicular chain is located medial to the insertion of the stapedius muscle on the head of stapes (e.g., on one or both crura toward the stapes footplate), the decreased admittance caused by stapedius muscle contraction will be transmitted through the incus and malleus to the tympanic membrane and will be detected by the immittance device. Because energy transmission is disrupted somewhere between the tympanic membrane and the inner ear, this patient may have a substantial conductive hearing loss despite the presence of acoustic reflexes. The good news is that this pattern of findings (highly compliant middle ear system, air-bone gap greater for the high frequencies, and the presence of acoustic reflexes with the probe in the involved ear) is highly site-specific for a stapes fracture/break. You might want to examine some of the figures illustrating ossicular anatomy, located in Chapter 1.

Technical Tip

How to describe and report acoustic reflex findings for ipsi- and contralateral stimulation.

Describe acoustic reflexes by the ear that was stimulated. For ipsilateral (uncrossed) acoustic reflexes, the stimulus ear is also the probe ear. For contralateral (crossed) acoustic reflexes, right ear acoustic reflexes are elicited with acoustic stimulation (sound) to the right ear (and the probe in the left ear). Conversely, left ear acoustic reflexes are elicited with acoustic stimulation (sound) to the left ear (and the probe in the right ear).

Plotting Acoustic Reflexes

Audiogram form showing acoustic reflex pattern (lower portion) in relation to results for pure tone audiometry in a patient with normal hearing sensitivity and normal middle ear function. See Jerger, S., & Jerger, J. (1977). Diagnostic value of crossed versus uncrossed acoustic reflexes. *Archives Otolaryngology, 103*, 445.

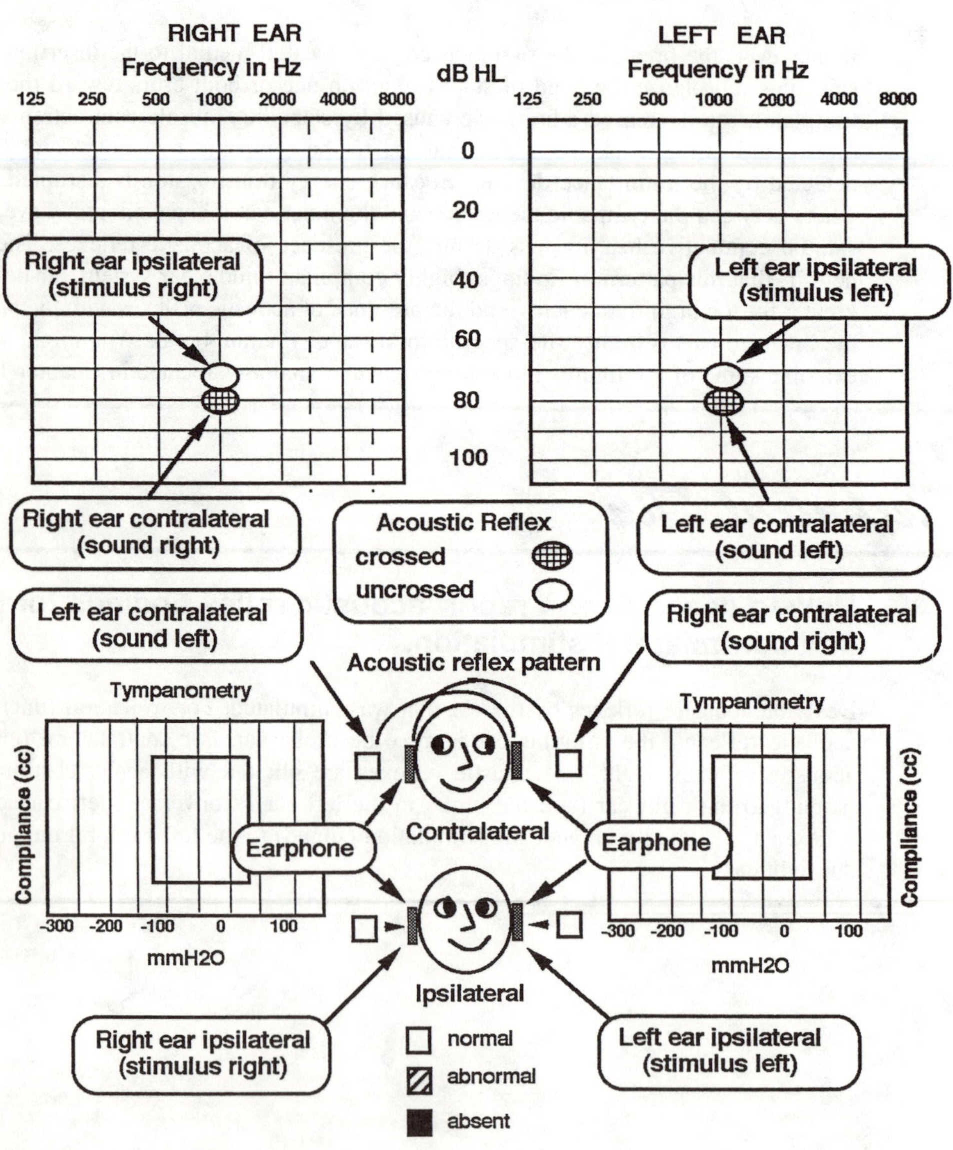

Plotting Acoustic Reflexes

Mild Conductive Hearing Loss

Audiogram form showing acoustic reflex pattern (lower portion) in relation to results for pure tone audiometry in a patient with middle ear dysfunction and *mild* conductive hearing loss. This is known as the "vertical" pattern in which abnormalities associated with middle ear dysfunction are common to the probe ear. See Jerger, S., and Jerger, J. (1977). Diagnostic value of crossed versus uncrossed acoustic reflexes. *Archives of Otolaryngol, 103*, 445, 1977.

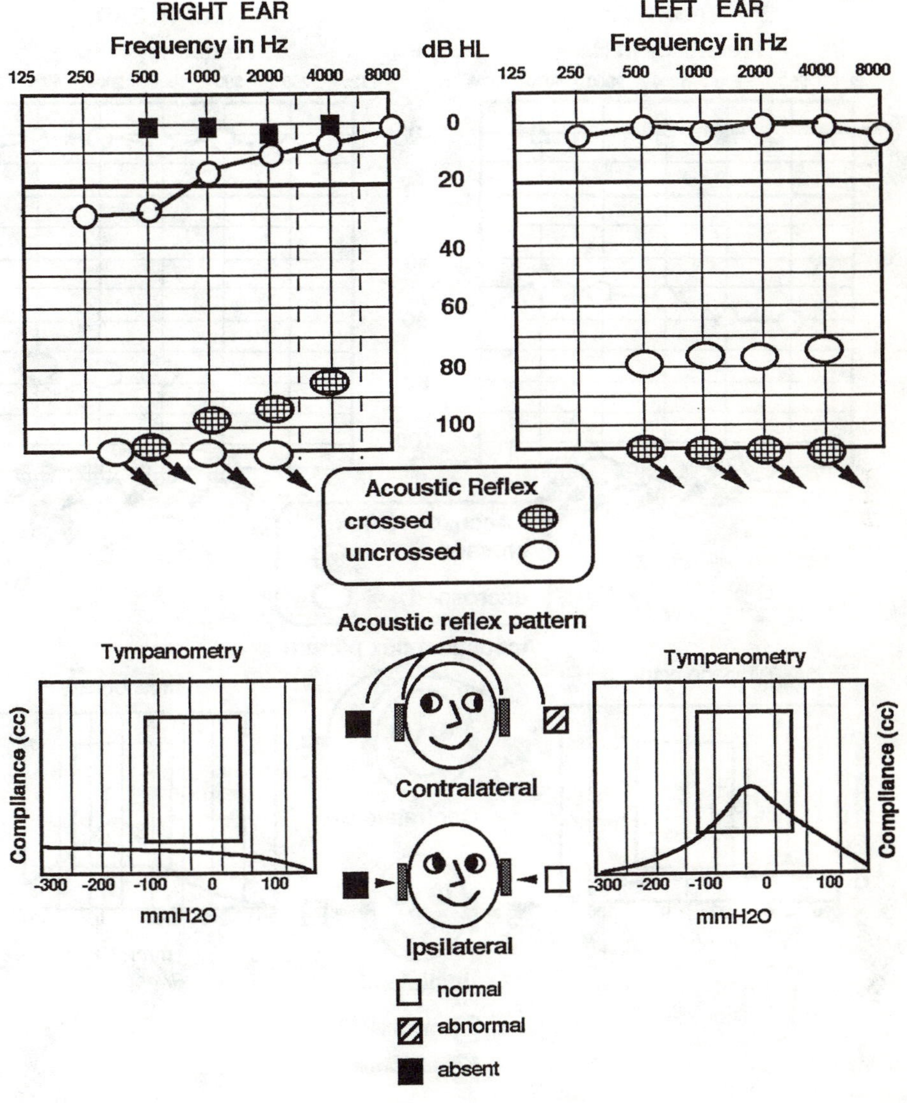

Plotting Acoustic Reflexes

Moderate Conductive Hearing Loss

Audiogram form showing acoustic reflex pattern (lower portion) in relation to results for pure tone audiometry in a patient with middle ear dysfunction and *moderate* or *severe* conductive hearing loss. This is known as the "inverted L" pattern in which abnormalities associated with middle ear dysfunction are common to the probe ear, plus stimulation of the ear with conductive hearing loss. See Jerger, S., and Jerger, J, Diagnostic value of crossed versus uncrossed acoustic reflexes. *Archives of Otolaryngol 103*, 445, 1977.

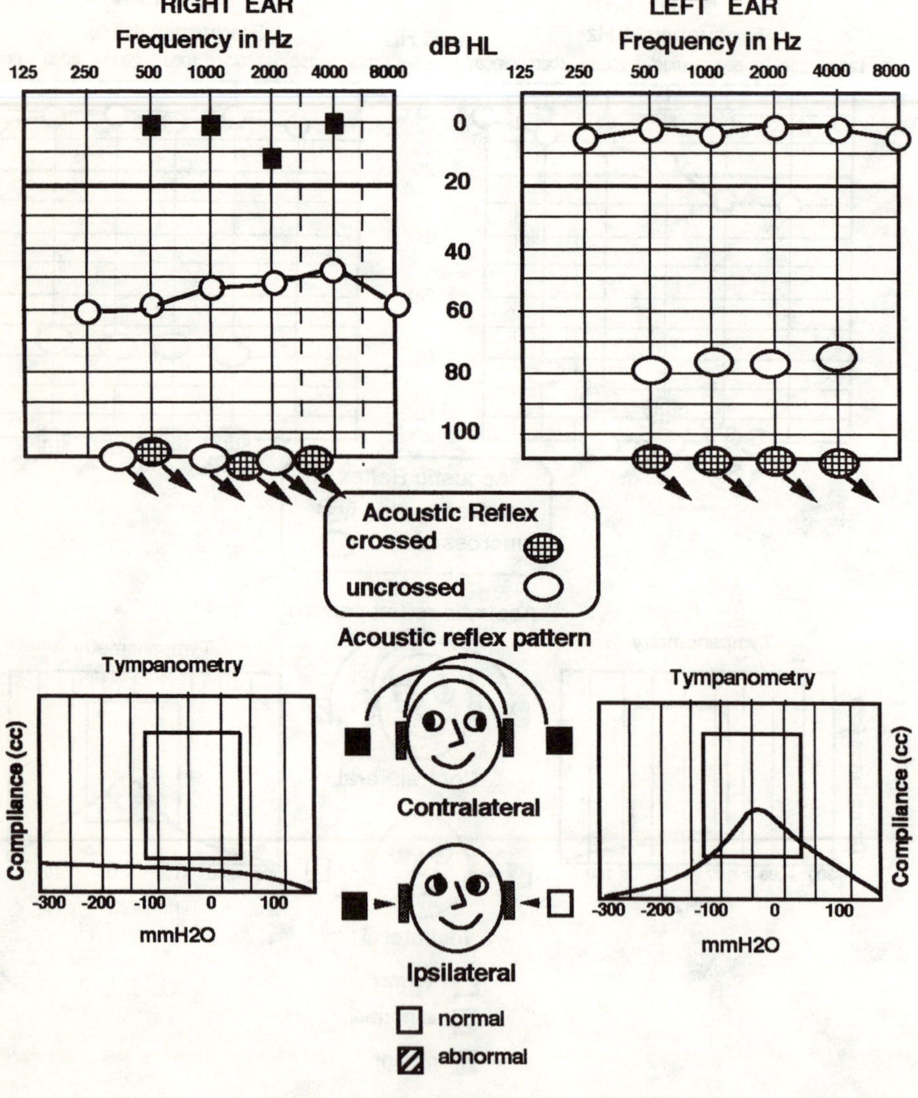

Plotting Acoustic Reflexes

Sensory Hearing Loss

Audiogram form showing acoustic reflex pattern (lower portion) in relation to results for pure tone audiometry in a patient with cochlear dysfunction and *severe sensory* hearing loss. This is known as the "diagonal" pattern in which abnormalities associated with cochlear dysfunction are common to the stimulus ear. See Jerger, S., and Jerger, J, Diagnostic value of crossed versus uncrossed acoustic reflexes. *Arch Otolaryngol 103*, 445, 1977.

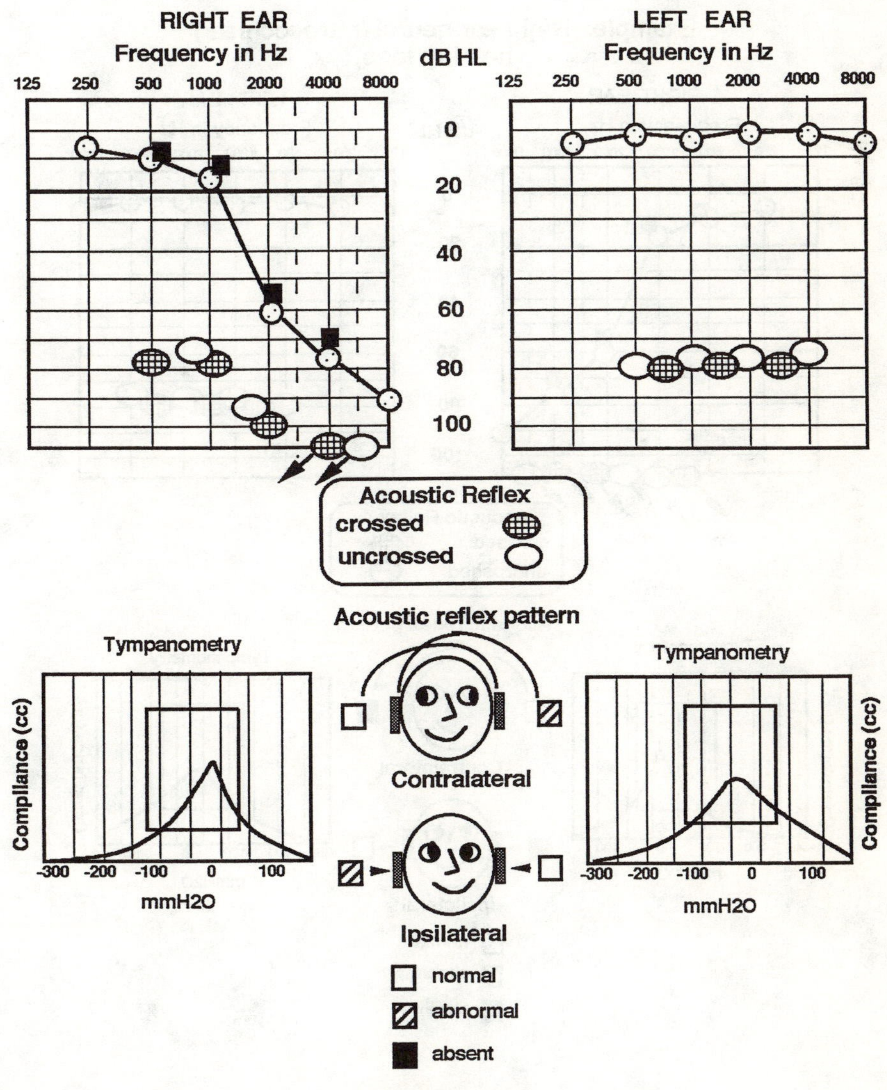

Plotting Acoustic Reflexes

Neural Hearing Loss

Audiogram form showing acoustic reflex pattern (lower portion) in relation to results for pure tone audiometry in a patient with retrocochlear dysfunction and a mild, but *neural*, hearing loss. This is known as the "diagonal" pattern in which abnormalities associated with neural dysfunction are common to the stimulus ear. See Jerger, S., and Jerger, J. Diagnostic value of crossed versus uncrossed acoustic reflexes. *Arch Otolaryngol 103*, 445, 1977.

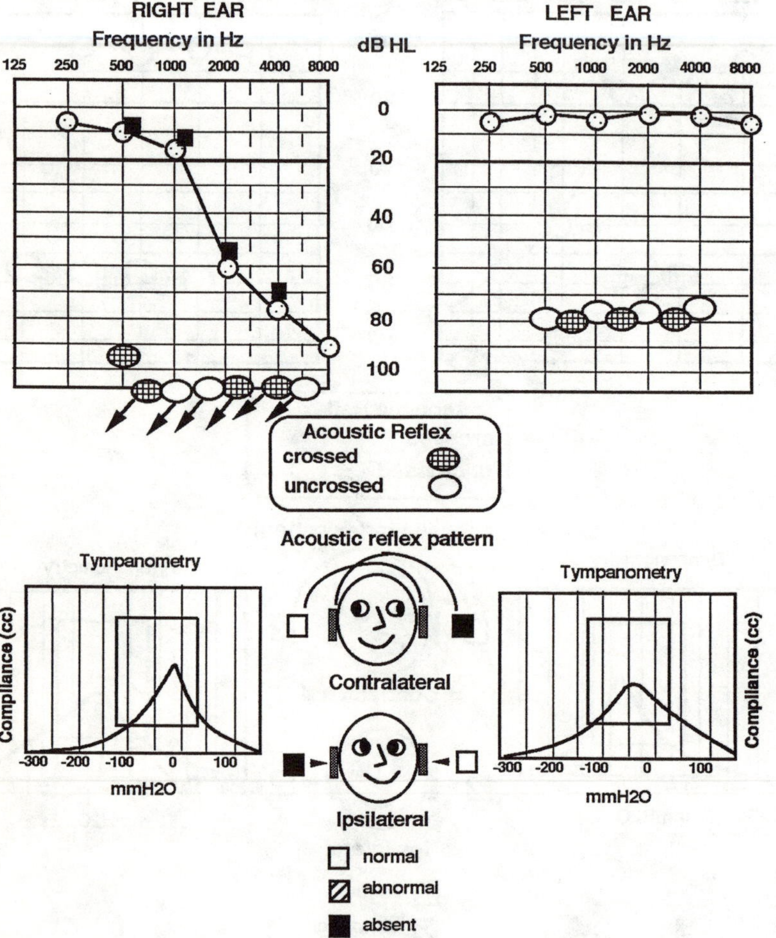

Plotting Acoustic Reflexes

Brainstem Auditory Dysfunction

Audiogram form showing acoustic reflex pattern (lower portion) in relation to results for pure tone audiometry in a patient with a low auditory brainstem dysfunction, abnormal speech audiometry, yet normal hearing sensitivity. This is known as the "horizontal" pattern in which abnormalities associated with neural dysfunction are common to contralateral (crossed) acoustic reflexes only. See Jerger, S., and Jerger, J. Diagnostic value of crossed versus uncrossed acoustic reflexes. *Archives of Otolaryngology 103,* 445, 1977.

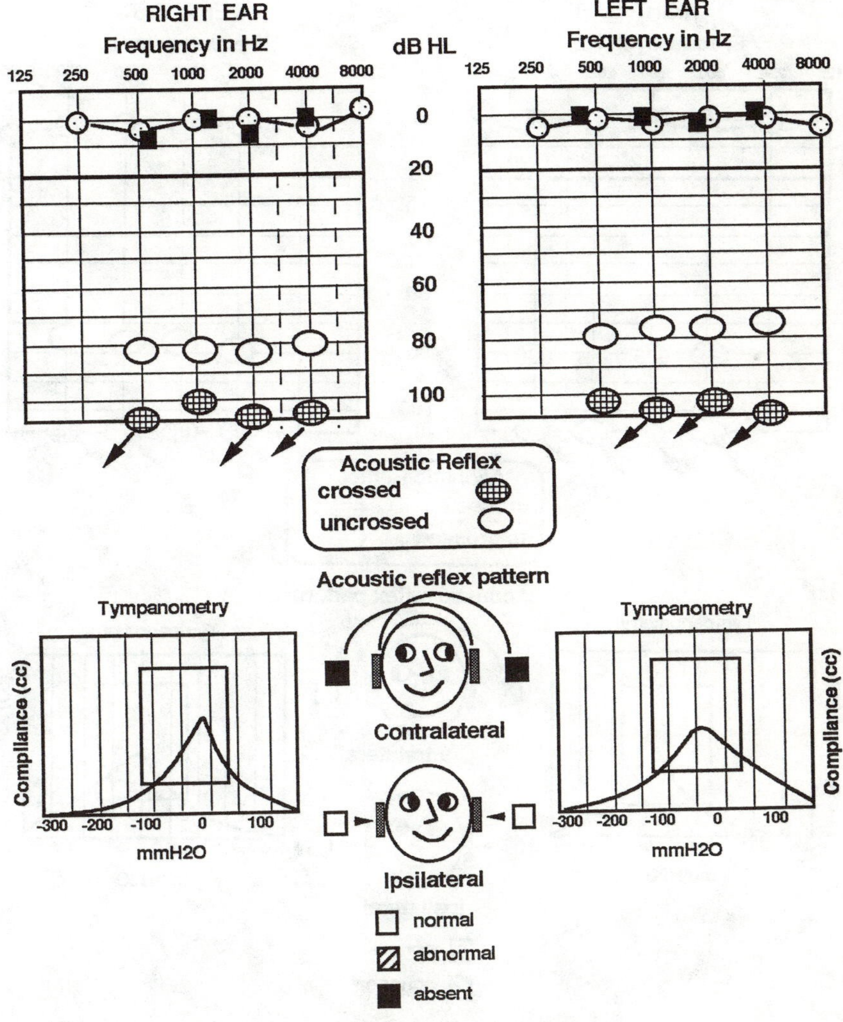

Plotting Acoustic Reflexes

Facial Nerve Dysfunction

Audiogram form showing acoustic reflex pattern (lower portion) in relation to results for pure tone audiometry in a patient with facial nerve disorder. This is also known as the "vertical" pattern in which abnormalities associated with the final efferent pathway (facial nerve) are common to the probe ear side with the facial nerve dysfunction. The audiogram and tympanograms are normal. See Jerger, S., and Jerger, J. (1977) Diagnostic value of crossed versus uncrossed acoustic reflexes. *Archives of Otolaryngology, 103*, 445, 1977.

Example: Right ear facial nerve dysfunction

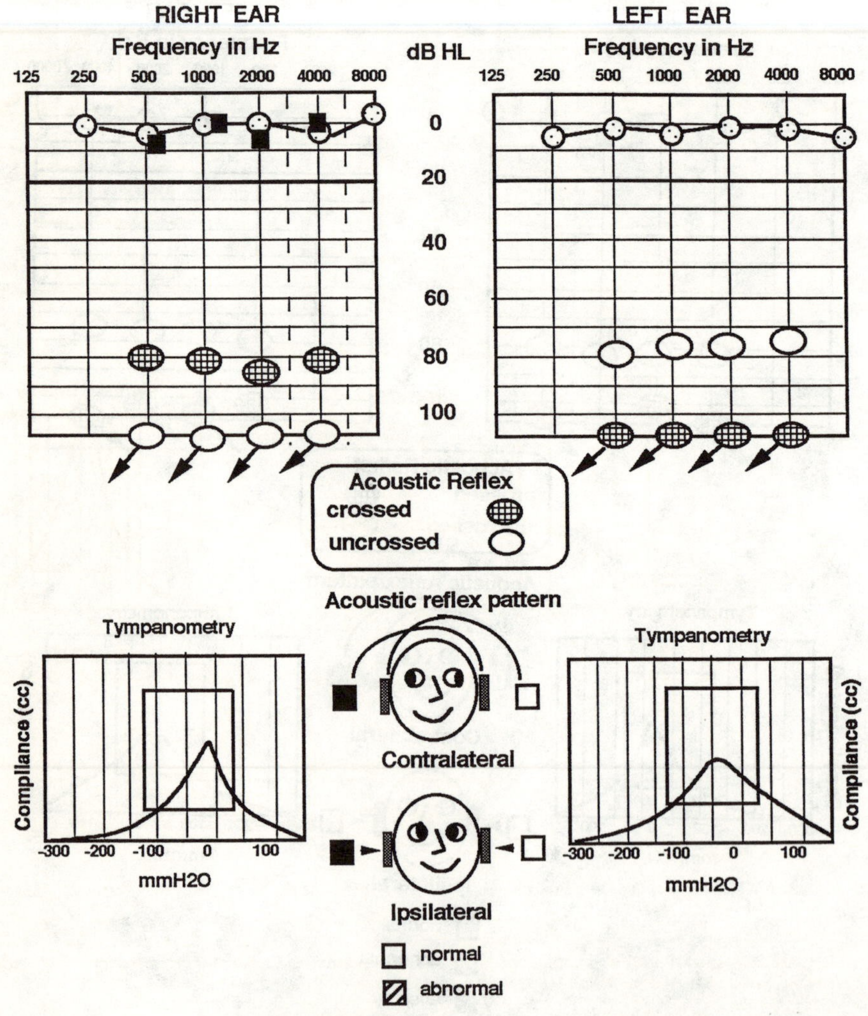

OTHER PRACTICAL IMMITANCE STUFF

Audiogram "Tilts"

Audiogram "tilts" or configurations associated with stiffness versus mass controlled middle ear dysfunctions. Respective tympanograms are shown in the lower portion.

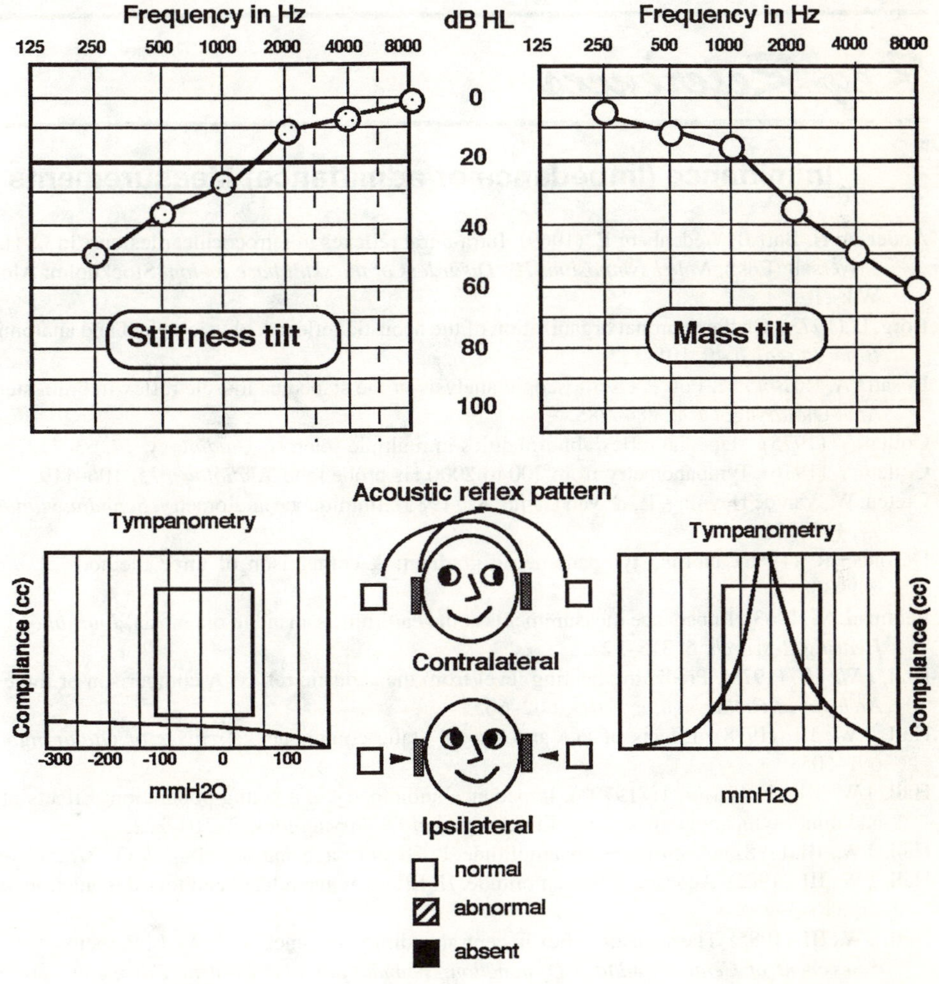

Terminology

Tubes

- ☐ A common surgical therapy to improve hearing in patients with otitis media with effusion is the insertion of small tubes or grommets into the tympanic membrane. These tubes are often referred to as:
  - ventilation tubes
  - pressure equalization (PE) tubes

Key References

Immittance (Impedance or admittance) Measurements

Anderson H, Barr B, Wedenberg E. (1969). Intra-aural reflexes in retrocochlear lesions. In C. Hamburg & J. Wersall (Eds.), *Nobel symposium 10: Disorders of the skull base region*. Stockholm: Almquist and Wiksell.

Borg, E. (1973). On the neuronal organization of the acoustic reflex: A physiological and anatomical study. *Brain Research 49,* 101–123.

Bosatra A, Russolo M, Poli P. Oscilloscopic analysis of the stapedius muscle reflex in brain stem lesions. *Arch Otolaryngol 102*, 284–285.

Colletti V. (1975). Stapedial reflex abnormalities in multiple sclerosis. *Audiology, 14*, 63–71.

Colletti V. (1976). Tympanometry from 200 to 2000 Hz probe tone. *Audiology, 15,* 106–119.

Creten, W., Van de Heyning, P., & Van Camp, K. (1985). Immittance audiometry. *Scandinavian Audiology, 14*, 115–121.

DeJonge, R. (1986). Normal tympanometric gradient: A comparison of three methods. *Audiology, 25,* 299–308.

Feldman, A. (1963). Impedance measurements at the eardrum as an aid to diagnosis. *Journal of Speech and Hearing Research, 6,* 315–327.

Hall, J.W., III. (1978). Predicting hearing level from the acoustic reflex: A comparison of three methods. *Archives of Otolaryngology, 104*, 602–605.

Hall, J.W., III. (1978). Effects of age and sex on static compliance. *Archives of Otolaryngology, 105*, 601–605.

Hall, J.W., III., & Weaver, T. (1979b). Impedance audiometry in a young population: Effects of age, sex, and minor tympanogram abnormality. *Journal of Otolaryngology, 8,* 210–222.

Hall, J.W., III. (1982). Acoustic reflex amplitude. I. Effect of age and sex. *Audiology, 21,* 294–309.

Hall, J.W., III. (1982). Acoustic reflex amplitude. II. Effect of age related auditory dysfunction. *Audiology, 21,* 386–399.

Hall, J.W., III. (1985). The acoustic reflex in central auditory dysfunction. In M. L. Pinheiro, & F. E. (Eds.). *Assessment of Central Auditory Dysfunction: Foundations and Clinical Correlates* (pp. 103–130). Baltimore: Williams & Wilkins.

Hall, J.W., III. & Chandler, D. (1994). Tympanometry in clinical audiology. In J. Katz (Ed.). *Handbook of clinical audiology* (4th ed) pp. 283–299). Baltimore: Williams & Wilkins.

Holmquist, J. (1969). Eustachian tube function assessed with tympanometry. *Acta Otolaryngologica, 68,* 501–508.

Holte L., Margolis, R.H., & Cavanaugh, R.M., Jr. (1991). Developmental changes in multifrequency tympanograms. *Audiology, 30,* 1–24.

Jeck L, Ruth R, Schoeny Z. High frequency sensitization of the acoustic reflex. *Ear and Hearing 4*: 98–101, 1983.

Jerger J. Clinical experience with impedance audiometry. *Arch Otolaryngol 92*: 311–324, 1970.

Jerger J, Anthony L, Jerger S, Mauldin L. Studies in impedance audiometry. III. Middle ear disorders. *Arch Otolaryngol 99*: 165–171, 1974.

Jerger J, Jerger S, Mauldin L. Studies in impedance audiometry. I. Normal and sensorineural ears. *Arch Otolaryngol 96*: 513–523, 1972.

Jerger J, Harford E, Clemis J, Alford B. The acoustic reflex in eighth nerve disorders. *Arch Otolaryngol 99*: 409–413, 1974.

Jerger J, Burney P, Mauldin L, Crump B. Predicting hearing loss from the acoustic reflex. *Arch Otolaryngol 99*: 11–22, 1974.

Jerger S, Jerger J. Diagnostic value of crossed vs. uncrossed acoustic reflexes. *Arch Otolaryngol 103*: 445–453, 1977.

Jerger J, Jerger S. Acoustic reflex decay: 10-second or 5-second criterion? *Ear and Hearing 4*: 70–71, 1983.

Jerger J, Hayes D. Latency of the acoustic reflex in eighth-nerve tumor. *Arch Otolaryngol 109*: 1–5, 1983.

Lilly D. Multiple frequency, multiple component tympanometry: New approaches to an old diagnostic problem. *Ear and Hearing 5*: 300–308, 1984.

Margolis RH, Van Camp KJ, Wilson RH, Creten WL. Multifrequency tympanometry in normal ears. *Audiology 24*: 44–53, 1985.

Margolis RH, Heller J. Screening tympanometry: Criteria for medical referral. *Audiology 26*: 197–208, 1987.

Metz O. The acoustic impedance measured on normal and pathologic ears. *Acta Otolaryngologica (Supplement) 63*: 1946.

Olsen W, Noffsinger D, Kurdziel S. Acoustic reflex and reflex decay. *Arch Otolaryngol 101*: 622–625, 1975.

Popelka G. Acoustic immittance measures: Terminology and instrumentation. *Ear and Hearing 5*: 262–267, 1984.

Riedel C, Wiley, T, Block M. Tympanometric measures of Eustachian tube function. *J Speech Hear Res 30*: 207–214, 1987.

Sesterhenn G, Breuninger H. The acoustic reflex at low sensation levels. *Audiology 15*: 523–533, 1976.

Shanks J. Tympanometry. Ear and Hearing 5: 268–280, 1984.

Shanks J, Lilly D. An evaluation of tympanometric estimates of ear canal volume. *J Speech Hear Res 24*: 557–566, 1981.

Van Camp K, Creten W, Van de Heyning P, Decraemer W, Vanpeperstraete P. A search for the most suitable immittance components and probe tone frequency in tympanometry. *Scandinavian Audiology 12*: 27–34, 1983.

Van Camp K, Vanpeperstraete P, Creten W, Vanhuyse V. On irregular acoustic reflex patterns. Scandinavian *Audiology 4*: 227–232, 1975.

Van Camp KJ, Margolis RH, Wilson RH, Creten WL, Shanks JE. Principles of Tympanometry. *ASHA Monographs No.* 24, 1986.

Weatherby L, Bennett, M. The neonatal acoustic reflex. *Audiology 9*: 103–10, 1980.

Wiley T, Goldstein R. Tympanometric and acoustic-reflex studies in neonates. *J Speech Hear Res 28*: 265–272, 1985.

Wilson RH, Shanks J, Kaplan S. Tympanometric changes at 226 Hz and 678 Hz across 10 trials and for two directions of ear canal pressure change. *J Speech Hear Res 27*: 257–266, 1984.

Zwislocki J. An acoustic method for clinical examination of the ear. *J Speech Hear Res 6*: 303–314, 1963.

Step-by-Step Protocol

Eustachian Tube Function Tests

☐ **Perforated tympanic membrane (TM) or patent PE (pressure equalization) tube.** When pressure is introduced into the external ear canal and the TM is not intact, air will fill the middle ear space. The air may also escape through the eustachian tube if it opens normally. Follow these steps to assess eustachian tube function. Have a glass of water handy before you start.

- ✔ Fit the probe in the ear canal properly (technique is described elsewhere in this ADR chapter).
- ✔ Increase air pressure slowly.
- ✔ If pressure is released before you reach +200 daPA (mmH_2O), note the pressure reading. This is the pressure that opens the eustachian tube. Report it as the opening pressure. This is evidence of good eustachian tube function.
- ✔ If the eustachian tube does not open by +200 daPA (mmH_2O), maintain the pressure at +200 daPA (mmH_2O), instruct the patient to take a sip of water. Alternatively, increase the pressure to +300 daPa or higher.
- ✔ If pressure is released by swallowing, then the eustachian tube is functioning poorly. If pressure is not released, the eustachian tube is malfunctioning (always closed).

☐ **Intact TM.** When functioning normally, the eustachian tube equalizes pressure between the middle ear and nasopharynx (outside or ambient pressure). This occurs during yawning or swallowing. If the eustachian tube doesn't open regularly, negative pressure (re: ambient or atmospheric pressure) will build up in the middle ear space. It may ultimately result in the effusion of fluid into the middle ear, and even infection.

Hearing loss is a common result of this process. When pressure is changed in the external ear canal, and the TM is intact, the TM will move. Positive air pressure moves the TM inward. Air within the middle ear is compressed and some may be forced out the eustachian tube. Negative air pressure moves the TM outward. Air within the middle ear is expanded and slight negative pressure is created in the middle ear space. This procedure forces the eustachian tube to open. Follow these steps to assess eustachian tube function. Have a glass of water handy before you start.

- ✔ Perform tympanometry as you normally do over the range of +200 daPA (mmH_2O) to –400 daPA. (See PROTOCOL, page 190.) Plot and/or save the tympanogram for comparison with subsequent tymps.
- ✔ Set the pressure at +400 daPA. This pushes the TM inward and reduces the volume, and increases the air pressure, within the middle ear space.
- ✔ Have the patient swallow a sip of water. If the eustachian tube opens, air under pressure escapes from the middle ear space through the

eustachian tube. The eustachian tube then closes. The tympanogram pressure peak will usually change.

- ✓ When you return air pressure in the ear canal to atmospheric pressure (0 daPA), there is less than normal air pressure within the middle ear space.
- ✓ Run another tympanogram as you typically do. The peak should be slightly to the negative (e.g., up to –75 daPa) in comparison to the pressure peak of the initial tympanogram.
- ✓ Repeat this process, but with negative pressure (–400 daPA). This pulls the TM outward, and produces a temporary increase in middle ear space volume. Since the same amount of air is within this space, air pressure is reduced.
- ✓ Have the patient swallow some water again. If the eustachian tube opens (as it should normally), air will flow into the middle ear space.
- ✓ Return air pressure in the air canal (on the dial) to normal. The air pressure in the patient's middle ear space should now be slightly positive.
- ✓ Record a third tympanogram. If the eustachian tube is functioning normally, a slightly positive pressure tympanogram peak will be recorded (to approximately +15 to 20 daPa), in comparison to the initial tympanogram.

Technical Tip

How (and Why) to Perform a Fistula Test

- ☐ Performed to confirm the presence of a fistula between the membranous labyrinth and the middle ear.
- ☐ Based on the assumption that a pressure change in the middle ear will be transmitted to the labyrinth and will be reflected in a vestibular sign (e.g., sensation of vestibular disturbance or observed nystagmus).
- ☐ Instruct patients to inform you if they experience any sensation of dizziness or vertigo at any time during the procedure.
- ☐ Insert the immittance probe as you normally do for tympanometry.
- ☐ Gradually, increase negative pressure to a maximum of –400 mmH_2O (daPa)
- ☐ Observe the patient's eyes for nystagmus. You might have the patient wear Frenzel glasses which magnify eyeball movements and eliminate the possibility of the patient fixating during the test. Or, alternatively, connect the patient via electrodes to ENG instrumentation and record eye movements (good documentation).
- ☐ Reduce the external ear canal pressure to atmospheric pressure (0 mm H_2O).
- ☐ Remove the probe from the patient's ear.
- ☐ Report findings of the fistula test. A "positive" fistula test is defined by nystagmus and/or a patient report of vertigo or dizziness as negative pressure was created in the ear canal.

Technical Tip

How immittance findings can save you lots of test time *or* when you don't need to perform bone conduction pure tone audiometry.

Immittance measurements are extremely sensitive to middle ear dysfunction. If all immittance measures are normal, middle ear function is normal. There is no clinical value in carrying out bone conduction pure tone audiometry (e.g., Why do it?) if:

- ☐ *Tympanometry.* Tympanograms are normal type A bilaterally (e.g., Not too shallow and not too deep—just right).
- ☐ *Acoustic reflexes.* Acoustic reflex thresholds are at expected intensity levels (about 85 dB) under all conditions (right and left ear, ipsilateral and contralateral).

Success of Impedance Measurement in Children

Impedance findings in 398 children less than 6 years old

Test Outcome	Number of Children	% of Children
Successful result	308	77.4
Unsuccessful result	90	22.6
Earphones not tolerated	35	8.8
Sedative	10	2.5
No seal	7	1.8
Uncooperative	12	3.0
Incomplete results	26	6.5

Source: Jerger, S., Jerger, J., Mauldin, L., & Segal, P. (1972). Studies in impedance audiometry. II. Children less than 6 years old. *Archives of Otolaryngology, 96.*

CHAPTER 5

Otoacoustic Emissions (OAE)

In This ADR Chapter

- Clinical Concept: Relation Between OAE and the Audiogram
- Abnormal OAE and Normal Audiograms
- Relationship Between Audiogram and DPOAE: Sensory Hearing Loss
- Relation Between Audiogram and DPOAE: Normal Hearing
- Relation Between Audiogram and DPOAE: Low Frequency Tinnitus
- Relation Between Audiogram and DPOAE: Very Mild High Frequency Sensory Deficit
- Relation Between Audiogram and DPOAE: Mild High Frequency Sensory Deficit
- Relation Between Audiogram and DPOAE: Mild Noise Induced Notching Sensory Deficit
- Relation Between Audiogram and DPOAE: Child with Pervasive Developmental Disorder and, Reportedly, Hyperacusis

Perspective

The theoretical concepts underlying our understanding of otoacoustic emissions (OAE) date back to the fascinating work of Thomas Gold in the late 1940s. An Englishman, Dr. Gold was involved in radar research for Great Britain during World War II. After the war, while studying cochlear function in a prestigious auditory laboratory, Dr. Gold developed a prophetic theory on inner ear mechanisms. In short, he described active and nonlinear cochlear processes. Unfortunately, his ideas were ahead of their time and, after a less-than-positive response from von Bekesy, Gold abandoned his auditory research. About 30 years later, this line of work was picked up by another English auditory scientist, Dr. David Kemp. In a now classic paper published in 1978, Dr. Kemp unequivocally identified a byproduct of the nonlinear and active processes that Gold had studied many years earlier. Kemp clearly showed that the ear, quite remarkably, was capable of producing, as well as receiving, sounds. These sounds produced by the cochlea became known as "evoked otoacoustic emissions."

Since 1978, OAE have been intensively investigated in the laboratory. There are well over 300 articles on OAE and related topics. However, because instrumentation for clinical measurement of OAE was lacking until the late 1980s and early 1990s, few audiologists had even heard of OAE, let alone applied them clinically. In fact, a variety of FDA-approved devices for clinical application of OAE has been available only since 1995. Now, however, OAE have captured the interest of clinical audiologists, much as audiologists took to ABR in the 1980s, immittance measurement in the 1970s, and the traditional diagnostic audiology test battery in the 1960s.

OAE are not a test of hearing, and they certainly will not supplant pure tone audiometry, immittance measures, or ABR. But, OAE do offer information on auditory function that is not available from any other measure—behavioral or electrophysiologic. Literature is rapidly accumulating on assorted clinical applications of OAE, ranging from newborn hearing screening to identification and differentiation of a host of auditory dysfunctions in children and adults. The emphasis of this ADR chapter is on principles and protocols, normative data, and trouble shooting. The reader is strongly encouraged to review selectively the rather vast literature on the topic—basic and applied—to gain an adequate background prior to clinical application of OAE. Also, textbooks on OAE will soon be forthcoming.

FOUNDATIONS OF OTOACOUSTIC EMISSIONS

Classic Quote

Thomas Gold on Cochlear Mechanisms (the foundations of otoacoustic emissions)

"Then I started to think—in my capacity as a tame physicist—I started to think 'well what could such a mechanism—the hardware of the ear—what could it do?' And I concluded very quickly that the degree of resonance that could be acheived in a passive system was of course limited." (Gold, 1989, p. 300)

"Well, I puzzled very much about that for some time, and then one day when I was sitting for a colloquium in the Cavendish—listening to an extremely dull physics colloquium—nothing to do with the subject—and my mind strayed, and I said to myself—'Boy! If the thing only had a positive feedback in it, all these problems would disappear wouldn't they." (Gold, 1989, p. 300)

"We had written in the 1948 paper on the physical basis of the action of the cochlea and we clearly spelled out that when you observed it on a live cochlea the frequency response curve you would see would be a curve that rises steeply and cuts off very steeply. I had discussed at length in 1948 with von Bekesy at Harvard, that the observations that he made on the dead cochlea were unrepresentative. But he wouldn't have that! He thought that there must have been some cunning neural mechanism that somehow steepens up the subjective response." (Gold, 1989, p. 301) "So I returned from my meeting with Bekesy even more convinced that I was correct because, before I met him, I may have had the viewpoint that well, maybe these great men they have something up their sleeve that we don't know about that I don't understand." (Gold, 1989, p. 302).

"It is shown that the assumption of a 'passive' cochlea, where elements are brought into mechanical oscillation solely by means of the incident sound, is not tenable. The degree of resonance of the elements of the cochlea can be measured, and the results are not compatible with the very heavy damping which must arise from the viscosity of the liquid. For this reason the 'regeneration hypothesis' is put forward, and it is suggested that an electro-mechanical action takes place whereby a supply of electrical energy is employed to counteract the damping" (Gold, 1948, p. 492) "The interposition

of a feedback stage . . . makes a construction possible where the nerve ending abstracts much energy from a mechanical resonator." (Gold, 1948, p. 498)

Sources: Gold T. Historical background to the proposal, 40 years ago, of an active model for cochlear frequency analysis. In JP Wilson, DT Kemp (eds). *Cochlear Mechanisms,* New York: Plenum, 1989.
Gold T. Hearing II. The physical basis of the action of the cochlea. *Proc Royal Soc Brit*: 135, 492–498, 1948.

Classic Quote

David Kemp in 1978 on OAE

"A new auditory phenomenon has been identified in the acoustic impulse of the human ear. Using a signal averaging technique, a study has been made of the response of the closed external acoustic meatus to acoustic impulses near to the threshold of audibility . . . . This component of the response appears to have its origin in some nonlinear mechanism probably located in the cochlea, responding mechanically to auditory stimulation, and dependent upon the normal functioning of the cochlea transduction process." (Kemp, 1978, p. 1386)

"No defect in or spurious behavior of the instrumentation has been found which in any way mimics phenomenon seen in the normal ears . . . It has not been possible to formulate a purely acoustic explanation . . . An origin in the middle ear itself is strongly counterindicated by the acoustic analyses performed by Zwislocki and others." (Kemp, 1978, p. 1389)

"Various physiological possibilities have been examined. Sound generation during acoustic reflex contractions of either the stapedius or post auricular muscles, cannot, for several reasons, account for the phenomenon . . . The possibility that electrophysiological signals of cochlear microphonic, neurogenic, or myogenic origin, were received and mistaken for acoustic signal was also rejected.

"To summarize, the cochlear reflection hypothesis receives support from the new evidence here and from existing psychoacoustical evidence (Kemp, 1978, p. 1390). "In the absence of a complete understanding of the mode of action of the sensory cells in the cochlea, it is tempting to suggest that one of the functions of the outer hair cell population is the generation of this mechanical energy. If a cochlear origin is confirmed by experiments currently in progress, the technique developed in this study will provide a new avenue for investigation of the auditory system, with applications in both research and audiological medicine." (Kemp, 1978, p. 1391) .

Source: Kemp DT. Stimulated acoustic emissions from within the human auditory system. *J Acoust Soc Amer 64:* 1386–1391, 1978.

Historical Developments

Evoked Otoacoustic Emissions (OAE)

- ☐ 1948: Thomas Gold describes “mechanical resonator” within cochlea
- ☐ 1978: David Kemp publishes the first of his numerous comprehensive descriptions of otoacoustic emissions
- ☐ 1982: N Johnsen and his Scandinavian colleagues publish a series of papers on transient evoked OAE, including findings in normal adults and newborn infants
- ☐ 1983: Hallowell Davis describes “cochlear amplifier” and hints at outer hair cells as the source of this active process
- ☐ 1983: F Grandori, of Italy, reviews characteristics of OAE
- ☐ 1985: WE Brownell discovers motility of outer hair cells
- ☐ 1988: Bannister et al. provide details on the unique subsurface cisternae of the outer hair cells
- ☐ 1988: Bonfils and French colleagues study transient evoked OAE in newborn infants, children, and adult patients with varying types and degrees of sensory hearing loss
- ☐ 1988: Introduction of the ILO 88 device for clinical measurement of transient evoked OAE by Otodynamics, Ltd. of Great Britain (designed by David Kemp and Peter Bray)
- ☐ 1989: Harris, Lonsbury-Martin, et al. systematically study influence of the f_2/f_1 ratio on distortion product OAE amplitude
- ☐ 1989 Increased experimental use of Etymotic Research DPOAE device with Ariel board
- ☐ 1990: Brenda Lonsbury-Martin summarizes various clinical applications of transient evoked and distortion product OAE
- ☐ 1991: Virtual Corporation introduce an FDA-approved device for measurement of distortion product OAE
- ☐ 1991: L Collet links stimulation of the efferent auditory system to suppression of OAE
- ☐ 1993: Karl White and colleagues report preliminary data on large-scale study of TEOAE in newborn hearing (the Rhode Island Infant Hearing Project)
- ☐ 1994: Siegel publishes data on the possibility of standing wave contamination in OAE measurement
- ☐ 1994: Grason Stadler, Inc. and Madsen, Inc. introduce FDA-approved devices for measurement of distortion product OAE

- ☐ 1994: Hall and colleagues report comparative newborn hearing screening findings for TEOAE, DPOAE, and automated ABR
- ☐ 1995: CPT (current procedural terminology) codes first assigned for otoacoustic emissions
- ☐ 1995: Bio-Logic Corporation introduces a FDA-approved device for measurement of distortion product OAE

Classic Quote

Hallowell Davis on Cochlear Mechanics (or on the possible source of otoacoustic emissions)

"In the proposed overall model the organ of Corti acts at low levels as a sharply tuned amplifier to enhance the vibration of a narrow segment of the basilar membrane. This segment acts as a high-Q acoustic resonator. The inner hair cells clearly increase the discharge of nerve impulses in their afferent fibers when the amplitude of the movement of the basilar membrane, with or without the assistance of the cochlear amplifier (CA) reaches a constant value of about 3×10^{-10} m. At middle frequencies the gain in sensitivity provided at threshold by a healthy CA is about 45 dB, which is the length of the 'tips' of the tuning curves of both neural output and mechanical vibration. The CA is vulnerable to mechanical insult, as by noise or experimental operative procedures, to anoxia, and to certain drugs. The outer hair cells are necessary for CA and their cochlear microphonic (CM), acting in a controlled positive feedback relation is a possible source of the energy needed for 'negative damping.'" (Davis, 1983, p. 81)

"What is the source of the energy for the CA? The best hint that we have is the requirement that the outer hair cells (OHC) be intact . . . This suggest [s] a motor function for OHC, with the efferent innervation providing a modulating influence, and perhaps a trophic function also . . . The large number of OHCs, three rows instead of one, may be an expression of the need for a large source of power." (Davis, 1983, p. 88)

Source: Davis H. An active process in cochlear mechanics. *Hearing Research 9:* 79–90, 1983.

Characteristics of Spontaneous Otoacoustic Emissions (SOAE)

- ☐ present in less than 50% of normal hearers
- ☐ more common in females than in males
- ☐ less common, and fewer in number, in persons over age 50 years (ADR note: may be largely due to presbycusis rather than simply age)
- ☐ comparable prevalence in infants, children, and young adults
- ☐ frequencies of SOAE are stable for long periods of time
- ☐ amplitudes of SOAE may fluctuate over time
- ☐ most often present in the 1000 to 2000 Hz region
- ☐ multiple SOAE frequencies are common in individuals
- ☐ if present in an individual, likely to be present in both ears
- ☐ there is no positive association between SOAE and tinnitus
- ☐ SOAE are not consistent with "objective tinnitus"

Otoacoustic Emissions (OAE) Categories

- ☐ **Spontaneous OAE (SOAE)**
- ☐ **Evoked OAE**
  - ✓ transient evoked OAE (TEOAE)
  - ✓ distortion product OAE (DPOAE)
  - ✓ stimulus frequency OAE

ANATOMIC AND PHYSIOLOGIC UNDERPINNINGS

See ADR Chapter 1 too.

Differences Between Inner and Outer Hair Cells

Inner Hair Cells	Outer Hair Cells
1 row	3 or 4 rows
N = 3500	*N* = 12,000 to 20,000
on spiral lamina	on basilar membrane
no contact between stereocilia and reticular membrane	tallest stereocilia contact tectorial membrane
95% of afferents synapse	5% of afferents synapse
not motile	motile
encompassed by support cells	supported on top and at bottom
central nucleus	nucleus at base of cell
wine bottle shape	test-tube shape
single layer endoplasmic reticulum	extensive subsurface cisternae in ER
mitochondria scattered	mitochondria along perimeter of cell
efferent fibers from lateral superior olive	efferents from medial superior olive

Source: Information contributed in part by Marleen T. Ochs, Ph.D.

Classic Quote

Harold Schuknecht on pathophysiology of loudness recruitment and outer hair cells

"The phenomenon of loudness recruitment appears to be the psychoacoustic expression of the loss of a large component of outer hair cells and the concurrent preservation of a large component of inner hair cells and type I cochlear neurons."

"It is well established that the outer hair cells are more susceptable than inner hair cells to almost all types of injury (e.g., inflammatory disease, trauma, ototoxic drugs) and that nerve fibers undergo degeneration only as a retrograde effect following injury to the sustenacular cells, particularly the inner pillar cells and the inner phalangeal cells."

Source: From Schuknecht HF. *Pathology of the Ear.* (2nd ed). Philadelphia: Williams & Wilkins, 1993, p. 91.

Major Anatomic Regions Involved in OAE Measurement

Schematic representation of the four main anatomic auditory regions involved in the generation and measurement of otoacoustic emissions, including: (1) the external ear canal, (2) the middle ear system, (3) the outer hair cells in the cochlea, and (4) the efferent (descending) auditory system. OAE generation is dependent on inward propagation of energy to the cochlea and outward propagation of energy from the cochlea.

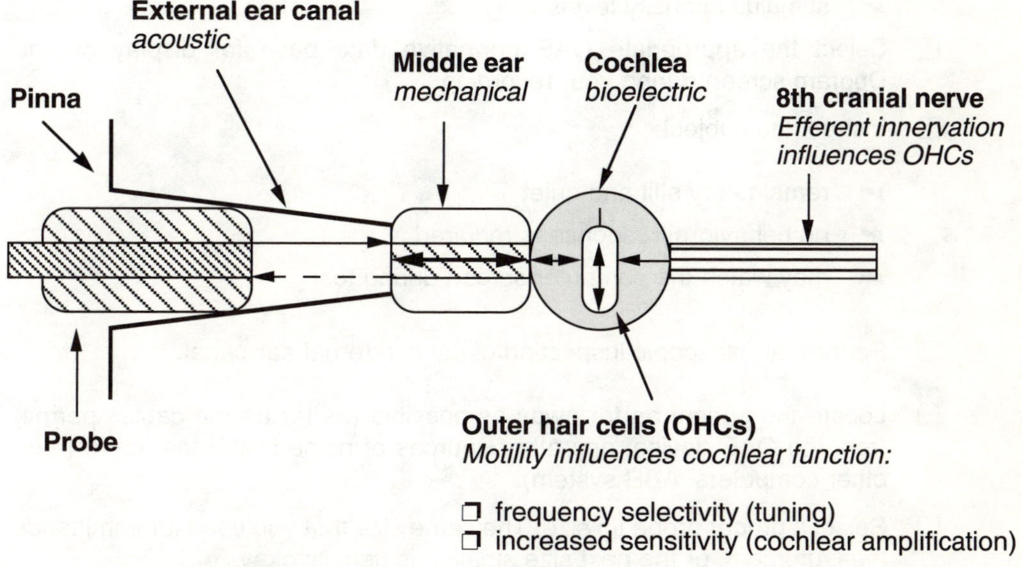

Inward propagation: acoustic - mechanical - bioelectric

Outward propagation: bioelectric - mechanical - acoustic

MEASUREMENT PROCEDURES, PROTOCOLS, AND PITFALLS

Step-by-Step

Preparation for OAE recording. Also, see OAE figures and tables in this ADR chapter.

- ☐ Log the patient (name, age, gender, etc.) into the computer.
- ☐ Select the desired test protocol.
  - ✔ diagnostic versus screening
  - ✔ stimulus intensity levels
- ☐ Select the appropriate OAE normative data base for display on the Dpgram screen during your recording.
- ☐ Instruct the subject:
  - ✔ remain very still and quiet
  - ✔ no behavioral response is required
  - ✔ may watch the computer screen during test
- ☐ Perform an otoscopic inspection of each external ear canal.
- ☐ Locate the patient as far away as possible (as far as the cables permit) from the OAE device, any other sources of noise in the test room (e.g., other computers, ABR system).
- ☐ Select a proper probe tip size. The same size that you used for immittance measurement, or the next size smaller, is usually okay.
- ☐ Fit the probe tip snugly, and deeply, into the external ear canal.
- ☐ Verify that the OAE device tubes (for the stimuli and the system microphone) are not rubbing.
- ☐ Peform a probe fit routine if recommended by the manufacturer (e.g., by Otodynamics for the ILO 88 transient evoked OAE device).

Protocol

Recording Diagnostic DPOAE Protocol (a diagnostic DPgram). Also, see other OAE figures and tables in this ADR chapter.

- ☐ f_2/f_1 = 1.2 (but vary as needed. See page 251).
- ☐ f_1 = 65 dB SPL; f_2 = 55 dB SPL (initially, then DPgrams at lower intensities as desired)
- ☐ f_2 of 500 through 8000 Hz
- ☐ 3 or more frequencies per octave
- ☐ Noise reduction algorithm or configuration appropriate for typical test setting. Consult with the manufacturer of your OAE system.

Protocol

Recording screening DPOAE data (a screening DPgram). Also, see other OAE figures and tables in this ADR chapter.

- ☐ f_2/f_1 = 1.2 (but vary as needed using optimal ratio for test frequency region. See page 251).
- ☐ f_1 = 65 dB SPL; f_2 = 55 dB SPL (don't worry—you won't be passing babies with communicatively significant sensory hearing loss).
- ☐ f_2 of 1000 through 4000 Hz or f_2 of 2000 through 4000 Hz
- ☐ 3 frequencies per octave
- ☐ noise reduction algorithm or configuration appropriate for typical nursery setting (i.e., use more time averages or frames and more strict criteria for noise floor reduction). Consult with the manufacturer of your OAE system.

Transient Evoked Otoacoustic Emissions Information

Transient evoked otoacoustic emissions (TEOAE) information as displayed on the screen and plot out of the Otodynamics ILO 88 device (Otodynamics is a company in the United Kingdom which maintains an exclusive license for TEOAE instrumention until the year 1999.) Information indicated by the circled numbers is as follows: (1) acoustic waveform of the click stimulus, (2) spectrum (0 to 6000 Hz) and average intensity level of the stimulus in the external ear canal, (3) peak stimulus intensity level within the ear canal (in dB SPL) and the agreement (correlation) in % of the intensity level for the first vs. last click presented in the TEOAE averaging process, (4) noise level within the ear canal during TEOAE recording (33.7 dB SPL in this case), and the noise cutoff level for rejection of averaging because of excessive noise (the manufacturer recommends that the noise rejection cutoff not exceed 52 dB SPL), (5) the number of stimuli, and percentage of total stimuli presented, when the noise floor was lower than the rejection cutoff (quiet) vs. the number of stimuli presented when noise was above this value (noisy), (6) two TEOAE waveforms (A and B) recorded in the ear canal as dB SPL over time for alternating stimuli (in this case there is clearly a high degree of similarity between the two waves). TEOAE generated in the basal (high frequency) regions of the cochlea are observed earlier in the waveform whereas lower frequency TEOAE are found later in the waveform, (7) spectrum of TEOAE amplitude (open line in dB SPL) over the maximum measurable region from 0 to 5000 Hz in comparison to noise (*shaded area*) over the same frequency region. In OAE recordings, noise from the environment and the patient (physiologic) is almost always greatest in the low (< 1500 Hz) frequency region, (8) from the upper to lower portion of this little box, overall ("whole") TEOAE ("response") amplitude in dB SPL, wave reproducibility ("repro") and, for each of five octave bands, the reproducibility in percent (%) between TEOAE "A" and "B" waveforms and the signal (TEOAE) to noise ratio (SNR) in dB SPL , and (9) test time. Manufacturer can supply more details on equipment operation.

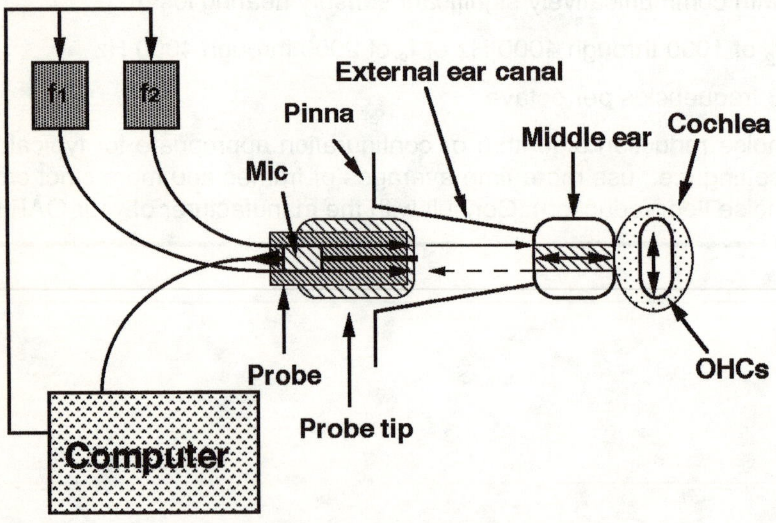

DPOAE Measurement Principles

Illustration of the measurement of distortion product otoacoustic emissions (DPOAE). The two boxes on the left represent transducers for the two stimulus frequencies (f_1 and f_2). Stimulus generation and the processing of DPOAE and noise energy are performed by the computer.

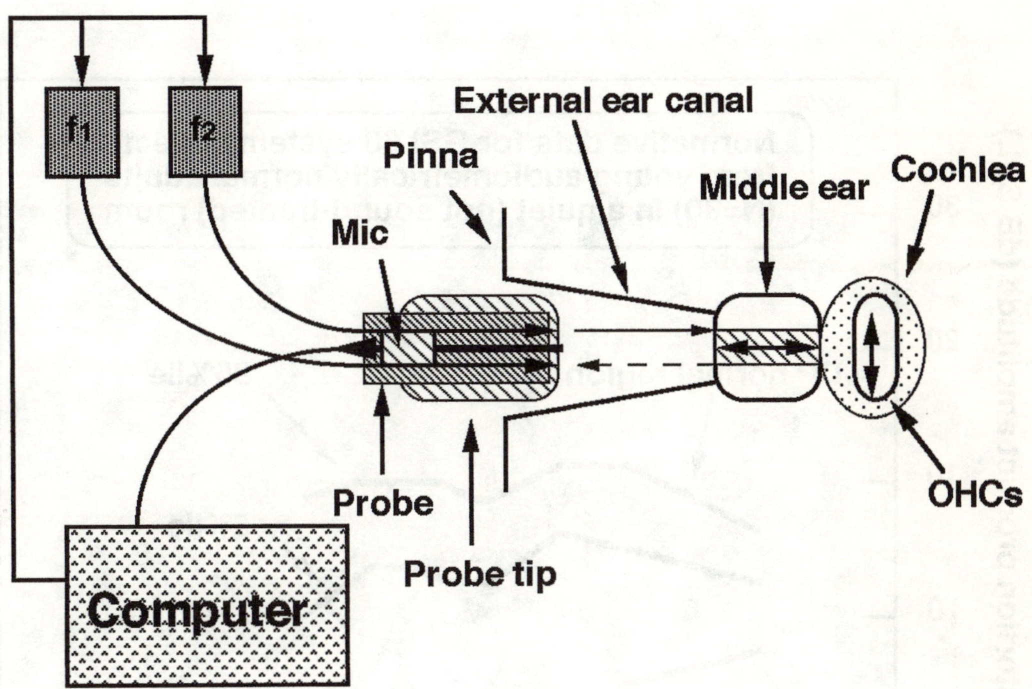

Example of DPOAEgram

Normal data

The normal region encompasses the region between the 5th and 95th percentiles for a group of 30 otologically and audiologically normal adult subjects. The line labeled "noise in ear canal" is drawn from measurement noise points at the 95th percentile for the normal group in a typical non-sound-treated room.

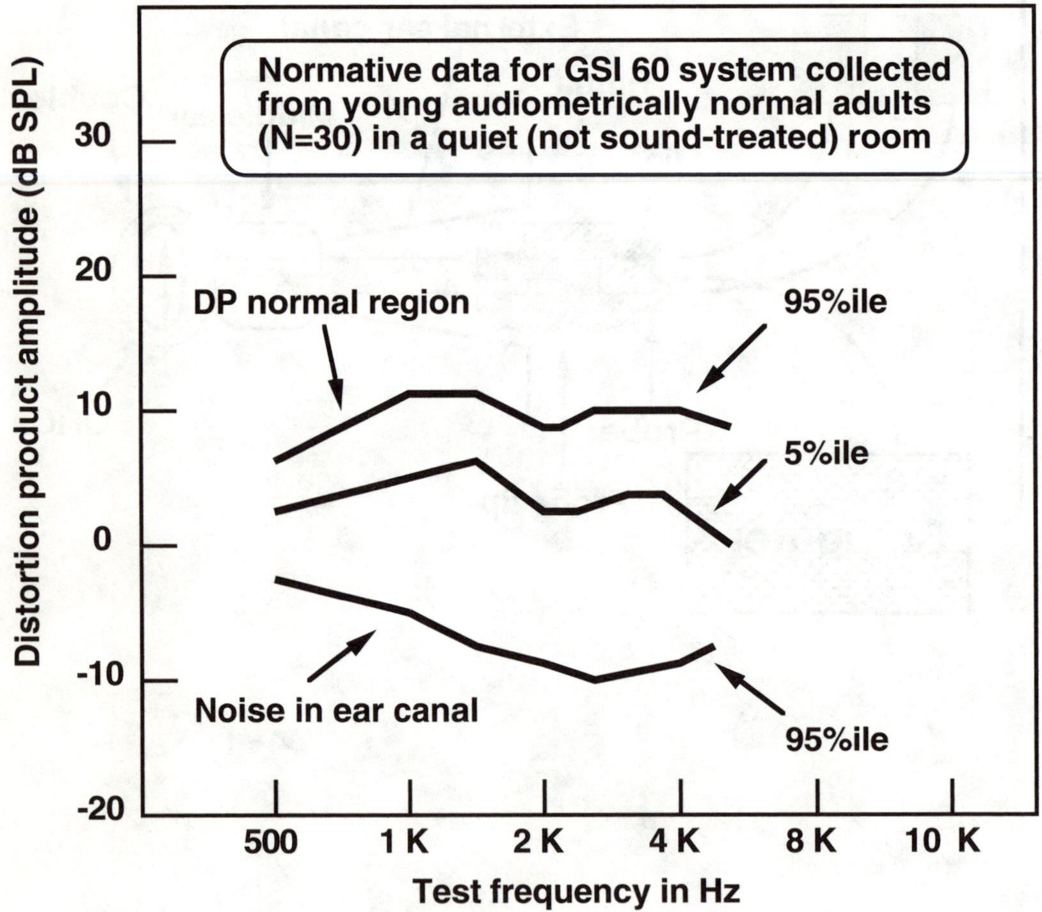

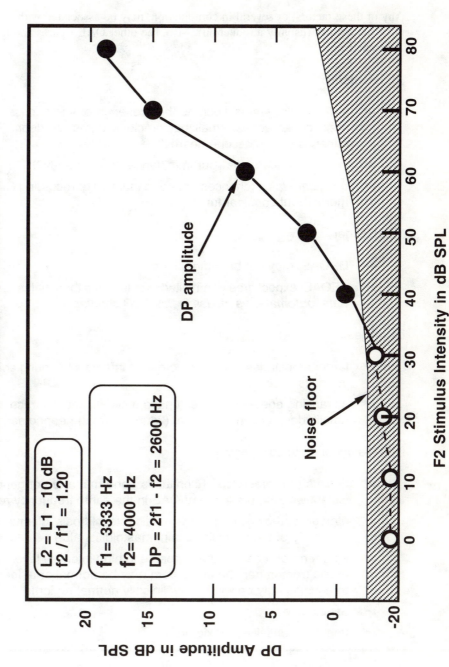

Illustration of DPOAE Input/Output (I/O) Function

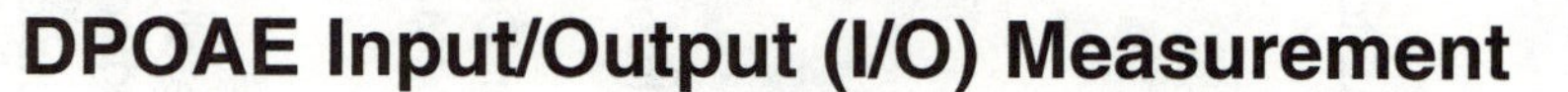

Subject Factors in OAE Interpretation

Any of these factors, or several in combination, may be associated with a deviation in OAE amplitudes (usually a reduction). Also, see other OAE figures and tables in this *ADR* chapter.

☐ Anatomic

- *external ear status*, such as the presence of vernix casseous, cerumen, cockroaches, small but precious gems, or debris in the ear canal. Is your otoscope nearby?
- *middle ear status* (is your immittance device handy?)
- *cochlear status* (chances are good that you're recording OAE to learn more about cochlear function)

☐ Gender

- DPOAE: may not be a big factor
- TEOAE: expect greater amplitudes in females than males. See *TEOAE data for females vs. males in this ADR chapter*.

☐ Age

- larger amplitudes may be recorded in infants and young children than in adults
- advancing age alone doesn't have a significant influence on DPOAE amplitudes, assuming normal (young normal) hearing sensitivity

☐ History and otologic findings

- tinnitus (the presence of tinnitus is abnormal and not generally consistent with the presence of OAE in the same frequency region)
- otologic pathology (e.g., otitis media, otosclerosis, glomus tumor, discontinuity of the ossicular chain, mastoiditis, etc.)
- long-term or recent acute exposure to high intensity levels of noise or music (remember, the audiogram may be normal or at least hearing thresholds may be within the clinically normal region)
- aspirin use
- use of potentially ototoxic drugs

Step-by-Step

Recording OAE in the Clinic (after OAE preparation Step-by-Step is complete). Also, see OAE figures and tables in this ADR chapter.

- ☐ Verify that the actual stimulus intensity level is within ± 1.5 to 3 dB of target intensity level.
- ☐ Verify that noise levels (noise floor or NF) are not excessive within the ear canal. Compare to normal expectations. **See DPOAE normative TABLES in this ADR chapter**.
- ☐ Monitor each of these parameters visually on computer screen as the DPgram is performed.
- ☐ Replicate (at least twice) the DPgram for each protocol in each ear. Superimpose the two DPgrams for rapid evaluation of replicability. **See STEP-BY-STEP: DPOAE Analysis in this ADR chapter**.
- ☐ Verify that you have stored the DPOAE data for each run on the computer hard or floppy disk.
- ☐ Analyze OAE data for amplitude and noise floor as a function of stimulus frequency. **See STEP-BY-STEP: DPOAE Analysis in this ADR chapte**r.
- ☐ Interpret OAE data versus normative data as a function of stimulus frequency. **See DPOAE normative TABLES in this ADR chapter**.

Trouble-Shooting

OAE recording. Also, see other OAE figures and tables in this ADR chapter.

☐ No stimulus?

- ✔ Verify that power for the stimulus external box is on
- ✔ Verify that all tubes and cords leading to/from the computer to the probe are completely plugged in.

☐ Very low stimulus intensity level (as detected by probe and displayed on computer screen)?

- ✔ Verify that you selected the appropriate stimulus intensity.
- ✔ Verify by ear check that a stimulus is present at the level of the probe.
- ✔ Make sure that the probe is fit properly in the ear canal.
- ✔ Inspect probe ports and tubes for debris (e.g., cerumen).
- ✔ Inspect the external ear canal for excessive cerumen.

☐ Excessive noise levels?

- ✔ Is the patient quiet, not moving, not chewing, etc.?
- ✔ Is the door to the test room closed?
- ✔ What is the typical ambient noise level in the test room?
- ✔ Is the test ear away from the OAE device and other sources of sound in the test room (e.g., ABR computer, door, air-conditioning vent)?
- ✔ Is the probe fit well and deeply into the external ear canal? Try inserting eeper to reduce noise levels.
- ✔ Are you averaging an adequate number of times per frequency? Maybe more processing is needed to reach a suitable noise level.
- ✔ If all else fails, you should consider only averaging OAE for test frequencies above 1000 Hz to avoid the frequency region where noise is greatest.

Neo-Classic Quote

J. H. Siegel on standing waves in otoacoustic emissions measurement

"Since the sound pressure at the eardrum near 5–7 KHz is underestimated by as much as 20 dB, the stimulus level actually delivered to the eardrum will exceed the desired level by the same value . . .

Individual differences in the standing wave patterns in a population of subjects will thus introduce a maximum error that will vary significantly in frequency and magnitude. Because of this variability, pooled emission data should reveal trends in the data for stimuli near 5–7 KHz that will be less pronounced than that seen in individual subjects. Superimposed on this variability will be systematic differences, due to differing canal lengths, between adult males and females and between infants and adults . . .

The upshot is that much of the existing high-frequency distortion product emission data in humans is likely to be inaccurate and unsuitable for adoption of normative standards."

Source: Siegel JH. Ear-canal standing waves and high-frequency sound calibration using otoacoustic emission probes. *J Acoustic Soc Amer* 95: 2589–2597, 1994.

Technical Tip

Distortion Product Otoacoustic Emissions (DPOAE) Analysis Strategy. Also, see other OAE figures and tables in this ADR chapter.

- ☐ Analyze each test frequency separately
- ☐ Is DP amplitude minus noise floor (DP − NF) difference >5 dB (or some might require 10 dB)?
- ☐ Is DP amplitude > −10 dB (e.g., −5 or 0 dB)?
- ☐ Are DPOAE data replicable (e.g., amplitude values within 3 to 5 dB)?
- ☐ Is DP amplitude within the normative region used by your clinic for the test protocol at the majority of frequencies per octave that you use in your criteria for DP presence (e.g., 4 out of 6 frequencies)?

OAE NORMATIVE DATA

Protocol

Vanderbilt DPOAE Normative Study. See Tables summarizing normative data for five commercially available systems in this ADR chapter.

☐ Data collected for five commercially available, FDA-approved DPOAE systems.

- Virtual 330
- Grason Stadler, Inc. (GSI) 60
- Etymotics Research/Mimosa Acoustics CUB^{e}DIS
- Madsen Celesta 501
- Bio-Logic Scout

☐ Subjects

- 30 young adults (60 ears) age 20 to 40 years
- audiometrically super-normal or semi-normal
- super-normal = pure tone hearing thresholds of 15 dB or better at frequencies of 250 to 8000 Hz
- no recent history of aspirin use, noise exposure, or otologic disease

☐ Test protocols

- f_2/f_1 ratio = 1.2
- Dpgram from 500 through 8000 Hz
- two stimulus intensity conditions:
  $L_1 = L_2 = 65$ dB SPL *and*
  $L_1 = 65$ dB SPL; $L_2 = 55$ dB SPL

☐ Test environment

- quiet, but not sound-treated, room
- 47 to 50 dBA
- 51 to 55 dBC

Equipment Parameters

DPOAE Amplitude and Noise Floor

Mean normal distortion product otoacoustic emission (DPOAE) amplitude values (open symbols) plotted as a function of stimulus frequency (for three frequencies per octave) for five different FDA-approved DPOAE devices. Filled symbols indicate noise values at each of the test frequencies. Note the considerable variability among devices at some test frequencies, especially the highest stimulus frequency recorded. See Tables and Lists for details on the subject population, and specific DP and noise values, with statistics.

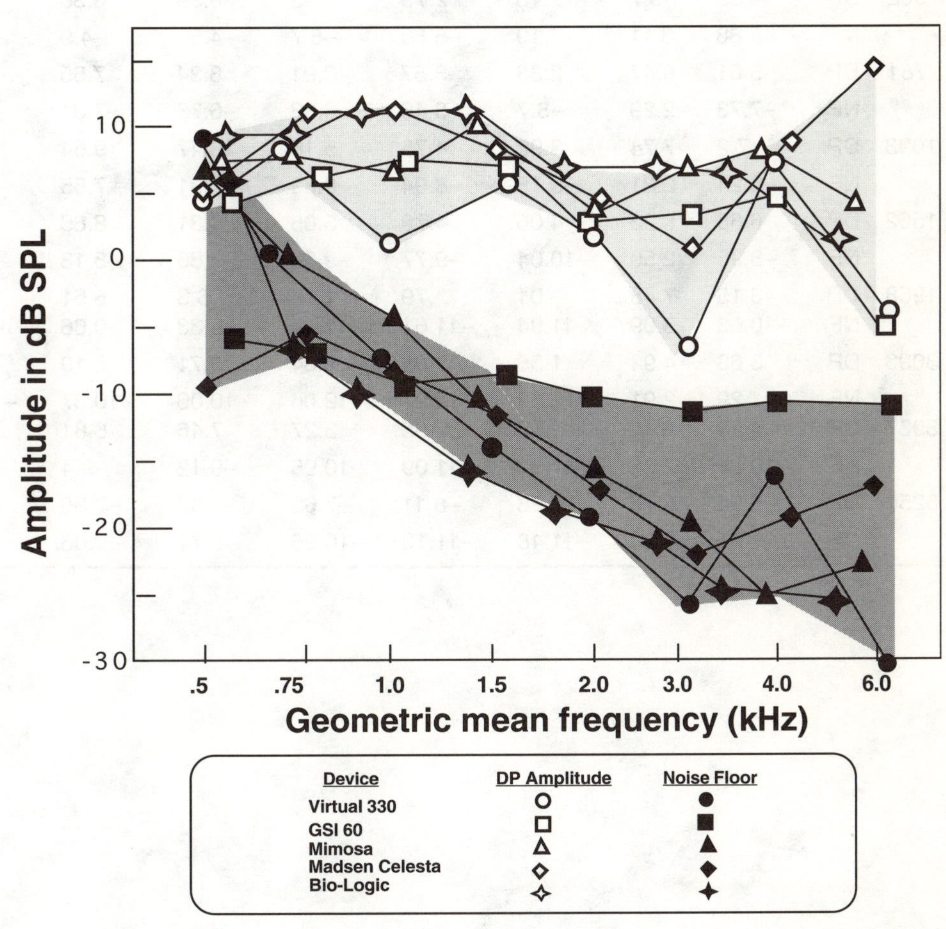

Normative Data

DPOAE for the Grason Stadler 60 DPOE

Normative DPOAE data in dB SPL for the GSI (*N* = 41 ears) collected from young audiometrically normal adults (hearing threshold levels 15 dB or better from 250 to 8000 Hz and type A tympanograms) in a quiet, non-sound-treated room. Test protocol includes: $f_1/f_2 = 1.2$; $L_1 = 65$ / $L_2 = 55$ dB SPL. Frequency is geometric mean of f_1 and f_2. DP = distortion product amplitude in dB SPL; NF = noise floor level in dB SPL. You can enter these normative data into your GSI 60.

Frequency		Mean	SD	1%ile	5%ile	10%ile	99%ile	95%ile	90%ile
562	DP	4.59	5.7	2.18	2.79	3.09	6.99	6.38	6.08
	NF	–5.88	3.11	–7.19	–6.86	–6.7	–4.57	–4.9	–5.06
781	DP	5.61	6.47	2.88	3.57	3.91	8.34	7.65	7.31
	NF	–7.73	2.29	–8.7	–8.46	–8.33	–6.76	–7.01	–7.13
1093	DP	7.2	7.74	3.92	4.75	5.16	10.47	9.64	9.23
	NF	–8.24	2.21	–9.18	–8.94	–8.83	–7.31	–7.55	–7.66
1562	DP	6.68	6.22	4.06	4.72	5.05	9.31	8.65	8.32
	NF	–8.95	2.59	–10.04	–9.77	–9.63	–7.86	–8.13	–8.27
1968	DP	3.15	7.48	–.01	.79	1.18	6.3	5.51	5.11
	NF	–10.63	3.09	–11.94	–11.61	–11.45	–9.33	–9.66	–9.82
3093	DP	3.63	4.92	1.55	2.08	2.34	5.71	5.19	4.93
	NF	–11.29	2.91	–12.52	–12.21	–12.06	–10.06	–10.37	–10.53
3937	DP	4.88	6.11	2.3	2.95	3.27	7.46	6.81	6.48
	NF	–10.24	2.67	–11.37	–11.09	–10.95	–9.12	–9.4	–9.54
6250	DP	–5.54	8.15	–8.98	–8.11	–7.68	–2.09	–2.96	–3.39
	NF	–10.1	3.28	–11.48	–11.13	–10.96	–8.71	–9.06	–9.24

Normative Data

DPOAE for the Virtual 330

Data are for N = 46 ears collected from young audiometrically normal adults (hearing threshold levels 15 dB or better from 250 to 8000 Hz and type A tympanograms) in a quiet, non-sound treated room. Test protocol includes: $f_2/f_1 = 1.2$; $L_1 = 65$; $L_2 = 55$ dB SPL. Frequency is geometric mean of f_1 and f_2.

Frequency		Mean	SD	1%ile	5%ile	10%ile	99%ile	95%ile	90%ile
500	DP	4.12	8.38	.54	1.44	1.89	7.71	6.81	6.36
	NF	9.06	7.55	5.83	6.65	7.05	12.3	11.48	11.08
700	DP	7.97	6.75	5.08	5.82	6.18	10.87	10.13	9.77
	NF	.38	6.26	-2.3	-1.62	-1.29	3.06	2.38	2.05
1000	DP	.48	6.81	-2.43	-1.7	-1.33	3.39	2.66	2.29
	NF	-7.42	6.98	-10.41	-9.65	-9.28	-4.43	-5.19	-5.56
1580	DP	5.19	6.63	2.35	3.07	3.42	8.03	7.31	6.96
	NF	-14.82	7.04	-17.83	-17.07	-16.69	-11.81	-12.57	-12.94
2000	DP	2.27	6.92	-.69	.06	.43	5.24	4.49	4.12
	NF	-19.72	6.45	-22.48	-21.78	-21.44	-16.96	-17.65	-18
3180	DP	-7.7	8.48	-11.33	-10.41	-9.96	-4.07	-4.99	-5.44
	NF	-25.63	5.95	-28.18	-27.54	-27.22	-23.09	-23.73	-24.05
4000	DP	7.32	9.69	3.18	4.23	4.74	11.47	10.42	9.91
	NF	-16.61	4.89	-18.71	-18.18	-17.92	-14.52	-15.05	-15.31
6350	DP	-4.2	9.15	-8.12	-7.13	-6.64	-.28	-1.27	-1.76
	NF	-31.72	4.33	-33.57	-33.1	-32.87	-29.87	-30.33	-30.57

*DP = amplitude of DP in dB SPL
NF = amplitude of noise floor in dB SPL

Normative Data

DPOAE for the Bio-Logic Scout

N = 40 ears collected from young audiometrically normal adults (hearing threshold levels 15 dB or better from 250 to 8000 Hz and type A tympanograms) in a quiet, non-sound-treated room. Test protocol includes: $f_2/f_1 = 1.2$; $L_1 = 65$; $L_2 = 55$ dB SPL. Frequency displayed is f_2.

Frequency		Mean	SD	1%ile	5%ile	10%ile	99%ile	95%ile	90%ile
634	DP	9.25	5.97	6.69	7.34	7.66	11.81	11.16	10.84
	NF	5.63	6.68	–8.49	–7.77	–7.41	–2.77	–3.5	–3.85
805	DP	9.01	6.39	6.27	6.96	7.31	11.74	11.05	10.71
	NF	–7.43	8.65	–11.14	–10.2	–9.74	–3.73	–4.67	–5.13
1001	DP	10.18	6.56	7.38	8.09	8.44	12.99	12.28	11.93
	NF	–11.28	7.72	–14.58	–13.75	–13.33	–7.97	–8.81	–9.22
1586	DP	10.65	6.63	7.81	8.53	8.88	13.48	12.76	12.41
	NF	–16.45	7.56	–19.69	–18.87	–18.47	–13.21	–14.03	–14.44
2002	DP	6.85	6.4	4.11	4.81	5.15	9.6	8.9	8.56
	NF	–19.41	6.07	–22.01	–21.35	–21.03	–16.81	–17.46	–17.79
3174	DP	6.1	5.18	3.88	4.44	4.71	8.31	7.75	7.48
	NF	–21.16	6.04	–23.74	–23.09	–22.77	–18.57	–19.23	–19.55
4003	DP	6.1	5.68	3.66	4.28	4.58	8.53	7.91	7.61
	NF	–24.65	7.08	–27.68	–26.92	–26.54	–21.62	–22.39	–22.77
6347	DP	1.22	8.51	–2.42	–1.5	–1.04	4.87	3.95	3.49
	NF	–25.24	6.38	–27.97	–27.28	–26.93	–22.5	–23.19	–23.54

*DP = amplitude of DP in dB SPL;
NF = amplitude of noise floor in dB SPL

Normative Data

DPOAE for the Madsen Celesta

N = 30 ears collected from young audiometrically normal adults (hearing threshold levels 15 dB or better from 250 to 8000 Hz and type A tympanograms) in a quiet, non-sound treated room. Test protocol includes: f_2/f_1 = 1.2; L_1 = 65; L_2 = 55 dB SPL. Frequency is geometric mean of f_1 and f_2.

Frequency		Mean	SD	1%ile	5%ile	10%ile	99%ile	95%ile	90%ile
500	DP	4.9	4.92	2.42	3.06	3.37	7.38	6.74	6.43
	NF	–9.97	4.33	–12.14	–11.58	–11.31	–7.79	–8.35	–8.62
753	DP	11.3	5.44	8.56	9.27	9.61	14.04	13.33	12.99
	NF	–5.63	6.08	–8.69	–7.9	–7.52	–2.57	–3.36	–3.75
1006	DP	11.9	6.98	8.39	9.29	9.73	15.41	14.51	14.07
	NF	–8.23	4.48	–10.49	–9.91	–9.62	–5.98	–6.56	–6.84
1512	DP	7.9	6.97	4.39	5.3	5.74	11.41	10.5	10.06
	NF	–11.43	6.59	–14.75	–13.89	–13.48	–8.12	–8.97	–9.39
2011	DP	4.8	5.39	2.09	2.79	3.13	7.51	6.81	6.47
	NF	–17.03	3.32	–18.7	–18.27	–18.06	–15.36	–15.79	–16
3023	DP	.6	4.5	–1.66	–1.08	–.8	2.86	2.28	2
	NF	–22.43	3.19	–24.04	–23.63	–23.42	–20.83	–21.24	–21.44
4036	DP	8.03	5.75	5.14	5.89	6.25	10.93	10.18	9.82
	NF	–19.3	3.72	–21.17	–20.69	–20.46	–17.43	–17.91	–18.14
6060	DP	14.17	8.03	10.12	11.17	11.67	18.21	17.17	16.66
	NF	–16.6	3.42	–18.32	–17.88	–17.66	–14.88	–15.32	–15.54

*DP = amplitude of DP in dB SPL
NF = amplitude of noise floor in dB SPL

Normative Data

DPOAE data in dB SPL for the Etymotics/Mimosa Acoustics

N = 40 ears collected from young audiometrically normal adults (hearing levels 15 dB or better from 250 to 8000 Hz & type A tympanograms) in a quiet, non-sound-treated room. Test protocol includes: $f_2/f_1 = 1.2$; $L_1 = 65$; $L_2 = 55$ dB SPL. Frequency is geometric mean of f_1 and f_2.

Frequency		Mean	SD	1%ile	5%ile	10%ile	99%ile	95%ile	90%ile
534	DP	6.78	5.74	4.17	4.84	5.16	9.39	8.72	8.40
	NF	6.29	6.69	3.25	4.02	4.40	9.32	8.55	8.17
704	DP	8.68	6.23	5.85	6.57	6.92	11.51	10.79	10.43
	NF	.31	6.27	–2.54	–1.82	–1.46	3.15	2.43	2.07
1070	DP	6.69	7.92	3.1	4.01	4.46	10.29	9.37	8.92
	NF	–4.34	8.63	–8.25	–7.26	—6.77	–.42	–1.42	–1.91
1408	DP	9.93	6.82	6.83	7.62	8.01	–7.09	–7.85	–8.22
	NF	–10.06	6.53	–13.02	–12.26	–11.89	–7.09	–7.85	–8.22
2113	DP	3.14	5.7	.55	1.21	1.53	5.73	5.07	4.74
	NF	–15.92	6.1	–18.69	–17.98	–17.63	–13.15	–13.85	–14.2
3084	DP	6.76	5.17	4.41	5.01	5.30	9.11	8.51	8.21
	NF	–19.65	10.05	–24.21	–23.05	–22.48	–15.08	–16.25	–16.82
3935	DP	7.48	4.67	5.36	5.9	6.16	9.59	9.05	8.79
	NF	–25.19	5.98	–27.9	–27.21	–26.87	–22.47	–23.17	–23.5
5710	DP	3.47	5.89	.79	1.47	1.81	6.14	5.46	5.12
	NF	–23.04	10.25	–27.7	–26.51	–25.93	–18.39	–19.58	–20.16

*DP = amplitude of DP in dB SPL
NF = amplitude of noise floor in dB SPL

Transient Evoked Otoacoustic Emissions (TEOAE)

Normal findings recorded from 20 audiologically normal females and males at Vanderbilt University Medical Center by Jane E. Baer, Ph.D. TEOAE amplitude ("echo") and reproducibility data are reported for octave bands for each gender, and each ear.

	Female (*N* = 20)				Male (*N* = 20)			
Parameter	**Mean**	**SD**	**10%ile**	**90%ile**	**Mean**	**SD**	**10%ile**	**90%ile**
Right Ear								
Echo (dB)								
Overall (whole)	12.49	3.46	8.65	17.95	8.74	3.07	4.2	12.65
1000 Hz	10.55	4.26	6	16.5	4.95	4.81	0	11.6
2000 Hz	14.1	5.07	6.5	21.5	8.58	5.78	.4	14.6
3000 Hz	12.4	6.53	5.5	21	6.84	5	0	14
4000 Hz	10.6	6	2	19	6.63	4.34	2	11
5000 Hz	4.1	6.21	-1	12	.42	2.27	−3.6	2
Reproducibility (%)								
Overall (whole)	92	4.67	85	98	75.85	17.65	53.5	93
1000 Hz	89	7.88	78	97	69.53	23.08	46.2	93.2
2000 Hz	93.35	6.75	82	99	80	24.62	47.6	96.6
3000 Hz	87.1	21.74	76.5	98.5	71.79	28.75	17.2	96
4000 Hz	80.3	29.12	31	98.5	66.26	36.07	0	92
5000 Hz	38.15	43.82	0.00	94	4	17.44	0	0
Low Noise Stimuli (%)	96.2	3.41	90.5	99.5	93.4	7	82.5	99
Noise Level (dB)	33.81	1.23	32.0	35.45	35.36	1.7	33.1	37.1
Stimulus Intensity (dB)	82.65	2.94	79.5	84.0	79.6	1.49	78	82
Stimulus Stability (%)	94	4.58	88.5	99	88.1	12.48	79.5	100
Test Time (sec)	.46	.01	.44	.48	.47	.04	.44	.53

(continued)

Parameter	Female (*N* = 20)				Male (*N* = 20)			
	Mean	SD	10%ile	90%ile	Mean	SD	10%ile	90%ile
Left Ear								
Echo (dB)								
Overall (whole)	11.68	2.8	8.6	15.85	6.72	3.3	2.85	12.65
1000 Hz	9.26	4.6	4	15.2	2.15	4.08	−2	7
2000 Hz					5.4	5.82	−2	13.5
3000 Hz	12	5.08	5.4	18	4.55	5.37	−1	11
4000 Hz	9.63	6.18	.4	16.2	3.5	5.71	−5	10
5000 Hz	3.26	6.01	−5	12.6	.3	5.02	−5	7
Reproducibility (%)								
Overall (whole)	90.2	5.36	81.5	96.5	62.95	22.61	32.5	91.5
1000 Hz	84.74	14.24	70.8	96.6	46.25	33.77	0	83
2000 Hz	91.74	7.19	81	98	62.65	35.44	0	95
3000 Hz	87	22.19	76.8	98	49.25	42.5	0	92.5
4000 Hz	79.53	29.76	23.2	97.6	48.2	41.02	0	90
5000 Hz	39.98	43.76	0	94	16.5	34.21	0	82.5
Low Noise Stimuli (%)	95.25	5.05	86.5	99	94.45	5.89	85.5	99
Noise Level (dB)	34.23	1.41	32.4	36.1	35.68	1.96	32.9	38.5
Stimulus Intensity (dB)	82.65	2.76	80	85.5	80.15	2.01	77.5	83
Stimulus Stability (%)	93.8	4.94	85.5	100	92.65	4.8	85	98.5
Test Time (sec)					.47	.04	.44	.52

CLINICAL APPLICATIONS

Clinical Applications of OAE and Their Rationale

Application	Rationale
☐ Newborn hearing screening	✓ OAE can be recorded reliably from newborn infants (see Chapter 10 on hearing screening) ✓ OAE recording can be performed in nursery setting (test performance may be affected by noise) ✓ Normal OAE are recorded in persons with normal sensory (cochlear) function ✓ OAE are abnormal in persons with even mild degrees of sensory hearing loss; the main objective of screening is to detect sensory hearing impairment ✓ OAE recording may require relatively brief test time ✓ OAE measurement may be performed by nonaudiologic personnel (e.g., at reduced cost)
☐ Pediatric audiometry	✓ OAE recording is electrophysiologic, and not dependent on patient behavioral response ✓ OAE assess cochlear function specifically (behavioral audiometry and ABR are also dependent on the status of the central auditory nervous system). See case reports in Chapter 9 Pediatric Audiometry. ✓ OAE can be recorded from sleeping or sedated children ✓ OAE recording requires relatively short test time ✓ OAE provide ear-specific audiologic information ✓ OAE provide frequency-specific audiologic information ✓ OAE are a valuable contribution to the "cross-check principle"
☐ Assessment in suspected functional hearing loss	✓ OAE recording is electrophysiologic and is not dependent on patient behavioral response ✓ Normal OAE invariably imply normal sensory function ✓ OAE provide frequency-specific audiologic information
☐ Differentiation of cochlear vs. retrocochlear auditory dysfunction	✓ OAE are site-specific for cochlear (sensory) auditory dysfunction

	✓ In combination with ABR, OAE can clearly distinguish sensory vs. neural auditory disorders
☐ Monitoring ototoxicity	✓ OAE are site-specific for cochlear (sensory) auditory dysfunction ✓ Ototoxic drugs exert their effect on outer hair cell function; OAE are dependent on outer hair cell integrity ✓ OAE recording is electrophysiologic and is not dependent on patient behavioral response; can be recorded from patients who, due to their medical condition, are unable to perform behavioral audiometry tasks, or from infants and young children ✓ OAE can detect cochlear dysfunction before it is evident by pure tone audiometry ✓ OAE provide frequency-specific audiologic information
☐ Tinnitus	✓ OAE are site-specific for cochlear (sensory) auditory dysfunction ✓ OAE can provide objective confirmation of cochlear dysfunction in patients with tinnitus and normal audiograms ✓ OAE provide frequency-specific audiologic information which may be associated with the frequency region of tinnitus
☐ Noise/music exposure	✓ OAE are site-specific for cochlear (sensory) auditory dysfunction ✓ Excessive noise/music intensity levels affect outer hair cell function; OAE are dependent on outer hair cell integrity ✓ OAE can provide objective confirmation of cochlear dysfunction in patients with normal audiograms ✓ OAE findings are associated with cochlear frequency specificity (i.e., "tuning"); musician complaints of auditory dysfunction can be confirmed by OAE findings, even with a normal audiogram ✓ OAE can provide an early and reliable "warning sign" of cochlear dysfunction due to noise/music exposure before any problem is evident in the audiogram

Clinical Measurement of DPOAE

Major steps in the clinical measurement of distortion product otoacoustic emissions (DPOAE). Information summarized in these steps is described in accompanying tables and text.

FUNCTIONAL ANATOMY OF OAE

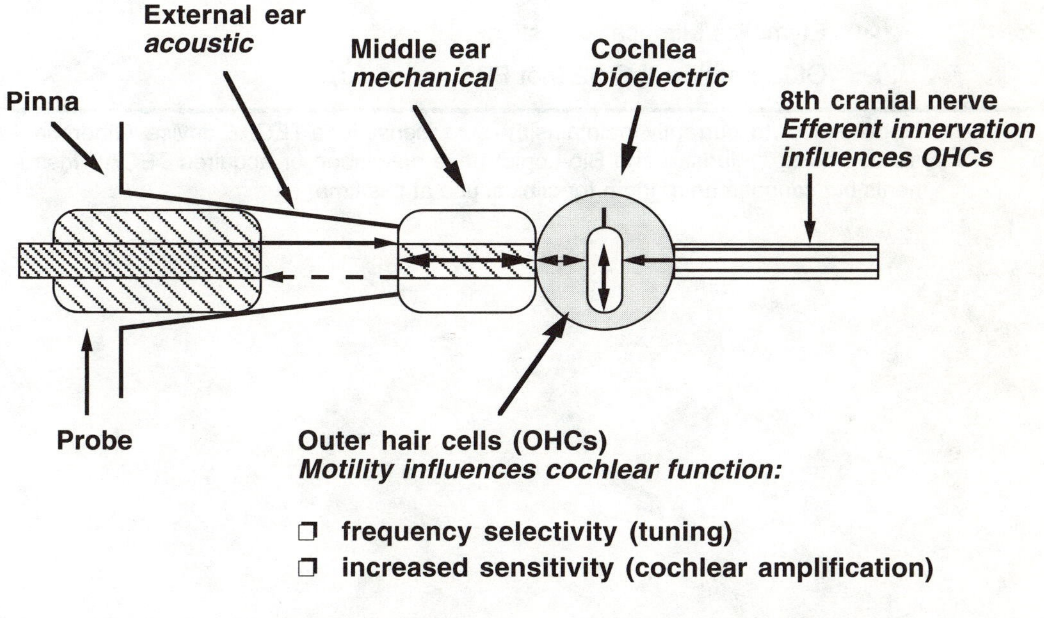

- ❐ frequency selectivity (tuning)
- ❐ increased sensitivity (cochlear amplification)

Inward propagation: *acoustic - mechanical - bioelectric*

Outward propagation: *bioelectric - mechanical - acoustic*

Manufacturers of OAE Instrumentation

- ☐ Transient evoked otoacoustic emissions (TEOAE)
  - ✔ Otodynamics: ILO 88 *
- ☐ Distortion product otoacoustic emissions (DPOAE)
  - ✔ Virtual Corporation: Virtual 330
  - ✔ Grason Stadler: GSI 60
  - ✔ Madsen: Celesta
  - ✔ Bio-Logic Corp.: Scout
  - ✔ Etymotics/Mimosa Acoustics
  - ✔ Otodynamics: ILO 92 (not FDA approved)

*Otodynamics Ltd. currently maintains the sole license for a TEOAE device. Other manufacturers (e.g., Madsen and Bio-Logic) have developed or acquired TEOAE instruments but cannot market them for clinical use at this time.

TEOAE Findings for a Neonate Recorded in a Sound-treated Room

See Figure 7 (and legend) for explanation of the components of the figure. TEOAE were recorded with the "Quickscreen" option which limits analysis to the higher frequencies (shorter analysis time) to reduce test time and minimize the effects of low frequency ambient and physiologic noise. Measurement noise was relatively low, TEOAE response amplitude and reproducibility was relatively high, and test time was quite short (only 27 secs) under these test conditions. Using published criteria (Kemp, 1993) for TEOAE screening analysis, this neonate would be a "pass" outcome.

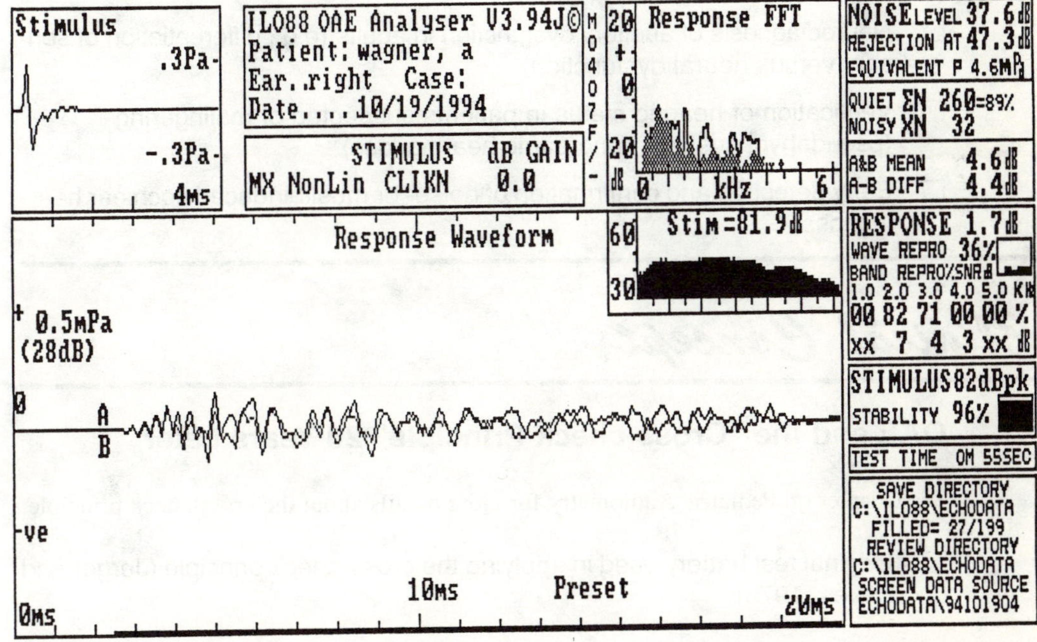

Clinical Applications of OAE

Also, see other OAE figures and tables in this ADR chapter.

- ☐ Diagnostic audiologic assessment in difficult-to-test, neurologically impaired developmentally delayed, or multiply involved children
- ☐ Newborn and infant hearing screening
- ☐ Monitoring hearing status during medical therapy with potentially ototoxic drugs
- ☐ Verification of normal cochlear function in patients undergoing central auditory processing assessment
- ☐ Neurodiagnosis of auditory dysfunction in adults (e.g., differentiation of sensory versus neural dysfunction)
- ☐ Verification of hearing status in patients suspected of malingering (pseudohypacusis or nonorganic hearing loss)
- ☐ Early detection and confirmation of noise- or music-induced cochlear hearing loss

Clinical Concept

OAE and the "Cross-check Principle" 20 Years Later

See Chapter on Pediatric Audiometry for more details about the cross-check principle.

- ☐ Original test battery used in applying the cross-check principle (Jerger and Hayes, 1976)
  - ✔ behavioral audiometry
  - ✔ immittance measurement: tympanometry and acoustic reflexes
  - ✔ auditory brainstem response (ABR): air- and bone-conduction click stimuli
- ☐ Current test battery used in applying the cross-check principle
  - ✔ behavioral audiometry
  - ✔ immittance measurement: tympanometry and acoustic reflexes
  - ✔ auditory brainstem response (ABR): air- and bone-conduction, click *and* tone burst stimuli
  - ✔ *otoacoustic emissions*

OAE and Pediatric Audiology Test Patterns

The role of otoacoustic emissions (OAE) in the audiometric test battery for diagnostic assessment of children. OAE contribute unique information, especially when interpreted with measures of middle ear and retrocochlear auditory function.

KEY:
- normal ○
- maybe abnormal ◍
- abnormal ●

PEDIATRIC AUDIOLOGY TEST BATTERY PATTERNS

TEST PROCEDURE	DISORDER / DISEASE					
	Otitis media	Meningitis	CMV	Hyper-bilirubinemia	Developmental Delay	Degenerative Disease
Aural Immittance						
Tympanometry	●	○	○	○	○	○
Acoustic reflexes	●	◍	●	◍	◍	◍
Pure tone audiometry	●	◍	◍	◍	◍	◍
Word recognition	◍	◍	◍	◍	◍	◍
Otoacoustic emissions	●	◍	◍	◍	○	○
Diagnostic speech audiometry	○	◍	●	●	●	●
Evoked Responses						
ABR	●	◍	●	●	●	●
AMLR	NA	◍	◍	◍	●	●
P300/MMN	NA	◍	◍	◍	●	●

OAE and Infant Hearing Screening

Limitations in existing published information on the performance of otoacoustic emissions in newborn hearing screening.

☐ Instrumentation

- TEOAE: Almost all data reported in the literature have been collected with a single instrument design and OAE processing algorithm, using manufacturer default stimulus and acquisition parameters.
- DPOAE: Most of data reported through 1995 were collected with experimental instrumentation that was not designed for clinical use.

☐ Population

- WBN: OAE data for healthy infants (e.g., well-baby nursery [WBN]) population not at risk for hearing impairment, were collected days or even weeks after birth. This strategy is not realistic as most babies are discharged from the hospital within 1 to 2 days after birth, and many don't return for follow-up appointments. Failure rates several days after birth are likely to be lower than within the first 48 hours after birth, due to fewer problems with vernix in the ear canal.
- ICU: Published OAE data for infants at risk for hearing impairment and initially managed in the intensive care unit (ICU) were collected after hospital discharge. In real-life screening programs these infants would be tested in the noisy nursery setting before discharge to maximize the proportion screened.

☐ Test Setting

- Most published OAE data were collected in a sound-treated room, whereas screening in the nursery is typically necessary in real-life.
- Some of the largest infant hearing screening studies were conducted in nursery settings especially constructed for hearing screening.
- Some recent infant hearing screening OAE data were collected with the infant in a specially designed mini sound-treated chamber which may not be feasible option in hospitals.

☐ Tester

- Most published OAE data were collected by hearing scientists (usually the authors of the papers) who have considerable experience in OAE recording.

- In some of the studies, the tester was a clinical research audiologist with extensive OAE experience
- In few of the studies OAE data were collected by trained nonprofessional personnel (e.g., technicians or volunteers).

DPOAE in Ménière's Disease

Distortion product otoacoustic emissions (DPOAE) findings for a group of subjects diagnosed with Ménière's disease in comparison with a group of normal subjects and subjects with non-Ménière's disease sensory (cochlear) hearing loss. On the average, patients with Ménière's disease cannot be distinguished from patients with other sensory hearing loss etiologies based on DPOAE findings alone. (Courtesy of Donna Schwaber.)

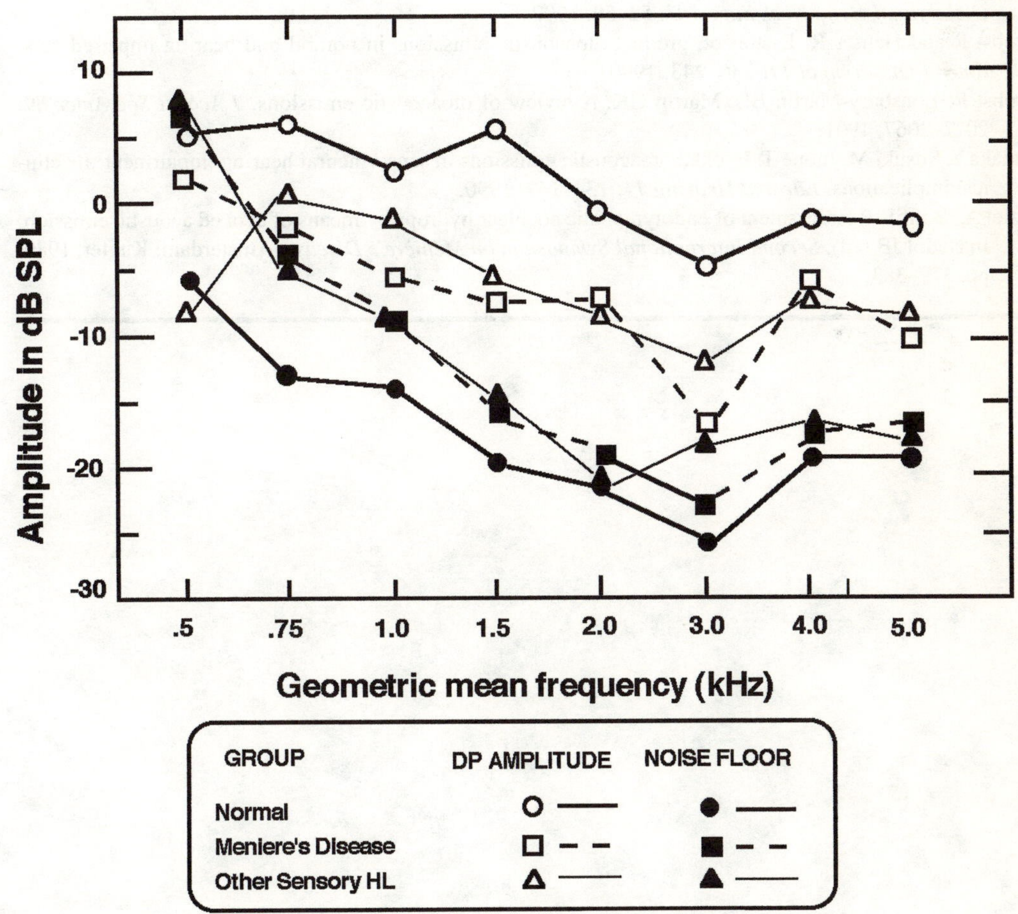

Key References

OAE in Ménière's Disease

Bonfils P, Uziel A, Pujol R. Evoked oto-acoustic emissions: A fundamental and clinical survey. *Acta Otolaryngologica 105*: 445–449, 1988

Harris FP, Probst R. Transiently evoked otoacoustic emissions in patients with Ménière's Disease. *Acta Otolaryngologica 112*: 36–44, 1992.

Horner K, Cazals Y. Rapidly fluctuating thresholds at the onset of experimentally-induced hydrops in the guinea pig. *Hearing Res 26*: 319–325, 1987.

Horner K, Cazals Y. Distortion products in early stage experimental hydrops in the guinea pig. *Hearing Res 43*: 71–80, 1989.

Martin GK, Ohlms LA, Franklin DJ, Harris FP, Lonsbury-Martin BL. Distortion product emissions in humans III. Influence of sensorineural hearing loss. *Ann Otol, Rhinol, and Laryngol 99*: 30–42, 1990.

Ohlms LA, Lonsbury-Martin BL, Martin GK. The clinical application of acoustic distortion products. *Otolaryngol-Head Neck Surg 103*: 52–59, 1990.

Probst R and Hauser R. Distortion product otoacoustic emissions in nomral and hearing impaired ears. *Amer J Otolaryngol 11*: 236–243, 1990.

Probst R, Lonsbury-Martin BL, Martin GK. A review of otoacoustic emissions. *J Acoust Soc Amer 89*: 2027–2067, 1991.

Tanaka Y, Susuki M, Inoue T. Evoked otoacoustic emissions in sensorineural hearing impairment: Its clinical implications. *Ear and Hearing 11*: 134–143, 1990.

Uziel A, Bonfils P. Assessment of endolymphatic cochlear hydrops by means of evoked acoustic emission. In Nadol JB (ed). *Second International Symposium on Ménière's Disease*. Amsterdam: Kugler, 1989, pp. 379–383.

OAE AND THE AUDIOGRAM

TEOAE Findings in Mild Middle Ear Dysfunction

Findings for an adult female patient with normal hearing sensitivity but mild long-standing middle ear dysfunction. Stimulus and noise conditions were good. These are abnormal TEOAE findings based on an analysis of amplitude and reproducibility for octave bands. See the figure (and legend) on p. 257 for an explanation of the components of the figure.

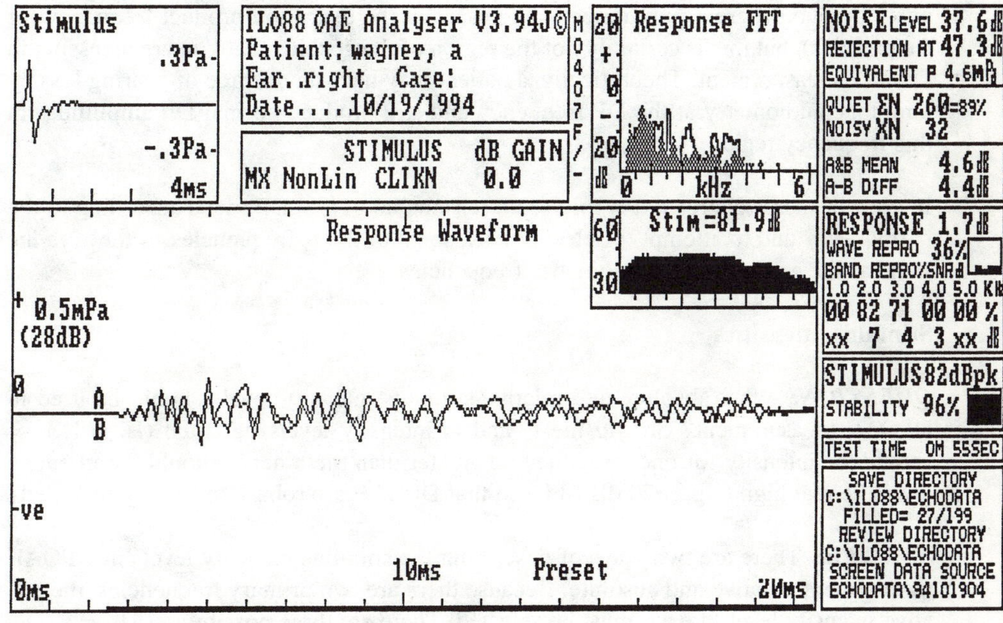

Questions and Answers

Relation Between DPOAE and the Audiogram

Stimulus frequencies

Question: In DPOAE measurement, there are two test (primary) frequencies—the f_1 and f_2—and then at least one distortion product frequency (e.g., $2f_1 - f_2$. What frequency region of the cochlea are we actually assessing?

Answer: Although initially, and intuitively, the region of stimulation was considered the frequency around the geometric mean between the two primary frequencies (between f_1 and f_2), the current thinking is that the cochlea is really being activated mostly at the f_2 frequency. The nonlinear cochlear "response" to activation simultaneously by two different pure tones is expressed at the distortion product frequency (or frequencies), but this is certainly not the region of the cochlea that you are assessing in DPOAE measurement. Theoretically, a patient may have any degree of hearing loss by pure tone audiometry at the DP frequency and still produce normal DP amplitudes in this frequency region.

In view of these relations, it would seem reasonable to plot DPgrams according to the f_2 frequency and to attempt to select at least some of the f_2 frequencies so they are the same as the conventional audiometric frequencies.

Stimulus intensities

QUESTION: What absolute and relative stimulus intensity levels should be used in DPOAE measurement? Should the f_1 and f_2 intensity levels be equal ($L_1 = L_2$), or should the intensity for one frequency be greater than the other? Should the intensity levels be real high (e.g., >70 dB SPL) so that DPOAE are robust and easily recorded?

ANSWER: There are two ways of describing the stimulus intensity levels in DPOAE meaurement: relative and absolute. Because there are two primary frequencies, the relative intensity level of each must be selected. There are three possibilities: $L_1 = L_2$, $L_1 > L_2$, and $L_1 < L_2$. Scratch the latter off your list immediately. DPOAE are clearly not optimally recorded when the amplitude for f_2 exceeds f_1 amplitude.

When recorded from entirely normal ears (cochleas), DPOAE amplitude is statistically similiar when $L_1 = L_2$, or when the intensity level of f_2 is 5 to 15 dB lower than the intensity level for f_1. Actually, slightly larger DP amplitudes may be recorded for this condition ($L_1 > L_2$), perhaps because the f_2 is less likely to influence the stimulation effectiveness of the f_1. However, in ears with cochlear dysfunction secondary, for example, to noise exposure or ototoxicity, DPOAE amplitudes are lower when $L_1 > L_2$, in comparison to $L_1 = L_2$ (Whitehead et al., 1995). Put another way, using a slighltly lower L_2 enhances the sensitivity of DPOAE to cochlear dysfunction.

Question: What about the absolute intensity level?

Answer: Avoid high intensity levels, exceeding 70 dB SPL. Technical problems may arise in measurement of DPOAE at these higher levels. One problem is contamination of DPOAE findings by standing waves, at least for stimulus frequencies above 5000 Hz (Siegal, 1994). Another is the possibility that you will record passive DPs which do not reflect outer hair cell motility and active processes within the cochlea. Passively generated DP-type responses and standing waves can even be recorded from cadavers!

Avoid very low absolute stimulus intensity levels as well. Very few persons with apparently normal cochlear function will consistently show robust DPOAE amplitudes (e.g., nonlinear cochlear function) for stimulus frequency levels below 45 dB SPL.

For recording Dpgrams, practical clinical intensity combinations are L_1 + and L_2 values of 65 + 55 dB, and 55 + 45 dB. Another approach is to record input-output DP functions to assure that the patient's maximum DP amplitude will be recorded for a given set of stimulus frequencies.

Clinical Concept

The relation between OAE and the audiogram, *or* "How come my patient has abnormal OAE when the audiogram is normal? What's wrong with my OAE technique?"

- ☐ OAE measurement is not a substitute for pure tone audiometry. Clinical audiologists should not be concerned or discouraged, but, rather, excited and encouraged by differences in patient findings for pure tone audiometry versus OAE. Indeed, if OAE and pure tone audiometry findings were consistently in agreement, there would be little clinical value in recording OAE.
- ☐ OAE findings are an almost direct measure of outer hair cell functional integrity "almost" because middle ear function is also a factor in OAE measurement, whereas pure tone audiometry is dependent on status of the cochlea, eighth nerve, central auditory system, and auditory perceptual factors, as well as the middle ear.
- ☐ OAE stimuli typically include many frequencies that are not assessed with pure tone audiometry. In fact, in comparing findings for OAE and pure tone audiometry, it is possible that none of the test frequencies are the same for both measures. For example, none of the OAE test frequencies (f_2 or geometric mean of f_1 and f_2) fall on an audiometric frequency (e.g., 1000 or 2000 Hz).
- ☐ Dysfunction (versus destruction) of some outer hair cells is likely to be reflected by less than normal motility and reduced OAE amplitude, without affecting hearing sensitivity for steady state (pure tone) signals at audiometric frequencies.
- ☐ Abnormal OAE findings may be recorded in a variety of patient populations with normal audiograms yet some cochlear dysfunction, including patients with:
  - ✔ tinnitus
  - ✔ excessive noise/music exposure
  - ✔ ototoxicity, including aspirin use
  - ✔ vestibular pathology
- ☐ Abnormal OAE findings may also be recorded in a very small proportion of persons with normal audiograms and no apparent history or clinical signs of cochlear dysfunction.
- ☐ Normal OAE may be recorded in patients with abnormal audiograms, including patients with:
  - ✔ functional or nonorganic hearing loss (malingerers)

- ✔ reduced attention or attention deficits
- ✔ psychogenic hearing loss (e.g. conversion hysteria)
- ✔ eighth nerve (neural) auditory dysfunction
- ✔ central auditory nervous system dysfunction

- ☐ The relation between OAE and pure tone audiometry findings is highly dependent on the intensity level of the stimuli used to evoke OAE.
- ☐ At this time, OAE findings cannot be reliably correlated with pure tone audiometric threshold levels.

Abnormal OAE and Normal Audiograms

Questions you might ask when you record abnormal OAE from a patient with a normal audiogram. Also, see figures in this ADR chapter which relate OAE and audiogram findings.

☐ Is the audiogram *really* normal?

- Any hearing thresholds that are poorer than about 15 dB HL may be associated with abnormally low OAE amplitude values, even though by clinical guidelines the patient is audiometrically normal.
- Cochlear function is different for the patient with hearing thresholds at 0 dB HL versus the patient with hearing thresholds at 15 or 20 dB HL. Remember the standard deviation for pure tone thresholds is about 5 dB.
- Since OAE reflect cochlear (outer hair cell) status, it is reasonable to expect reduced OAE amplitudes for patients with hearing thresholds at the low end of the audiometrical normal region.

☐ Is the patient *really* otologically normal, even though he has a normal audiogram?

- *Tinnitus.* Does the patient have tinnitus? This is a sign of cochlear dysfunction, and could be related to reduced OAE amplitude values.
- *Middle ear status.* Is middle ear function entirely normal? Obtain a detailed otologic history, and closely examine tympanometry findings, to verify that the middle ear is not involved. Remember, OAE are dependent on the transmission of stimulus energy inward through the middle ear system, and OAE energy outward through the middle ear system. Even under the best of middle ear conditions, energy will be lost coming and going.
- *Ototoxic medications.* Is the patient taking any drugs that could be affecting cochlear (outer hair cell) function, even slightly. Ask about antibiotics, diuretics, and aspirin use.
- *Noise/music exposure.* Does the patient have a history of exposure to high levels of any kind of sound (noise or music)? Cochlear deficits associated with noise/music exposure may produce dramatically reduced OAE amplitudes, or no OAE activity, even though the audiogram is still within the clinically normal region. Be suspicious of noise/music exposure when pure tone audiometry for a patient shows a very slight notch (e.g. 10 to 15 dB) in the 4000 Hz region.

Relationship Between Audiogram and DPOAE

Pure Sensory Hearing Loss

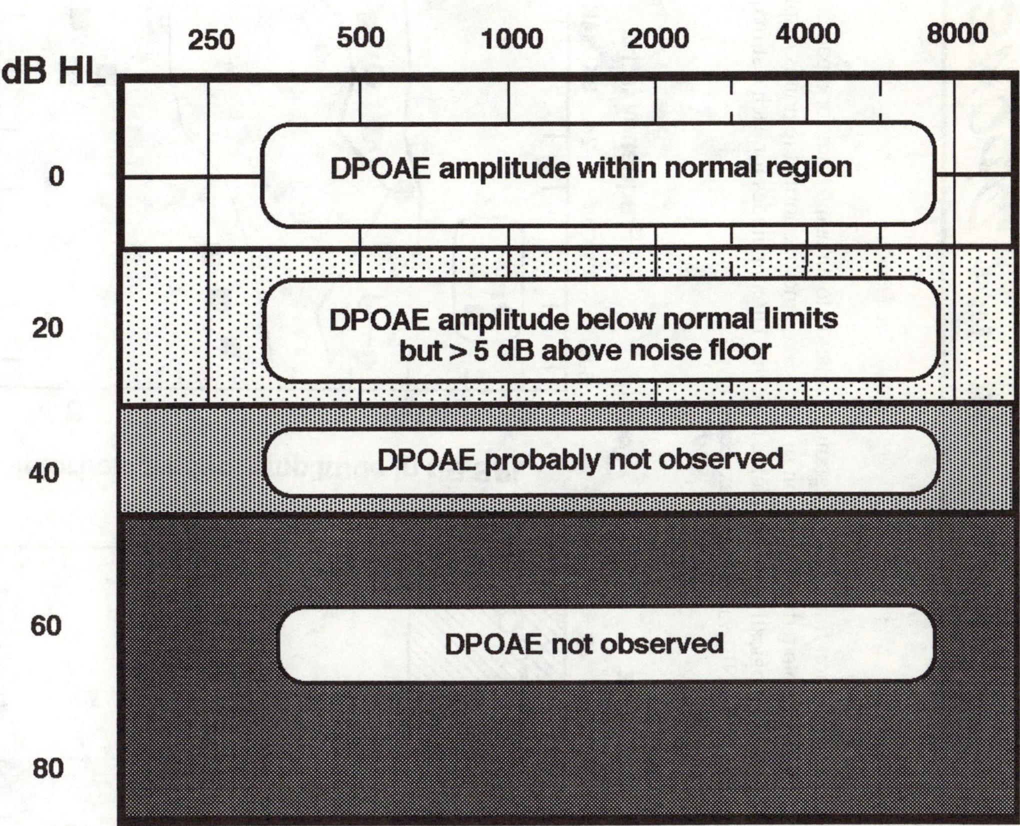

Relationship Between Audiogram and DPOAE

Normal Hearing

An example of distortion product otoacoustic emission findings, a DPgram, in relation to an audiogram for a patient with entirely normal hearing sensivity and otologic function. DP amplitudes are plotted as a function of the f_2 frequency. A normal region is displayed representing the 10th to 90th percentile for 30 young audiologically and otologically normal adults. Note that DP amplitudes for each test frequency (f_2 and f_1 combination) are within the clinic normal region and noise floor (NF) values are at expected levels.

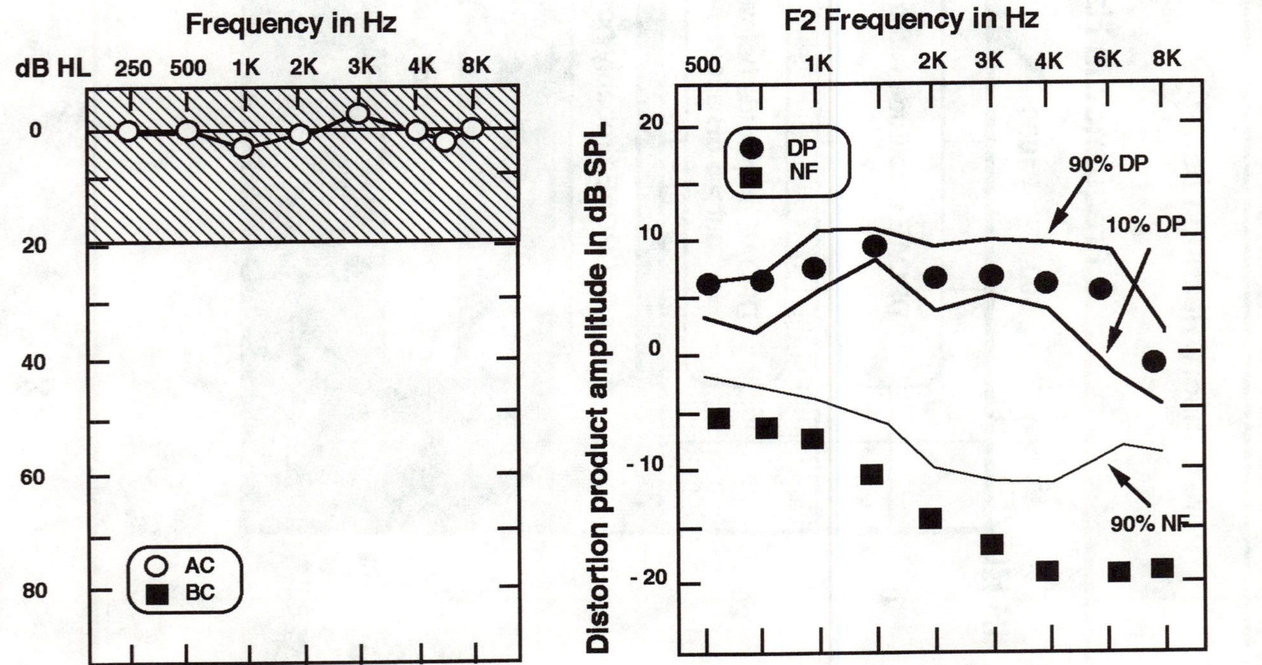

Relationship Between Audiogram and DPOAE

Low Frequency Tinnitus

An example of distortion product otoacoustic emission findings, a DPgram, in relation to an audiogram for a patient with the chief complaint (CC) of low frequency tinnitus that sounded like a motor running. DP amplitudes are plotted as a function of the f_2 frequency. A normal region is displayed representing the 10th to 90th percentile for 30 young audiologically and otologically normal adults. Hearing sensivity was within normal limits, but the audiogram showed a rising configuration. Note that DP amplitudes for lower test frequencies (1000 Hz and below) are equivalent to the noise floor (NF) values (i.e., no DP was recorded). DP amplitude is below the normal region for mid-frequencies, and at the lower limit of the clinical normal region and noise floor (NF) values are at expected levels. Abnormal DP amplitudes may be recorded in persons with hearing levels of 15 dB HL, or worse.

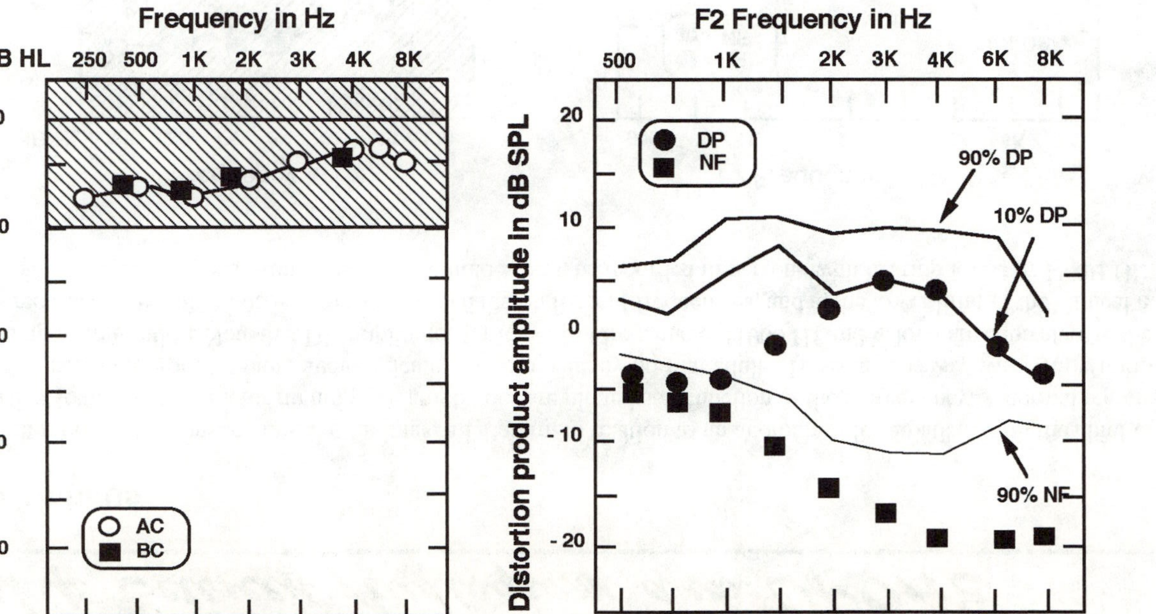

Relationship Between Audiogram and DPOAE

Low Frequency Tinnitus

An example of distortion product otoacoustic emission findings, a DPgram, in relation to an audiogram for a patient with the chief complaint (CC) of low frequency tinnitus that sounded like a motor running. DP amplitudes are plotted as a function of the f_2 frequency. A normal region is displayed representing the 10th to 90th percentile for 30 young audiologically and otologically normal adults. Hearing sensivity was within normal limits, but the audiogram showed a rising configuration. Note that DP amplitudes for lower test frequencies (1000 Hz and below) are equivalent to the noise floor (NF) values (i.e., no DP was recorded). DP amplitude is below the normal region for mid-frequencies, and at the lower limit of the clinical normal region and noise floor (NF) values are at expected levels. Abnormal DP amplitudes may be recorded in persons with hearing levels of 15 dB HL, or worse.

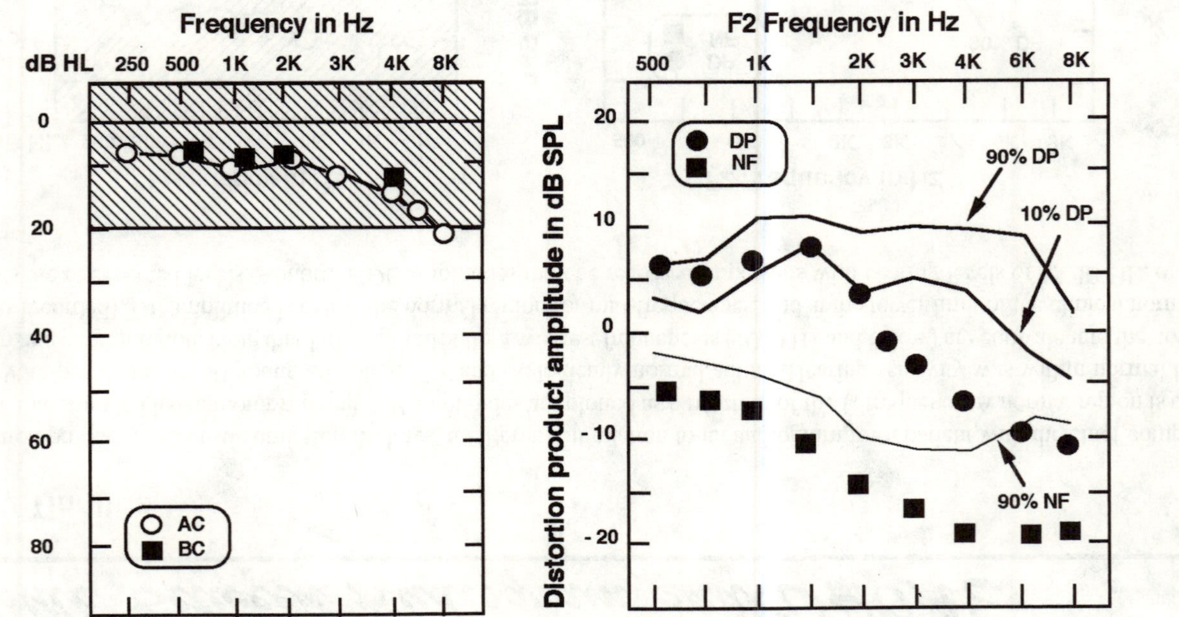

Relationship Between Audiogram and DPOAE

Low Frequency Tinnitus

An example of distortion product otoacoustic emission findings, a DPgram, in relation to an audiogram for a patient with the chief complaint (CC) of low frequency tinnitus that sounded like a motor running. DP amplitudes are plotted as a function of the f_2 frequency. A normal region is displayed representing the 10th to 90th percentile for 30 young audiologically and otologically normal adults. Hearing sensivity was within normal limits, but the audiogram showed a rising configuration. Note that DP amplitudes for lower test frequencies (1000 Hz and below) are equivalent to the noise floor (NF) values (i.e., no DP was recorded). DP amplitude is below the normal region for mid-frequencies, and at the lower limit of the clinical normal region and noise floor (NF) values are at expected levels. Abnormal DP amplitudes may be recorded in persons with hearing levels of 15 dB HL, or worse.

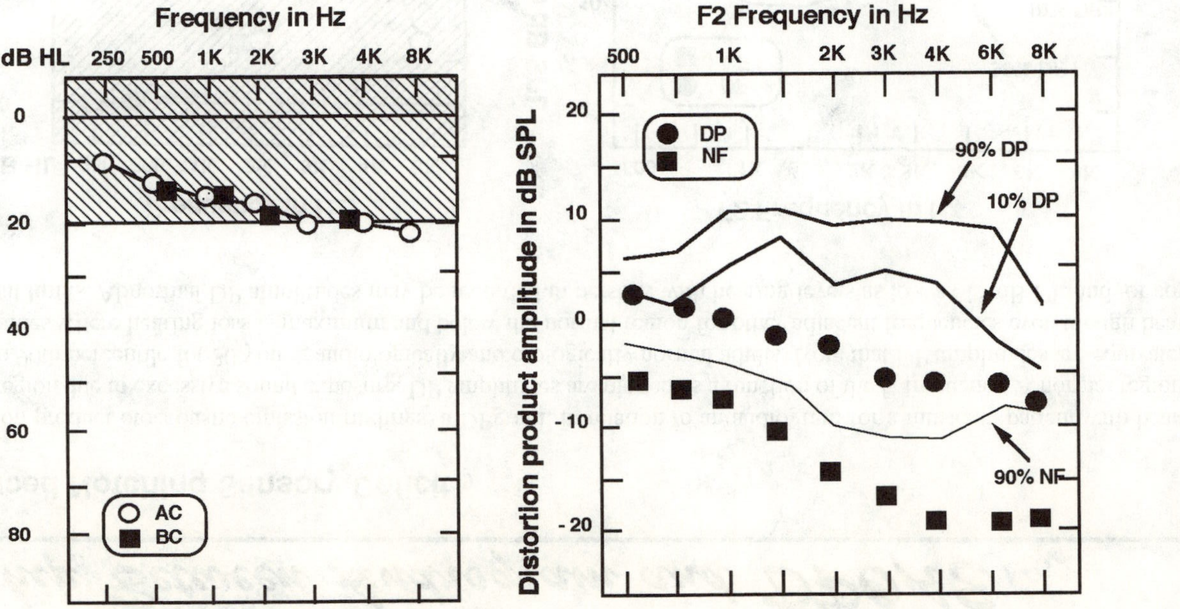

Relationship Between Androgram and DPOAE

Mild Noise-induced Notching Sensory Deficit

An example of distortion product otoacoustic emission findings, a DPgram, in relation to an audiogram for a musician patient with hearing sensivity deficit in the 4000 Hz region due to excessive sound exposure. DP amplitudes are plotted as a function of the f_2 frequency. A normal region is displayed representing the 10th to 90th percentile for 30 young audiologically and otologically normal adults. Note that DP amplitudes are equivalent to the normal noise floor (NF) values where hearing loss is maximum and below the normal region for other adjacent frequencies even though hearing sensitivity is well within normal limits. Abnormal DP amplitudes may be recorded in persons with hearing levels as low as 15 dB HL and, of course, worse.

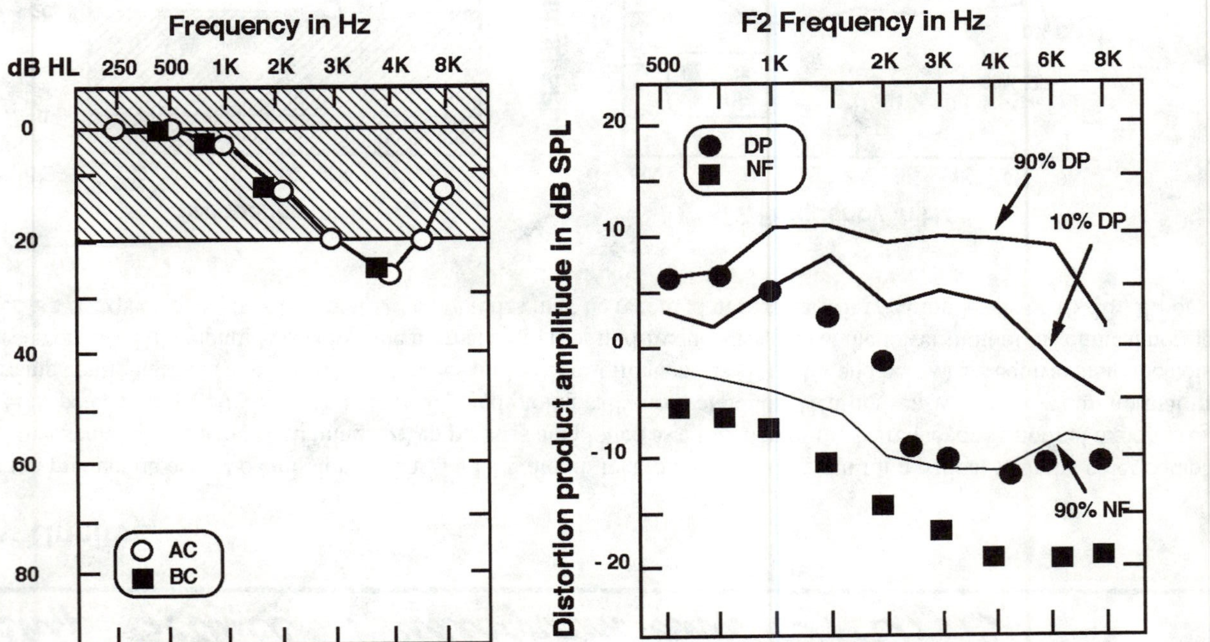

Relationship Between Audiogram and DPOAE

Child with Pervasive Developmental Disorder and Hyperacusis

An example of distortion product otoacoustic emission findings, a DPgram, in relation to an audiogram for a 16-year-old male evaluated for central auditory processing disorder (CAPD) with the complaint of hypersensitivity to sounds and "auditory defensiveness." DP amplitudes are plotted as a function of the f_2 frequency. Note that DP amplitudes are extremely high (greater than normal limits) for stimulus frequencies above 4000 Hz.

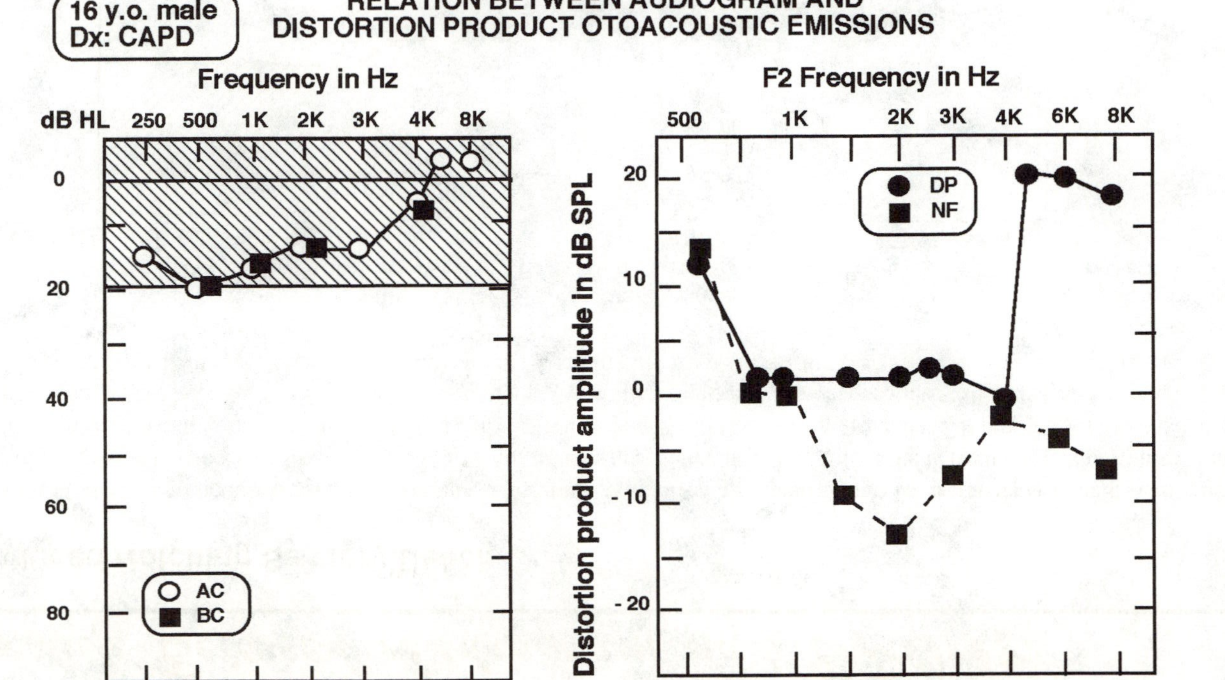

CHAPTER 6

Electrocochleography (ECochG)

In This ADR Chapter

Perspective

The first of the auditory evoked responses to be "discovered," electrocochleography, has, during the past 60-plus years, gone through cycles of clinical popularity and, conversely, confinement to the laboratory. Today, many audiologists apply ECochG in the neurodiagnostic evaluation of Ménièr's disease, during neurophysiologic monitoring of auditory system function intraoperatively, and as an adjunct to ABR in neurodiagnosis of cochlear and retrocochlear disorders of the auditory system.

Most of the principles of ECochG measurement have changed little since the 1940s and 1950s. Electrode design has, however, improved and the commercial availability of electrodes has expanded in recent years. This is fortuitous for clinical applications, because the inverting (ear level) electrode is the most important component of successful ECochG recording. Audiologists now have easy access to extratympanic, tympanic membrane, and transtympanic electrode options, and a variety of evoked systems for recording auditory evoked responses, including ECochG. Clinical uses of ECochG are clearly defined. An ECochG CPT code is recognized by third-party payors. All of these factors have contributed to the inclusion of ECochG in the diagnostic audiology test battery of the 1990s.

FOUNDATIONS OF ECochG

Classic Quote

Wever and Bray on ECochG

In 1930, Ernest Glen Wever and Charles W. Bray, both of Princeton University, published the following paper (yes, this is the whole paper . . . you have time to read it all) entitled "Auditory Nerve Impulses." It describes the ECochG.

"By placing an electrode on the cat's auditory nerve near the medulla, with a grounded electrode elsewhere on the body, and leading the action currents through an amplifier to a telephone receiver, the writers have found that sound stimuli applied to the ear of the animal are reproduced in the receiver with great fidelity. Speech is easily understandable. Simple tones, as from tuning forks, are received at frequencies which, so far as the observer can determine by ear, are identical with the original. Frequencies as high as 3000 cycles per second are audible.

"Numerous checks have been used to guard against the possibility of artifact. No response was obtained when the active electrode was placed on any other tissue. After destruction by pithing of the cochlea on the electrode side, the intensity of the response was diminished; after destruction of the cochlea on the other side as well, the response ceased. However, the possibility is still conceivable that these results are due to purely mechanical action of the nerve, which is brought about by mechanical vibrations transmitted from the cochlear structure acting as a special receptor and transmitter. Further experiments are in progress."

Source: Wever EG & Bray CW. (1930) *Science 71:* p. 215.

Clinical Concept

ECochG Applications

Application	Rationale
☐ Enhancement of ABR wave I	✔ ECochG parameters maximize the AP (wave I) amplitude ✔ A clear wave I is very important in neurodiagnostic ABR recordings ✔ Wave I permits calculation of interwave latency values ✔ Interwave latencies are not seriously influenced by peripheral hearing status
☐ Diagnosis of Ménière's disease	✔ Ménière's disease is characterized by an abnormally large ECochG SP component ✔ A clear and repeatable SP and AP are recorded ✔ SP and AP amplitudes are calculated from a common baseline ✔ The SP/AP ratio is calculated ✔ The patient's SP/AP ratio is compared for the ear suspected of Ménière's involved vs. the opposite ear ✔ The patient's SP/AP ratio is compared for the ear suspected of Ménière's involved vs. normative data
☐ Intraoperative monitoring	✔ ECochG parameters maximize the AP (wave I) amplitude ✔ A clear wave I is very important in intraoperative ABR recordings ✔ The AP (wave I) component is a measure of peripheral (cochlear) status ✔ A large wave I (e.g., > 0.5 μV) can be recorded quickly (< 1 minute) in patients with serious hearing loss ✔ Wave I permits calculation of interwave latency values ✔ Interwave latencies are not seriously influenced by peripheral hearing status ✔ A transtympanic technique (Schwaber & Hall, 1990) is optimal for the intraoperative application of ECochG

Classic Quote

Lempert on ECochG

As early as 1947 and 1950, Julius Lempert (an otologist) and colleagues, among them two prominent auditory physiologists from Princeton (Ernest Glen Wever and Merle Lawrence), recognized the optimal site for ECochG recordings and wisely predicted the clinical value of ECochG. Also, see Classic Quote: Wever and Bray on ECochG in this ADR chapter and Mover and Oscillator: Merle Lawrence in ADR Chapter 1.

"Our observations thus confirm those previously reported that the round window membrane is the only suitable location for the electrode." (Lempert et al., 1947, p. 67) . . . . Here we envisage their being used both for general diagnosis and for surgical guidance." (Lempert et al., 1947, p. 65)

"It is possible, as we have found, to pass a needle electrode through the tympanic membrane and to make contact with the bony promontory beyond. The needle electrode then may be maintained safely in position for the time necessary for a series of cochlear response tests. After the needle is withdrawn, the drum membrane heals perfectly in a short time." (Lempert et al., 1947, p. 310)

Source: Lempert J, Wever EG, Lawrence M. The cochleogram and its clinical application. (1959) *Arch Otolaryngol 51:* 307–311.

Historical Perspective

Important Developments and Discoveries in ECochG

Year	Investigator(s)	Finding
1930	Wever & Bray	Cochlear microphonic (CM) discovered in animal
1935	Fromm et al.	CM recorded from round window in human through tympanic membrane (TM) perforation
1935	Davis & Derbyshire	Action potential (AP) recorded from round window in animal and analyzed by superposition
1939	Andreev et al.	CM recorded from round window in human through TM perforation
1941	Perlman & Case	CM recorded from round window in human through TM perforation and photographed
1947	Lempert et al.	CM recorded from round window in human through TM perforation
1950	Davis	Summating potential (SP) discovered in animal
1951	Dawson	Averager for evoked responses
1953	Tasaki	Action potentials (APs) in single fibers of auditory nerve in animal
1954	Goldstein (Robert)	SP in animal
1954	Tasaki et al.	SP in animal
1959	Ruben, Berlin, et al.	Round window CM in human with hearing impairment (first real clinical application of EcochG, but restricted to operating room setting)
1960	Ruben et al.	Round window AP in human with ear pathology
1961	Clark	Description of average response computer (ARC) which was a forerunner of later evoked response systems
1963	Ruben et al.	Direct 8th nerve AP recorded in human patients
1965	Kiang	Classic monograph on discharge patterns of auditory nerve
1967	Yoshie et al.	Promontory CM in human with transtympanic (TT) electrode (application of ECochG in the clinic vs. operating room setting)
1967	Yoshie et al.	AP with ear canal electrode (an extratympanic, noninvasive ECochG technique)
1967	Portmann et al.	Promontory AP with TT electrode averaged in human
1967	Sohmer & Feinmesser	AP with earlobe electrode (the ABR was also described as an aside, and not really "discovered")
1968	Aran et al.	Promontory AP recorded in human with TT electrode (some clinicians still use their technique)
1968	Yoshie promontory	AP recorded in human with TT electrode (normative data become available)

1969	Aran, Portmann, et al.	Promontory AP recorded in children with TT electrode (remember, the ABR had not quite been discovered at this time)
1970	Coats	AP recorded in human with external ear canal electrode (you can still purchase the "Coats butterfly electrode")
1971	Salomon, Elberling	AP recorded in human with external ear canal electrode
1971	Jewett & Williston	ABR discovered but confirmation of clinical application as an electrophysiologic audiologic procedure still a few years off so excitement about EcochG in hearing assessment continues
1972	Cullen, Berlin et al.	AP recorded in human with tympanic membrane (TM) electrode
1974	Coats	CM, SP, and AP recorded in human with ear canal electrode
1974	Eggermont	ECochG applied in the diagnosis of Ménière's disease
1974	Eggermont	Frequency-specific response with masking
1974	Berlin et al.	ECochG recorded from TM in human patients
1974	Hecox, Galambos	Description of ABR in infants and children
1977	Gibson et al.	Further description of ECochG in diagnosis of Ménière's disease
1977	Arlinger	Responses recorded with bone conduction stimulation
1979	Eggermont	Another report of ECochG in Méinère's disease
1981	Coats	A series of articles in *Archives of Otolaryngology* on ECochG in Ménière's disease with normative data
1985	Ferraro et al.	Applied in management of Ménière's disease
1985	Mori et al.	Management of Ménière's disease
1985	Yanz, Dodds	Improved ear canal electrode for use in human recordings
1987	Stypulkowski & Staller	A TM electrode for use in humans late 1980s TIPtrode™ becomes commercially available
1988	Ruth et al.	Ear canal vs. TM electrodes in human
1990	Schwaber & Hall	A simple TT electrode technique
1995	Bio-Logic, Inc.	An FDA-approved tympanic membrane electrode
1996	Durrant et al.	Sensitivity and specificity of ECochG in Ménière's disease

Historical Biographical Sketch

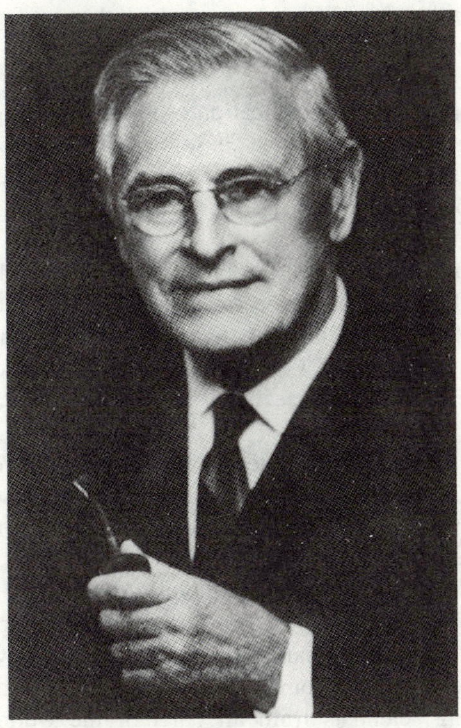

Hallowell Davis, M.D.

HALLOWELL DAVIS, "the Father of Auditory Evoked Responses"

"Hallowell Davis, M.D., former director of Research at Central Institute for the Deaf and Professor at Washington University, died Saturday (August 22, 1992 . . . He was 96).

After graduating from Harvard College in 1918 and earning his M.D. From Harvard Medical School in 1922, he [Dr. Davis] spent a year at Cambridge University (England) where, in the pioneering laboratory of Lord Adrian, he became an electrophysiologist. From 1923 to 1946 he held various appointments at Harvard College and Harvard Medical School. During this period he studied the electrical properties of the basic nerve impulse, the electrical responses of the inner ear and auditory nerve, and rhythmic electrical activity of the human brain.

He played a key role in the development of the electroencephalogram (EEG) in the period 1934 to 1941. The first unmistakable EEG activity seen in this country was recorded from Dr. Davis's scalp by his students using amplifiers modified from his other electrophysiological equipment.

From the beginning he was relating his physiological findings on the inner ear and auditory nerve to our ability to hear. In 1938 with S.S. Stevens he published the book, *Hearing: Its Psychology and Physiology,* in which they set forth as many such relations as were then known.

Dr. Davis was a pioneer in the application of rapidly developing electronic amplifiers to other problems related to hearing. These included the measurement of normal and impaired hearing, the assessment of the effects of noise on hearing, the design of hearing aids, and various problems in speech communication.

Dr. Davis came to St. Louis from the faculty of Harvard Medical School in 1946 to establish a research program and research department at Central Institute. He also held appointments at Washington University School of Medicine as Professor of Physiology and as Research Professor of Otolaryngology, with an additional appointment as Lecturer in the Department of Speech and Hearing.

Dr. Davis brought to Central Institute a new concept for a research program oriented toward problems of hearing and deafness. It combined the scientific methods of electrophysiology, behavioral psychology, and electroacoustic engineering in such a way that the respective specialists could complement each other's knowledge and experience to find new solutions to these problems. At the same time he edited the book *Hearing and Deafness: A Guide for Laymen*, which also employed a multidisciplinary approach. With co-editor S. Richard Silverman, the book grew in three subsequent editions to be a popular textbook for students in the new para-medical specialty of audiology. Many young scientists from all parts of the world learned of Dr. Davis's research, and a steady stream during the subsequent years came to St. Louis to study this approach by observing and assisting in the research program.

A memorial service was held for Dr. Davis on Sunday, September 13, 1992 in Graham Chapel at Washington University. He has donated his inner ears to medical science as part of the 'old time ears' program and was cremated. Burial of his ashes was in the State of Maine.

He is survived by his wife, Nancy Vose Davis, a brother Horace Davis, sisters Sarah Pope and Esther Brown, a son Allen Y. Davis of Colorado Springs, a daughter Anna N. Hessey of Bronxville, New York, a son Rowland H. Davis of Laguna Beach, California, four grandchildren and four great-grandchildren."

Source: Reprinted from *Aro News*, Fall 1992, with permission.

ADR Note: The first ADR author used the third edition of *Hearing and Deafness* (1970) in his Introduction to Audiology class at Northwestern University, taught by Earl Harford.

ECochG RECORDING

ECochG Measurement Strategy

Flowchart summarizing a clinical electrocochleography (ECochG) measurement strategy.

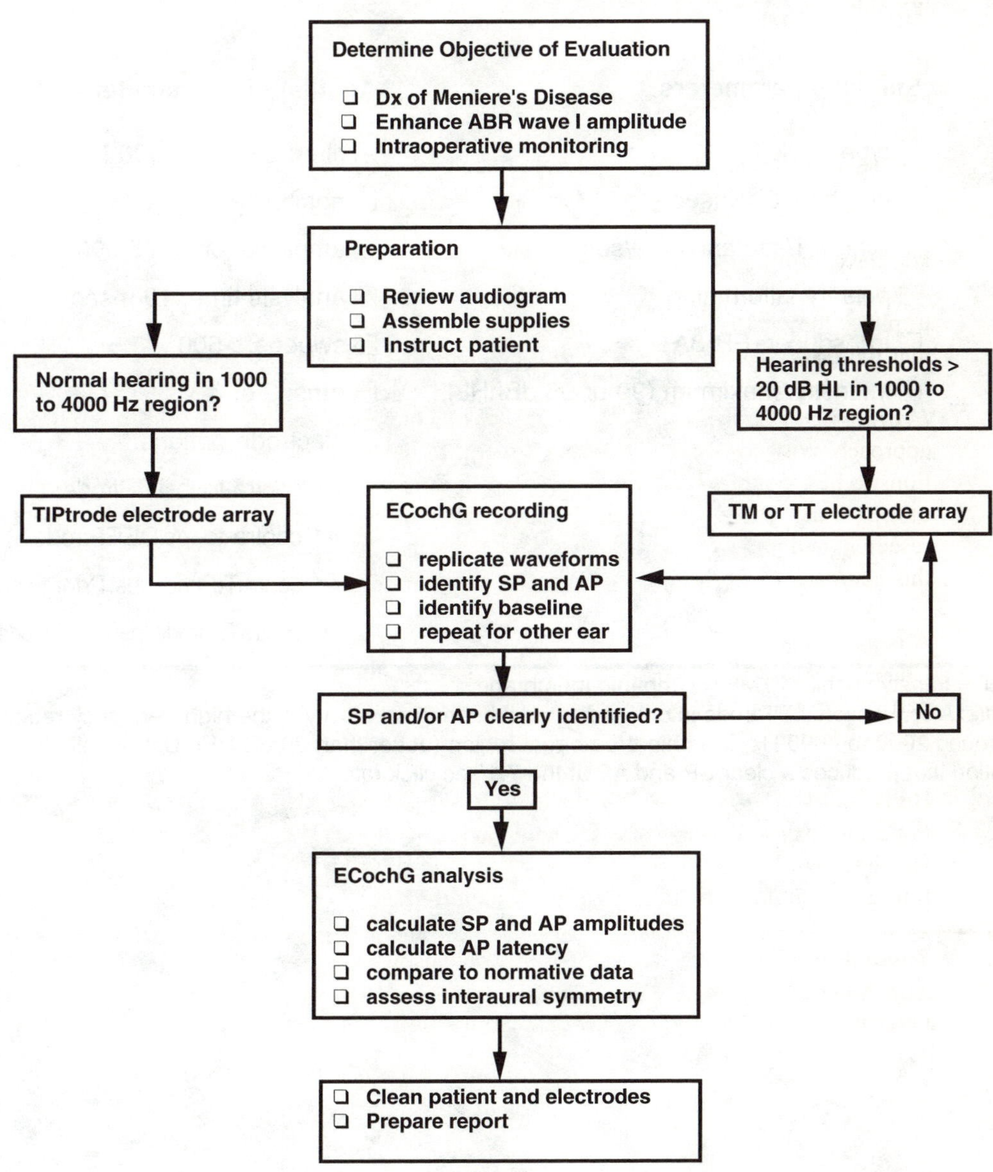

Protocol

Electrocochleography (ECochG) Protocol at the Vanderbilt Audiology Clinics

OBJECTIVE: To record a clear and reliable summating potential (SP) and action potential (AP) for right and left ear stimulation, to calculate the SP/AP ratio for each ear, and to categorize the SP/AP ratio as normal versus abnormal based on symmetrical and normal expectations.

PROTOCOL

Stimulus parameters

- ☐ type: click
- ☐ duration: 0.1 msec
- ☐ rate: 7.1/sec *and* 99.9/sec
- ☐ polarity: alternating
- ☐ transducer: ER-3A
- ☐ intensity: maximum (90 or 95 dBnHL)

Acquisition parameters

- ☐ filter: 5 or 10–1500 Hz
- ☐ notch filter: none
- ☐ amplification: ×75,000
- ☐ analysis time: 10 msec
- ☐ sweeps: >500
- ☐ runs: 3 or 4
- ☐ electrode options:*
  - ✓ contra-to-ipsiTIPtrode
  - ✓ contra-to-ipsiDEEPtrode
  - ✓ contraTIPtrode-ipsiTYMPtrode
  - ✓ contraTIPtrode-ipsiTT electrode

*TT = transtympanic; TYMP = tympanic membrane

Note: A conventional TIPtrode is only indicated if hearing sensitivity in the high-frequency region (around 2000 to 4000 Hz) is within the normal region (better than 30 dB HL). Use an electrode option that produces a clear SP and AP at the 7.1/sec click rate.

Protocol

Electrocochleography (ECochG) Protocol and Rationale

Measurement Parameter	Rationale
Stimulus parameters	
☐ type: click	Abrupt onset for synchronous response
☐ duration: 0.1 msec	Onset response; duration is not important
☐ rate: 7.1/sec *and* 99.9/sec	Slow rate for enhanced AP component; fast rate to differentiate SP (still robust) from AP (deteriorated by rate increase)
☐ polarity: alternating	Minimizes the cochlear microphonic
☐ transducer: ER-3A	The usual advantages of insert earphones (see another table in this ADR chapter) plus TIPtrode™ is an insert earphone, and insert earplug keeps the TYMPtrode and transtympanic needle electrode wire in place
☐ intensity: maximum (90 or 95 dBnHL)	Response is largest; SP component is not detectable at intensities levels below about 50 dB
Acquisition parameters	
☐ filter: 5 or 10–1500 Hz	Low frequencies included to enhance the DC potential contributing to the SP component; don't need the real high frequencies to resolve response
☐ notch filter: none	Never really filters out 60 Hz electrical interference and higher frequency harmonics of 60 Hz
☐ amplification: ×75,000 or less	The higher the ECochG amplitude (e.g., with a TT electrode) the less amplification
☐ runs: 3 or 4	Must verify repeatablity of the sometimes somewhat elusive SP component
☐ analysis time: 5 msec usually	Need to capture only the first few wave components (mostly SP and AP); short time offers better resolution of SP vs. AP
☐ sweeps: 50 to >500	Few sweeps usually needed for TT electrode (large response) and more responses for TIPtrode™ technique
☐ electrodes	
✓ contraTIPtrode-ipsiTT electrode	Records the best possible ECochG
✓ contraTIPtrode-ipsiTYMPtrode	Ideal choice (noninvasive) for audiologist
✓ contraDEEPtrode-ipsiDEEPtrode	Uses regular TIPtrode, but deeper in EAC
✓ contraTIPtrode-ipsiTIPtrode	Easy to get and easy to use

Insert Earphone and TIPtrode-type Electrode

Components of the ER-3A "insert" earphone (*top*) from the audiometer or evoked response system (*left*) to the patient (*right*). Modification of the ER-3A as TIPtrode™ for ECochG or ABR recording. The stimulus is delivered as usual. In addition, gold foil covering the foam insert contacting the wall of the external ear canal detects the evoked response. An electrode wire is coupled to the gold foil with a specially designed alligator clip, and then leads to an electrode box or strip.

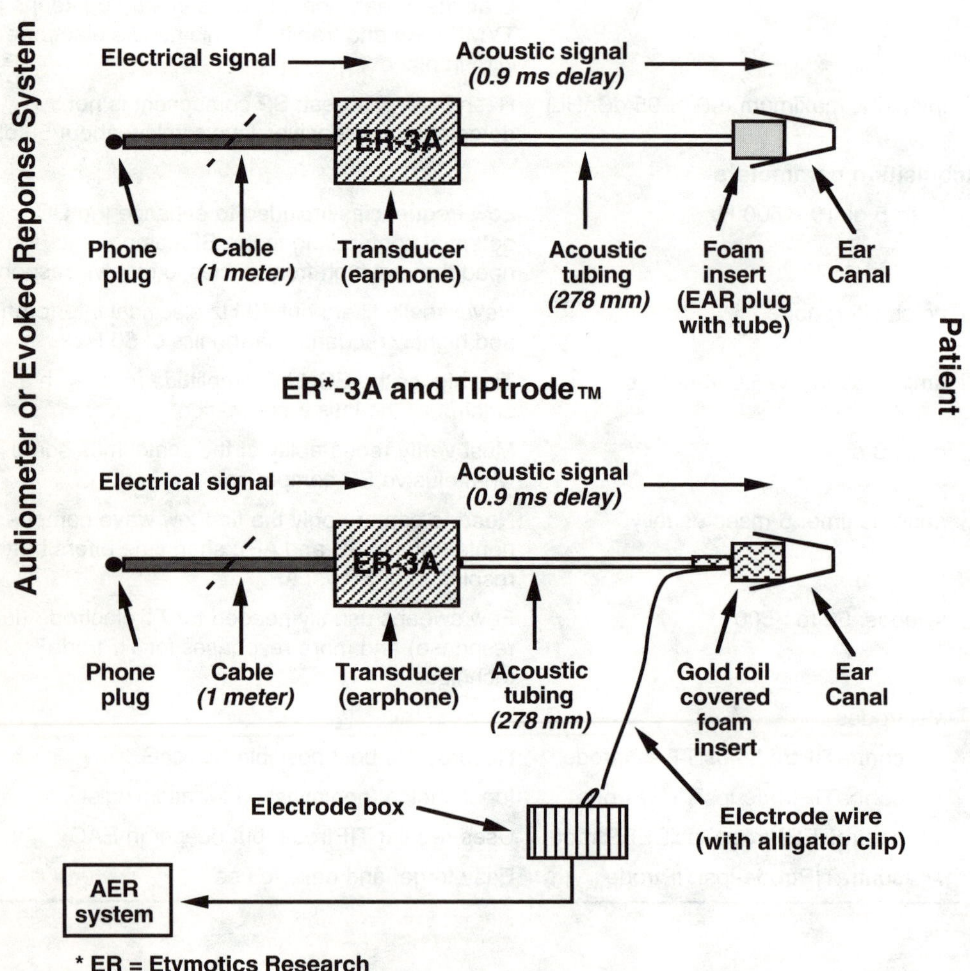

* ER = Etymotics Research

Technical Tip

ECochG Measurement

MEASUREMENT

- ☐ Obtain at least three replicated waveforms for better hearing or "uninvolved" ear at rate of 7.1/sec. Verify the presence of the SP component at 99.9/sec if necessary.
- ☐ Repeat for poorer hearing or "suspect" ear.

ANALYSIS

- ☐ Assure replicability of SP and AP among 3 or 4 runs of at least 500 stimuli each.
- ☐ Verify SP presence and amplitude with fast click rate (99.0/sec).
- ☐ For each rate, add all waveforms together digitally.
- ☐ Calculate SP and AP amplitude from common stable baseline.
- ☐ Calculate SP and AP ratio.
- ☐ Assess interaural asymmetry in SP/AP ratio (report difference of >10%).
- ☐ Assess SP/AP value at 7.1/sec rate versus normative expectations.
- ☐ TIPtrode: normative value = <50%
- ☐ DEEPtrode: normative value = <45%
- ☐ TYMPtrode: normative value = <35%
- ☐ Transtympanic (TT) electrode: normative value = <30%

Step-by-Step

Protocol for Recording ECochG in the Clinic

☐ Assemble all supplies

- electrodes (sterilized for transtympanic needles)
- tape, conducting paste or gel, light source

☐ Review patient's audiogram

- is there hearing loss in the 2000 to 4000 Hz region?
- is there asymmetry or an "involved" ear?

☐ Instruct the patient

- briefly explain reason for assessment
- describe electrode placement
- encourage the patient to relax during the test

☐ Select inverting electrode type (see figures in this ADR chapter)

- *TIPtrode* is an option if hearing is normal in the 2000 to 4000 Hz region.
- *Tympanic membrane (TM) electrode* if there is a hearing loss in the 2000 to 4000 Hz region, or if a clear SP and/or AP component is not recorded with a TIPtrode. A transtympanic membrane electrode is an option if otologic support is handy.
- *Transtympanic (TT) electrode* if there is a hearing loss in the 2000 to 4000 Hz region, and if an AP and/or SP component is not recorded with the tympanic membrane electrode. Use a tympanic membrane electrode if there is no otologic support handy.

☐ Select measurement protocol

- Decide whether you will record a combined ABR/ECochG or just an ECochG.
- Verify stimulus and acquisition parameters (see tables in this ADR chapter).

☐ Data collection

- Record ECochG from normal, or least involved, ear first.
- Keep record of ECochG files.
- Attempt to identify SP and AP components while averaging first run.

- Modify test protocol immediately if either SP and/or AP is not identified. See ECochG Troubleshooting in this ADR chapter.
- Record at least two, and preferably three or four, replications of ECochG for first test ear.
- Repeat this process for the second ear.
- Superimpose all waveforms for each ear.

☐ Data analyses

- Verify presence of SP and AP components.
- Sum replicated waveforms, keeping all replications intact.
- Calculate SP and AP amplitudes. See figure in this ADR chapter.
- Calculate SP/AP ratio for each ear.
- Analyze SP/AP ratio for interaural asymmetry.
- Compare patient's SP/AP ratio with normative data.
- Mark all ECochG components.

☐ Post-test duties

- Clean and discharge patient. This should be done as soon as usable ECochG data are confirmed for each ear.
- Print all waveforms (replicated and summed).
- Prepare report.
- Clean (or dispose of) electrodes and clean the test area.

ECochG Recording Electrode Options

Noninvasive Electrodes

Illustration of two noninvasive electrode options for electrocochleography (ECochG) recording. The TIPtrode™ is shown in the top portion, whereas a tympanic membrane electrode (TYMPtrode) is shown in the lower portion. The TYMPtrode makes direct contact with the tympanic membrane. It is held in place with an ER-3A foam insert, and connected via a wire to a conventional electrode pin. The ratio of the ECochG summating potential (SP) to action potential (AP), the SP/AP ratio, varies depending on the electrode type. The ratio is larger as the electrode is located farther away from the cochlea.

Recording electrode options: noninvasive

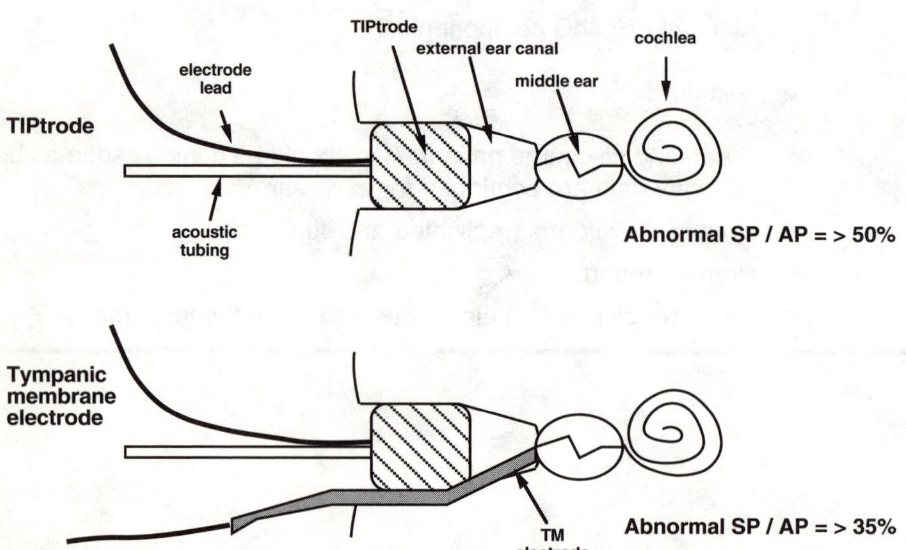

ECochG Recording Electrode Options

Invasive Electrodes

Illustration of a transtympanic (TT) needle electrode option for electrocochleography (ECochG) recording. A commercially available, noninsulated, subdermal, needle electrode (with a needle shaft of about 14 mm) is ideal. Using bayonette forceps with an operating microscope view, the TT electrode is inserted through the inferior portion of the tympanic membrane, with the tip placed on the promontory on the medial wall of the middle ear. In the clinic, the tympanic membrane is numbed with a local anesthetic. This is not necessary in the operating room after general anesthesia is administered. The TT electrode wire is held in place with a compressed ER-3A foam insert and connected via the wire to a conventional electrode pin. ECochG recordings have optimal quality and amplitude with this TT technique. See Schwaber and Hall (1990) for details on placement.

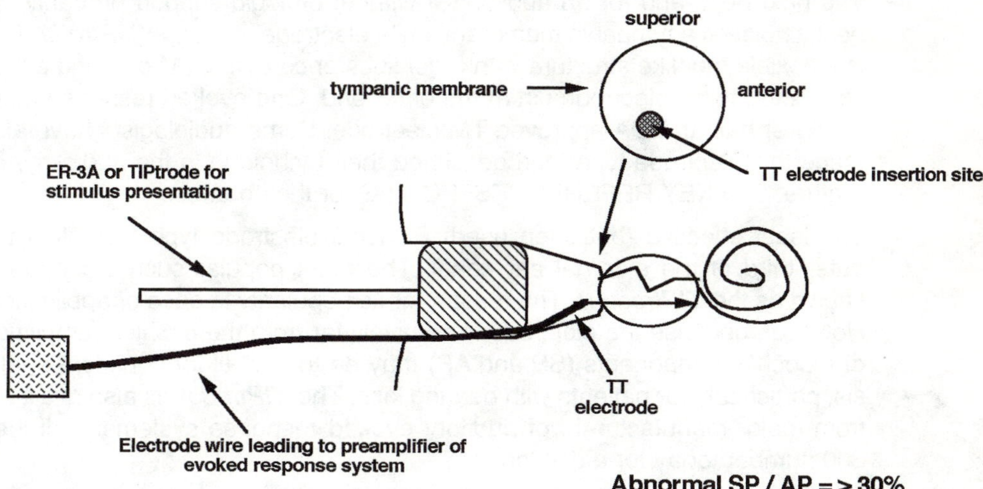

* uninsulated subdermal needle (approximately 14 mm in length) available from evoked response manufacturers

Technical Tip

ECochG Electrodes

Also, see Advantages and Disadvantages of ECochG Electrodes in this ADR chapter.

The noninverting electrode for ECochG recording is often a disc-type electrode located on the forehead, or a spring-loaded earclip disc electrode located on both sides of the earlobe of the ear contralateral to the stimulus.

There are three inverting electrode options.

- The best possible choice for a robust and reliable ECochG is a *transtympanic needle* placed onto the promontory. Use an uninsulated stainless steel needle electrode with a shaft of about 14 mm. This electrode type is available from major evoked response manufacturers. Check out their catalogs. See Schwaber and Hall (1990) for details on recording ECochG with a simplified TT electrode technique.
- The next best, and for an audiologist without otologic support probably the best, choice is a tympanic membrane style electrode, or the *TYMPtrode*. This is a flexible tubelike structure with a gel substance at the TM end and a wire connected to an electrode pin at the other end. One evoked response manufacturer has an FDA-approved TM electrode. Some audiologists have also made this electrode type, and described their technique in the audiology literature. See KEY REFERENCES: ECochG for their names.
- The least effective (but often used) ECochG electrode type fits within the outer third of the external ear canal. The most popular such electrode is known as the *TIPtrode*™. The reason for its popularity is ease of application. However, because the electrode is relatively far from the cochlea, amplitude of ECochG components (SP and AP) may be too small for confident analysis, particularly for patients with hearing loss. The *TIPtrode*™is also available from major manufacturers of auditory evoked response systems. Call their 800 number today for a catalog.

Step-by-Step

ECochG Recording with TIPtrode™ Electrode Technique

- ☐ Follow general test protocol for preparation, patient instruction, and test parameters.
- ☐ Closely inspect the ear canal for debris and any evidence of pathology.
- ☐ Apply all electrodes (discs) except the TIPtrode™.
- ☐ Apply a small amount of abrasive (e.g., OmniPrep) onto a cue tip.
- ☐ Gently but firmly abrade the ear canal meatus in a circular manner, never letting the cotton on the cue tip get out of sight within the ear canal.
- ☐ No conducting gel is required on the TIPtrode™.
- ☐ Compress a fresh TIPtrode™.
- ☐ Use a pediatric sized TIPtrode™ for female, or otherwise small, ears.
- ☐ Insert a fresh compressed TIPtrode™ into the ear canal attempting to make the lateral end of the TIPtrode™ flush with the outer edge of the external ear canal meatus.
- ☐ Plug the acoustic tubing from the ER-3A transducer into the stalk tube of the TIPtrode™.
- ☐ Plug the TIPtrode™ pin into the appropriate electrode box recepticle.
- ☐ Immediately verify electrode impedance for all electrodes.
- ☐ Impedance for all electrodes, including the TIPtrode™, should be less than 5 K ohms.
- ☐ Begin presenting stimulation to TIPtrode™ ear.
- ☐ Inspect waveform for AP component in the 1.5 to 2.0 msec region.
- ☐ AP amplitude should be about 0.5 μV in normal hearing (at least in the 1000 to 4000 Hz region, or even in mild hearing loss).
- ☐ If a reliable AP component is not observed, verify all electrode connections and reinspect the patient's audiogram.
- ☐ If no AP is observed after appropriate trouble-shooting, consider using a TM or TT electrode design.
- ☐ Proceed with ECochG measurement and analysis.

Step-by-Step

EcochG Recording with a Tympanic Membrane (TMPtrode) Electrode Technique

- ☐ Follow general test protocol for preparation, patient instruction, and test parameters.
- ☐ Closely inspect the ear canal for debris and any evidence of pathology.
- ☐ Apply all electrodes (discs) except the tympanic membrane electrode, and plug these electrode pins into the appropriate electrode box receptacles.
- ☐ Instruct the patient on the proposed procedure, and ask him to report whatever sensation he has (e.g., tickle, discomfort, coughing reflex, pain, pressure).
- ☐ Ask the patient to report when he senses that the electrode is resting on the TM.
- ☐ Have the patient turn onto his side with the test ear upward (employ the force of gravity as you insert the electrode).
- ☐ Apply conducting gel to the TM end of the electrode, if recommended by the manufacturer.
- ☐ Begin inserting a clean TM electrode gradually down the ear canal.
- ☐ Continue to insert the TM electrode as you question the patient on his or her sensations, and you note any changes in the "feel" of the electrode.
- ☐ Once you and/or the patient sense that the electrode is resting on the TM, secure the electrode lead temporarily with a finger.
- ☐ Grasp a compressed foam insert plug, or TIPtrode™, perhaps with bayonette forceps, and insert into the ear canal. Pediatric-sized foam inserts fit best with women and other persons with small ear canals.
- ☐ Allow the foam insert earplug to expand against the electrode lead.
- ☐ Tap the electrode lead and ask the patient to report any sensation. The patient should hear a sound associated with the tapping if the electrode is resting on the TM.
- ☐ Plug the acoustic tubing from the ER-3A transducer into the stalk tube of the insert earplug (or TIPtrode™).
- ☐ Plug the tympanic membrane electrode pin into the appropriate electrode box recepticle.
- ☐ Immediately verify electrode impedance for all electrodes.
- ☐ Don't be alarmed if the impedance for the TM electrode is excessively high (>20 K ohms).
- ☐ Begin presenting stimulation to tympanic membrane electrode ear.
- ☐ Inspect waveform for AP component in the 1.5 to 2.0 msec region.
- ☐ AP amplitude should exceed 1.0 μV, even in mild to moderate hearing loss.
- ☐ If a reliable AP component is not observed, withdraw the TM electrode and reinsert as described above.
- ☐ If no AP is observed on the second attempt, remove TM electrode and inspect closely for any evidence of damage. Replace if condition is in doubt.
- ☐ Proceed with ECochG measurement and analysis.

Step-by-Step

ECochG Recording with a Transtympanic (TT) Electrode Technique

- ☐ Follow general test protocol for preparation, patient instruction, and test parameters.
- ☐ Apply all electrodes (discs) except the transtympanic electrode, and plug into the appropriate electrode box receptacles.
- ☐ Under microscope, apply anesthetic (phenol) to the region of the tympanic membrane that will receive the needle.
- ☐ Grasp a short, stainless steel, uninsulated, subdermal needle electrode (available from most manufacturers) at the needle end of the electrode cable with bayonette forceps.
- ☐ Insert the tip of the needle through the inferior posterior portion of the tympanic membrane and place against the promontory.
- ☐ Secure the electrode lead temporarily with a finger.
- ☐ Grasp a compressed foam insert plug, or TIPtrode™, with bayonette forceps and insert into the ear canal.
- ☐ Allow the foam insert earplug to expand against the electrode lead.
- ☐ Plug the acoustic tubing from the ER-3A transducer into the stalk tube of the insert earplug (or TIPtrode™).
- ☐ Plug the transtympanic needle electrode pin into the appropriate electrode box recepticle.
- ☐ Immediately verify electrode impedance for all electrodes.
- ☐ Transtympanic electrode impedance should be about 12 K ohms or lower, and impedance for other electrodes should be less than 5 K ohms.
- ☐ Begin presenting stimulation to transtympanic electrode ear.
- ☐ Inspect waveform for AP component in the 1.5 to 2.0 msec region.
- ☐ AP amplitude should be robust (as high as 10 μV in mild-to-moderate hearing loss).
- ☐ Proceed with ECochG measurement and analysis.

ECochG ANALYSIS AND INTERPRETATION

Normative Data

Normal cutoff values for the ECochG summating potential to action potential (SP/AP) ratio.

	Finding	
Electrode location (type)	Normal	Abnormal
Ear canal (TIPtrode™)	0 to 50%	> 50%
Tympanic membrane	0 to 35%	> 35%
Promontory (transtympanic needle)	0 to 30%	> 30%

ECochG Analysis Strategy

Simple technique for analysis of the ratio of the amplitude of the electrocochleography (ECochG) summating potential (SP) versus action potential (AP), as measured from a common baseline. See nearby tables for guidelines on the interpretation of SP/AP amplitude relations.

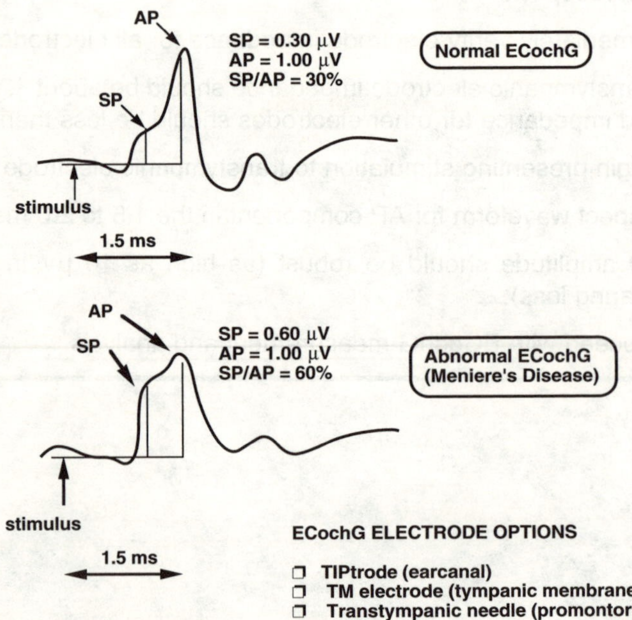

ECochG Analysis

Verification of the SP Component

Two techniques for verifying the presence of the summating potential (SP) component of the ECochG. The top portion shows the prolongation of the SP component with tone burst stimulation. The action potential (AP) occurs only at stimulus onset, whereas the SP component is maintained during stimulation. In the lower portion, the SP is verified by dramatically increasing click stimulus rate. At very high stimulus rates, the AP component is small and delayed in latency, whereas the SP component remains relatively unaffected and, therefore, more easily detected.

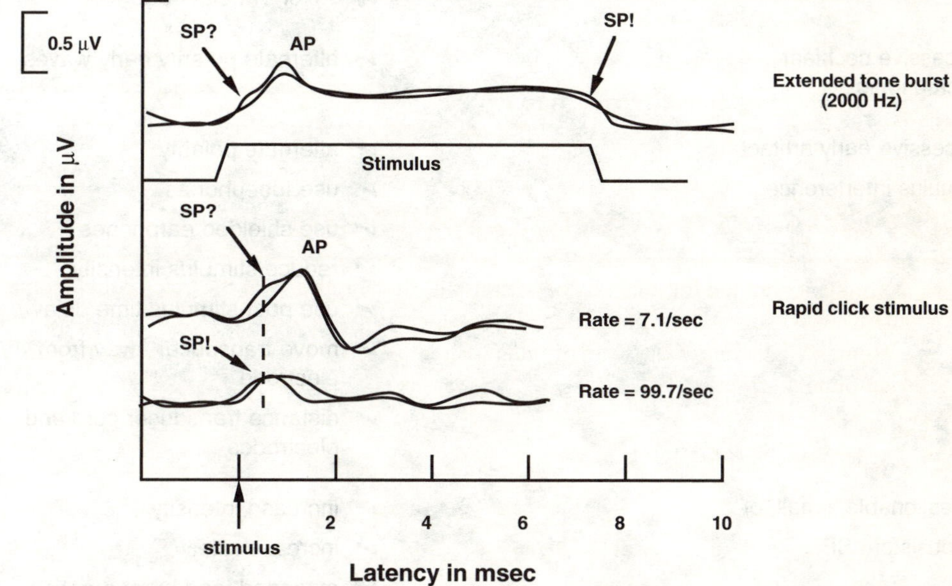

Trouble-Shooting

Electrocochleography (ECochG) Measurement Problems and Solutions

Symptom	Possible Problems	Possible Solutions
No response	No stimulus	✓ listening check
		✓ verify correct transducer
		✓ verify test ear
	Improper electrode	✓ obtain audiogram
		✓ increase stimulus intensity
		✓ TT or TM electrode
Excessive cochlear microphonic		✓ alternate polarity early waves
Excessive early artifact stimulus interference		✓ alternate polarity
		✓ use tubephones
		✓ use shielded earphones
		✓ reduce stimulus intensity
		✓ use post-stimulus time delay
		✓ move transducer away from electrode
		✓ distance transducer cord and electrodes
Questionable, small, or inconsistent SP		✓ increase intensity
		✓ increase rate
		✓ extended tone burst duration
		✓ TT or TM electrode
		✓ lower high-pass filter setting
Questionable, small, or inconsistent AP		✓ increase intensity
		✓ decrease rate
		✓ TT or TM electrode
		✓ additional sweeps
Noisy waveform	Excessive electrical artifact	✓ verify impedance of each electrode
		✓ alter stimulus rate
		✓ increase distance between patient and electrical devices
		✓ lower low-pass filter setting

Electrode Advantages and Disadvantages

Electrode type	Advantages	Disadvantages
Transtympanic needle	✓ very large amplitude for SP and AP components (AP usually > 5 μV)	✓ invasive
	✓ SP and AP reliably recorded even in patients with hearing loss	✓ requires otologic support
	✓ interelectrode impedance fair (usually less than 10K ohms)	✓ placement requires microscope
	✓ rapid test time (large amplitude means few responses need to be averaged)	✓ placement requires TM anesthesic
	✓ clear cutoff for normal vs. abnormal due to invariability in location relative to cochlea	✓ needle should be sterilized
	✓ stable placement when used with insert ear phone E.A.R. Plug (see diagram in this ADR chapter)	
	✓ excellent choice for intraoperative ECochG	
	✓ commercially available from several manufacturers	
Tympanic membrane	✓ large amplitude for SP and AP components (AP usually >1 μV)	✓ limited commercial availability
	✓ SP and AP usually reliably recorded in patients with mild-moderate hearing loss	✓ interelectrode impedance high (can't scrub TM surface . . . don't try!)
	✓ generally reliable cutoff for normal vs. abnormal due to invariability in location relative to cochlea	✓ placement not always stable (may rest on EAC wall, and not TM)
	✓ can be placed by an experienced audiologist	✓ requires some technical skill
	✓ doesn't require otologic support	✓ may cause patient some discomfort
	✓ doesn't require TM anesthesia	✓ some patients may not comply with test
TIPtrode™	✓ easy placement without much experience	✓ small AP amplitude in patients with hearing loss (< 0.5 μV)
	✓ doesn't require much technical ability	✓ SP component may not be detectable
	✓ commercially available	✓ doesn't record a near-field response
	✓ doesn't cause patient much or any discomfort	
	✓ enhances ECochG AP component in normal hearers	

ECochG IN MÉNIÈRE'S DISEASE

ECochG SP/AP Relations for Different Electrodes

The relation of electrocochleography (ECochG) summating potential (SP) versus action potential (AP) amplitudes for three different types of ECochG electrodes. The SP amplitude increases directly with AP amplitude, but the specific ratio (in %) varies depending on the electrode site relative to the cochlea. An electrode closer to the cochlea produces a smaller ratio than an electrode relatively farther from the cochlea.

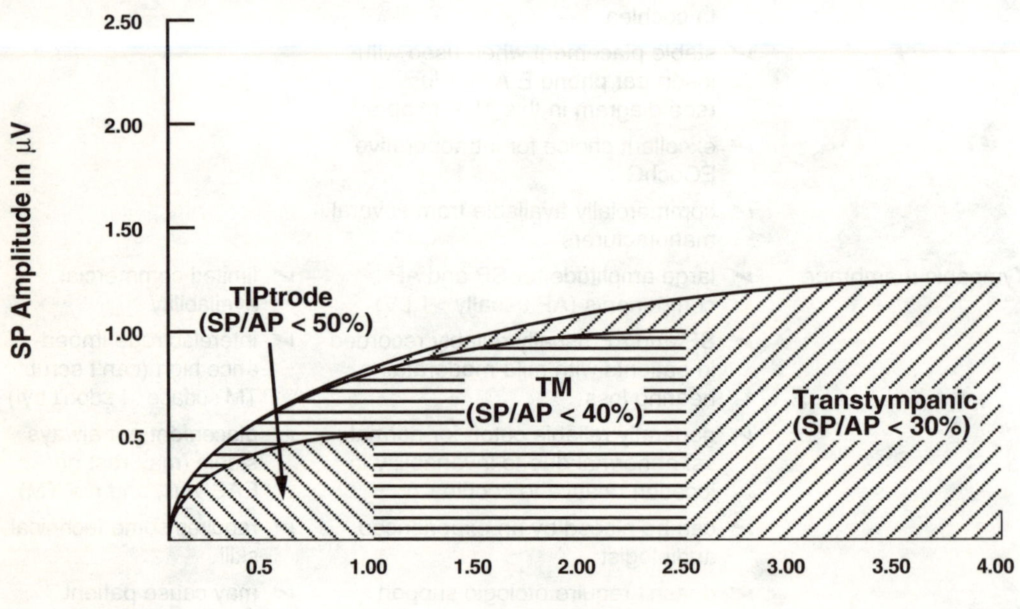

Diagnosis of Ménière's Disease

Certain Ménière's disease

- ☐ Definite Ménière's disease, plus histopathologic confirmation

Definite Ménière's disease

- ☐ Two or more definitive spontaneous episodes of vertigo lasting 20 minutes or longer
- ☐ Audiometrically documented hearing loss on at least one occasion
- ☐ Tinnitus or aural fullness in the treated ear
- ☐ Other causes excluded

Probable Ménière's disease

- ☐ One definitive episode of vertigo
- ☐ Audiometrically documented hearing loss on at least one occasion
- ☐ Tinnitus or aural fullness in the treated ear
- ☐ Other causes excluded

Possible Ménière's disease

- ☐ Episodic vertigo of the Ménière type without documented hearing loss, or
- ☐ Sensorineural hearing loss, fluctuating or fixed, with dysequilibrium, but without definitive episodes
- ☐ Other causes excluded

Source: Committee on Hearing and Equilibrium. *Otolaryngology—Head and Neck Surgery 113*: 181–185, 1995.

Staging of Ménière's Disease

Stage	Four frequency pure tone average (500, 1000, 2000, and 3000 Hz)
1	< 25 dB
2	26 to 40
3	41 to 70
4	> 70

Source: Committee on Hearing and Equilibrium. *Otolaryngology—Head and Neck Surgery 113:* 181–185, 1995.

KEY REFERENCES

Electrocochleography (ECochG)

Arenberg IK, Ackley RS, Ferraro J. EcoG results in perilymph fistula: clinical and experimental studies. *Otolaryngol Head Neck Surg 99*: 435–443, 1988.

Berlin CI, Cullen JK, Jr, Ellis MS, Lousteau RJ, Yarbrough WM, Lyons GD, Jr. Clinical application of recording human VIIIth nerve action potentials from the tympanic membrane. *Trans Amer Acad Ophthalmol Otolaryngol 87*: 401–410, 1974.

Coats A. On electrocochleographic electrode design. *J Acoust Soc Am 56*: 708–711, 1974.

Davis H, Deatherage BH, Eldredge DH, Smith CA. Summating potentials of the cochlea. *Amer J Physiol 195*: 251–261, 1958.

Durrant JD. Extratympanic electrode support via vented earmold. *Ear and Hearing 11*: 468–469, 1990.

Ferraro J, Best LG, Arenberg IK. The use of electrocochleography in the diagnosis, assessment, and management of endolymphatic hydrops. *Otol Clinics North Amer 16*: 69–82, 1983.

Ferraro J, Murphy G, Ruth R. A comparative study of primary electrodes used in extratympanic electrocochleography. *Seminars in Hearing 7*: 279–287, 1986.

Gibson WRP, Moffat DA, Ramsden RT. Clinical electrocochleography in diagnosis and management of Meniere's disease. *Audiology 16*: 389–401, 1977.

Goin DW, Staller SJ, Asher DL, Mischkle RE. Summating potential in Ménière's disease. *Laryngoscope 92*: 1383–1389, 1982.

Hall JW III. *Handbook of Auditory Evoked Responses*. Needham, MA: Allyn & Bacon, 1992.

Meyerhoff WL, Yellin MW. Summating potential/action potential ratio in perilymph fistula. *Otolaryngol Head Neck Surg 102*: 678–682, 1990.

Portmann M, Aran JM. Electro-cochleography. *Laryngoscope 81*: 899–910, 1971.

Rubin RJ, Bordley JE, Lieberman AT. Cochlear potentials in man. *Laryngoscope 71*: 1141–1164, 1961.

Ruth RA, Lambert PR. Comparison of tympanic membrane to promontory electrode recordings of electrocochleographic responses in patients with Meniere's disease. *Otolaryngol Head Neck Surg 100*: 546–552, 1989.

Schwaber MK, Hall JW III. A simplified approach for transtympanic electrocochleography. *Amer J Otol 11*: 260–265, 1990.

Stypulkowski PH, Staller SJ. Clinical evaluation of a new ECoG recording electrode. *Ear and Hearing 8*: 304–310, 1987.

van Deelen GW, Ruding PRJW, Veldman JE, Huizing EH, Smoorenburg GF. Electrocochleographic study of experimentally induced endolymphatic hydrops. *Arch Otol Rhinol Laryngol 244*: 167–173, 1987.

Wever E, Bray C. Auditory nerve impulses. *Science 71*: 215, 1930.

CHAPTER 7

Auditory Brainstem Response (ABR)

In This ADR Chapter

Perspective

The auditory brainstem response (ABR) was discovered officially by Jewett and Williston, at the beginning of the 1970s. The term "ABR" was coined by Hallowell Davis at the end of the decade, in 1979. In between, multiple clinical applications of the technique were described and confirmed independently by numerous investigators in the audiologic, otolaryngologic, and neurologic literature. ABR during this period became the procedure of choice for newborn hearing screening in the nursery setting, diagnostic assessment of the muliply involved and the difficult-to-test child, differentiation of cochlear versus retrocochlear auditory dysfunction, and monitoring neurophysiologic status in the operating room and intensive care unit.

During the decade of the 1980s, several evoked response systems were introduced to the marketplace, and ABR was embraced by clinicians as an essential component of the audiologic test battery. With automated ABR algorithms, infant hearing screening became clinically feasible for nonaudiologic personnel. Although investigations of newer, faster, and more accurate strategies for ABR measurement and analysis continue, we have to a large extent reached a plateau in ABR application. Perhaps the most important objective at this time is to bring all audiologists to a uniformly high level of clinical competence with ABR. This chapter includes the essential concepts and principles for everyday clinical application of ABR. The reader is referred to other textbooks (e.g., Hall, 1992) for comprehensive coverage of the topic.

FOUNDATIONS OF ABR

Historical Perspective

Important Developments and Discoveries in ABR

Year	Investigator(s)	Finding
1951	Dawson	Rudimentary signal averager for evoked responses
1961	Clark	Description of average response computer (ARC)
1967	Sohmer & Feinmesser	A brainstem response first shown in human subjects but described as ECochG
1970	Jewett & Romano	Response first described in animal
1971	Jewett & Williston	Systematic study in humans which marks the true "discovery" of ABR for clinical purposes
1971	Moore E	Unpublished Ph.D. study
1973	Terkildsen, Osterhammel et al.	Series of studies on stimulus and acquisition parameters
1974	Hecox & Galambos	Description in infants and children (probably the first real clinical paper)
1975	Schulman-Galambos & Galambos	Response reliably recorded in premature infants
1975	Starr	Response described in patients with varied CNS pathology
1976	Salamy	Description of the development of the response in neonates
1976	Robinson, Rudge	Abnormal response described in patients with multiple sclerosis
1977	Selters & Brackmann	Response applied in acoustic tumor detection
1977	Clemis	Response applied in acoustic tumor detection
1977	Terkildsen et al.	Response applied in acoustic tumor detection
1977	Stockard & Rossiter	Findings in patients with varied CNS pathology
1977	Arlinger	Responses recorded with bone stimulation
1977	Robinson & Rudge	Further findings in multiple sclerosis
1978	Stockard, Stockard & Sharbrough	Monograph on measurement techniques and variables
1978	Don & Eggermont	High-pass masking for frequency specific response
1979	Jerger & Mauldin	Clinical study of ABR with bone conduction stimulation
1979	Yamada	Effects of cochlear hearing impairment described
1979	Chiappa	Normal variations in waveforms

1979	Dobie & Berlin	Binaural response investigated
1979	Don	Frequency-specific response with masking paradigms
1980	Jerger & Hall et al.	Effects of age and gender on responser
1981	Moller	Neural generators studied with depth electrodes from human eighth nerve and brain resulting in reappraisal of the anatomic generators of ABR
1981	Hashimoto	Neural generators studied with depth electrodes from human eighth nerve and brain
1981	Borg	Effects of recording parameters, cochlear hearing impairment, bone conduction stimulation
1981	Grundy	Application in intraoperative monitoring
1981	Rosenhamer et al.	Systematic study in peripheral auditory pathology
1982	Hall et al.	Systematic application in monitoring of head injured patients in the intensive care unit
1984	Pratt et al.	Lissajous multichannel geometric vector analysis
1984	Burkhard	Effect of stimulus parameters and ipsilateral noise
1984	Elberling	Computerized analysis of response
1985	Hall et al.	Determination of brain death
1986	Thornton (Aaron)	Automated ABR technique and algorithm field tested in neonatal screening (ALGO 1)
1987	Gorga et al.	Comprehensive neonatal and pediatric normative data
1987	Martin W	3-channel Lissajous trajectory analysis investigations
1988	Kileny et al.	Electrically elicited response
1988	Hall	Spectral analysis of ABR applied clinically
1991	Hammill et al.	Chained stimuli technique for rapid threshold estimation
1991	Fausti et al.	High-frequency (>8000 Hz) stimulation of ABR
1992	Picton	Maximum length sequence (MLS) stimulation strategy for rapid measurement
1992	Hall	Publication of the *Handbook of Auditory Evoked Responses*
1993	Thorton (ARD)	Maximum length sequence (MLS) stimulation strategy for rapid measurement
1994	Nicolet Biomedical	MLS and Fsp features incorporated into a clinical evoked response system
1993	Marsh	Simultaneous binaural stimulation strategy
1993	Intelligent Hearing Systems	Automated ABR device involving cross-correlation technique
1994	Bio-Logic	Evoked response system with built in neonatal normative data base and statistical waveform analysis feature
1994	Natus, Inc.	Automated ABR technique employing simultaneous binaural stimulation

Clinical Concept

Why the ABR Is Not a Test of Hearing

Selected anatomic and clinical reasons why the auditory brainstem response (ABR) to click stimuli should not be relied on as a measure of "hearing."

ANATOMIC

- ☐ ABR is generated by activation of the cochlea in the 2000 to 4000 Hz region, not for lower frequencies.
- ☐ ABR is an onset response (a "time keeper"), probably dependent only on a subset of onset sensitive neurons in the auditory brain stem. The different structural and functional types of auditory system neurons are described pictorially in Chapter 1.
- ☐ ABR does not involve auditory regions above the level of rostral brainstem (e.g., the lateral lemniscus to inferior colliculus level). ABR provides no information on status of the all-important cortical auditory centers.

CLINICAL

- ☐ A normal appearing ABR can be recorded in persons with clinically important low-frequency hearing impairment when high-frequency hearing is normal.
- ☐ ABR may be absent in severe high-frequency hearing impairment, even when hearing is normal for the low-frequency region which is so important for communication.
- ☐ ABR may be absent in the presence of a normal audiogram or very mild hearing impairment in patients with diseases that result in desynchrony in firing of neurons in the auditory pathways.
- ☐ ABR is not correlated with perception of loudness.
- ☐ ABR is not consistently correlated with speech understanding performance.
- ☐ Normal ABR can be recorded in severe and debilitating cerebral pathology, such as severe traumatic head injury and stroke.
- ☐ A normal ABR can be recorded in deep drug-induced and natural sleep, anesthesia, and coma.

ABR Facts and Features

BACKGROUND

- ☐ Term "ABR" coined by Hallowell Davis, the "Father of Auditory Evoked Responses" in 1979
- ☐ Other terms and abbreviations for auditory brainstem response (ABR) include:
  - ✔ brainstem auditory evoked response (BAER)
  - ✔ brain stem evoked response (BSER)
  - ✔ brainstem auditory evoked potential (BAEP)
  - ✔ early response, fast response, or short latency response
- ☐ First thorough description was by Jewett and Williston in 1971. Jewett was a prodigy of the well-known auditory neurophysiologist Robert Galambos who, in turn, had been associated with Hallowell Davis and other notables in auditory science in his earlier days at Harvard. Both Galambos and Jewett went west young men (and women), stopping in California in the late 1960s.
- ☐ Hundreds of, maybe even a thousand or more, published clinical studies on myriad applications in auditory assessment and neurodiagnosis have appeared since mid-1970s.
- ☐ A more recent application was neuromonitoring of auditory system integrity in the operating room and intensive care unit.
- ☐ **WARNING**: *Do not sell your ABR system* just because otoacoustic emissions have arrived on the scene. OAE will complement, not supplant, ABR in clinical audiology.

ANATOMIC GENERATORS

- ☐ Major peaks in waveform are labeled by Roman numerals (i.e., Waves I, II, III, IV, V and VI) following recommendations of Jewett & Williston. Back in the old days, the waves were actually referred to as "Jewett bumps."
- ☐ The response occurs within a 5.5 to 6 msec period following presentation of a high-intensity acoustic stimulus.
- ☐ Evidence from human investigations by Moller, Hashimoto, and others indicates that the *anatomic generators* are:
  - ✔ distal eighth nerve for wave I
  - ✔ proximal (brainstem portion) of the eighth nerve for wave II

- ✓ auditory pathways and structures in pons for wave III, (e.g., trapezoid body, superior olivary complex)
- ✓ auditory pathways and structures more rostral brainstem for wave V (e.g., lateral lemniscus near entry to inferior colliculus).

- ☐ Waves I and II arise on the side of the auditory system ipsilateral to the stimulus, whereas wave III and later components probably receive bilateral contributions (maybe more contralateral, however).
- ☐ Response presumably reflects synchronous activation primarily of onset-type neurons within the auditory system (only one of the six structural and functional subtypes of neurons in the auditory brain stem).
- ☐ Waves I and II are action potentials, whereas later waves may reflect post-synaptic activity in major brain stem auditory regions.
- ☐ Click-generated response dependent on activation of basal (vs. apical) portion of the cochlea, mainly in the 2000 to 4000 Hz region.

STIMULUS FEATURES

- ☐ Optimal *stimulus* is a brief duration electrical pulse (e.g., 0.1 msec) which is transduced by the earphone into a click and enhances synchronous neural activity.
- ☐ A stimulus rate of 20/sec or even faster is appropriate for ABR. (Don't try these fast rates with longer latency AERS.)
- ☐ Up to about 70 dB nHL, an increase in stimulus intensity produces a decrease in response latency values and increased response amplitude; above this level, latency remains stable whereas amplitude continues to increase.

ACQUISITION FEATURES

- ☐ One electrode is typically located at the top of the head (vertex) or high on the forehead with another electrode on the ear lobe or within the ear canal of the stimulated side (other electrode arrays may also be useful).
- ☐ Bandpass filter settings of 30 or 100 to 3000 Hz are appropriate to encompass spectrum of response while reducing undesirable electrical activity.

OTHER FACTORS TO CONSIDER IN ANALYSIS AND INTERPRETATION

- ☐ ABR is influenced by subject age (under age 18 months and over age 60 years), gender, and body temperature.
- ☐ The response is not seriously affected by subject state of arousal (including sleep) or most drugs, including sedatives and anesthetic agents; this is a major clinical advantage.

CLINICAL APPLICATIONS

- ☐ Newborn infant auditory screening with conventional operator controlled evoked response systems or automated infants hearing screeners.
- ☐ Estimation of auditory sensitivity in very young or difficult-to-test children with air conduction click stimuli and, as indicated, bone conduction and tone burst stimulation.
- ☐ Neurodiagnosis of eighth nerve or auditory brainstem dysfunction.
- ☐ Monitoring eighth nerve and auditory brainstem status intraoperatively during posterior fossa surgery.

CLINICAL LIMITATIONS

- ☐ With click stimulus, response estimates hearing sensitivity only in 2000 to 4000 Hz region, not for lower frequencies.
- ☐ ABR is not a test of hearing, as it can be recorded in patients with significant dysfunction at more rostral auditory regions of the central nervous system. It can be recorded in comatose and anesthetized patients, and it may be not be recorded in persons with demyelinating diseases with otherwise apparently normal auditory findings.

Technical Tip

The JWH III Motto for Successful Auditory Evoked Response Measurement

- ☐ **Adult version**

  Whatever works—do it!

- ☐ **Pediatric version**

  Whatever works—do it quickly!

Clinical Concept

Generators of Auditory Evoked Responses

- ☐ Auditory brain stem response (ABR)
  - wave I = distal end of the eighth nerve (near cochlea)
  - wave II = proximal end of the eighth nerve (near brain stem)
  - wave III = caudal (lower) brain stem near trapezoid body and superior olivary complex
  - wave V = lateral lemniscus as it enters the inferior colliculus
  - trough after wave V = inferior colliculus (?)
- ☐ Auditory middle latency response (AMLR)
  - Na component = thalamus (?)
  - Pa component = primary auditory cortex (measured over temporal-parietal lobe)
  - Pa component = subcortical generator (as measured with a midline electrode)
- ☐ Auditory late response (ALR)
  - P2 component = primary or secondary auditory cortex
- ☐ Auditory P_{300} response
  - P3 component = auditory regions of hippocampus in medial temporal lobe
- ☐ Mismatch negativity (MMN) response
  - subcortical and primary cortical auditory regions

Audiometric Region Important in Generation of ABR with Click Stimulus

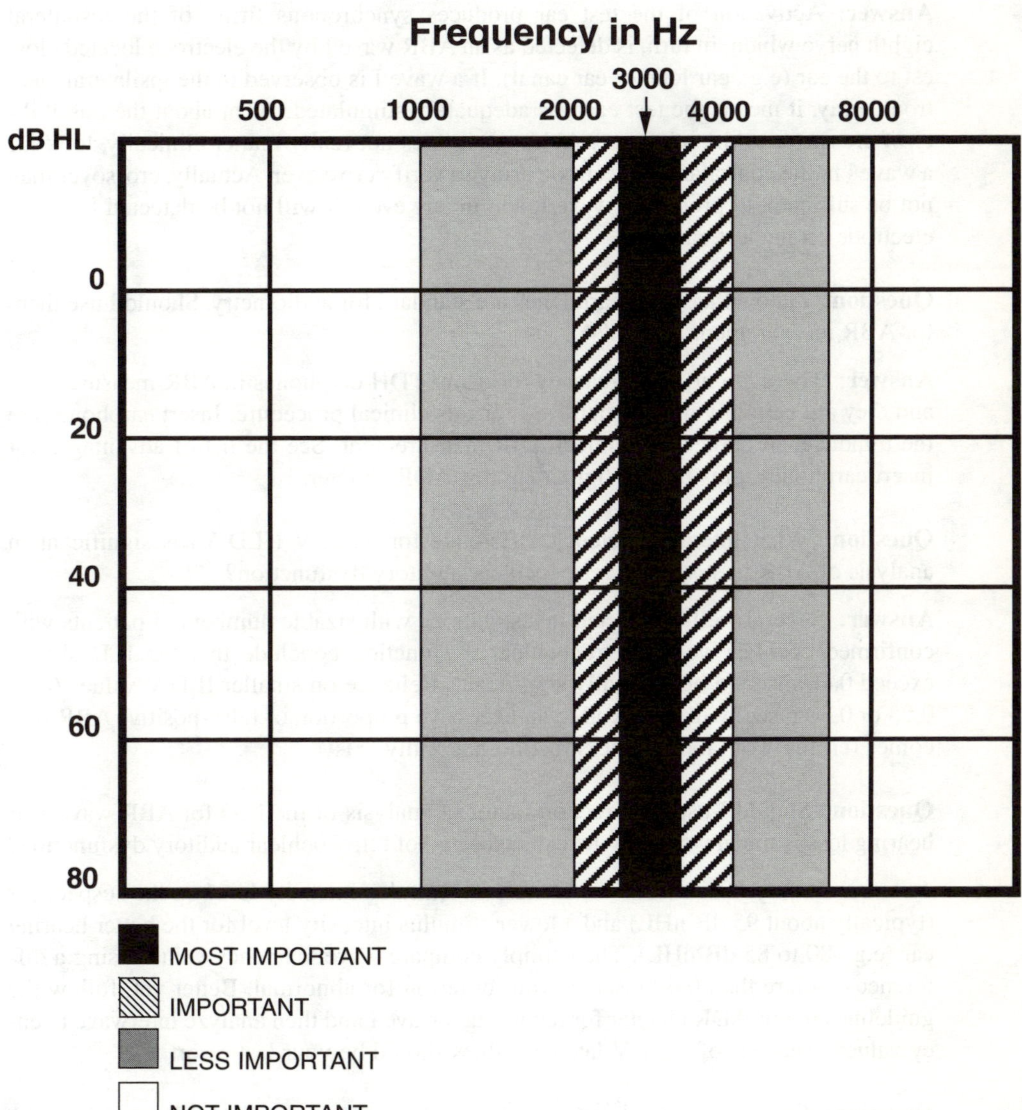

Clinical Concepts

Answers to six common questions about ABR measurement

Question: How can I be sure that my bone-conduction ABR is due to activation of the test ear, and not crossover to the nontest ear?

Answer: Activation of the test ear produces synchronous firing of the ipsilateral eighth nerve which, in turn, is detected as an ABR wave I by the electrode located closest to the ear (e.g., ear lobe or ear canal). If a wave I is observed in the ipsilateral electrode array, it means the test ear was adequately stimulated. What about the possibility of crossover to the other ear? Although it does not really matter clinically, look for a wave I in the contralateral electrode array to verify crossover. Actually, crossover may not be sufficient to produce a wave I, and in any event it will not be detected from the electrode on the test ear.

Question: I know that TDH earphones are standard for audiometry. Should I use them for ABR measurement as well?

Answer: There are no good reasons for using TDH earphones in ABR measurement, and they are certainly not standardized for this clinical procedure. Insert earphones are the tranducer of choice for clinical ABR measurement. See the list of advantages for insert earphones, plus related figures, in this ADR chapter.

Question: What interaural latency difference for wave V (ILD V) is significant in analysis of ABR in suspected retrocochlear auditory dysfunction?

Answer: Several well-conducted investigations with sizable numbers of patients with confirmed cochlear versus retrocochlear dysfunction conclude that the ILD should exceed 0.40 msec to be clinically significant. Reliance on smaller ILD V values (e.g., 0.25 or 0.30 msec) will only lead to an excessive proportion of false-positive ABR outcomes (crying wolf about tumors that do not really exist).

Question: Should I use a correction factor in analysis of the ILD for ABR wave V if hearing loss is much worse on the ear suspected of retrocochlear auditory dysfunction?

Answer: Rarely, if ever. Use the maximum stimulus intensity level on the suspect ear (typically about 95 dB nHL) and a lower stimulus intensity level for the better hearing ear (e.g., 80 to 85 dB nHL). Then simply compare wave V latency values using a difference of more than 0.40 msec as your criterion for abnormal. Better yet, follow the guidelines in this ADR chapter for recording a wave I and then analyze interwave latency values. Analysis of wave V latency values should be your last resort.

Question: Can I use a tone burst stimulus for frequency-specific ABR recording with commercially available equipment?

Answer: Absolutely. Follow the guidelines in this ADR chapter. You should not expect, however, the same waveform morphology for low frequency tone burst stimulated ABRs as you would for a click stimulus. The emphasis is on estimating auditory threshold in the stimulus frequency region by analysis of response presence, rather than close calculation of ABR wave V latency.

Question: Should I use a fast stimulus rate to increase the sensitivity of ABR to retrocochlear auditory dysfunction?

Answer: It probably will add little to sensitivity of the ABR, especially if you were successful in recording a wave I and analyzing interwave latency values. If you do employ faster stimulus rates, go to a really fast rate (e.g., 91.1 or 99.9 per sec) and expect a wave V latency shift of about 0.6 msec for normal or sensory ears (more for neural disorders). Do not pussyfoot around at modest stimulus rates, such as 50 or 60 per sec.

Thanks to Jennifer Anderson and Mandy Lamb for prompting these questions and answers.

ABR RECORDING

Technical Tips

Patient Instructions for ABR

WHAT IS AN ABR?

An ABR is a computerized hearing test, used to measure the "brain waves" your ear produces when it hears sounds. Sometimes an ABR is called a BAER (brainstem auditory evoked response). An ABR test is indicated when complete results cannot be obtained with routine audiometry (hearing tests). For adults, an ABR is often needed when a simple hearing test shows a certain type of hearing loss pattern. An ABR is usually required also for hearing assessment of infants and young children less than 6 years old, or those with developmental delays. An ABR for children is referred to as a pediatric ABR or PABR.

WHERE IS IT DONE?

The test is performed by an audiologist at The Vanderbilt Balance and Hearing Center. The center is located at The Village at Vanderbilt, 1500 21st Avenue South, Suite 2600, Nashville, Tennessee.

HOW LONG DOES IT TAKE?

The test usually takes an hour or, for children, up to an hour and a half.

WHAT PREPARATION IS REQUIRED?

This test requires that the patient lie very still, so that any muscle movement will not be picked up by the computer. In the case of an infant or small child (under the age of 5 years), the patient should be asleep. No other preparation is required. Patients may take their typical medicine and follow their normal routine on the day of the ABR evaluation.

WHAT SHOULD BE EXPECTED BEFORE THE TEST?

Flat electrodes (wires) will be taped to the patient's forehead and ears. These electrodes will measure the response to sound from the ears and the brain. An adult does not have to prepare for the test in any way.

WHAT SHOULD BE EXPECTED DURING THE TEST?

There will not be any discomfort during the test. While the patient sleeps or rests quietly, he or she will hear clicking sounds through earplugs, and the brain's response to the sound will be recorded by a computer and analyzed by the audiologist.

WHAT CAN BE EXPECTED IMMEDIATELY AFTER THE TEST?

Adult patients will experience no discomfort after the test and are free to return to their daily activities. Children who are sedated during the test will be aroused and monitored in the clinic until they are fully awake.

For both children and adults, the audiologist usually will completely analyze and interpret the ABR results after the patient has left the clinic. A written report of the results is mailed within a day after the testing.

If you have any other questions regarding this test, you can speak with an audiologist by calling 615-322-HEAR (4327).

Technical Tips

Do's and Don'ts for AER Measurement

☐ **DO:**

- Make sure that the evoked response system has been inspected and approved by certified safety engineering or biomedical engineering personnel according to hospital safety standards
- Replace immediately any defective or faulty electrical wiring, plugs, or components
- Verify that the evoked response system is properly grounded
- Always use hospital-grade, three-prong plugs for the evoked response system power

☐ **DON'T:**

- Use extension cords to power the evoked response system. They are O.K. for printers, etc.
- Use three-prong to two-prong couplers or adapters for the evoked response system power system
- Turn the evoked response system power off or on while the patient is connected to the electrodes. There is a slim chance that the patient could be shocked.
- Place drinks or food on or near the evoked response system. A spill could be dangerous and expensive.

Protocol

Auditory Brainstem Response (ABR)

Parameters	Suggestion	Rationale/Comment
Stimulus		
transducer	ER-3A	For comfort, no EAC collapse, reduced stimulus artifact (with adequate distancing between transducer box and electrodes and the electrode vs. transducer cables), accurate placement with infants without hand-holding
	B-70	For bone conduction stimulation
type	click	Produces robust response/only evaluates basal turn of cochlea and 1K to 4K Hz region
	tone bursts	As indicated; use Blackman ramping
duration		
click	0.1 ms	ABR is onset response
tones	2-1-2 cycles	Other durations are useful too
polarity	rarefaction	Usually clearest wave I/use condensation if response not optimal; use alternating with excessive stimulus artifact
rate	21.1/sec	Relatively fast data acquisition without response deterioration, but use a slower rate (e.g., 7.1/sec) to enhance wave I
intensity	80 to 95 dB nHL	Produces robust response for neurodiagnosis
	95 dB nHL down to 0 dB nHL	Vary for threshold in 10or 5 dB increments
masking	occasional	50 dB white noise to nontest ear when stimulus is >70 dB and ABR shows no wave I and delayed latency for wave V
presentation ear	monaural	For ear-specific findings
Acquisition		
electrode arrays *		
	Ch 1: Fz-A1	Forehead (vs. vertex) for convenience
	Ch 2: Fz-A2	Ear lobe vs. mastoid for > wave I amplitude
	Ch 3: Fz-NC	Ch 3 (noncephalic) optional for better definition of all waves
	Fpz ground	Convenient; no electrode changing
filter	30–3000 Hz	Encompasses response, including low-frequency energy; less filter distortion (e.g., latency alterations) and greater wave I and V amplitude

Parameters	Suggestion	Rationale/Comment
notch filter	none	Introduces latency distortion and rarely eliminates all 60 Hz related electrical interference
amplification	×100,000	Usually necessary for the small ABR amplitude
sensitivity	±25μv	Not a setting for all equipment; the smaller this number is, the higher the amplification
analysis time		
overall	15 msec	Encompasses response, including wave V, for low intensities, in newborns, with most tone burst stimuli, and in conductive loss. Try 20 msec for a 500 Hz tone burst.
prestimulus	1 msec	For estimation of background noise
sample points	512	Minimally 256 with 10 msec analysis time
sweeps	500 to 4000	Less needed with normal hearing, quiet patient and high intensity and vice versa; dependent on signal-to-noise ratio. There is no magical number of stimuli. It's simply a matter of detecting the desired signal in the presence of undesirable noise.

*Noninverting-inverting electrode according to International 10-20 Electrode System

Insert Earphone and TIPtrode Type Electrode

Components of the ER-3A "insert" earphone (top) from the audiometer or evoked response system (left) to the patient (right). Modification of the ER-3A as TIPtrode™ for ECochG or ABR recording. The stimulus is delivered as usual. In addition, gold foil covering the foam insert contacting the wall of the external ear canal detects the evoked response. An electrode wire is coupled to the gold foil with a specially designed alligator clip, and then leads to an electrode box or strip. TIPtrode™ ABR recordings enhance wave I amplitude without influencing latency of any ABR components.

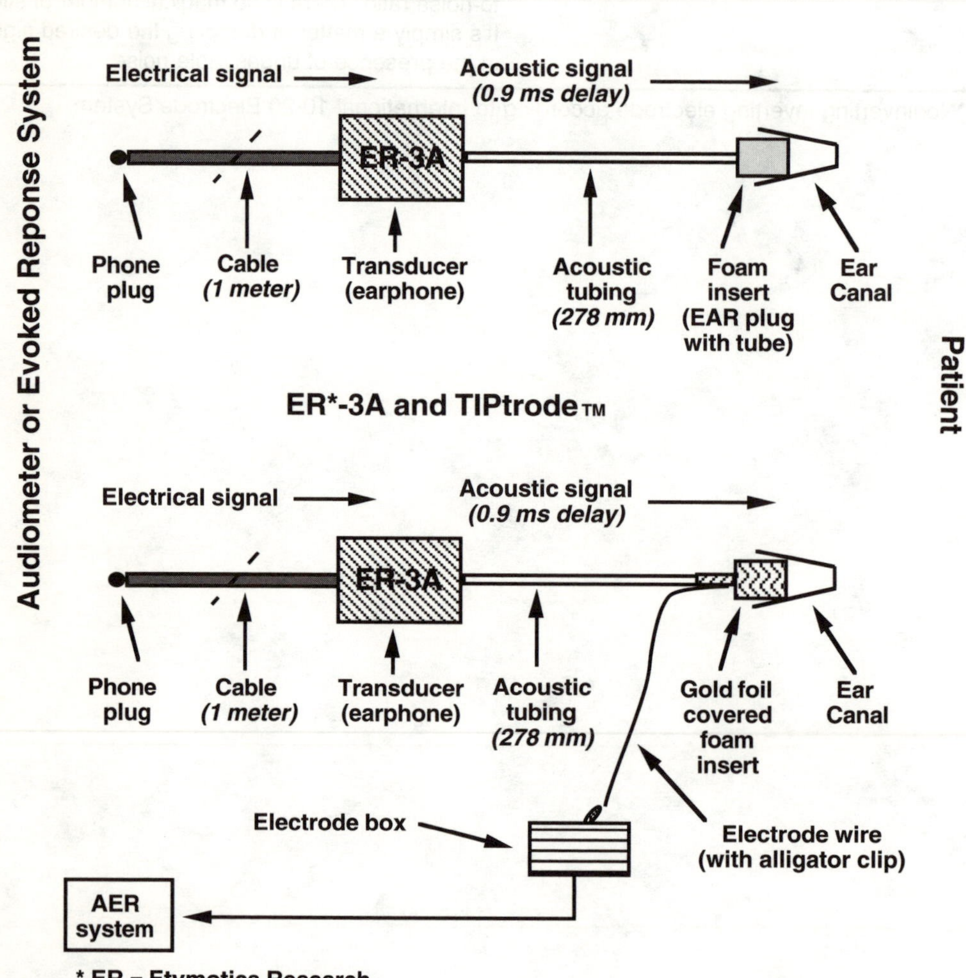

Advantages Cited for Insert (ER-3A) Earphones

General

- increased interaural attenuation
- increased ambient noise attenuation
- elimination of ear canal collapse
- increased patient comfort

Auditory evoked response stimulation

- reduced transducer ringing
- reduced electrical (stimulus) artifact with separation of transducer and inverting electrode

Temporal Waveforms and Spectral Characteristics of Supra-aural Versus Insert Earphones

Three types of transducers typically used in ABR stimulation

In addition to the other advantages of "insert earphones" in ABR measurement (see nearby List), with a transient (e.g., click) stimulus, the ER-3A produces less ringing and a flatter frequency response. The ER-3A is, therefore, the transducer of choice for ABR (and ECochG) measurement.

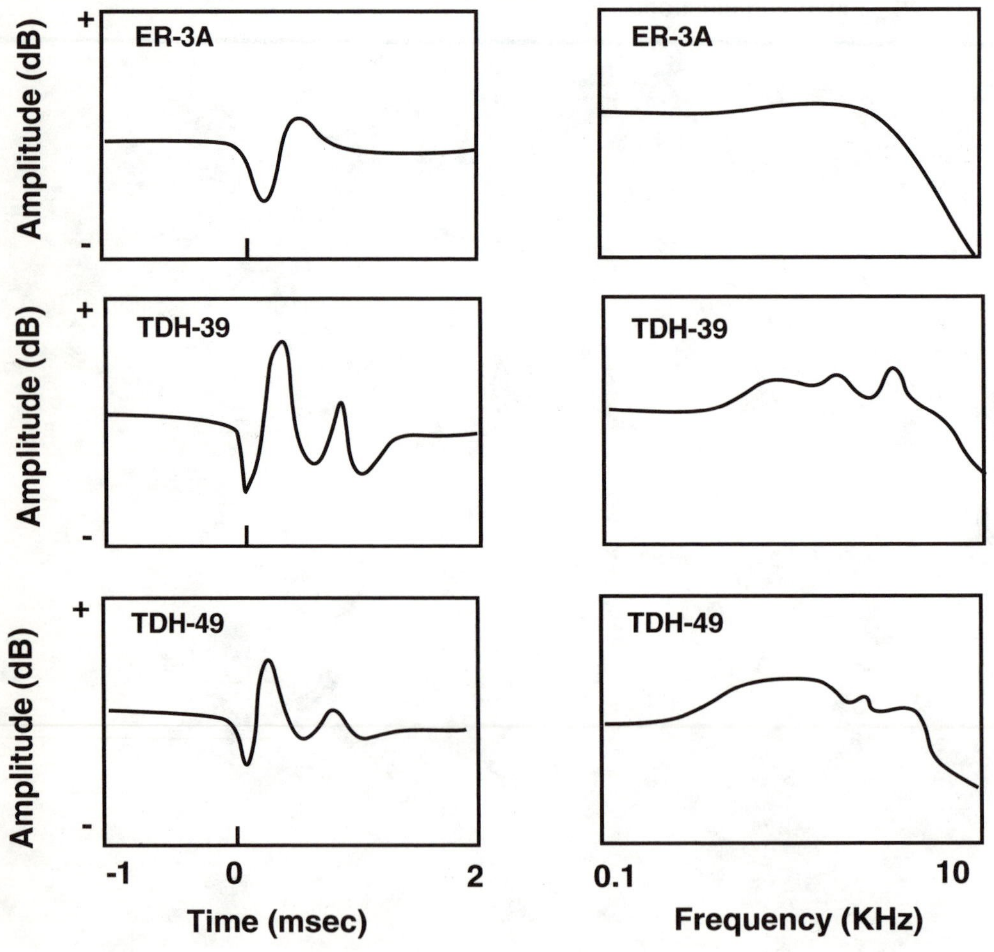

Technical Tip

ABR and Stimulus Durations

Trick questions:

- ☐ Which weighs more: 100 pounds of beer or 100 pounds of pretzels?
- ☐ What's the difference in duration between an ABR click stimulus of 0.1 msec and a click stimulus of 100 µsec?

Answer to both questions:

- ☐ There is no difference.

ABR Electrode Terminology

Locations of the electrodes in a conventional auditory brainstem response (ABR) recording array. A common (ground) electrode is located on the low forehead, approximately between the eyebrows. The "ipsilateral" array consists of a noninverting electrode on the high forehead (close to the Fz site) and an inverting electrode on the earlobe (or the ear canal if a TIPtrode™ is used). The "contralateral" array also consists of a noninverting electrode on the high forehead but the inverting electrode on the earlobe on the side opposite from stimulation. The "horizontal" array consists of an inverting electrode on lobe of the stimulated ear, and the noninverting electrode on the earlobe on the side opposite from stimulation. A "derived" ipsilateral array can be generated by digitally subtracting the contralaterally recorded waveform from the ipsilaterally recorded waveform.

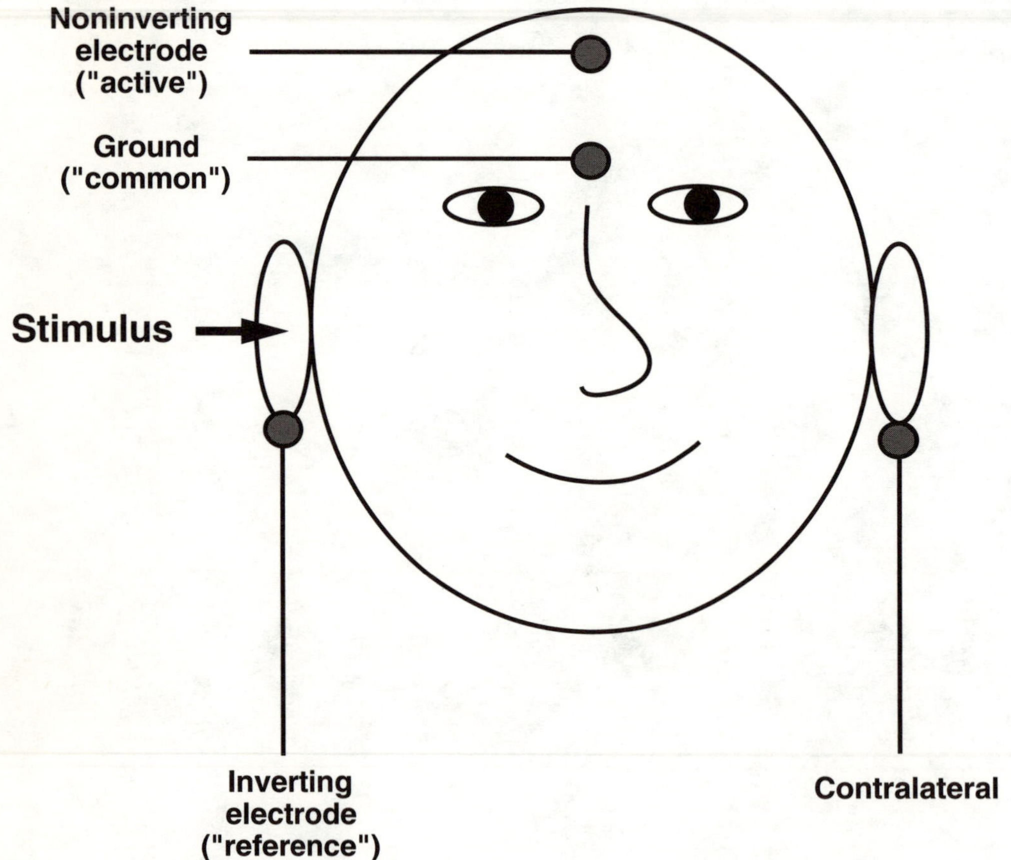

ABR Electrode Array

An auditory brainstem response (ABR) waveform recorded with the conventional ipsilateral electrode array (see previous figure). Typical absolute (for each wave) and interwave (between major waves) latency values (in milliseconds) are also shown.

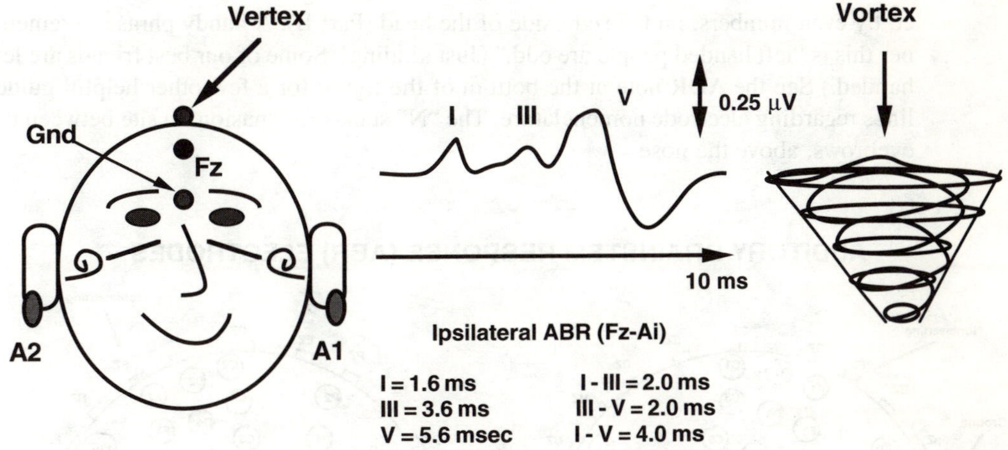

KEY TO SYMBOLS:

Fz = mid frontal (forehead)
Gnd = ground (common)
A1 = left ear lobe (A = auris = Latin. ear)
A2 = right ear lobe (A = auris = Latin. ear)

International 10-20 Electrode Array System

Illustration of some of the electrode sites of the 10-20 International System (Jasper, 1958). The sites typically used in auditory brainstem response (ABR) recording are shaded. Part A shows electrodes and symbols for the left side of the head. Odd numbers indicate the left side of the head. There is an analogous set of electrodes, indicated by even numbers, on the right side of the head (Part B). A handy phrase to remember this is "left handed people are odd." (Just kidding! Some of our best friends are left handed.) See the ADR note at the bottom of the figure for a few other helpful guidelines regarding electrode nomenclature. The "N" stands for "nasion," a site between the eyebrows, above the nose.

AUDITORY BRAINSTEM RESPONSE (ABR) ELECTRODES

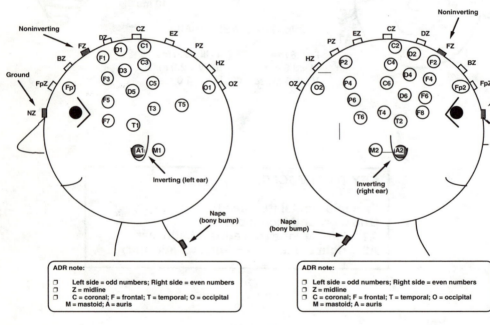

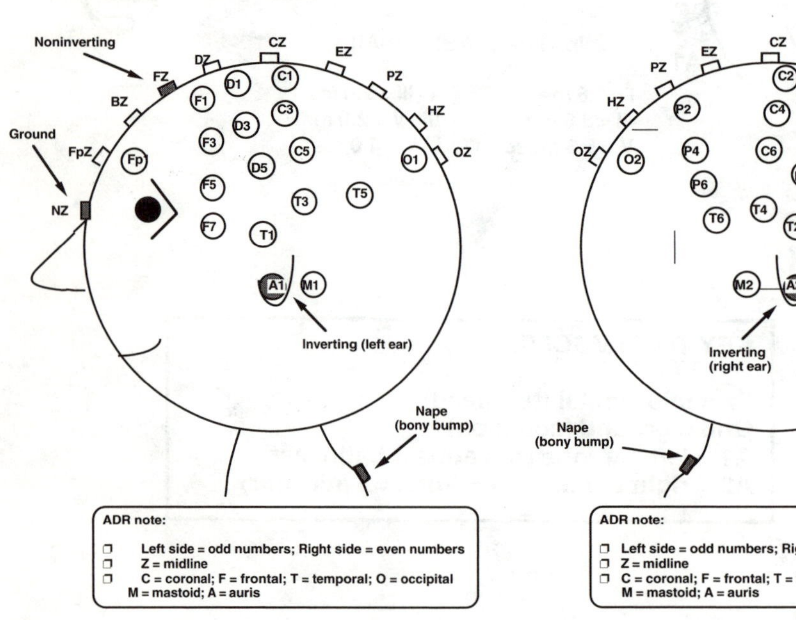

Trouble-shooting

ABR Measurement Problems and Solutions

Symptom	Possible Problems	Possible Solutions
No display	Technical error	✔ verify system power on ✔ verify monitor(screen) power on ✔ verify monitor intensity adequate ✔ verify evoked program loaded ✔ consult equipment manual
	Equipment set-up error	✔ verify stimulus won't average repetitions (sweeps) not set at "0" ✔ verify stimulus duration not set at "0" ✔ verify adequate memory (memories) for number of channels ✔ verify stimulus rate not too fast for analysis time ✔ verify all measurement parameters ✔ turn power off, wait, then power on *or* perform "warm boot" ✔ consult equipment manual
More than one response in analysis time	Stimulus rate vs. analysis time incompatible	✔ slow rate so that the ISI is longer than analysis time ✔ shorten analysis time to less than ISI ✔ ISI (for click) is analysis time/rate
No response	No stimulus	✔ listening check or ask the patient if he or she hears the stimulus ✔ verify correct transducer ✔ verify test ear
	Improper electrode	✔ verify correct site electrode sites
	Severe hearing loss	✔ obtain audiogram ✔ increase stimulus intensity ✔ attempt bone conduction stimulation
	Inadequate amplification	✔ check gain/ amplification
Excessive early artifact	Stimulus interference	✔ alternate polarity ✔ use tubephones ✔ reduce stimulus intensity ✔ move transducer away from electrode ✔ avoid contact and proximity of transducer cord and electrodes ✔ use poststimulus time delay ✔ use shielded earphones ✔ not unexpected for bone conduction stimulation
Large, slow, artifact	Muscle interference	✔ attempt to relax patient ✔ attempt to make the patient comfortable

(continued)

(continued)

Symptom	Possible Problems	Possible Solutions
		✔ does the patient need to use the restroom? ✔ encourage the patient to sleep ✔ check sleep status (suspect sleep EEG waves) ✔ sedate the patient lightly (e.g., Valium with adults) ✔ raise high-pass filter cutoff frequency ✔ verify that artifact rejection is on
Poor waveform morphology	High frequency sensory (cochlear) hearing loss	✔ increase stimulus intensity to maximum ✔ slow the stimulus rate ✔ change stimulus polarity (e.g., rarefaction to condensation) ✔ increase the number of sweeps ✔ record multiple replications of waveforms ✔ sum the replicated waveforms ✔ use click vs. tone burst stimuli ✔ open up filter settings ✔ analyze pre- vs. poststimulus baseline ✔ verify that the artifact reject option is on
Excessive high frequency noise or spikes	Electrical interference	✔ make sure that all unecessary electrical devices are off ✔ is the cleaning crew outside the room with their buffer? ✔ verify a good ground electrode and check impedance ✔ lower the low pass filter setting (e.g., to 1500 Hz) ✔ alter the electrode array ✔ increase the number of sweeps ✔ alter stimulus rate (e.g., from 21.1/sec to 17.9/sec) ✔ is a physiologic monitor with O_2 saturation transducer on? ✔ smoothe (digitally) the waveform after averaging
Small, or no, wave I	High frequency sensory (cochlear) hearing loss	✔ increase intensity to maximum ✔ decrease stimulus rate ✔ do a listening check or ask the patient if he or she hears stimulus ✔ verify the ipsilateral inverting electrode site ✔ make sure you're not recording a contralateral ABR ✔ change the stimulus polarity (whatever it is) ✔ use an ear lobe vs. mastoid

Symptom	Possible Problems	Possible Solutions
		✔ use an ear canal electrode (e.g., TIPtrode™) ✔ use a TM or even a TT electrode ✔ try a horizontal electrode array ✔ use a click vs. tone burst stimulus ✔ lower the high-pass filter (e.g., from 100 to 30 Hz) ✔ increase the number of sweeps ✔ obtain an audiogram ✔ perform OAE recording
Bifid (twin peaked) wave I	You might use the wrong peak for interwave latency calculations	✔ decrease stimulus intensity slightly ✔ change stimulus polarity (even try alternating) ✔ try an ECochG electrode type ✔ use a horizontal electrode array
Delayed wave I latency	Conductive hearing loss	✔ obtain air- vs. bone conduction pure tone audiogram ✔ complete bone-conduction stimulus ABR ✔ perform tympanometry ✔ perform otoscopy ✔ increase stimulus intensity to maximum
No wave II and/or III	Hearing loss or brainstem dysfunction	✔ increase stimulus intensity ✔ use horizontal array or noncephalic inverting electrode ✔ change stimulus polarity ✔ try a TIPtrode™ or TM electrode ✔ notch in 3000 to 6000 Hz region in the audiogram?
Indistinct wave V	Imprecise absolute and interwave latency calculations, and threshold estimations	✔ obtain audiogram, if possible ✔ increase stimulus intensity ✔ decrease the high-pass filter setting ✔ raise the low-pass filter setting ✔ use a noncephalic inverting electrode ✔ analyze latency as a function of intensity ✔ rule out inadvertent ipsilateral masking ✔ record multiple waveform replications ✔ change stimulus polarity
Delayed wave V latency	Peripheral or brainstem auditory dysfunction	✔ obtain audiogram, if possible ✔ increase stimulus intensity to maximum ✔ rule out stimulus crossover ✔ mask nontest ear ✔ document age in young patient (less than 18 months) ✔ see wave I enhancement techniques listed above

(continued)

continued)

Symptom	Possible Problems	Possible Solutions
Prominent wave VI (or is it really a V?)	Error in latency calculation and ABR interpretation	✔ lower stimulus intensity level by 10 to 20 dB ✔ use contralateral masking (it may be a contra wave V) ✔ use a horizontal array or a non-cephalic inverting electrode
Is it wave IV or V?	Error in latency calculation and ABR interpretation	✔ use a noncephalic or contralateral inverting electrode ✔ compare morphology with ABR for the other ear ✔ use horizontal array (wave V will be small or disappear)
Delayed wave I–V latency	Brainstem dysfunction?	✔ rule out hypothermia ✔ consider age if patient is less than 18 months old ✔ calculate the interear difference for I–V latency ✔ verify wave V and I identification (see lists above) ✔ use gender-matched normative data ✔ obtain diagnostic audiometry findings
Short wave I–V latency	Brainstem function?	✔ is the patient a young female? ✔ use gender and age-matched norms ✔ rule out high frequency hearing loss ✔ rule out *hyper*thermia ✔ is wave I delayed or wave V too short? ✔ verify the real wave I and wave V ✔ is there a bifid wave I (see above)?
Small wave V/I amplitude ratio	Brainstem dysfunction?	✔ verify real wave V (see above) ✔ are you using a TIPtrode™ (with a larger wave I)? ✔ verify reliability (amplitude is highly variable) ✔ is the wave I too large or the wave V too small?

Source: Hall JW III. *Handbook of Auditory Evoked Responses*. Needham, MA: Allyn & Bacon, 1992.

Pseudo-Classic Quote

How to almost always record a high quality ABR

"Whatever works in auditory evoked response measurement . . . .

DO IT!"

ABR ANALYSIS AND INTERPRETATION

ABR Analysis

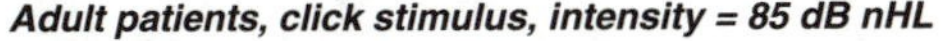

Waveform Patterns

Patterns of auditory brainstem response (ABR) waveforms, largely based on analysis of latencies and morphology (shape), associated with major types of peripheral hearing loss. These patterns are appropriate only for a high intensity (e.g., 85 dB nHL click stimulus) and a patient with hearing thresholds of about 60 dB HL or better in the 2000 to 4000 Hz region.

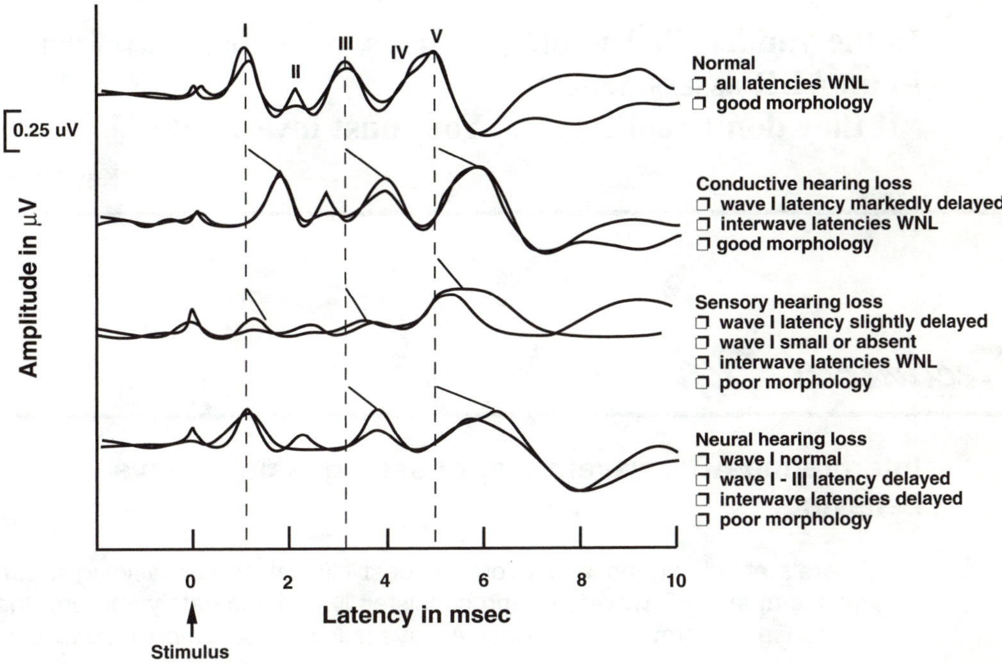

Pseudo-Classic Quote

Catchy Couplets on the Repeatability of ABRs

In the trial of you-know-who, regarding guilt:
"If it doesn't fit . . . you must acquit!"

Johnnie Cochran

In the Vanderbilt Audiology Clinics, regarding waveforms in an AER assessment:
"If they don't repeat . . . It's not complete."

Jay Hall

In the Vanderbilt Audiology Clinics, regarding waveforms in an AER assessment:
"If they don't replicate . . . You must investigate."

Kay Rupp

Technical Tip

Interpreting ABR waveforms, *or* seeing is not always believing.

- ☐ There's absolutely no way even the best clinical neurophysiologist can glance at an ABR waveform and consistently and accurately interpret the response as normal or abnormal. Always follow these simple guidelines:
  - ✓ Calculate latency values for wave I and wave V (preferrably as the averaging continues) after replicable waveforms are confirmed.
  - ✓ Compare these values to age-corrected normative data.
  - ✓ For auditory threshold estimation, always calculate wave V latency values for all stimulus intensity levels, and then plot these values on an appropriate latency-intensity form (see an example of a latency-intensity form in this ADR chapter).

- ☐ Remember, all absolute and interwave latency values at all stimulus intensity levels must be within age-corrected normal regions before you can interprete the ABR as "normal."

- ☐ When you're using a high-powered computer in evoked response measurement, there is no excuse for "eyeballing" ABR waveforms.

Technical Tips

Differentiating ABR Wave V from VI

How you differentiate the real ABR wave V from a "wave V wannabe," such as a wave VI doing a real good wave V impression

- ☐ At high intensity levels, the stimulus might produce the usual ipsilateral ABR and also crossover to the nontest ear and generate an ABR, or at least a delayed wave V component (remember that the crossover reduces stimulus intensity by 40 or 50 dB and delays the latency by 1 or 2 msec). This delayed contralaterally stimulated wave V may appear just slightly later than the ipsilaterally stimulated wave V.

- ☐ To distinguish wave V from wave VI, try these techniques:

  - ✓ lower the stimulus intensity level (e.g., from 85 to 65 dB nHL). The real wave V will remain prominent, whereas the contralateral wave V or a wave VI will become very small or disappear.
  - ✓ Apply some contralateral masking noise. About 50 dB nHL should do it.
  - ✓ Use a horizontal electrode array. With an adult patient, wave V and wave VI are rarely recorded using this array.

- ☐ Use a noncephalic (true reference electrode on the nape of the neck). The real wave V will be very distinct.

Enhancinc ABR Wave I

Things to do when ABR wave I is too small, or not there at all

- ☐ Verify that you're really using an ipsilateral (versus contralateral) site for the inverting ("reference," but not really) electrode.
- ☐ Use a "near-field" ECochG-type electrode placement.
    - ✔ A tympanic membrane site is the optimal noninvasive option.
    - ✔ A deep-seated TIPtrode™ is the next best choice.
    - ✔ If you must, use an ear lobe but definitely not a mastoid electrode site.
    - ✔ A mastoid electrode site has lots of clinical disadvantages. A 30% reduction in amplitude versus an ear lobe site is one of them.
- ☐ Increase stimulus intensity to maximum (usually 95 dB nHL). Don't pussy-foot around at 70 to 80 dB nHL.
- ☐ Change stimulus polarity. If you're using rarefaction (a good first choice), change to condensation. Only use alternating if there are several bumps in the general region of wave.
- ☐ Decrease stimulus rate (go down to 11.1/sec or even slower).
- ☐ A horizontal electrode array might help, although not very often.
- ☐ Use a click versus a tone burst stimulus (for a clearer wave I)
- ☐ Increase the number of sweeps (e.g., 2000 versus 1000 Hz).

Technical Tip

The FIVE (5) principles ABR for remembering important ABR response parameters *or* keep the number 5 in mind and you'll do O.K.

At a high click stimulus intensity, such as 85 dB nHL:

- ☐ wave V latency is normally about 5.5 msec
- ☐ wave V amplitude is about 0.5 μV (microvolts)
- ☐ the upper end of the adult normal region for the wave I–V latency interval is 4.50 msec
- ☐ the upper end of the term neonate normal region for the wave I–V latency interval is 5.00 msec

Key References

New Strategies for ABR Stimulation, Acquisition, and Analysis

Stimulus

Fausti SA, Gray PS, Frey RH, Mitchell CR. Rise time and center-frequency effects on auditory brainstem responses to high-frequency tone bursts. *Journal of American Academy of Audiology 2:* 24–31, 1991.

Fausti SA, Rappaport BZ, Frey RH, Henry JA, Phillips, DS, Mitchell CR, Olson DJ. Reliability of evoked responses to high-frequency (8–14 KHz) tone bursts. *Journal of American Academy of Audiology 2:* 105–114, 1991.

Fausti SA, Mitchell CR, Frey RH, Henry JA, O'Connor JL. Multiple-stimulus method for rapid collection of auditory brainstem responses using high-frequency (> or = 8k Hz) tone bursts. *Journal of American Academy of Audiology 5*: 119–126, 1994.

Hammill TA, Hussung RA, Sammeth CA. Rapid threshold estimation using the "chained-stimuli" technique for auditory brain stem response threshold. *Ear and Hearing 12*: 229–234, 1991.

Hoke M, Pantev C, Ansa L, Lutkenhoner B, Herrmann E. A timesaving BERA technique for frequency-specific assessment of auditory threshhold through tone-pulse series stimulation (TOPSTIM) with simultaneous gliding high-pass noise masking (GHINOMA). *Acta Oto-Laryngologica, Supplement 482:* 45–56, 1991.

Kim Y, Aoyagi M, Koike Y. Measurement of cochlear basilar membrane traveling wave velocity by derived ABR. *Acta Otolaryngologica, 511(Suppl.)*: 71–76, 1994.

Kramer SJ. Frequency-specific auditory brainstem responses to bone-conducted stimuli. *Audiology 31*: 61–71, 1992.

Lina-Granade G, Collet L, Morgon A. Auditory-evoked brainstem responses elicited by maximum-length sequences in normal and sensorineural ears. *Audiology 33:* 218–236, 1994.

Marsh RR. Signal to noise constraints on maximum length sequence auditory brain stem responses. *Ear and Hearing 13*: 396–400, 1991.

Marsh RR. Concurrent right and left ear auditory brain stem response recording. *Ear and Hearing 14:* 169–174, 1993.

Picton TW, Champagne SC, Kellett AJ. Human auditory evoked potentials recorded using maximum length sequences. *Electroencephalography and Clinical Neurophysiology 84*: 90–100, 1992.

Thornton ARD, Slaven A. Auditory brainstem responses recorded at fast stimulation rates using maximum length sequences. *British Journal of Audiology 27*: 205–210, 1993.

Van Campen LE, Sammeth CA, Hall JW III, Peek BF. Comparison of Etymotic insert and TDH supra-aural earphones in auditory brainstem response measurement. *Journal of the American Academy of Audiology 3:* 315–323, 1992.

Acquisition

Frijns JH, van Wijngaarden A, Peeters S. A multi-channel simultaneous data acquisition and waveform generation system designed for medical applications. *Journal of Medical Engineering & Technology 18*: 54–60,1994.

Analysis

Moore EJ, Semela JJ, Rakerd B, Robb RC, Ananthanarayan AK. The I' potential of the brainstem auditory-evoked potential. *Scandinavian Audiology 21:* 153–156, 1992.

Pratt H, Martin WH, Schwegler JW, Rosenwasser RH, Rosenberg SI, Flamm ES. Temporal correspondence of intracranial, cochlear and scalp-recor

ABR IN ESTIMATION OF HEARING SENSITIVITY

Normative Data

Comparison of ECochG and ABR click-stimulus intensity levels for 0 dB Re: normal hearing level expressed in dB SPL for different stimulus presentation rates.

Study, year	Rate	peak SPL	peSPL*
Burkard & Hecox, 1983	27	40.0	—
Campbell et al., 1981	10	40.0	34.0
Hood & Berlin, 1986	27.7	36.0	—
Ozdamar & Stein, 1981	20	—	32.0
Selters & Brackmann, 1977	20	38.0	—

*pe = peak equivalent (i.e., with reference to a sustained tone stimulus)

Latency-Intensity Function for Plotting ABR Findings

An example of a clinical form for recording auditory brainstem response wave V latency as a function of stimulus intensity (i.e., plotting an ABR latency-intensity function). Feel free to copy and modify this form for use in your clinic.

Vanderbilt Balance & Hearing Center

NAME ______________________________ DATE ____________

AUDITORY BRAINSTEM RESPONSE (ABR)
Latency / intensity function

Wave V latency in msec

10.0
9.0
8.0
7.0
6.0
5.0

Age-corrected normal region

20 40 60 80 100

Click intensity level in dB nHL

	Right ear	Left ear
Air conduction	○	□
Bone conduction	●	■

Latencies in msec at 85 dB nHL *

	I	III	V	I - III	III - V	I - V
Right ear						
Left ear						

** value exceeds normal region*

COMMENTS ____

____

Audiologist ______________________________

Flowchart of ABR in Estimating Hearing Sensitivity

Flowchart summarizing the steps in auditory brainstem response (ABR) measurement and analysis when the clinical objective is estimation of hearing sensitivity levels.

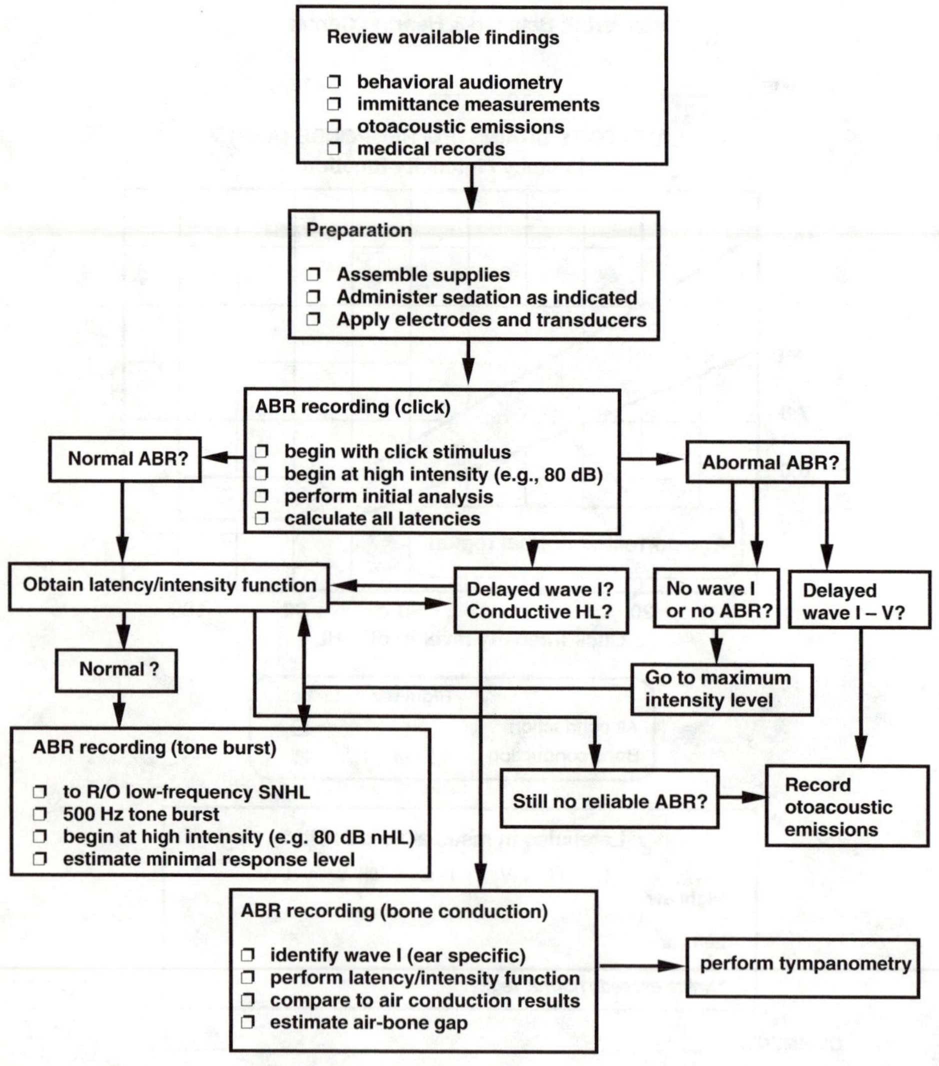

Classic Quote

Benjamin Franklin on being as quick as you can in performing audiologic services

"Remember that time is money."

Benjamin Franklin (1706-1790)
Advice to a Young Tradesman [1748]

Maturation of the ABR

Also, see normative neonatal and infant ABR data in this chapter.

- ☐ First measured at about 27 or 28 weeks gestational age
- ☐ Waveform initially is characterized by reliable wave I and V, whereas other wave components usually not observed
- ☐ ABR threshold (minimum intensity level at which a reliable response is recorded) appears to improve from prematurity until term (40 weeks gestational age)
- ☐ Maturational changes in ABR continue until approximately 18 months after term birth. These include:
  - ✔ improvement in waveform morphology (synchrony)
  - ✔ appearance of wave III, then wave II and IV
  - ✔ decrease in latency values for later waves (III and V)
  - ✔ decrease in interwave latency values (e.g., I–V)
  - ✔ increase in high frequency spectral energy

Bone-Conduction ABR

Auditory brainstem response (ABR) measurement with bone-conduction stimulation. Effective bone conduction stimulation produces an ABR wave I (generated by the ipsilateral eighth nerve) which is detected by the ipsilateral electrode array (particularly the inverting electrode on the stimulated ear lobe), as illustrated by the lower left waveform. Generally, the contralateral waveform will not show a distinct wave I, confirming that the bone conduction stimulation is ear-specific. For these anatomic reasons, contralateral masking is rarely indicated or needed in bone conduction ABR recording. When considering ear-specific ABR measurement, forget what you learned about the indications for masking during pure tone audiometry with air- or bone-conduction stimuli.

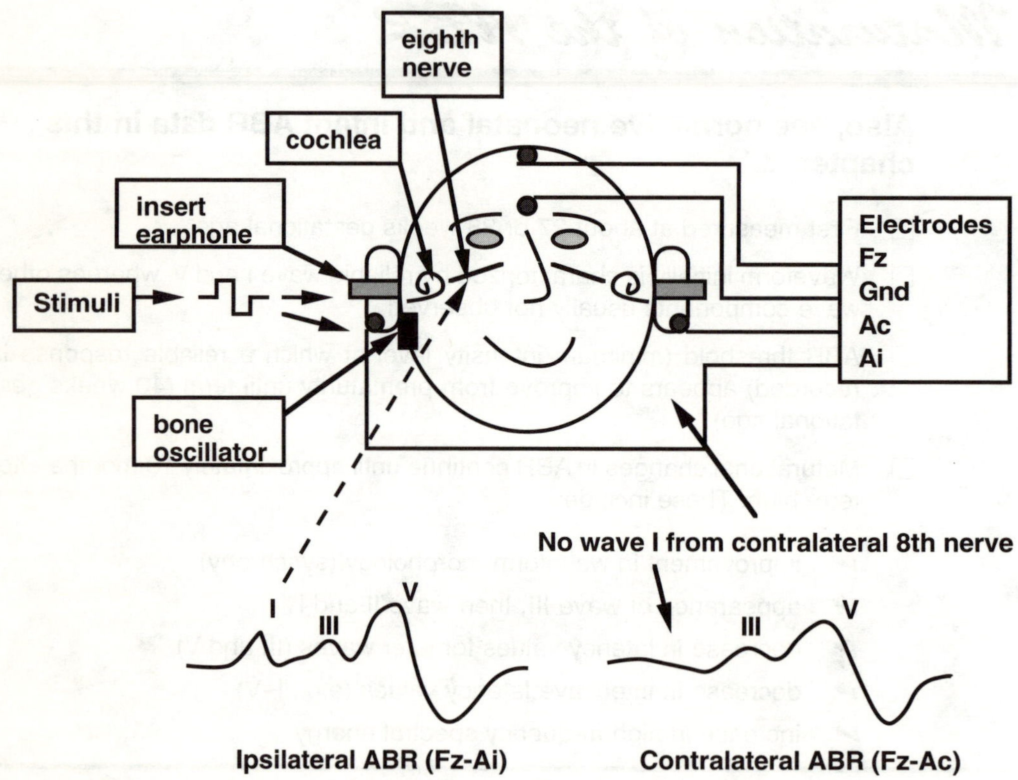

Protocol

Bone-Conduction ABR

The conventional ABR protocol for air conduction click stimuli must be modified to record ABRs successfully for bone conduction stimuli. Here are the main differences between protocols. Also, see PROTOCOL: ABR and FIGURES.

Parameters	Suggestions	Rationale/Comment
Stimulus		
Transducer	B-70	Apply the bone vibrator for bone conduction ABR on the mastoid
Polarity	Alternating	Instead of the usual rarefaction polarity, use a alternating polarity to minimize the stimulus artifact that produced by the close proximity of the bone vibrator and the inverting electrode on the ipsilateral ear lobe
Rate	7.1/sec	A slower rate helps to enhance identification of wave I which is essential to assure that the response is ear-specific, even without masking the contralateral ear
Intensity	< 55 dB nHL	This is about the maximum intensity that can be reached with the relatively inefficient bone conduction mode of stimulus presentation. That is, at maximum intensity settings for the ABR equipment (e.g., 95 dB), the effective stimulus level is only about 50 to 55 dB nHL. Put another way, behavioral threshold for the bone conduction click stimulus for a normal hearer is approximately 40 to 45 dB on the dial.
Masking	Occasional	If you can observe a clear and reliable wave I component in the ipsilateral electrode array (the inverting electrode is on the stimulus ear), then the cochlea of the test ear is being activated, and is producing an eighth nerve AP plus the ABR, and no masking is needed. If there is no clear wave I, then apply 50 to 60 dB white noise to nontest ear (via insert earphones) and reanalyze the ABR.
Acquisition		
Electrode arrays*		
	Ch 1: Fz-Ai	Forehead (vs. vertex) noninverting electrode site (for convenience) with the noninverting electrode on the ipsilateral (I) earlobe, making sure to distance the electrode from the bone vibrator as far as possible

(continued)

(continued)

Parameters	Suggestions	Rationale/Comment
	Ch 2: Fz-Ac	Use this contralateral channel as a "control" when you examine the ipsilateral channel for the presence of a wave I. If you see a bump in both channels where wave I should be, it may not be wave I.
Filter	30-3000 Hz	Keep the high pass filter cutoff this low (30 Hz) because the bone conduction ABR consists of plenty of low-frequency energy
Sweeps	500 to 4000	More may be needed because the stimulus intensity isn't very high, and the response reliability may be poor due to the less than ideal stimulus delivery via BC, and difficulties with consistent bone vibrator placement site and pressure.

*Noninverting-inverting electrode according to International 10-20 Electrode System

Clinical Concept

Four Excuses for Why Bone-Conduction ABR Is Not Done

Bone-conduction ABR is clinically feasible and valuable. Here are four reasons (excuses) for why many audiologists don't use a bone-conduction ABR technique clinically.

- ☐ Test protocols which are appropriate for air-conduction stimuli will not produce quality bone-conduction ABR recordings. It is necessary to modify these test protocols to record reliable bone-conduction ABR waveforms.
- ☐ Strategies for analysis and interpretation of ABR waveforms and latency intensity functions are distinctly different for bone- vs. air-conduction stimuli.
- ☐ Most clinicians probably attempt to record bone conduction ABRs initially from adult patients, although it is actually much easier to record quality bone-conduction ABR recordings from infants and children.
- ☐ It is generally assumed, incorrectly, that the same bothersome masking problems associated with bone-conduction pure tone audiometry are encountered in bone conduction ABR measurement. In fact, with a proper use of inverting electrodes, and an understanding of the generation of wave I, masking is rarely required for ear specific bone conduction ABR measurement.

Clinical Concept

Masking and Bone-Conduction ABR

If masking is not used, or effective masking cannot be applied, in bone-conduction ABR, then how do you know the ABR findings are ear-specific?

There is one main reason why identification of an ear-specific response is easier for bone-conduction ABR than for bone-conduction pure tone audiometry. With pure tone audiometry, the behavioral responses for the test ear versus the nontest ear are indistinguishable. For bone-conduction ABR, however, the generator for the response (test ear versus nontest ear) often can be unequivocally determined. The ABR wave I is near-field response. It is detected best with an electrode located as close as possible to its generator (i.e., the distal, or cochlear, end of the eighth cranial nerve). If the ABR wave I can be clearly observed in the waveform recorded with an ipsilateral electrode array (see Figure in this ADR chapter), then the response is unequivocally arising from the test ear. Any manipulations of measurement parameters which increase wave I amplitude are therefore useful in confirming an ear-specific bone-conduction ABR. If only an ABR wave V component is observed in the waveform, however, it is not possible to determine test ear confidently without applying adequate masking to the nontest ear. Observation of a wave I component in both the ipsilateral and contralateral electrode arrays confirms direct stimulation of the test ear, and also crossover stimulation of the nontest ear.

Protocol

Tone-burst ABR Recording

The conventional ABR protocol for air conduction click stimuli must be modified to record ABRs successfully for tone burst stimuli. Here are the main differences between protocols. Also, see PROTOCOL: ABR and FIGURES, and TECHNICAL TIP: BONE CONDUCTION AND TONE BURST ABR ANALYSIS.

Parameters	Suggestions	Rationale/Comment
Stimulus		
polarity	alternating	Instead of the usual rarefaction polarity, you may want to use a alternating polarity to minimize the possibility of a frequency-following type response.
ramping	Blackman	This is how the rise/fall portions of the tone burst are shaped. Certain nonlinear ramping or windowing techniques reduce spectral splatter and increase frequency specificity of tone burst stimulation. Blackman windowing is the best, and most modern AER systems include it in their stimulus package.
duration	variable	The rise/fall, and plateau, times for the tone burst stimuli vary depending on the frequency. As a rule, it's desirable to use longer times for lower frequencies so as to include more cycles. This increases the chances that the stimulus sounds like the desired frequency, and not a click. Here are some suggestions: ✔ 500 Hz: 4 msec rise/fall and 0 msec plateau ✔ 1000 Hz: 2 msec rise/fall and 0 or 1 msec plateau ✔ 2000 Hz: 1 msec rise/fall and 0 or 0.5 msec plateau ✔ 4000 Hz: 0.5 msec rise/fall and 0 msec plateau
intensity	variable	Keep in mind that the intensity levels "on the dial" for your ABR system will usually not be defined in dB nHL, as they are for a click. That is, you may select 95 dB on the dial, but the intensity range for the tone burst frequency may go as high as 115 dB. Always get behavioral threshold data for each tone burst stimulus you intend to use for ABR recording (with the earphones you'll use and in the ABR test room), and then develop a "correction factor" for tone burst intensity. For example, if your maximum dial setting for a 500 Hz tone burst is 115 dB, but your normal subjects have an average threshold of 30 dB for this stimulus, then at 115 dB on the dial you're really presenting an intensity level of 85 dB nHL. You may also want to record ABRs for this 500 Hz stimulus from a few of these normal-hearing subjects to estimate the lowest intensity level that produces an observable and reliable ABR wave V.
Acquisition		
filter	30–3000 Hz	It is essential that you keep the high-pass filter cut-off this low (30 Hz) because the tone burst ABR is dominated by low-frequency energy

*Noninverting-inverting electrode according to International 10-20 Electrode System

Sedation Personnel and Procedures

Conscious sedation of patients, as in pedatric ABR assessment. Also, see other lists related to sedation in this ADR chapter.

Personnel

☐ The physician responsible for the patient or supervising the procedure should be present at the procedure or within the procedure area during the entire sedation period.

☐ A registered or licensed practical nurse or other appropriately qualified professional must be present to monitor and document the patient's physiologic parameters and assist in any supportive or resuscitative measures. This person should be trained in basic life support and anesthesia recovery principles.

Procedures

☐ Obtain informed consent for conscious sedation, as well as the procedure (e.g., ABR) as indicated.

☐ Perform a health evaluation prior to sedation on the same day, or within recent days, to include:

- age and weight
- medical history, including drug allergies, current medications, relevant diseases, adverse drug reactions (e.g. paradoxical reaction to the planned sedative), and any relevant family history
- review of systems, especially any airway or respiratory problems
- history of specific drug, dosage, and time of any medications taken on the day of the procedure
- history of food or fluid intake within the past 8 hours
- vital signs, including heart rate, blood pressure, respiratory rate, level of consciousness, and temperature

☐ Conscious sedation orders for patients must be written. Prescriptions or orders from areas outside the area where conscious sedation is administered are not acceptable.

☐ All medication is administered by a physician or nurse.

☐ Physicians or their designee will maintain a time-based record including the name, route, site, time, dosage, and patient effects of any drugs administered during the procedure.

- ☐ The patient's vital signs and oxygen saturation will be monitored by the physician or nursing staff during the procedure and documented in the record at intervals.
- ☐ After the procedure, the patient must be observed in a facility appropriately staffed and equipped (see Sedation Equipment in this chapter).
- ☐ If a patient is discharged following completion of the procedure, the physician or designee will identify a person responsible for the patient, and provide verbal and written instructions and information about limitations of activity, anticipated changes in behavior, and so on, to this person.
- ☐ Discharge criteria must be met and documented prior to discharging a patient following sedation.
  - ✔ Vital signs are stable and within the preprocedure range.
  - ✔ The patient has returned to his or her presedation level of consciousness.
  - ✔ The patient has written instructions for post-procedure care.

Source: Adapted from Vanderbilt University Medical Center policy for conscious sedation of patients.

Sedation

Emergency equipment and supplies that should be available and in good working order in the location where conscious sedation takes place.

- ✔ An emergency cart with supplemental equipment to handle both adult and pediatric emergencies. The cart should be checked daily by a designated individual and maintained as per hospital policy.
- ✔ Oral suction equipment and a variety of suction catheter sizes.
- ✔ A portable cardiac monitor and defibrillator with cardioversion capability.
- ✔ A pulse oximeter suitable for monitoring every sedated adult and pediatric patient.
- ✔ Oxygen with positive pressure delivery system capable of delivering 90% O_2.
- ✔ Sphygmomanometer or automated blood pressure monitor with adult and/or pediatric cuff sizes.

Source: Adapted from Vanderbilt University Medical Center policy for conscious sedation of patients.

Sedation Strategies and Responsibilities

Important things to do when administering chloral hydrate sedation for patients undergoing ABR assessment. Also, see Sedation: Emergency Equipment in this chapter.

- Give instructions in advance to parent or caregiver on clinic policy for obtaining prescription, sleep deprivation, and eating and/or drinking before sedation.
- Inquire about any prior experience with chloral hydrate sedation. If chloral hydrate sedation failed previously for ABR or another diagnostic procedure, such as computerized tomography. If so, consider IM injection of Demerol, Phenargan, Thorazine combination (a "pediatric cocktail").
- Verify prescription from referring physician for proper dosage.
- Document the referring physician's complete name, office address, telephone number, and page number.
- Document (or have nurse document) any possible contraindications to sedation, any other medications or any pertinent medical history (e.g., allergies, seizures, respiratory, or heart disorders).
- Contact medical support personnel (nurse or physician) upon patient arrival, and closely follow hospital or facility procedures and policy for conscious sedation.
- Weigh the patient (note: patient plus caregiver weight minus caregiver weight = patient weight).
- Convert patient's weight from pounds to kilograms. Remember 1000 grams (1 Kg) is equivalent to 2.2 lb.
- Verify the availability and accessability (e.g., unlocked) of stocked emergency kit or cart and other required monitoring devices (e.g., pulse oximeter).
- Unless contraindicated or previously unsuccessful, administer chloral hydrate. Recommended dosage is either 50 mg/kg (milligram of drug per kilogram of body weight or 75 mg/kg. With referring physician written approval, a one-half dose may be repeated in 45 minutes. Dosage should not exceed 100 mg/kg of body weight or a total of 1000 mg (1gram). Any discrepancies between written prescription and chloral hydrate supplied are discussed with referring physician or on call attending or resident physician.
- Chloral hydrate is typically adminstered orally (drinking from cup or injected from syringe without needle into mouth) by nurse.
- Amount of sedations ingested is documented in writing.

- Vital signs (respiration, heart rate, pulse oximetry) are evaluated and monitored before, periodically or continuously during, and always immediately after sedation by a nurse, or a physician
- After testing, nurse or physician examines the patient (vital signs, state of arousal) and otains vital signs every 15 minutes until the patient is stable and responds readily to stimulation.
- Nurse or tester counsels parent or caregiver about post sedation care of patient (according to clinic policy for sedation precautions), and documents this in the medical record. The parent or caregiver is given the telephone number of personnel accepting responsibility for subsequent treatment of patient.
- Post sedation status of the patient is documented in medical records.

ABR Latency–Intensity (L-I) Function

Normal, Conductive, and Sensory-impaired Ears

Examples of auditory brainstem response (ABR) wave V latency versus click stimulus intensity functions for patients over 18 months of age with three different categories of hearing status: normal hearing, conductive hearing loss, and high frequency sensorineural (really sensory). Some typical ABR latency values (at an intensity level of 85 dB nHL) are shown in the lower portion. The normal L-I function is within normal limits for latency. The conductive L-I function has delayed latencies at all intensities. The sensorineural L-I function is within normal limits at high intensity levels (well above audiometric thresholds in the 2000 to 4000 Hz region). As the click intensity level approaches audiometric threshold in this frequency region, latency rapidly increases as the ABR is generated by lower frequencies. The delay is caused by increased traveling wave time along the basilar membrane until a region of adequate cochlear function is reached.

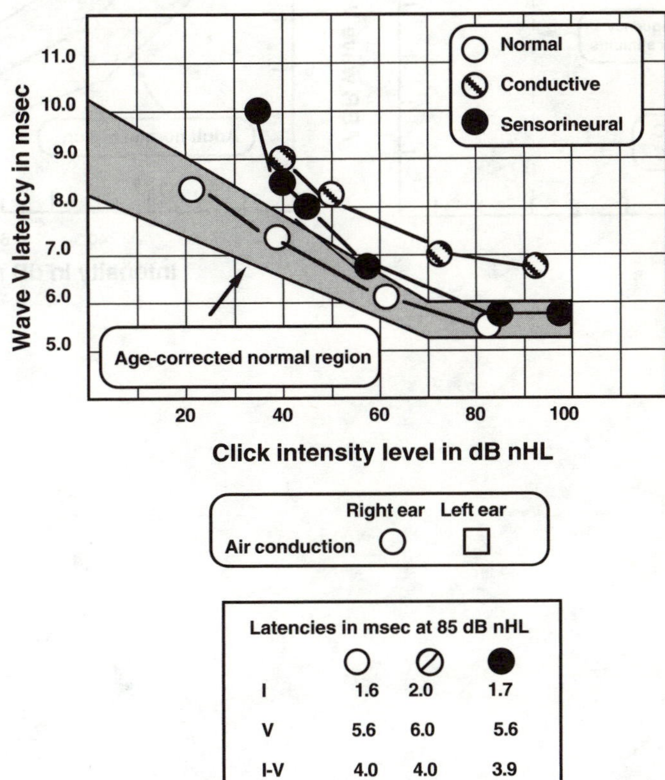

Latencies in msec at 85 dB nHL

	○ (Normal)	⊘ (Conductive)	● (Sensorineural)
I	1.6	2.0	1.7
V	5.6	6.0	5.6
I-V	4.0	4.0	3.9

Audiogram and ABR L-I Function

Normal Hearing

Auditory brainstem response (ABR) wave V latency versus click stimulus intensity function for a patient over 18 months of age with normal hearing sensitivity in the 2000 to 4000 Hz region, and normal auditory brainstem function.

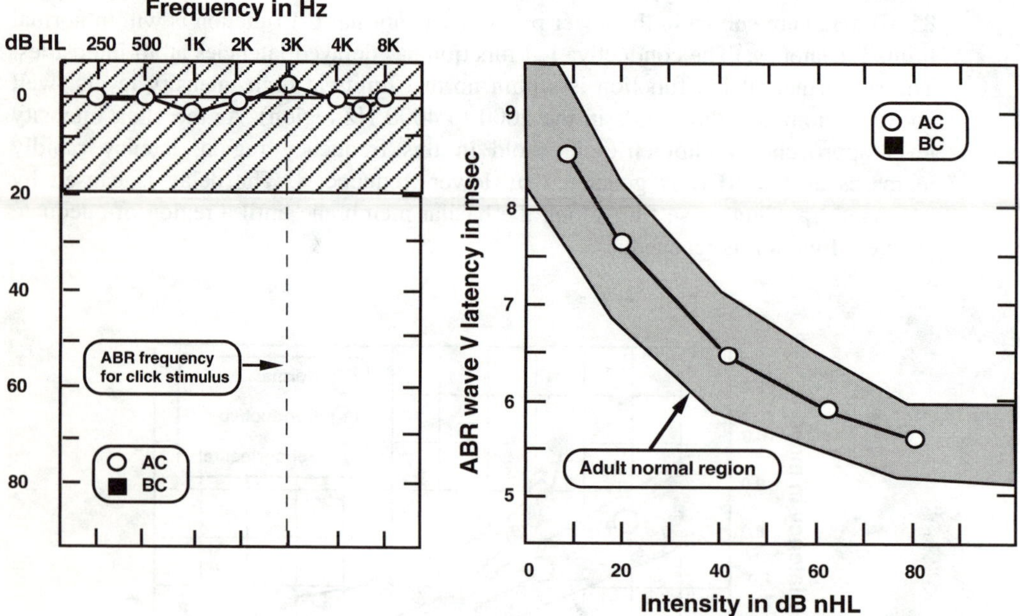

Audiogram and ABR L-I Function

Conductive Hearing Loss

Auditory brainstem response (ABR) wave V latency versus click stimulus intensity function for a patient over 18 months of age with conductive hearing loss (and normal auditory brainstem function). The conductive component attenuates the stimulus intensity level and causes a latency shift. The amount of the shift approximately what would be expected by attenuating the stimulus by the amount of the conductive component. In such cases, bone-conduction stimulation produces an ABR with wave V latency that is within normal limits (WNL).

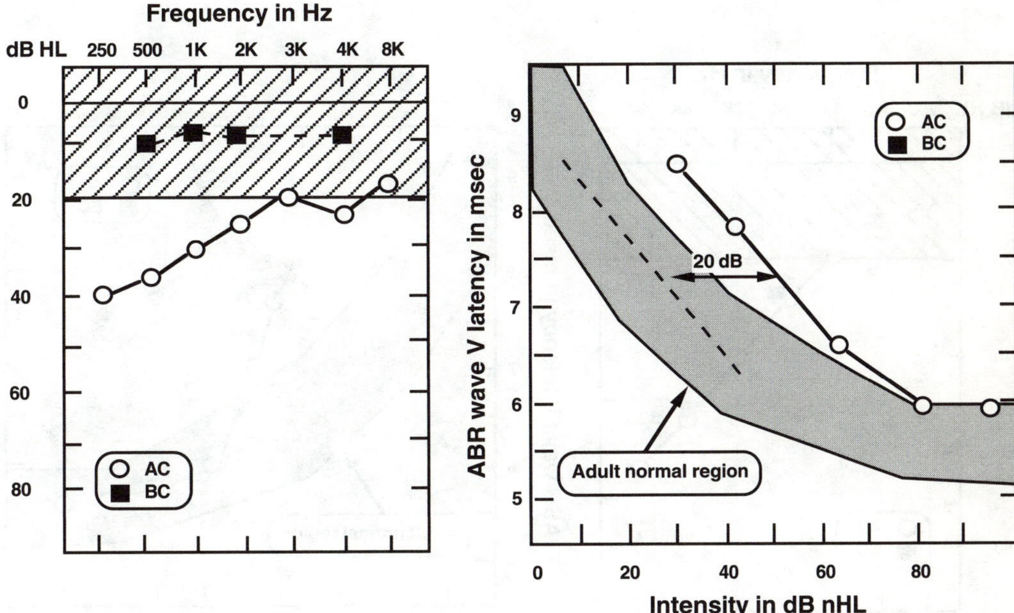

Audiogram and ABR L-I Function

High-frequency Sensory Hearing Loss

Auditory brainstem response (ABR) wave V latency versus click stimulus intensity function for a patient over 18 months of age with mild-to-moderate, high frequency sensory (cochlear) hearing loss (and normal auditory brainstem function). The sensorineural L-I function is within normal limits at high intensity levels (well above audiometric thresholds in the 2000 to 4000 Hz region). As the click intensity level approaches audiometric threshold in this frequency region, latency rapidly increases as the ABR is generated by lower frequencies. The delay is caused by increased traveling wave time along the basilar membrane until a region of adequate cochlear function is reached.

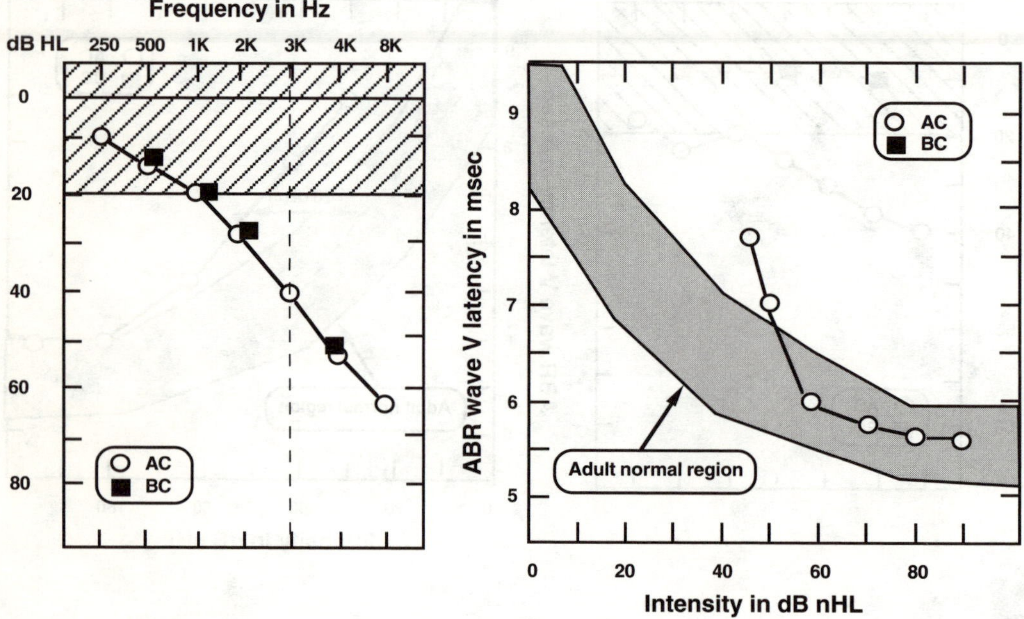

Audiogram and ABR L-I Function

Low-frequency Sensory Hearing Loss

Auditory brainstem response (ABR) wave V latency versus click stimulus intensity function for a patient over 18 months of age with low-frequency sensory (cochlear) hearing loss (and normal auditory brainstem function). Since hearing sensitivity is within normal limits in the frequency region most important for generation of the ABR (see page ___ in this ADR chapter), the click-evoked ABR lacks sensitivity to the hearing loss. If this were a neonate undergoing ABR hearing screening, the outcome would be a "pass". A low frequency sensory hearing loss can be detected with a low frequency (e.g., 500 Hz) tone burst stimulus.

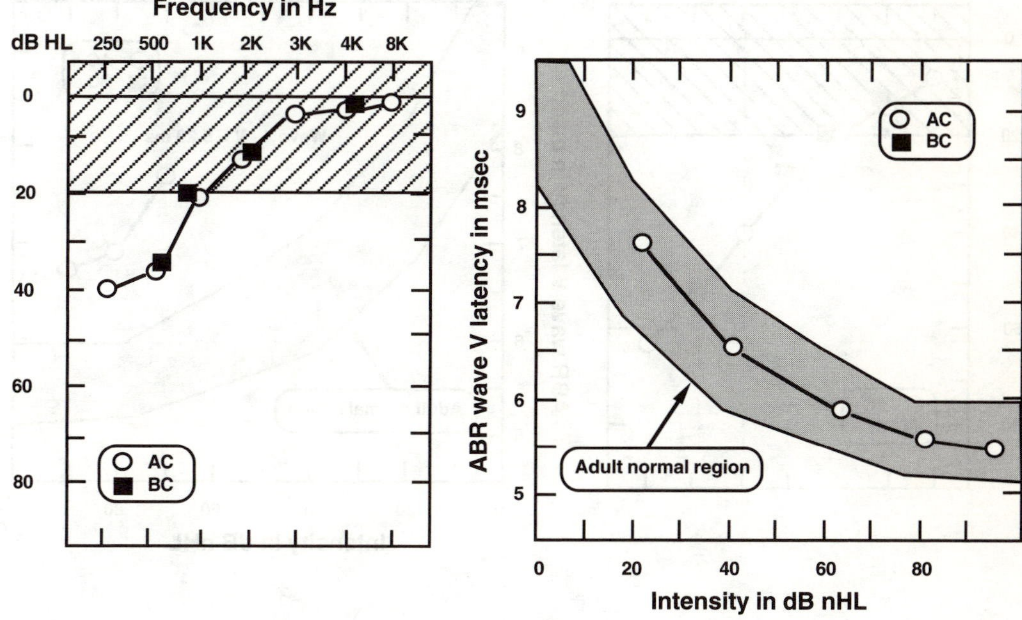

Audiogram and ABR L-I Function

Retrocochlear Hearing Loss

Auditory brainstem response (ABR) wave V latency versus click stimulus intensity function for a patient over 18 months of age with mild-to-moderate, high frequency neural (retrocochlear) hearing loss. The sensorineural L-I function is far outside normal limits at all intensity levels, even well above audiometric thresholds in the 2000 to 4000 Hz region. The wave I-V latency value is markedly abnormal (the upper limit of normal is 4.50 msec).

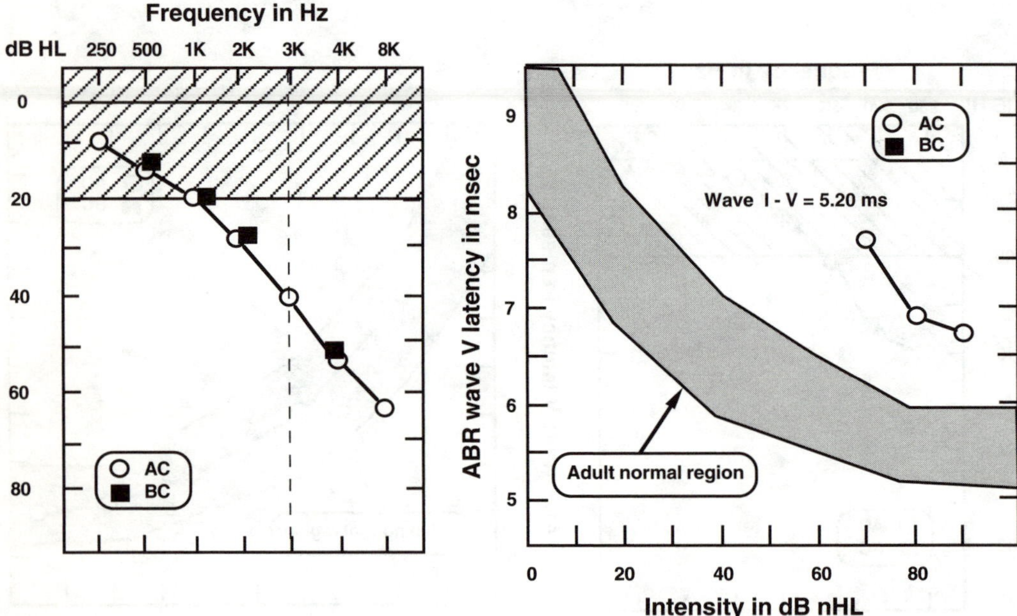

Audiogram and ABR L-I Function

Severe High-frequency Hearing Loss

Auditory brainstem response (ABR) wave V latency versus click stimulus intensity function for a patient over 18 months of age with severe high frequency sensory (cochlear) hearing loss (and normal auditory brainstem function). Since hearing sensitivity approaches the upper limits of a click stimulus in the frequency region most important for generation of the ABR (see page ___ in this ADR chapter), the click-evoked ABR wave V latency is markedly delayed. The longer latency values at lower intensity levels are because the ABR is then generated at lower frequencies. A low frequency (e.g., 500 Hz) tone burst stimulus might be useful to better estimate audiogram configuration.

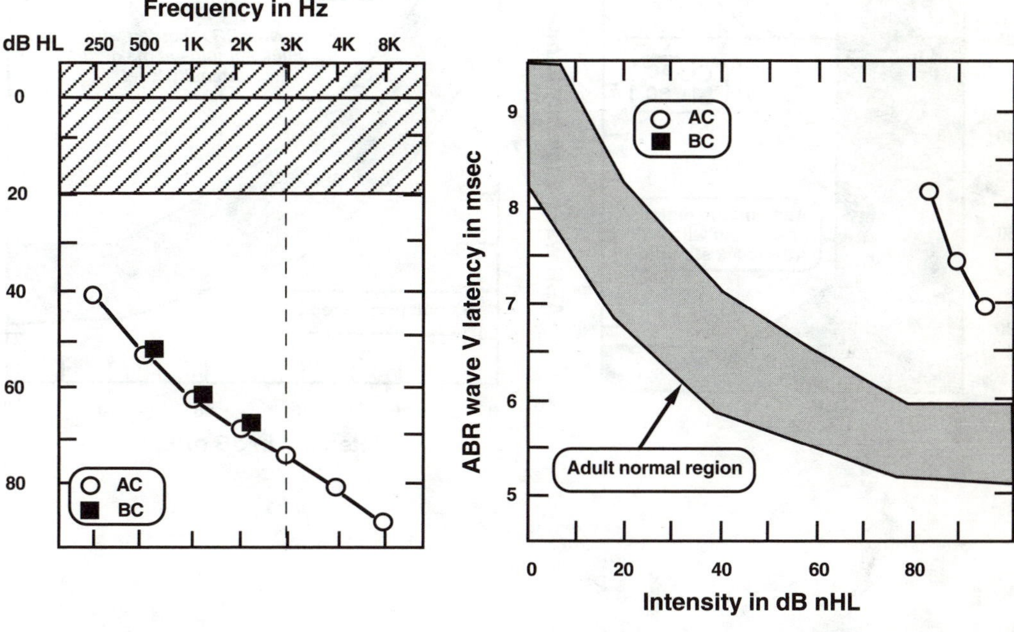

Audiogram and ABR L-I Function

Severe-to-Profound Hearing Loss

Audiometric region (*shaded*) that is associated with an absent auditory brainstem response (ABR). That is, if hearing thresholds are within the shaded area, no ABR are likely to be generated by click stimuli, even at maximum intensity levels.

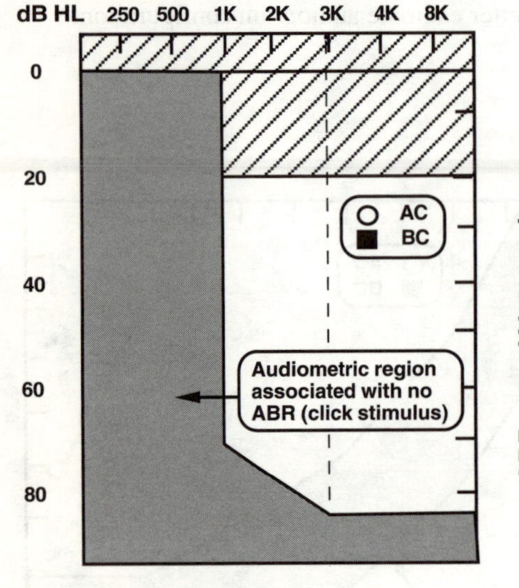

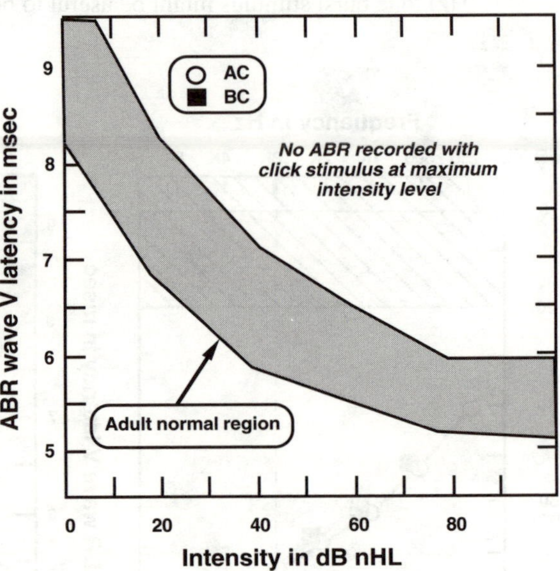

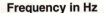

ABR IN NEURODIAGNOSIS

Flowchart

ABR in Neurodiagnosis

Flowchart summarizing the steps in auditory brainstem response (ABR) measurement and analysis when the clinical objective is neurodiagnostic (e.g., differentiation and localization of cochlear versus retrocochlear auditory dysfunction).

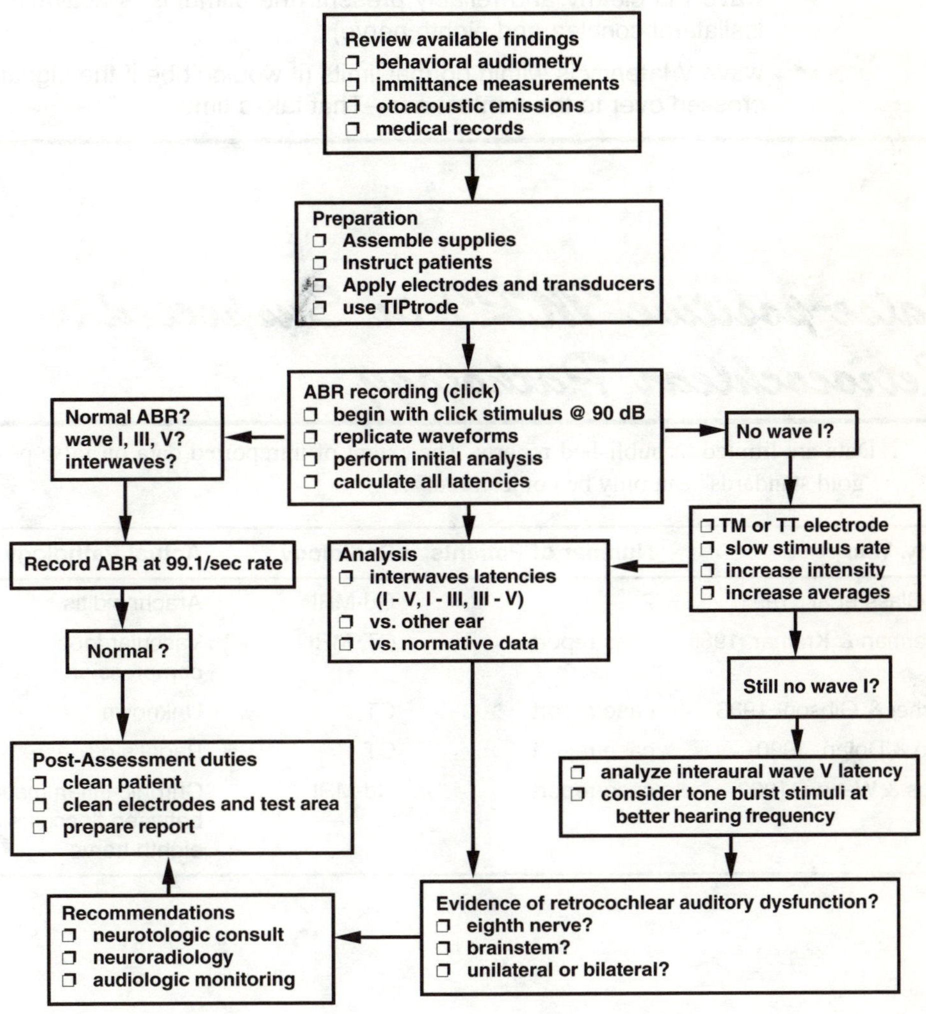

Technical Tip

ABR Measurement: When you need to use masking in ABR measurement, and when you don't.

- ☐ Masking is only needed when:
  - ✔ wave I is not present
  - ✔ wave V latency is abnormally delayed
- ☐ Masking is not needed when:
  - ✔ wave I is clearly and reliably present (the stimulus is activating the ipsilateral cochlea and eighth nerve)
  - ✔ wave V latency is within normal limits (it wouldn't be if the signal had crossed over to the nontest ear—That takes time)

False-positive MRI in Suspected Retrocochlear Pathology

Data are limited to published reports. The extent of unreported data on false-positive "gold standards" can only be conjectured.

Study, Year	Number of Patients	Radiology	Actual Pathology
von Glass et al., 1991	2	Gd-MRI	Arachnoiditis
Haberman & Kramer, 1989	case report	CT, MRI	Vascular loop compression
Prasher & Gibson, 1983	case report	CT	Unknown
Crain & Dolan, 1990	case report	CT	Paget's disease
Loftus & Wazen, 1990	case report	Gd-MRI	Chronic inflammation between flocculus and eighth nerve

ABR in Retrocochlear Pathology

Optimal criteria which most efficiently differentiate patients at low risk for retrocochlear pathology (normal audiometry and radiology) versus those with confirmed retrocochlear pathology.

ABR Variable	Criterion (in msec)	95% Confidence Limit* (in msec)
Waves I–III	2.65	2.52
Waves I–V (female)	4.69	4.34
Waves –V (male)	4.68	4.46
Interaural latency difference (ILD) for wave V	0.43	0.37
Rate latency shift for wave V (11/sec to 44/sec)	0.45	0.44
Rate latency shift for wave V (11/sec to 88/sec)	0.75	0.81

Source: Data from Lightfoot G. R. ABR screening for acoustic neuromata: the role of rate-induced latency shift measurements. *British Journal of Audiology 26*: 217–227, 1992, with permission.
*Derived from the group without confirmed retrocochlear pathology

Clinical Concept

Effect of Body Temperature on the ABR

See the figure illustrating temperature effects on ABR waveforms in this ADR chapter.

- ☐ Normal body temperature is 37° Centigrade, or 98.6° Fahrenheit.
- ☐ Body temperature for a patient may be different when recorded orally, rectally, at the tympanic membrane, or with a central line transducer.
- ☐ Hypothermia (low) body temperature prolongs ABR latencies, especially for later waves and the wave I–V latency interval.
- ☐ Hyperthermia (high) body temperature shortens ABR latencies, especially for later waves and the wave I–V latency interval.
- ☐ Use the following simple guideline to "correct" or adjust for the effects of body temperature on the ABR wave I–V latency value.
  - ✓ In *hypo*thermia, subtract **0.2 msec** from the wave I–V latency value for every degree of temperature below 37° Centigrade.
  - ✓ In *hyper*thermia, add **0.2 msec** to the wave I–V latency value for every degree of temperature above 37° Centigrade.

Technical Tips

Effects of Gender and Age on the ABR

- ☐ ABR latency is longer in males than females.
- ☐ ABR latency is longer in older adult patients (>60 years) than younger adult patients.
- ☐ ABR latency values (especially wave I–V) are shortest in young females and longest in older adult males.
- ☐ The ABR is mature in latency, amplitude, and morphology for children older than 1.5 years (18 months) chronological age.
- ☐ There is no major gender influence on the ABR in children.
- ☐ In infants, start calculating chronologic age after 40 weeks gestational age (e.g., be cautious about age calculations in premature infants).

ABR NORMATIVE DATA

Normative ABR Data for Neonates

ABR latency and amplitude values for 80 dB HL click intensity level in newborns

Chronologic Age (N) (in weeks)	Latency (in msec)				
	I	V	I–III	III–V	I–V
33–34 (38)					
Mean	1.78	7.05	2.86	2.41	5.27
SD	0.30	0.39	0.28	0.26	0.36
35–36 (150)					
Mean	1.78	7.02	2.84	2.39	5.24
SD	0.26	0.38	0.27	0.25	0.36
37–38 (158)					
Mean	1.74	6.94	2.80	2.34	5.17
SD	0.21	0.42	0.31	0.26	0.40
39–40 (111)					
Mean	1.72	6.82	2.70	2.38	5.09
SD	0.23	0.38	0.27	0.25	0.36
41–42 (74)					
Mean	1.69	6.69	2.74	2.24	5.00
SD	0.19	0.29	0.22	0.21	0.30
43–44 (35)					
Mean	1.65	6.53	2.65	2.21	4.88
SD	0.15	0.32	0.26	0.21	0.31

Source: Gorga et al. (1987).

Measurement parameters: stimulus = click; duration = 0.1 msec, intensity = 80 dB HL (110 dB peSPL); rate = 13/sec; mode = monaural; transducers = Beyer DT48 earphone; filters = 100–3,000 Hz; amplification = 100,000; sweeps = 1,024; analysis time = 15 msec; electrodes = Cz-Mi; CA = conceptional age in weeks; N = number of infants.

Normative Data for Children 3 Months–3 Years

ABR latency values as a function of intensity level in children ages 3 months to 3 years

		Latency (msec)				
		Wave V				Wave I
Age (in mos.)	*N*	80 dB	60 dB	40 dB	20 dB	80 dB
3–6	79					
Mean		6.25	6.73	7.43	8.72	1.59
SD		0.32	0.33	0.36	0.53	0.17
6–9	68					
Mean		6.10	6.56	7.28	8.59	1.59
SD		0.26	0.29	0.38	0.61	0.16
9–12	88					
Mean		5.90	6.31	7.05	8.31	1.59
SD		0.27	0.29	0.37	0.54	0.18
12–15	44					
Mean		5.91	6.30	7.10	8.28	1.59
SD		0.27	0.33	0.45	0.60	0.17
15–8	48					
Mean		5.84	6.24	7.00	8.33	1.58
SD		0.27	0.24	0.38	0.61	0.14
18–21	23					
Mean		5.74	6.19	6.95	8.22	1.55
SD		0.19	0.18	0.36	0.62	0.12
21–24	23					
Mean		5.71	6.14	6.79	8.05	1.57
SD		0.26	0.29	0.33	0.58	0.17
24–27	15					
Mean		5.71	6.09	6.89	8.30	1.53
SD		0.19	0.22	0.29	0.46	0.14
27–30	13					
Mean		5.60	6.08	6.75	7.98	1.59
SD		0.22	0.28	0.33	0.42	0.19
30–33	45					
Mean		5.68	6.07	6.79	8.12	1.56
SD		0.27	0.31	0.32	0.53	0.16
33–36	21					
Mean		5.68	6.06	6.82	8.10	1.56
SD		0.27	0.31	0.38	0.68	0.15

Source: Gorga et al. (1987).

Measurement parameters: stimulus = click; duration = 0.1 msec, intensity = 80 dB HL (110 dB peSPL); rate = 13/sec; mode = monaural; transducers = Beyer DT48 earphone; filters = 100–3,000 Hz; amplification = 100,000; sweeps = 1,024; analysis time = 15 msec; electrodes = Cz-Mi; CA = conceptional age in weeks; *N* = number.

Normative ABR Data

Neonates and Children to Age 5

ABR latency values at 60 dB HL as a function of age in children through age 5 years

Age	*N*	Latency (msec)						Amplitude (mV)	
		Preterm			Term			Preterm	Term
(in wks)*	(preterm/term)	I	V	I–V	I	V	I–V	V/I	V/I
33	52								
Mean		2.57	8.21	5.64	—	—	—	1.30	—
SD		0.54	0.79	0.70	—	—	—	1.13	—
36	62								
Mean		2.41	7.83	5.32	—	—	—	1.29	—
SD		0.38	0.59	0.55	—	—	—	0.58	—
40	36/161								
Mean		2.34	7.54	5.20	2.00	7.14	5.14	1.41	1.31
SD		0.44	0.62	0.60	0.31	0.43	0.40	0.86	1.55
43	13/57								
Mean		2.01	7.07	5.07	1.80	6.93	5.13	1.16	1.52
SD		0.24	0.23	0.33	0.24	0.37	0.35	0.53	0.83
46	7/57								
Mean		2.16	6.72	4.56	1.68	6.64	4.96	1.40	1.30
SD		0.28	0.28	0.13	0.19	0.26	0.27	0.52	0.63
53	86/34								
Mean		1.95	6.60	4.64	1.69	6.40	4.71	1.74	1.43
SD		0.38	0.46	0.37	0.22	0.22	0.27	1.52	0.75
66	20/43								
Mean		2.02	6.42	4.40	1.70	6.15	4.45	1.69	1.78
SD		0.39	0.34	0.39	0.17	0.23	0.21	0.94	1.22
70	70/35								
Mean		1.86	6.23	4.38	1.68	6.01	4.32	1.81	1.81
SD		0.30	0.45	0.40	0.24	0.26	0.20	1.20	0.79
144	41/19								
Mean		1.78	5.97	4.19	1.66	5.86	4.21	1.55	1.72
SD		0.25	0.32	0.26	0.12	0.19	0.21	0.63	0.47
196	23/14								
Mean		1.71	5.74	4.02	1.66	5.81	4.16	1.55	2.63
SD		0.17	0.21	0.23	0.11	0.32	0.29	0.62	2.35
248	12/16								
Mean		1.77	5.84	4.07	1.67	5.80	4.14	1.48	1.90
SD		0.20	0.31	0.26	0.15	0.25	0.21	0.43	0.61
300	2/5								
Mean		1.76	5.69	3.93	1.66	5.68	4.02	2.13	1.91
SD		0.17	0.06	0.25	0.09	0.21	0.16	1.26	0.58

Adult	33								
Mean		—	—	—	1.70	5.66	4.08	—	2.13
SD		—	—	—	0.16	0.23	0.25	—	1.26

Source: Eggermont & Salamy (1988).
Measurement parameters: stimulus = click; duration = 0.1 msec; rate = 15/sec; intensity = 60dB HL; transducer = Sennheiser HD-414 earphone= masking = white noise masking;filters, = 100-3000 Hz; electrodes = Cz-Ai.
*Postconceptional age in weeks (40 weeks = term).

Normative Data

Neurodiagnostic ABR data used at the Vanderbilt Audiology Clinics

PARAMETERS

Stimulus

- ☐ 0.1 msec click
- ☐ intensity = >80 dB nHL
- ☐ rate = 21.1/sec
- ☐ polarity = rarefaction
- ☐ transducer = ER 3A

Acquisition

- ☐ filter settings = 30–3000 Hz
- ☐ electrodes = Fz-to-Apsi and Fz-to-Acontra
- ☐ gain = 100,000
- ☐ analysis time = 15 msec with 1 msec prestimulus time
- ☐ sample points = 512

NEURODIAGNOSTIC NORMATIVE RETION (85 dB nHL click stimulus)

Absolute latencies

I = < 1.90 msec
V = < 6.25 msec

Interwave latencies

I–III = < 2.55 msec
III–V = < 2.35 msec
I–V = < 4.60 msec

Interwave amplitudes

V/I = > 0.5

ALWAYS:

1. correct for age under 18 months
2. account for gender in interpretation
3. account for age in interpretation for >60 years
4. account for asymmetry in hearing thresholds in 2K - 4K hZ region
5. account for possible conductive hearing loss component
6. adjust protocol to whatever yields the highest quality, most reliable ABR waveform

ABR IN NEUROPHYSIOLOGIC MONITORING

Flowchart

The Role of Audiologists in the Evaluation and Management of Patients with Auditory System or Facial Nerve Dysfunction, Including Intraoperative Neurophysiologic Monitoring

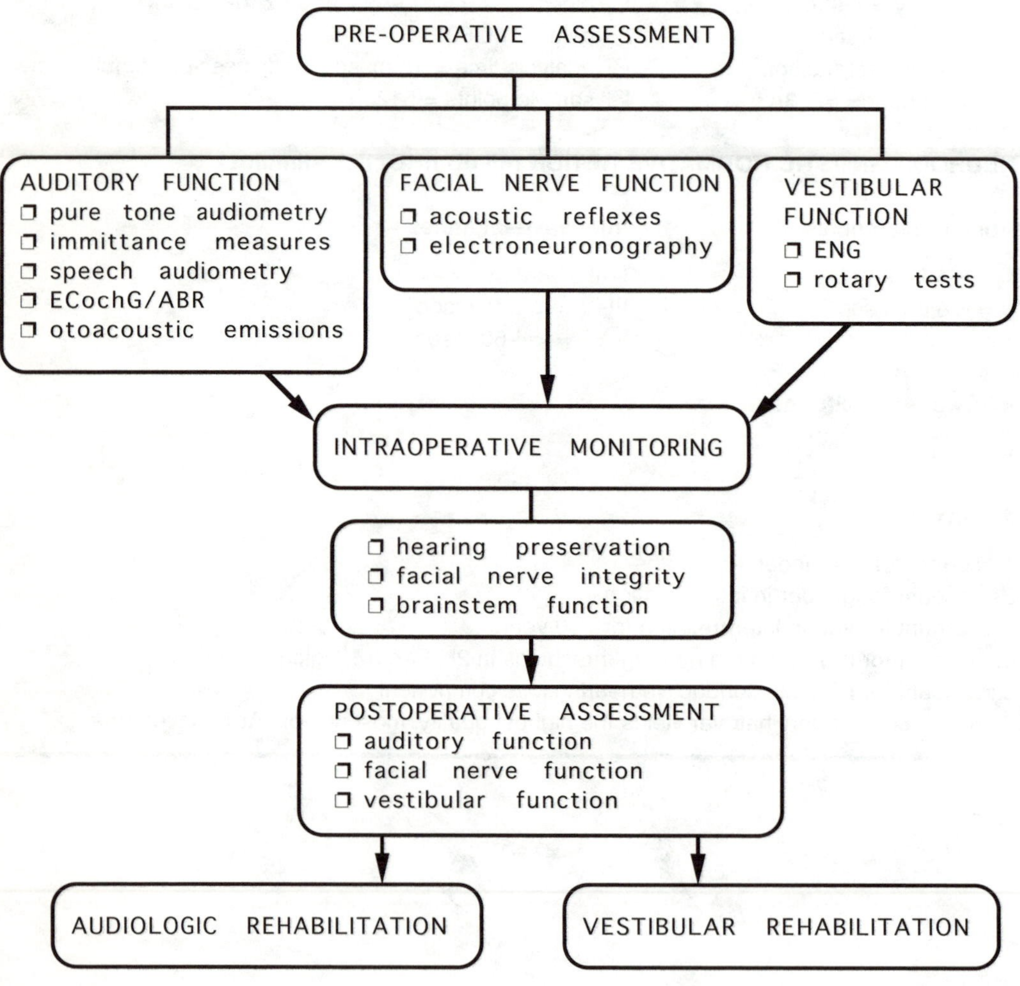

Facial Nerve Monitoring

Artifacts and Nonsurgical Stimuli in the Operating Room

Stimulus	EMG	Acoustic representation
Stimulator charged by prior cautery use	DC offset of EMG baseline even though stimulator placed distant from nerve	Machine gun
Static discharge	Single polyphasic response	Synchronous click
Too little anesthetic	Multiple asynchronous responses	Popping corn
Electrocautery	Multiple asynchronous responses	Silent if muting detector used
Peripheral nerve stimulator	Precisely timed responses	Machine gun

EMG and Acoustic Representation of Surgical Stimuli

Stimulus	EMG	Acoustic representation
Electrical	Precisely timed responses	Machine gun
Mechanical	Single polyphasic response (burst)	Synchronous click
Traction	Multiple asynchronous responses (train)	Popping corn, possibly delayed
Thermal	Initially: widened baseline Later: multiple asynchronous responses	Initially: silent Later: popping corn

Effects of Pharmacologic Agents on the ABR

- No effect
  - Althesin
  - Anticholinergics
  - Etomidate
  - Fentanyl
  - Ketamine
  - Nitrous oxide
  - Pentobarbital *
- Adverse Effects

Enflurane:	Up to 1 msec wave V latency change
Halothane:	Up to 0.5 msec delay in wave V latency
Isoflurane:	Beyond 1.5% end-tidal concentration over 0.5 msec increase in I–V interpeak latency
Lidocaine:	Reduction of the amplitude and delay in the latency of wave V
Sodium thiopental:	At very high doses (77.5 mg/l kg), a 0.5 msec increase in wave V latency was documented

*Hall (1992) reported a significant increase in wave I amplitude during barbiturate coma.

Checklist

Intraoperative Facial Nerve Monitoring Problems

Problem	Possible Solution
Current jump	Bipolar stimulator
Current shunting	Insulated stimulator
Cautery artifact noise	Muting Circuit
Cautery precludes monitoring	Visualize face
Laser heating effect	Monitor baseline amplitude
Saline cooling	Heat saline with "blood warmer"
Stimulus artifact	Increase "stimulus ignore" time
Static discharge	Insulated instruments
No response to stimulation	1. Power off
	2. Current intensity too low
	3. Current measured too low
	4. Electrode impedance too high
	5. Electrode disconnect
	6. Current shunting
	7. Threshold setting too high
	8. Volume too low
	9. Muscle relaxant used
	10. "Stimulus ignore" too long
	11. Seventh nerve not contacted
	12. Other cranial nerve/tissue
	13. Facial nerve injured

Strategies for Decreasing Artifacts

Auditory Evoked Responses Recorded Intraoperatively

- Remove debris and film from skin, and abrade skin before applying scalp electrodes.
- Keep electrode impedances at or below approximately 2,000 ohms.
- Use short electrode wires.
- Limit interelectrode distances between pairs of recording electrodes.
- Braid the recording electrode wires.
- Insert backup recording electrodes on the patient preoperatively.
- Keep recording versus stimulating wires and cords separated.
- Separate transducer(s) from recording electrodes as much as possible.
- Do not cross cables or wires over other cables, especially power cables.
- Do not touch or bump the wires; separate them from ventilation tubes and anesthesia lines.
- Unplug unused equipment.
- Never use two-pronged power plugs (ungrounded).
- Pause signal averaging whenever amplifiers are blocking (e.g., after electrocautery).
- Adjust amplifier sensitivity to produce some artifact rejection.
- Advice anesthesiology to use neuromuscular junction blocking agents.

Source: Adapted from: Kartush J, Bouchard, K. *Neuromonitoring in otology and head and neck surgery.* New York: Raven, 1992.

Sound Levels in the Operating Room

Sound levels (specified in dBA) generated by several surgical tools as measured at the level of the surgical tools, at the ear of the surgeon, and at the ear of the monitoring personnel during surgery.

	Location of Sound Level Meter		
Surgical Tool	**Surgeon**	**Tool**	**Monitor**
Pneumatic drill	83 dBA	85 dBA	78 dBA
CUSA	73 dBA	78 dBA	73 dBA
CO_2 Laser	71 dBA	79 dBA	74 dBA
PD and CUSA	85 dBA	79 dBA	
CUSA and Laser	86 dBA	80 dBA	

Source: Kartush J, Bouchard K. *Neuromonitoring in otology and head and neck surgery.* New York: Raven, 199, with permission.
CUSA = Cavitron Ultrasonic Surgical Aspirator; PD = Pneumatic drill

CHAPTER 8

Cortical Auditory Evoked Responses

In This ADR Chapter

Perspective

Literally dozens of cortical auditory evoked responses are described in a vast literature of scientific journal articles, monographs, and textbooks. Investigation of cortical AERs dates back to the 1930s and has not abated even today.

What's been reported during this span of over 60 years? We know much about the test protocols that should be followed to consistently record the response, where they are generated within the central auditory nervous system (usually in rather vague terms), which clinical populations are appropriate candidates for AER measurement, and which clinical applications should be attempted and avoided.

At this time, however, audiologists rely on just a handful of responses that arise above, or rostral to, the ABR. The auditory middle latency response (AMLR), first described in 1958, is probably recorded most often in audiology clinics, although still rarely in comparison to the ABR. The auditory late response (ALR) and P_{300} response also have enjoyed a measure of clinical use and have been reported in a variety of clinical populations. Computerized topographic analysis (brain mapping) has been employed with all of the cortical AERs in most clinical populations. The mismatch negativity (MMN) response is one of the most recent, and potentially most usefull clinically. These four cortical AERs—AMLR, ALR, P_{300}, and MMN—are cited, albeit superficially, in this chapter. The interested reader will find numerous sources of information on these responses in the library (e.g., Hall, 1992; Jacobson, 1994) and the audiologic, psychologic, and electrophysiologic literature.

FOUNDATIONS OF CORTICAL AUDITORY EVOKED RESPONSES

Historical Perspective

Overview of important developments and discoveries in AMLR

Year	Investigator(s)	Finding
1951	Dawson	Averager for evoked responses
1958	Rosenblith	Computer averager for evoked reponses
1958	Geisler	Response first recorded in man (with Rosenblith)
1964	Bickford et al.	Response described as myogenic
1965	Mast	Further evidence of a neurogenic origin
1967	Goldstein & Rodman	First of many papers on response, including introduction of labeling system for components
1968	Celesia	Identified in exposed human cortex
1982	Kraus et al.	Multichannel hemisphere recordings in cortical pathology in humans
1984	Lee, Leuders et al.	Neural generators studied with electrodes on surface of exposed brain of epileptic patients undergoing surgery
1987	Kileny et al.	Neural generators and findings in cortical pathology
1987	Woods, Knight, Clayworth et al.	Generators of responses in patients with CNS pathology
1988	Kraus et al.	Computed topography in normal humans
1988	Kileny et al.	Electrically elicited response in animal and human

AMLR Facts and Features

Background

- ☐ Initially described by Dan Geisler in 1958 while he was a doctoral student at M.I.T., before moving on to the University of Wisconsin (where he is even today).
- ☐ Extensively studied by Robert Goldstein and colleagues in late 1960s and during 1970s at the University of Wisconsin. Earlier in his career, Goldstein had come under the professional influence of Hallowell Davis while working in St. Louis.
- ☐ Recent renewed interest in measurement of response with multiple electrode arrays, including application of computed evoked potential topography techniques.

Waveform

- ☐ Major sequential peaks are labeled N (negative voltage waves) and P (positive voltage waves) with typical electrode arrangement. They are Na, Pa, Nb, and Pb, according to the widely accepted nomenclature introduced by Goldstein.
- ☐ Response occurs within the interval of 15 to 50 msec after presentation of a high intensity acoustic stimulus.
- ☐ Major peak is the Pa component which occurs about 25 msec after a relatively brief stimulus.

Anatomic Generators

- ☐ Recent evidence in humans suggests that generators in the auditory thalamus and primary auditory cortex contribute to the Pa component of the response.
- ☐ Anatomy of the response recorded with midline electrode vs. electrodes over the temporal-parietal hemispheres may differ.
- ☐ Anatomy probably includes reticular formation, in addition to lemniscal auditory pathways.

Stimulus Features

- ☐ A click or tone burst stimulus is appropriate. In fact, AMLR is a good choice for frequency-specific estimation of hearing sensitivity in certain patient populations (e.g., malingerers).
- ☐ Stimulus rate less than 11/sec (e.g., 7.1/sec) is optimal, and even slower rates are typically required to:
  - ✓ record a Pa component in young children
  - ✓ record an optimal response in patients with primary auditory cortex pathology

- record a clear Pb component

☐ High stimulus intensity may produce postauricular artifact.

☐ Response to electrical (vs. acoustic) stimulation of auditory system recently reported.

Acquisition Features

☐ Electrodes located over left and right hemispheres are indicated for neurodiagnostic application.

☐ A high-pass filter setting of 10 Hz or lower is necessary to encompass response spectrum and minimize filter artifact components in waveform.

Factors to consider in analysis and interpretation

☐ Response is often not adultlike ("mature") until age 8 to 10 years of age.

☐ There is an interaction between age (under 10 years) and stimulus rate (i.e., slower rates are needed for younger children).

☐ The Pa response amplitude may be influenced (reduced in amplitude and less reliably recorded) by sleep and sedation.

☐ Anesthetic agents and other CNS suppressants seriously alter or abolish response.

Clinical Applications

☐ Electrophysiologic documentation of auditory CNS dysfunction above level of brainstem, especially in patients who cannot be adequately evaluated with behavioral measures of auditory CNS function.

☐ Frequency-specific estimation of auditory sensitivity in older children and adults (e.g., malingerers).

Clinical Concept

AERs Compared and Contrasted

	Latency range		
	Early	**Middle**	**Later Latency**
Examples	ECochG, ABR	AMLR	ALR, P_{300}, MMN
Stimulus rate	faster (<30/sec)	<10/sec	slower (<2/sec)
Stimulus type	transient	transient	tonal
Stimulus duration	very brief (<5 msec)	brief (5 msec)	longer (>10 msec)
Spectral content	high (100 to 2000 Hz)	20 to 40 Hz	low (<30 Hz)
Filter settings	30 to 3000 Hz	10 to 200 Hz	1 to 30 Hz
Amplitude	0.5 microvolts	about 1 microvolt	> 5 microvolts
Number of repetitions averaged (typically)	>1000	about 500	<250
Pre-amplification	>75,000	about 75,000	<50,000
Effect of sedation	none	slight	pronounced

Clinical Concept

Generators of Auditory Evoked Responses

- ☐ Auditory brainstem response (ABR)
  - wave I = distal end of the eighth nerve (near cochlea)
  - wave II = proximal end of the eighth nerve (near brainstem)
  - wave III = caudal (lower) brainstem near trapezoid body and superior olivary complex
  - wave V = lateral lemniscus as it enters the inferior colliculus
  - trough after wave V = inferior colliculus (?)
- ☐ Auditory middle latency response (AMLR)
  - Na component = thalamus (?)
  - Pa component = primary auditory cortex (measured over temporal-parietal lobe)
  - Pa component = subcortical generator (as measured with a midline electrode)
- ☐ Auditory late response (ALR)
  - P2 component = primary or secondary auditory cortex
- ☐ Auditory P_{300} response
  - P3 component = auditory regions of hippocampus in medial temporal lobe
- ☐ Mismatch negativity (MMN) response
  - subcortical and primary cortical auditory regions

Near vs. Far-field AERs

Illustration of the concept of near-field versus far-field recording of auditory evoked responses.

With a near-field response, increasing the distance between the response generator (dipole) even slightly produces a big reduction in response amplitude. With a far-field response, in contrast, electrode distance from the generator has little or no effect on response amplitude. The ABR is an example of a far-field response, whereas electrocochleography (ECochG) or auditory middle latency response (AMLR) recorded with hemisphere electrodes, are examples of near-field responses.

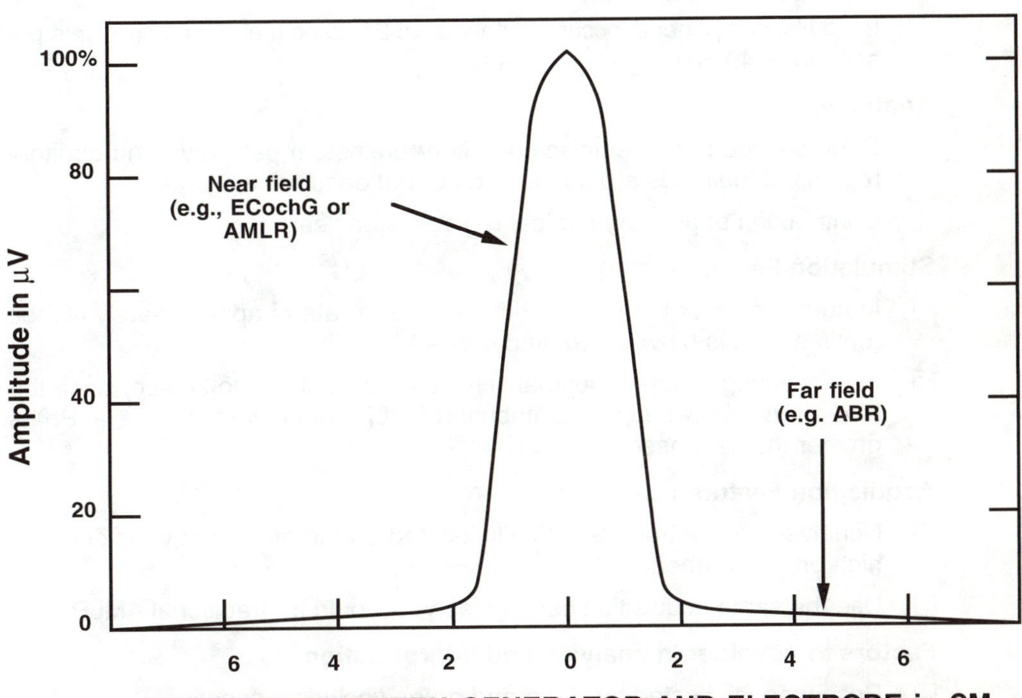

40 Hz Facts and Features

Background

- ☐ Intense interest in the response followed the modern-day description by Galambos and colleagues in 1981
- ☐ Clinical interest was high because the 40 Hz response could be averaged relatively quickly. The two main reasons were:
  - ✓ amplitude was rather high (1 μvolt or larger)
  - ✓ stimulus rate was rather fast (about 40/sec)

Components

- ☐ There is no accepted nomenclature for labeling components in the sinusoidal appearing waveform
- ☐ In adults, components occur at intervals of 25 msec (i.e., 40 components per second or 40 Hz)

Anatomy

- ☐ Contributions of nonlemniscal auditory brainstem pathways and auditory regions of thalamus are suspected but not documented
- ☐ Contribution of auditory cortical regions is unclear

Stimulation Features

- ☐ In adults, click or tone burst stimulation at a rate of approximately 40/sec (optimal rate is between 37 and 40/sec)
- ☐ In very young children, optimal stimulus rate is closer to 20/sec, since the time interval between the contributing AMLR components (e.g., Pa, Pb) is greater than 25 msec

Acquisition Features

- ☐ Noninverting electrode is typically located on the midline at vertex or high on the forehead
- ☐ Use the same acquisition settings as you would for traditional AMLR

Factors to consider in analysis and interpretation

- ☐ Response *is* affected by sleep and drugs (including sedatives)
- ☐ Response may occur at slower stimulus rate (e.g., 20/sec) in young children, and may not be optimally recorded at a rate of 40/sec in most patients

Clinical Applications

- ☐ Frequency-specific estimation of auditory sensitivity with tone burst stimulation in older children and adults

Clinical Limitations

- ☐ Anatomic origin is not clear
- ☐ Response not reliably recorded in young children
- ☐ Susceptible to influences of subject state of arousal and drugs; these factors may confound auditory threshold estimation

Historical Perspective

Overview of Important Developments and Discoveries in ALR and P_{300}

Year	Investigator(s)	Finding
1929	Berger	Human EEG discovered
1939	Davis (Pauline)	Alteration in EEG with auditory stimulation in human
1939	Davis H, Davis P, Loomis, et al.	"K-complex" observed in EEG of human during auditory stimuluation
1942	Woolsey & Walzl	Auditory evoked responses from animal cortex
1961	Kiang	Cortical evoked response in animal
1962	Williams et al.	Response in sleep; components labeled in lower case (p1, n1, p2, n2)
1963	Davis & Yoshie	Among first of many studies of stimulus parameters; components labeled in uppercase (P1, N1, P2, N2)
1964	Davis	P300 response first noted in ALR
1965	Sutton et al.	P300 response first investigated
1966	Davis et al.	Further study of effects of stimulus parameters
1967	Rapin, Graziani	Response applied in normal, brain damaged, and hearing-impaired infants
1968	Davis et al.	Further study of effect of stimulus parameters
1969	Jerger	Findings in temporal lobe pathology in human
1970	Vaughan & Ritter	Scalp topography and generators studied in human
1971	Kooi et al.	Scalp topography restudied
1973	Hillyard	Systematic study of P_{300} measurement factors
1975	Barnet et al.	Age effects described in infants and young children (ABR not yet commonly applied clinically in this population)
1977	Squires	Effect of stimulus parameters
1978	Goodin & Squires	Effects of aging on P_{300}, and clinical findings in dementia
1979	Ford & Pfefferbaum	Effects of aging, dementia, and alcohol on P_{300}
1980	Knight & Hillyard	Application in cortical pathology
1980	Halgren et al.	P_{300} neural generators described in humans
1980	Roth et al.	P_{300} findings in schizophrenia
1982	Wood & Wolpaw	Scalp topography and neural generators in human
1987	Woods, Knight, Clayworth et al.	Generators of responses in patients with CNS pathology
1995	Kraus et al.	Supplement of *Ear and Hearing* on mismatch negativity response

ALR Facts and Features

Background

- ☐ Over the years, the auditory late response has also been referred to as the:
  - ✓ vertex (V) response
  - ✓ vertex (V) potential
  - ✓ auditory cortical response (ACR)
  - ✓ auditory evoked potential (AEP)
  - ✓ averaged electroencephalic response (AER)
  - ✓ slow averaged evoked potential or response
  - ✓ cortical evoked response audiometry (ERA)
  - ✓ electroencephalic response (EER)
  - ✓ electric response audiometry (ERA)
- ☐ Auditory component in the EEG was noted as early as 1939 by Pauline Davis (first wife of Hallowell Davis) and Dr. Davis
- ☐ Systematic investigations of the effects of measurement parameters on the response were conducted by Hallowell Davis and colleagues at Central Institute for the Deaf in St. Louis from mid-1960s into the 1970s
- ☐ The classic early investigation of topographic mapping of the response was conducted by Vaughan and Ritter in 1970

Waveform

- ☐ Sequential peaks labeled by N (negative voltage) or P (positive voltage), including P1, N1, P2, N2, as recorded with vertex electrode
- ☐ Major components occur within 75 to 200 msec after moderate intensity stimulus (e.g., N1 in the range of 75 to 150 msec and P2 in the range of 150 to 200 msec)

Anatomical Generators

- ☐ Precise anatomic generators are not known, but N1 and P2 components presumably arise from auditory cortex
- ☐ Response reflects dendritic neural activity (vs. action potentials), as evidenced by their leisurely appearance and dependence on relatively slow stimulus presentation rates and long duration stimuli

Stimulation Features

- ☐ Optimally evoked by tone burst stimuli of relatively long duration (greater than 5 msec)
- ☐ Stimulus rates of 2/sec or less are appropriate

- ☐ Maximum response typically obtained for moderate (50 to 60 dB) vs. high-intensity stimuli

Acquisition Features

- ☐ Optimally, noninverting recording electrode site is midline at high forehead or vertex
- ☐ High-pass filter settings as low as 1 Hz are required to record this low-frequency response, and the entire response falls within a frequency region well below 30 Hz

Factor to consider in analysis and interpretation

- ☐ Response is highly susceptible to alterations in state of arousal (sleep stages) and to effects of drugs, such as sedatives

Clinical Applications

- ☐ Electrophysiologic assessment of higher level auditory CNS functioning, but other electrophysiologic measures such the AMLR or mismatch negativity may be more useful clinically
- ☐ Frequency-specific estimation of hearing sensitivity in cooperative children and adults, but if the patients are so cooperative why not just perform behavioral audiometry?

Clinical Limitations

- ☐ Considerable intra- and intersubject variability
- ☐ Susceptability to subject state and drugs
- ☐ Neuroanatomy not precisely defined

P300 Facts and Features

Background

- ☐ The auditory P_{300} response has at some point also been referred to as the:
  - ✔ P3 response
  - ✔ endogenous auditory evoked potential (AEP)
  - ✔ cognitive auditory evoked response
  - ✔ event related potential (ERP)
  - ✔ late potential complex
  - ✔ late or very late auditory evoked potential
- ☐ First described by Hallowell Davis in 1964 and, independently, by Samuel Sutton and colleagues in 1965

- ☐ Extensive investigation of test paradigm influences on P_{300} and other endogenous responses began during late 1960s and continues today
- ☐ There is substantial research on the clinical value of P_{300} in electrophysiologic assessment of higher level auditory processing, with a resultant large body of literature (hundreds of articles, a monograph or two, and more than a few books)
- ☐ Recent applications of computer evoked potential topography technology include the P_{300} response
- ☐ The P_{300} response research, and recognition of limitations in the P_{300} paradigm, have led to current interest in a related (close cousin or maybe sibling response), the mismatch negativity (MMN) response

Components

- ☐ Major peak is a large positive voltage wave (5 microvolts or greater) occuring at approximately 300 msec after a rare (oddball) auditory stimulus
- ☐ The P3 label often used for major component because it is the third positive-going wave in late response time frame
- ☐ The term "endogenous" is often used to describe the P_{300} response and other auditory evoked response components that are highly dependent on subject attention to certain auditory stimuli (vs. exogenous responses)

Anatomical Generators

- ☐ Human depth electrode studies provide evidence of medial temporal lobe (hippocampus) contribution to the response
- ☐ The P300 response reflects dendritic (vs. axonic) brain activity

Stimulus Factors

- ☐ The P_{300} response is optimally evoked by unpredictable, infrequent acoustic stimuli presented randomly with a probability of 15 to 20% in an "oddball" or unpredictable-presentation test paradigm
- ☐ A relatively slow rate of stimulation (2/sec or less) is appropriate

Acquisition Factors

- ☐ Acquisition factors are generally equivalent to those for ALR

Factors in analysis and interpretation

- ☐ Subject attention to the "oddball," but not the frequent, stimuli is an important feature in the measurement of the conventional P_{300} response, but not essential for measurement of the so-called P3a (earlier) response
- ☐ The response is profoundly affected by alterations in subject state of arousal, by sleep stage, and by drugs
- ☐ Instructions to the subject regarding the listening task produce marked effects on the type of response recorded. More than a dozen types of endogenous AERs can be recorded within the 200 to 500 msec latency region, depending on measurement parameters and subject tasks

- ☐ Response latency decreases and amplitude increases during childhood and then the process reverses in aging during adulthood

Clinical Application and Limitation (not an exhaustive list)

- ☐ Electrophysiologic assessment of higher level auditory processing
- ☐ Minor, perhaps unappreciated, alterations in attention or the listening task produce marked effects on the response

Historical Perspective

Development of Computed (Cortical) Evoked Response Topography

Year	Investigator(s)	Event
1939	P Davis et al.	Discovery of auditory late response
1965	H Davis et al. Sutton et al.	Discovery of P_{300} response
1970	Vaughan & Ritter	Topographical (noncomputerized) display of late responses
1978	Naatanen et al.	Description of the mismatch negativity (MMN) response
1979	Duffy et al.	Report of BEAM (brain electrical activity mapping) technique
1988	G Jacobson et al. Kraus et al.	Auditory middle latency response (AMLR) mapped
1989	Pool et al.	Auditory late response (ALR) mapped
1990	Giard et al.	Mismatch negativity (MNR) mapped

Clinical Concept

Categories of Cortical Evoked Responses

- **Exogenous**: responses that are directly dependent on stimulus characteristics (e.g., polarity) and are independent of whether the patient is attending, processing, or discriminating the stimulus
  - electrocochleography (ECochG)
  - auditory brainstem response (ABR)
  - auditory middle latency response (AMLR)
- **Endogenous**: responses that are dependent on subject state (e.g., attention) and/or on discrimination of some aspect of the stimulus
  - P_{300} (P_{3a} and P_{3b})
  - N2
  - mismatch negativity (MMN) response

Key References

Cortical Evoked Responses

Auditory middle latency response

Geisler CD, Frishkopf LS, Rosenblith WA. Extracranial responses to acoustic clicks in man. *Science 128: 1210–1211, 1958.*

Goldstein R, Rodman LB. Early components of averaged evoked responses to rapidly repeated auditory stimuli. *J Speech Hearing Research 10*: 697–705, 1967.

Hall JW III. *Handbook of Auditory Evoked Responses*. Needham, MA: Allyn & Bacon, 1992.

Jacobson GP, Privitera M, Neils JR, Grayson AS, Yeh H-S. The effects of anterior termporal lobectomy (ATL) on the middle-latency auditory evoked potential (MLAEP). *Electroencephalography and Clinical Neurophysiology 75*: 230–241, 1990.

Kileny PR, Paccioretti D, Wilson AF. Effects of cortical lesions in middle-latency auditory evoked responses (MLR). *Electroencephalography and Clinical Neurophysiology 66*: 108–120, 1987.

Kraus N, Ozdamar O, Hier D, Stein L. Auditory middle latency responses (MLRs) in patients with cortical lesions. *Electroencephalography and Clinical Neurophysiology 54*: 275–297, 1982.

Lee YS, Lueders H, Dinner DS, Lesser RP, Hahn J, Klemm G. Recording of auditory evoked potentials in man using chronic subdural electrodes. *Brain 107*: 115–131, 1984.

Woods PL, Clayworth CC, Knight RT, Simpson GV, Naeser MA. Generators of middle and long latency auditory evoked potentials: Implications from studies of patients with bitemporal lesions. *Electroencephalography and Clinical Neurophysiology 68*: 132–148, 1987.

Mismatch negativity (MMN) response

Alho K, Sainio K, Sajaniemi N, Reinikainen K, Naatanen R. Event-related brain potential of human newborns to pitch change of an acoustic stimulus. *Electroencephalography and Clinical Neurophysiology 77*: 151–155, 1990.

Csepe V. On the origin and development of the mismatch negativity. *Ear and Hearing 16*: 90–103, 1995.

Kraus N, Micco A, Koch D, McGee T, Carrell T, Sharma A. Wiet R, Weingarten C. The mismatch negativity cortical evoked potential evoked by speech stimuli. *Ear and Hearing 13*: 158–164, 1992.

Kraus N. Mismatch negativity in the assessment of central auditory function. *American Journal of Audiology 3*: 139–151, 1994.

Kraus N (ed). Special issue: Mismatch negativity as an index of central auditory function. E*ar and Hearing 16*: 1995

Naatanen R. The mismatch negativity: A powerful tool for cognitive neuroscience. *Ear and Hearing 16*: 6–18, 1995.

Naatanen R. Selective attention and evoked potentials in humans: A critical review. *Biological Review 2*: 237–307, 1975.

AMLR RECORDING

Classic Quote

Geisler on AMLR

ADR Note: Studies of human cortical auditory evoked responses were underway at M.I.T. by Rosenblith and colleagues with a digital device designed by Clark, the ARC (average response computer). Dan Geisler, a student in this laboratory, conducted doctoral research on the topic which led to the first published account of the human AMLR in 1958 (Geisler, Frishkopf, & Rosenblith, 1958).

The following passage is taken from this pioneering work:

"We have observed responses to acoustic clicks from ordinary scalp electrodes in man. These average responses . . . are characterized by onset latencies of approximately 30 msec and peak latencies of approximately 30 msec and by response amplitudes and latencies that depend upon the intensity and the rate of presentation of the stimulus. The threshold for the appearance of a detectable average response agrees closely with the minimum intensity at which the subject reports that he hears clicks . . . The response to monaural clicks is bilateral: electrodes placed symmetrically about the midline record virtually the same response . . . These data, and the latency of the surface-negative component of evoked responses to clicks, in cats and monkeys, suggest that the responses which we obtain are cortical in origin (Geisler, Frishkopf, Rosenblith, 1958)."

Source: From Geisler CD, Frishkopf LS, Rosenblith WA. Extracranial responses to acoustic clicks in man. *Science 128*: 1210–1211, 1958.

Protocol

Auditory Middle Latency Response (AMLR)

Parameter	Suggestion	Comment
Stimulus		
Transducer	ER-3A	Supra-aural is O.K. for AMLR
Type	click	For neurodiagnosis
	tone burst	For audiometry
Duration	0.1 ms	For click only
Rise/fall	2 cycle	For tone burst only
Plateau	1 cycle or 0 msec	For tone burst only
Rate	7.1/sec	Slower as indicated by age or pathology
Polarity	alternating	
Intensity	70 dB HL	For neurodiagnosis, but variable for audiometry. Use moderate, and avoid high, intensity levels.
Number	1000	Variable depending on size of response and background noise. Remember the signal-to-noise ratio is the key.
Presentation ear(s)	monaural	
Masking	50 dB	Only if stimulus intensity exceeds 70 dB HL, which it rarely should
Acquisition		
Amplification	75,000	
Sensitivity	50 μvolts	
Analysis time	overall100 ms	To encompass the Pa and the Pb component
Prestimulus time	10%	Gives a good estimate of background noise
Data points	512	
Sweeps	1000	See stimulus number just above
Filters		
bandpass	10 to 1500 Hz or 10 to about 200 Hz	Don't overfilter (e.g., 30–100 Hz); it may produce a misleading filter artifact
notch	none	Never indicated, and a very bad idea because the important frequencies in the response (around 40 Hz) may be removed
Electrodes		
Channel 1	C5-Ai/Ac	Hemispheric electrode for neurodiagnosis
Channel 2	C6-Ai/Ac	Hemispheric electrode for neurodiagnosis
Channel 3	Fz-Ai/Ac	Channel 3 for neurodiagnosis; only Channel 3 is needed for audiometry (estimation of hearing sensitivity)
Ground Fpz		

*NA = not applicable

**Noninverting-to-inverting electrode according to 10-20 International Electrode System; Ai/Ac = linked earlobes

AMLR Electrodes

Illustration of some of the electrode sites of the 10-20 International System (Jasper, 1958). Sites typically used in auditory middle latency response (AMLR) recording are shaded. This figure only shows electrodes and symbols for the left side of the head. Odd numbers indicate the left side of the head. There is an analogous set of electrodes, indicated by even numbers, on the right side of the head. A handy phrase to remember this is "left handed people are odd." See the ADR note at the bottom of the figure for a few other helpful guidelines regarding electrode nominclature. The "N" stands for "nasion," a site between the eyebrows, above the nose.

For neurodiagnostic purposes, it is appropriate to record the AMLR with a three channel electrode array. The noninverting electrode sites are shown in the figure for each channel, and include electrode site "C5" for channel 1, site "C4" (same location but on the right side) for channel 2, and a high forehead (almost "Fz") site for channel 3. Inverting electrodes can be located on the earlobes and connected or "linked" by a short jumper wire connecting each electrode input, or a single inverting electrode located at a noncephalic location (nape of the neck where most people have a small bump) for all of the electrode arrays.

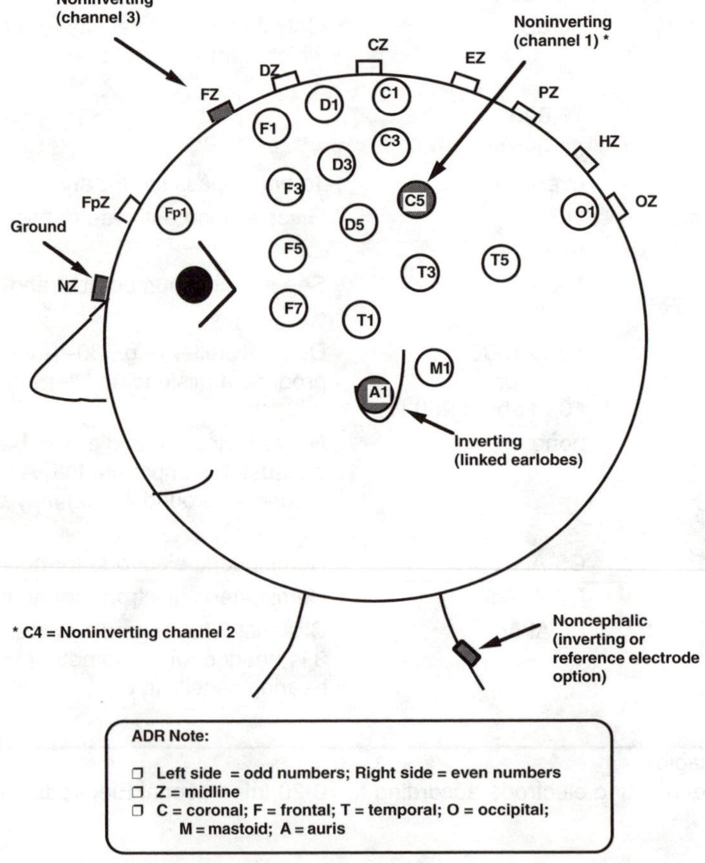

Technical Tip

How to Record an AMLR Pb Component Consistently

- ☐ The AMLR Pb component is not consistently recorded with a conventional AMLR test protocol. Actually, it corresponds to the ALR P1 component. The Pb component will be typically observed in the 45 msec region after the stimulus with modification of the test protocol, including:
  - ✔ slow stimulus rate down to approximately 1.1/sec
  - ✔ increase stimulus duration (e.g., 60 msec)
  - ✔ use a lower frequency tone burst stimulus (e.g., 500 Hz or 1000 Hz), rather than a click stimulus
  - ✔ increase analysis time to about 100 msec to encompass this 45 msec component
  - ✔ use a high-pass filter setting of as low as 1 Hz, to include the low-frequency energy contributing to the Pb component
  - ✔ use a noncephalic inverting electrode site (e.g., nape of the neck) rather than linked earlobes.

Source: Nelson MD. Doctoral dissertation thesis, Vanderbilt University, 1994.

Technical Tip

Electrode Sites for AMLR Recording

- ☐ There are three noninverting (scalp) electrodes.
  - ✔ *Left hemisphere at C5 site.* This is approximately halfway between the vertex (Cz) and the ear canal, and about 1 cm posterior.
  - ✔ *Right hemisphere at C4 site.* This is also approximately halfway between the vertex (Cz) and the ear canal, and about 1 cm posterior.
  - ✔ *Midline at Fz site.* This is approximately halfway between the bridge of the nose and the vertex (near the hair line for most folks).
- ☐ There are two typical choices for inverting electrode sites.
  - ✔ *Linked earlobes.* Connect the two earlobe electrode inputs with a "jumper cable" and then plug the electrode from each ear lobe into each end. This balances the earlobe sites across all inverting electrodes, preventing ipsilateral and contralateral electrode effects in hemisphere recordings.
  - ✔ *Noncephalic.* A single electrode for all three inverting electrodes—a true reference that is inactive to brain activity—located on the nape of the neck at about C7 (that little bump in the back of the neck down near your shoulders).

Classic Quote

Robert Galambos on the 40 Hz auditory response

"This phenomenon, the 40-Hz event related potential (ERP), displays several properties of theoretical and practical interest.

First, it reportedly disappears with surgical anesthesia, and it resembles similar phenomena in the visual and olfactory system, facts which suggest that adequate processing of sensory information may require cyclical brain events in the 30- to 50-Hz range.

Second, latency and amplitude measurements on the 40-Hz ERP indicate it may contain useful information on the number and basilar membrane location of the auditory nerve fibers a given tone excites.

Third, the response is present at sound intensities very close to normal adult thresholds for the audiometric frequencies, a fact that could have application in clinical hearing testing."

Source: From Galambos R, Makeig S, Talmachoff PJ. A 40-Hz auditory potential recorded from the human scalp. *Proceedings of the National Academy of Science U.S.A. 78:* 1981, p. 263

Mover and Oscillator

Robert Galambos, "Doctor of Auditory Neurophysiology"

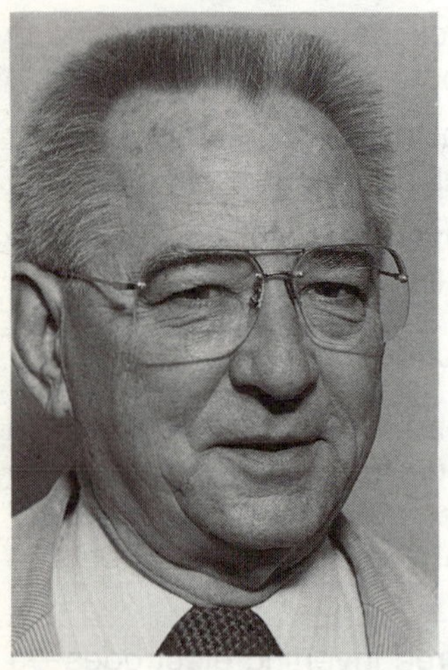

Robert Galambos, a pioneering auditory neurophysiologist whose important works have included germinal papers on such diverse topics as the efferent auditory system, the auditory brainstem response, and the 40 Hz response.

Dr. Galambos' initial contributions to auditory physiology began in 1939 with microelectrode recordings of cat single auditory neurons with Hallowell Davis, and doctoral thesis experiments on bat echolocation with Dr. D. R. Griffin. During the next quarter of a century, he published with collaborators about 30 papers reporting microelectrode auditory studies. Among the most notable, published in 1939 with colleagues David Hubel, C. O. Henson and Allen Rupert, was a paper describing cat auditory cortical cells that respond only when the animal pays attention to stimuli. Dr. Galambos performed pioneering experiments on the efferent olivocochlear bundle in 1955.

In the mid-1950s, the laboratory directed by Dr. Galambos began phasing out microelectrode experiments and phasing in the study, using unanesthetized animals, of what would come to be called cognitive evoked potentials. With laboratory co-workers Rupert and Guy Sheatz, he published one of the first examples of computer-averaged cognitive evoked potentials, recorded from monkey, in 1961. Ten years later, the laboratory no longer used animal subjects and, by 1995, Dr. Galambos and numerous collaborators had published some 35 reports on human cognitive potentials, and almost the same number of papers on the auditory brainstem response (ABR).

Don Jewett discovered the cat ABR in 1963 during a postdoctoral year with Dr. Galambos. When a preprint of the soon-to-be classic Jewett and Williston *Brain* paper on the human ABR reached Dr. Galambos in 1970, he began at once to look into its possible application to infant hearing testing. By 1977, the information from these early investigations had been published, with a variety of co-authors such as Paul Despland, Kurt Hecox, Steve Hillyard, Barbara Mokotoff, Terry Picton and, especially, Carol Schulman, in 15 papers on the ABR. This information convinced the San Diego Children's Hospital administration to require ABR screening for all graduates of the Intensive Care Nursery (ICN). Three interim accounts on the progress of this enterprise were published with Gayle Hicks and Mary-Jo Wilson, and a 20-year summary (with Mary-Jo Wilson and P. D. Silva) appeared in 1994. Dr. Galambos and associates continue to screen all second and third level ICN graduates at the hospital following the original protocol.

In 1978, when no commercial ABR instrumentation was as yet for sale, a doctoral candidate of Dr. Galambos, Peter Talmachoff, designed and built one as his thesis project. In his first tests on human volunteers in 1980, he delivered clicks at a rate of 40 Hz. What appeared to be an artifact in the recordings turned out to be the 40 Hz response which Dr. Galambos described in 1981 with Scott Makeig. An attempt to develop an infant audiometer using 40-Hz tone bursts at the audiometric frequencies was abandoned when Dr. Galambos and colleagues (J. A. Costello, Makeig, and David R. Stapells) discovered that newborns do not reliably produce 40-Hz responses.

Dr. Galambos is now conducting research on the role that glial cells play in the generation of evoked potentials, such as the ABR and the P_{300} response, a problem that is not likely to be of primary interest to clinical audiologists.

Source: The information in this narration was kindly supplied upon request by Dr. Galambos in December 1995.

AMLR ANALYSIS AND INTERPRETATION

AMLR Waveform Analysis

Typical auditory middle latency response (AMLR) waveform (*top portion*) showing major components. The symbol "P" refers to positive voltage, whereas the symbol "N" refers to negative voltage. Expected normal latency and amplitude values are noted. One of the potential problems in AMLR measurement, the dreaded postauricular muscle (PAM) artifact, is illustrated in the lower portion of the figure. This myogenic response usually has a peak with latency well before the Pa component (usually in the 13 to 20 msec region) and may be extremely large in amplitude. See Technical Tips and Trouble-shooting for more information on PAM artifact and how to avoid recording it.

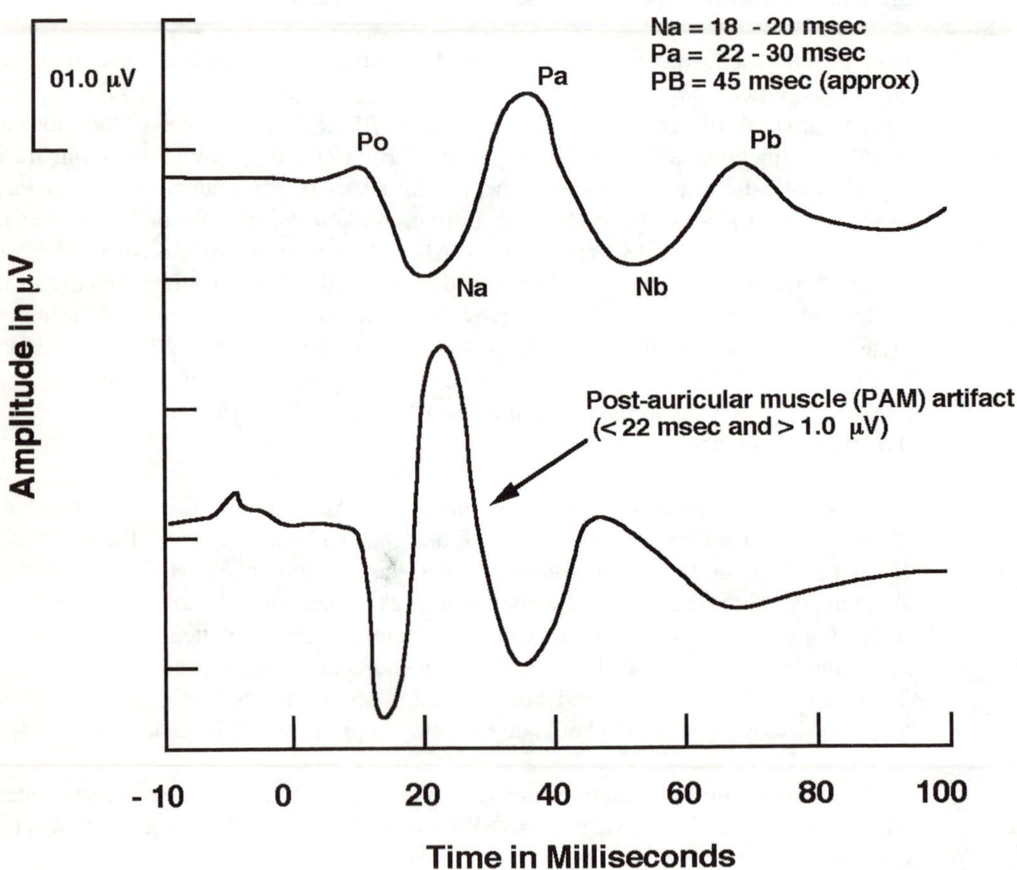

Clinical Concept

Analysis of the AMLR (versus ABR) in Neurodiagnosis

ABR	AMLR
☐ Analyze latency parameters	☐ Analyze amplitude parameters
☐ Latency is highly repeatable	☐ Latency is variable
☐ Amplitude is variable	☐ Amplitude is more repeatable
☐ Auditory dysfunction delays latency	☐ Auditory dysfunction reduces amplitude
☐ One electrode array is often adequate ("ipsilateral array")	☐ Multiple (3) electrode arrays are needed (each hemisphere and a midline electrode)
☐ Not influenced by sedatives and CNS suppressants	☐ Influenced by sedatives and CNS suppressants
☐ Gender influences adult responses	☐ Gender does not influence adult responses

Click Stimulus Intensity Levels in dB SPL Corresponding to 0 dB Normal Hearing Level (nHL).

	Stimulus Rate	Peak SPL	pe SPL*
Burkard & Hecox, 1983	27	40.0	—
Campbell et al., 1981	10	40.0	34.0
Hood & Berlin, 1986	27.7	36.0	—
Ozdamar & Stein, 1981	20	—	32.0
Selters & Brackmann, 1977	20	38.0	—

*pe SPL = peak equivalent sound pressure level

Source: Hall JW III. *Handbook of auditory evoked responses*. Needham, MA: Allyn & Bacon, 1992.

Technical Tip

Two Good Clinical Applications of AMLR

Application	Rationale
☐ Neurodiagnosis of auditory dysfunction	✔ electrophysiologic assessment of supra-brainstem auditory function not reached by ABR assessment
	✔ can be recorded with clinical evoked response system used for ABR measurement
	✔ is found in young children (with slower than usual stimulus rate)
	✔ is not suppressed by sedatives or coma
	✔ relative site specificity (each temporal hemisphere) with a three-channel electrode array
	✔ provides measure of auditory regions than are vital to auditory language functioning
☐ Frequency-specific hearing assessment	✔ doesn't require behavioral response or participation
	✔ useful in assessment of malingerers (functional hearing loss)
	✔ useful in differentiation of cochlear vs. retrocochlear auditory dysfunction when ABR is compromised by severe high-frequency sensorineural hearing loss. Record AMLR with tone burst at frequency with symmetric hearing sensitivity.
	✔ best evoked by frequency-specific tone burst (vs. click) stimuli
	✔ is not suppressed by sedatives or coma
	✔ is not seriously influenced by mild conductive hearing loss (vs. otoacoustic emissions)

Trouble-shooting

Problems in AMLR and ALR Measurement and Possible Solutions

Symptom	Possible Problems	Possible Solutions
No display	Technical error	✔ verify system power is on ✔ verify that the monitor screen is on ✔ verify that the monitor intensity is adequate ✔ verify that the evoked program is loaded ✔ verify that the program, file, or data requested are on disc ✔ consult equipment manual
Equipment setup error	Equipment won't average	✔ verify that stimulus repetitions are not set at "0" ✔ verify that the stimulus duration is not set at "0" ✔ verify adequate memory ✔ verify that the stimulus rate is not too fast for the analysis time ✔ verify all measurement parameters ✔ turn power off, wait a minute, then power on or perform warm boot
More than one stimulus in analysis time	Stimulus rate incompatible with analysis time	✔ slow the stimulus rate so that ISI is longer than analysis time ✔ shorten the analysis time to less than ISI ✔ Note: ISI = analysis time/rate (for a click)
No response	No stimulus	✔ listening check ✔ verify correct transducer (e.g. air or bone) ✔ verify test ear
	Improper electrode site	✔ verify correct electrode site
	Severe hearing loss	✔ obtain an audiogram ✔ increase the stimulus intensity ✔ use a tone burst (with frequency in region of good hearing)

(continued)

(continued)

Symptom	Possible Problems	Possible Solutions
	Inadequate amplification	✔ check gain ✔ check sensitivity
	Effect of drugs	✔ document CNS depressants
	Young age	✔ document age ✔ use a slower stimulus rate
Large, slow artifact	Movement or EEG artifact	✔ attempt to relax patient ✔ encourage sleep if necessary ✔ raise high-pass filter ✔ assess sleep status
Large peak at 10 to 15 msec	Postauricular muscle (PAM) in AMLR	✔ attempt to relax patient ✔ decrease stimulus intensity ✔ use a noncephalic electrode site for the inverting electrode ✔ reduce neck muscle tension ✔ offer the patient some George Dickel Tennessee Sipping Whiskey
Poor waveform morphology	Peripheral or central auditory dysfunction?	✔ increase the stimulus intensity ✔ slow the stimulus rate ✔ increase the number of sweeps ✔ raise the highpass filter to 10 Hz ✔ verify that the notch filter is OFF ✔ verify the highpass filter is less than 30 Hz ✔ record multiple replicated waveforms ✔ sum the replicated waveforms ✔ use a click vs. tone burst stimulus ✔ employ, and analyze, a prestimulus baseline ✔ is patient falling asleep . . . keep awake?
Excessive noise, spikes, or small fluctuations in waveform	High-frequency electrical interference	✔ rule out electrical devices and lines near electrodes and wires ✔ verify a good ground electrode ✔ alter the stimulus rate slightly ✔ lower the low pass filter ✔ increase the number of sweeps ✔ verify electrode impedance
Small or no Pa component (for AMLR)	Peripheral or central auditory dysfunction?	✔ increase stimulus intensity ✔ decrease stimulus rate

Symptom	Possible Problems	Possible Solutions
		✔ verify each electrode site (e.g., relocate C3 and/or C4 site)
		✔ use a low-frequency tone burst
		✔ document the patient's age (less than 10 years?)
		✔ document patient sleep status
		✔ document CNS depressant drugs
		✔ lower the high pass filter setting
		✔ increase the number of sweeps
		✔ obtain an audiogram
Small or no P_{300} component (for P_{300} response)	Inadequate subject attention	✔ reinstruct patient about attending to rare stimuli
		✔ request documentation of attention to rare stimuli
		✔ verify that the patient is alert
		✔ verify patient can distinguish between frequent and rare stimuli
		✔ verify the presence of rare vs. frequent stimuli
		✔ verify the rare vs. frequent ratio
		✔ verify the intensity of the rare stimulus
		✔ verify the randomness of rare stimulus presentation
	Poor hearing sensitivity in rare frequency region	✔ obtain audiogram
		✔ verify comparable hearing for rare vs. frequent stimuli
Delayed Pa component latency	Conductive hearing loss	✔ air vs. bone conduction audiogram
		✔ bone conduction AMLR
		✔ perform immittance measurement
		✔ increase stimulus intensity
	Young age	✔ slow the stimulus rate
		✔ document patient sleep status
Bifid Pa component	Which peak is used for analysis of AMLR?	✔ decrease stimulus intensity
		✔ use hemisphere electrodes
		✔ compare with opposite ear stimulation
		✔ use contralateral masking
		✔ normal variant; calculate latency for each component
Asymmetric Pa component	Peripheral or central auditory dysfunction?	✔ obtain audiogram
		✔ increase stimulus intensity

(continued)

(continued)

Symptom	Possible Problems	Possible Solutions
		✔ use tone burst stimuli ✔ verify transducer placement ✔ is ABR wave V latency asymmetric too? ✔ verify that stimulus intensity is the same for each ear
Very large Pa component amplitude	Real or artifact?	✔ If latency is too short (e.g., < 22 msec), consider PAM? ✔ open up filter settings ✔ is it present at fast vs. slow rates as well? ✔ could the patient be having a seizure?

P_{300} AND MISMATCHED NEGATIVITY (MMN) RESPONSE

Classic Quote:

Pauline Davis in 1939 on Cortical Auditory Evoked Responses

"In the human, the checking of the alpha rhythm by the opening of the eyes, and, less regularly, by a sudden sound, was described by Berger (1929) and widely confirmed by others. But immediate positive responses in the human to sounds or other stimuli have received only scant attention, partly because they do not appear under all conditions and partly because observers have feared being misled by artefacts due to muscular movement and particularly movement of the eyes. The present observations, made in 1935 - 1936, now take on a special interest because of their close relationship to responses of the human brain during sleep which are described in another paper [by Davis et al., 1939]."(Davis, 1939, p. 494)

"Acoustic stimuli cause electrical on-effects and off-effects in the waking human brain . . . The on-effect, composed of a diphasic and sometimes triphasic wave, was most prominent at the vertex . . . 'anticipatory' on-effects or off-effects appeared at an appropriate interval when a regularly spaced sequence of tones was unexpectedly stopped or prolonged." (Davis, 1939, p. 498).

Source: Davis PA. Effects of acoustic stimuli on the waking human brain. *J Neurophysiol 2:* 494–499, 1939.

Cited reference: Davis H, Davis PA, Loomis AL, Harvey EN, Hobart G. Electrical reactions of the human brain to auditory stimulation during sleep. *J Neurophysiol 2*: 129–135, 1939.

Classic Quote:

Hallowell Davis on the P_{300} Response

"The averaged, slow response evoked by auditory stimuli and recorded from the vertex of the human skull can usually be enhanced by requiring the listener to make a rather difficult auditory discrimination. An easy routine reaction is not effective."

Source: Davis H. Enhancement of evoked cortical potentials in humans related to a task requiring a decision. *Science 145:* 182–183, 1964, p. 182.

Protocol

Auditory Late Response (ALR) and P_{300}

Parameter	Suggestion	Comment
Stimulus		
type	tone burst	Click can be used
duration		
rise/fall	10 msec	Vary as indicated
plateau	30 msec	Vary as indicated
frequency		
frequent	1000 Hz	Vary as indicated
rare	2000 Hz	Vary as indicated
rate	1.1/sec	
polarity	alternating	Not important
intensity	70 dB	For neurodiagnosis
number	250	
probability of rare	15%	Presented randomly
presentation		
ear(s)	monaural	Binaural can be used
transducer	insert	
masking	rarely needed	
Acquisition		
Analysis time		
overall	600	To encompass the ALR and P3 components
prestimulus	10%	
Sample points	512	
Amplification	50,000	Less than for ABR, but the response is much bigger
Sensitivity	100 µvolts	
Filters		
bandpass	1–30 Hz	This is a very slow (low frequency) response
notch	none	Don't run the risk of filtering away the response
Electrodes		
Channel 1	Fz–Ai/Ac	Three-channel array as for AMLR can be used
Ground	Fpz	

Clinical Concept

Distinction Between P_{300} and (MMN) Responses

P_{300} (P3b) Response	MMN Response
☐ attention to rare stimuli required	attention to rare stimuli not required
☐ reflects conscious discrimation of stimuli	automatic discrimation of stimuli
☐ large differences in rare vs. frequent stimuli produce largest response	small differences between rare vs. frequent stimuli produce largest response

Typical ALR and P_{300} Waveforms

Typical auditory late response (ALR) waveform (*top*) and P300 waveform (*bottom*) showing major components.

The symbol "P" refers to positive voltage, whereas the symbol "N" refers to negative voltage. Expected normal latency and amplitude values are noted. A test protocol for recording the ALR and the P300 response is located in this ADR chapter.

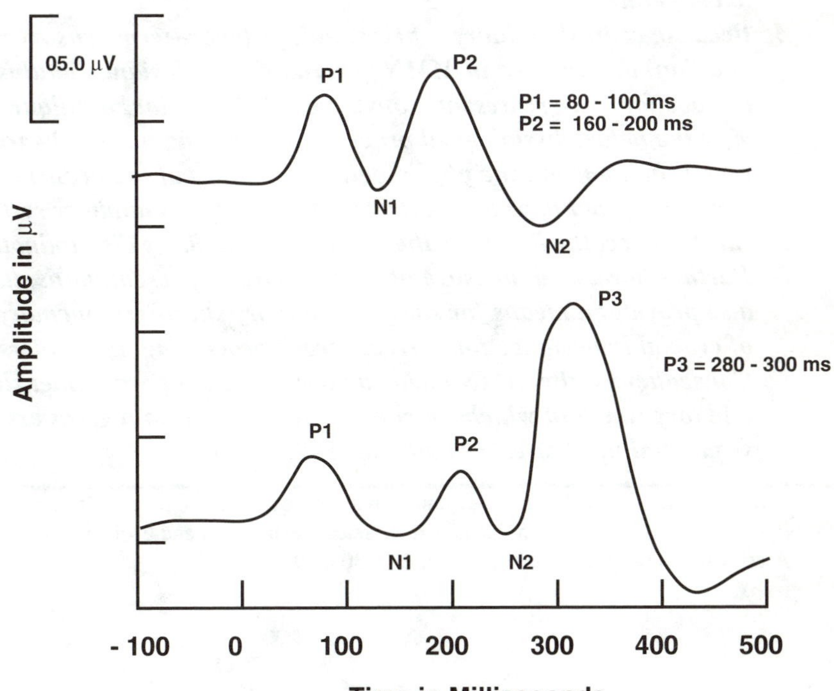

Classic Quote:

Risto Naatanen on the MMN

"The MMN is obtained by presenting the subject or patient with a block of several hundred identical stimuli ('standards') which are occasionally replaced by acoustically deviant stimuli, and thereafter subtracting the response elicited by standards from that elicited by the deviants. This difference wave shows a negativity that, depending on the magnitude of stimulus derivation, peaks at 100 to 200 msec after stimulus onset. This negativity is generated by a change-discrimination process that mainly occurs in auditory cortex. Several features make this response a specially attractive tool for auditory research and clinical practice.

1. ***The MMN is elicited by any discriminable change of a repetitive sound and can be elicited by stimulus differences that approximate the behavioral discrimination threshold.***
2. ***The MMN provides an objective measure of individual discrimination ability for different simple and complex (such as phonemic) sound features.***
3. ***Because it can be elicited without attention, the MMN if free from attentional variations that contaminate behavioral measures and attention-dependent physiological measures of auditory function. In addition, auditory function can be studied even in individuals unable or unwilling to cooperate.***
4. ***Because central auditory representations (short-term sensory memory in audition) are involved in MMN generation (the deviant stimulus acting as a probe for these representations), the MMN provides a unique window to view the neurophysiological processes underlying normal hearing. These representations are the physiological substrates of the acoustic stimulus parameters that have been extracted by the central auditory system. Those substrates set the limits for the precision of auditory discrimination.***
5. ***Furthermore, as a measure of these central representations, the MMN also provides a means for studying auditory short-term memory, which is of crucial importance for correct speech processing and understanding. Consequently, the MMN opens a view to the temporal dimension of auditory function which, in contrast to vision, is to a great extent sequential in nature." (Naatanen, 1995, p. 6)***

Sources: Naatanen R. The mismatch negativity: A powerful tool for cognitive neuroscience. *Ear and Hearing 16*: 6–18, 1995; Naatanen R. Selective attention and evoked potentials in humans: A critical review. *Biological Review 2*: 237–307, 1975.

Mismatch Negativity (MMN) Waveform

Recordings are made simultaneously for frequent (standard) stimuli and rare (deviant) stimuli. In this case, the standard stimulus is /da/ and the deviant stimulus is another consonant-vowel combination, such as /ga/ or /ta/. Once these waveforms have been averaged, the standard waveform is digitally subtracted from the frequent waveform, leaving a difference wave, or the MMN. The MMN is a negative voltage trough in the 200 msec region (after the stimuli are presented). See Lists, Tables, Key References, and other information on the MMN in this chapter.

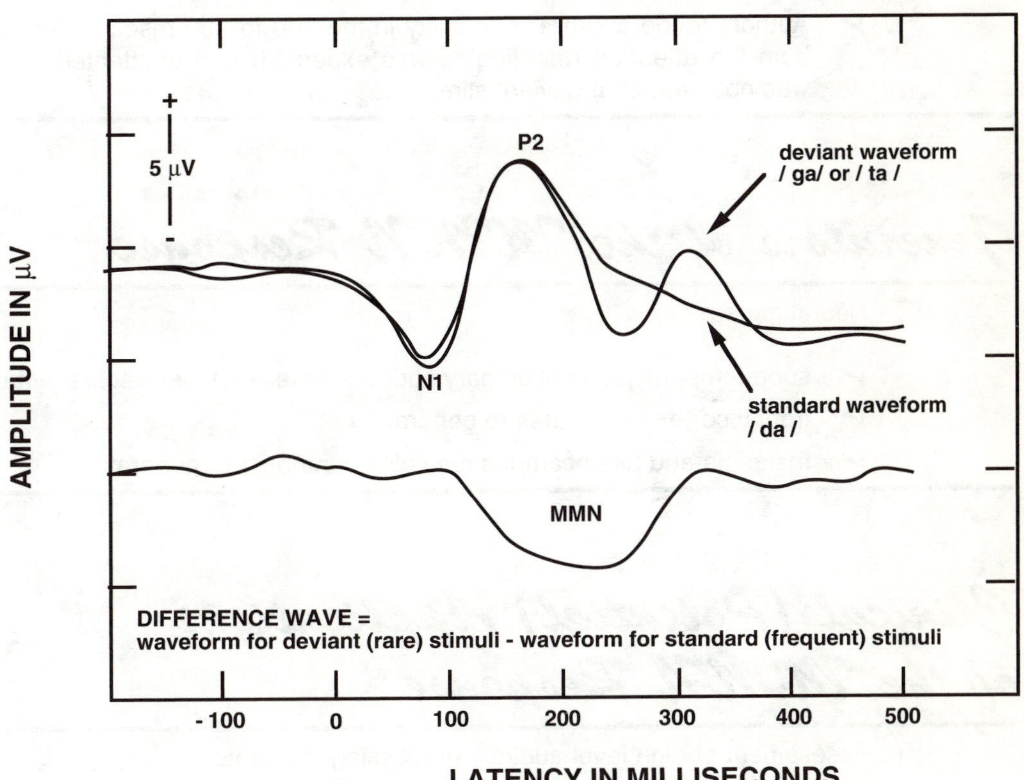

Historical Summary

Background on the Discovery of the Mismatch Negativity (MMN) Response

- ☐ Naatanen R, Gaillard AWK, Mantysalo S. Early selective-attention effect on evoked potential reinterpreted. *Acta Psychologica 42*: 313–329, 1979.
  - ✔ Outgrowth of experiments conducted on P_{300} response by the authors during a summer research project at the Institute for Perception in Soesterberg, The Netherlands
  - ✔ Task required attention to deviant stimuli in one ear while ignoring deviant stimuli presented to the other ear
  - ✔ Authors found a similar negativity in the 100 to 200 msec region to both the attended (this finding was expected) and unattented (this was not expected) deviant stimuli

Generators of the MMN Response

- ☐ Neural generators
  - ✔ supratemporal plane of primary auditory cortex (AI), or Heschl's gyrus
  - ✔ frontal cortex contributes to generation
  - ✔ thalamus and hippocampus may also contribute to generation

Clinical (Potential) Applications of the MMN Response

- ☐ Assessment of high level auditory processing in infants
- ☐ Description of cortical auditory organization
- ☐ Confirmation of neural dysfunction in clinical populations, including:
  - ✔ Parkinson's disease
  - ✔ dementia/Alzheimer's disease
  - ✔ stroke
  - ✔ schizophrenia

- dysphagia
- cochlear implant users
- hearing aid users
- central auditory processing disorders (CAPD)

☐ Studies of learning

☐ Study of speech perception in persons of all ages and mental states

- processing of fine acoustic differences
- plasticity of speech discrimination
- central auditory processing disorders
- neuroanatomy of speech perception

Stimulus Parameters

Eliciting the Mismatch Negativity (MMN) Response

☐ Frequency differences (smaller differences are better)

☐ Intensity differences

☐ Duration differences

☐ Location of sound in space

☐ Interstimulus interval

☐ Phonetic differences and cues

- voice-onset time (e.g., da vs. ta)
- formant-transition-duration contrasts
- formant-frequency contrasts (e.g., da vs. ga)
- acoustic differences (within phoneme categories)

☐ Abstract differences

Analysis of MMN Waveform Parameters

Illustration of four different strategies for mismatch negativity (MMN) analysis, including: (a) a simple measurement of the latency of the onset of the MMN, (b) absolute MMN amplitude from baseline to maximum negativity, (c) MMN duration from onset to the return to baseline, and (d) the area under the MMN wave.

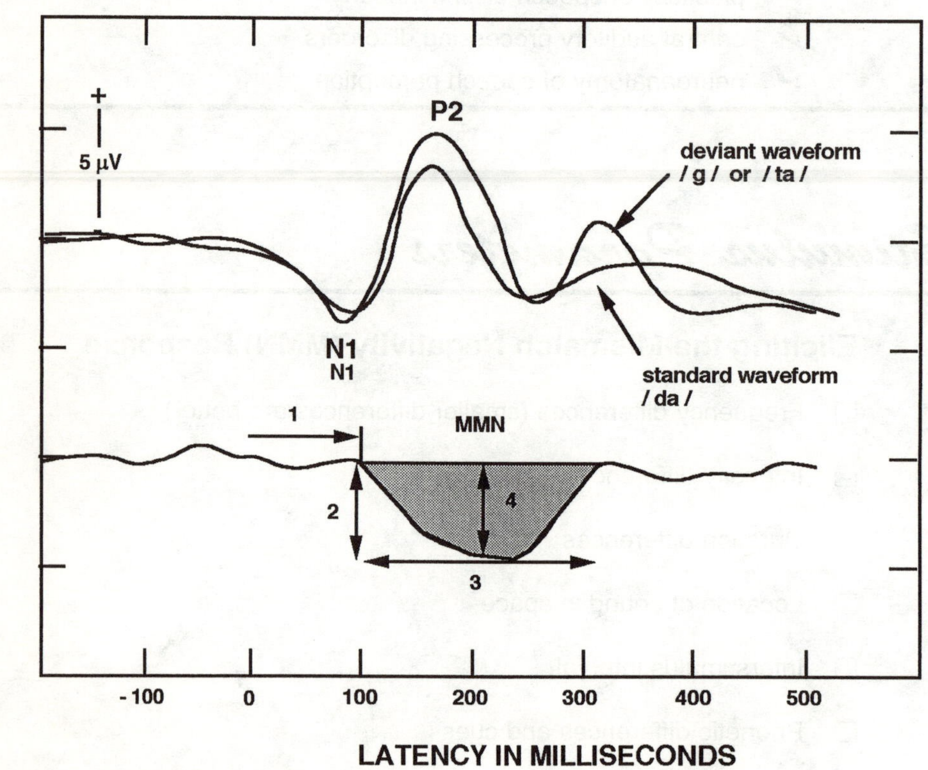

Point-by-Point Statistical Analysis of MMN

Illustration of a statistically-based, point-by-point analysis of the mismatch negativity response (MMN). MMN presence can be verified by statistical comparison with a non-MMN waveform, rather than simple visual inspection and analysis of latency and amplitude response parameters.

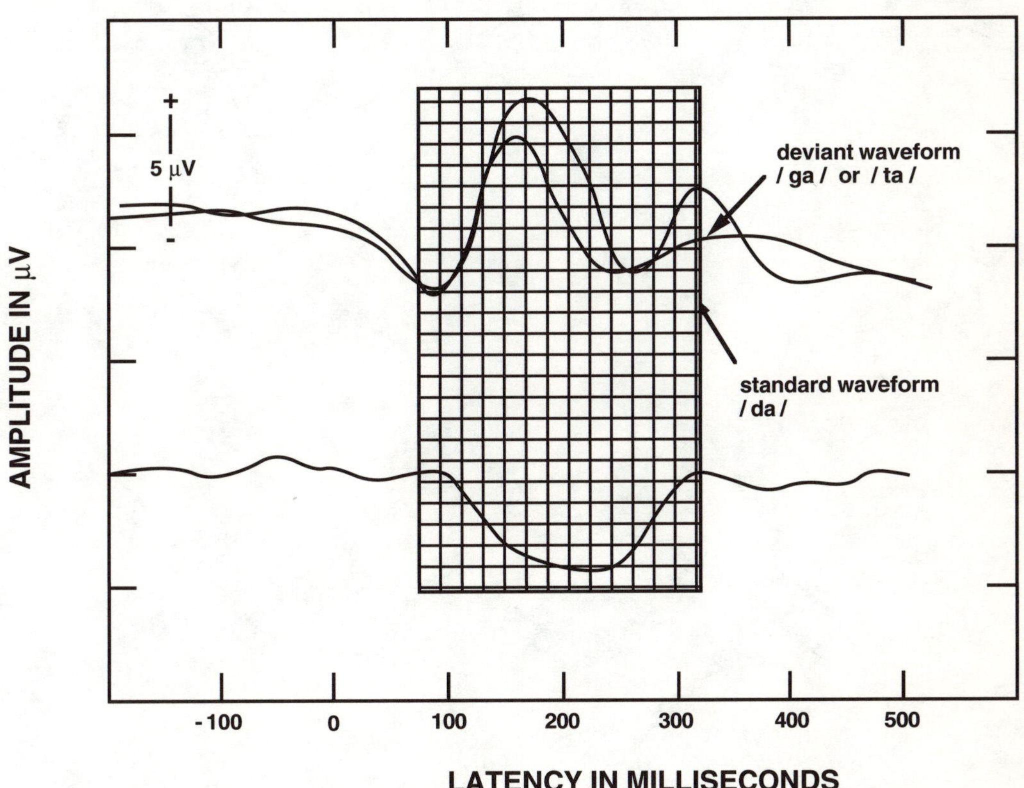

CHAPTER 9

Pediatric Audiology

In This ADR Chapter

Perspective

Pediatric audiology is almost a subspecialty within the profession. There are a handful of well-known, and a few new, textbooks devoted to the general topic. Actually, in its broadest sense, the practice of pediatric audiology requires application of almost all the clinical knowledge and technical expertise that any audiologist could hope to have. The pediatric audiologist must be able to record simplified auditory brainstem response (ABR) or otoacoustic emission (OAE) techniques in neonatal hearing screening. In diagnostic assessments, to confirm the type, degree, and configuration of hearing loss in each ear, and to differentiate peripheral versus central auditory dysfunction, the audiologist must apply aural immittance measures, OAE procedures, sophisticated ABR protocols, including the use of bone conduction and tone burst stimulation, and a variety of age-appropriate behavioral audiometry strategies. Of course, all of the above must be done with far greater test speed than is necessary in an adult population. Then, the audiologist must have a firm grasp of available management resources and options, ranging from amplification, to aural habilitation, to parent-infant stimulation, to counseling, to cochlear implants. Many of these audiologic assessment and management topics are addressed elsewhere in the ADR, and of course in hundreds of other references. What follows in this ADR chapter is simply information to augment and facilitate your practice of pediatric audiology.

FOUNDATIONS OF PEDIATRIC AUDIOLOGY

Components of Auditory System Development

- ☐ Improvement in the *threshold* (minimum response level) for different types of signals (e.g., pure tones, speech, noise).
- ☐ Development of *temporal (timing) resolution* (i.e., the detection of gaps between sounds).
- ☐ Improved detection of *sounds* (target signals) *in* the presence of *noise* or masking.
- ☐ Sharpening of *frequency discrimination* (smaller difference limens or just-noticable-differences between two frequencies).
- ☐ Development of *frequency resolution* (sharper tuning curves).

Developmental Changes

Neonatal MIDDLE EAR Structure and Function

- ☐ Vernix casseous in external ear canal dissipates within days after birth. Vernix is a lotionlike substance that covers the neonate's body at birth, and may remain in some cracks and crevices (e.g., the external ear canal) for awhile.
- ☐ Mesenchyme, present in the middle ear of some term neonates, dissipates within days after birth.
- ☐ Efficiency of the middle ear in transmitting acoustical energy to mechanical energy improves.
- ☐ Areal ratio of tympanic membrane (TM) to stapes footplate increases.
- ☐ TM curvature increases which increases lever function of the middle ear system and produces more efficiency in vibrational energy.
- ☐ TM thickness decreases.
- ☐ Lever function of the ossicles improves.

Important Principles

COCHLEAR and EIGHTH NERVE Maturation (before and soon after term birth)

General

- ☐ There are three general developmental factors to consider, including maturation of:
  - ✓ structure
  - ✓ physiology
  - ✓ biochemistry
- ☐ Afferent innervation (hair cell to to auditory nerve) precedes efferent innervation.
- ☐ The basal region (high-frequency region in the mature cochlea) of the cochlea matures earlier than the apical region (low-frequency region in the mature cochlea) by 1 to 2 weeks.

Stria Vascularis

- ☐ Stria vascularis increases in volume.
- ☐ Three cell types of the stria differentiate:
  - ✓ marginal cells (they face the endolymph)
  - ✓ intermediate cells (a layer between marginal cells)
  - ✓ basal cells (dividing stria from spiral ligament)
- ☐ Stria matures from the base to the apex.
- ☐ Melanin in the stria vascularis increases with development. Melanin may play a role in:
  - ✓ energy conversion
  - ✓ energy storage
  - ✓ energy release which probably generates the endocochlear potential

Endocochlear Potential (EP)

- ☐ Adult mammals have a positive electrical polarization of 80 to 90 mV in endolymph versus the perilymph (in the scala vestibuli and scala tympani). See the Cochlear Battery in Chapter 1.
- ☐ Endolymph ionic composition is similar to intracellular fluids in K+ (potassium) and Na+ (sodium) concentration.

- ☐ Perilymph ionic composition resembles extracellular fluids.
- ☐ Maintenance of EP dependent on stria vascularis activity.
- ☐ EP development is most rapid in the first 2 weeks after birth.
- ☐ EP development is dependent on the maturation of the stria.

Eighth Nerve

- ☐ There are two types of eighth nerve fibers (afferent and efferent).
- ☐ Afferent fibers lead proximally (centrally) to the spiral ganglion.
  - ✓ Type I: innervate inner hair cells (IHC)
  - ✓ Type II: innervate outer hair cells (OHC)
- ☐ Efferent fibers project distally (peripherally) from the brainstem down to the cochlea.
  - ✓ Lateral system: runs from the lateral olivary nuclei to innervate IHCs via synapses on afferent auditory dentrites.
  - ✓ Medial system: runs from the ventro-medial nuclei of the trapezoid body to direct synapses with OHCs.
  - ✓ Lateral efferent maturation preceeds the medial efferents

Maturation of the ABR

Also, see normative neonatal and infant data in Chapter 7.

- ☐ First measured at about 27 or 28 weeks gestational age
- ☐ Waveform initially is characterized by reliable wave I and V, whereas other wave components usually not observed
- ☐ ABR threshold (minimum intensity level at which a reliable response is recorded) appears to improve from prematurity until term (40 weeks gestational age)
- ☐ Maturational changes in ABR continue until approximately 18 months after term birth. These include:
  - ✓ improvement in waveform morphology (synchrony)
  - ✓ appearance of wave III, then wave II and IV
  - ✓ decrease in latency values for later waves (III andV)
  - ✓ decrease in interwave latency values (e.g., I–V)
  - ✓ increase in high-frequency spectral energy content

Classic Quote

Marion Downs on 20th-Century Pediatric Audiology

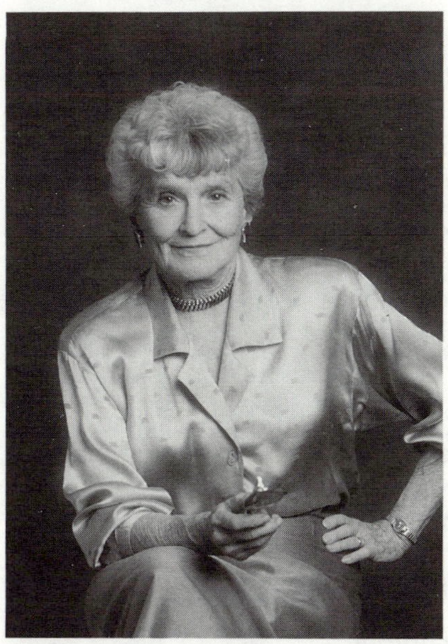

Marion Downs, the "Mother of Pediatric Audiology"

"Pediatric audiology came quietly into being in the early 1940s, spurred by dedicated educators of the deaf who studied the auditory behaviors of normal children. These educators were Alexander and Irene Ewing in England. They combined the use of gross noisemakers with their own sophisticated skills of observation, developing these simple techniques into an art."

"The full 20th-century response to the need for . . . pediatric audiology . . . utilizes a state-of-the-art technology to ensure that **all** ***children will have available to them the identification of their problems at the earliest possible moment. For the goal is all. Not just the children with parents who can afford testing and monitoring; not just those who happen to fall into a category that places them at risk for deafness; not just the ones who happen to be in the right place at the right time to be screened, but all children. They are all entitled to be touched by the screening hand of modern technology."***

Source: Downs. Twentieth century pediatric audiology: Prologue to the 21st. *Seminars in Hearing 11*: 408–411, 1990.

Pediatric Medical Referral Criteria

History

- ☐ Otalgia
- ☐ Otorrhea

Visual Inspection of the Ear

- ☐ Structural defect of the ear, head, or neck
- ☐ Ear canal abnormalities
  - ✔ blood or effusion
  - ✔ occlusion
  - ✔ inflammation
  - ✔ excessive cerumen, tumor, foreign material
- ☐ Eardrum abnormalities
  - ✔ abnormal color
  - ✔ bulging eardrum
  - ✔ fluid line or bubbles
  - ✔ perforation
  - ✔ retraction

Identification Audiometry

- ☐ Fail air conduction screening at 20 dB HL at 1, 2, or 4 kHz in either ear (ASHA, 1985)
- ☐ These criteria may require alteration for various clinical settings and populations.

Tympanometry

- ☐ Flat tympanogram and equivalent ear canal volume (Vec) outside normal range.
- ☐ Low static admittance (Peak Y) on two successive occurrences in a 4–6 week interval.
- ☐ Abnormally wide tympanometric width (TW) on two successive occurrences in a 4–6 week interval.

Source: ASHA (1990).

Etiology of Hearing Loss of Deaf Adults

As expressed by manually communi-cating deaf adults. Data in percent.

	Study	
Etiology	**Northern et al. (1971)**	**Schein (1965)**
Unknown	35.8	32.2
Congenital	25.5	10.5
Meningitis	13.1	12.7
Scarlet fever	9.5	4.6
Result of a fall	8.1	7.7
Whooping cough	3.6	2.3
Measles	2.2	3.4
Pneumonia		2.3
Mastoiditis		1.9
Other	2.2	16.7
	N = 137	*132*

Source: Northern JL, Downs MP. *Hearing in children* (4th ed.). Baltimore: Williams & Wilkins, 1991. Reprinted with permission.

Summary of Known Exogenous Causes of Prelingual Deafness

Preconception and Prenatal Causes

- ☐ Rubella
- ☐ CMV (cytomegalovirus)
- ☐ Ototoxic and other drugs, maternal alcoholism
- ☐ Hypoxia
- ☐ Syphilis
- ☐ Toxemia, diabetes, other severe systemic maternal illness
- ☐ Parental irradiation
- ☐ Toxoplasmosis

Perinatal Causes

- ☐ Hypoxia
- ☐ Traumatic delivery
- ☐ Maternal infection
- ☐ Ototoxic drugs
- ☐ Premature delivery

Neonatal and Postnatal Causes

- ☐ Hypoxia
- ☐ Infection
- ☐ Ototoxic drugs
- ☐ Erythroblastosis fetalis
- ☐ Infantile measles or mumps
- ☐ Otitis media (acute, chronic, serous)
- ☐ Noise-induced
- ☐ Meningitis
- ☐ Encephalitis

Source: Northern JL, Downs MP. *Hearing in children* (4th ed). Baltimore: Williams & Wilkins, 1991. Reprinted with permission.

Joint Committee on Infant Hearing

1994 Member Organizations

- ☐ American Academy of Audiology
- ☐ American Academy of Otolaryngology—Head and Neck Surgery
- ☐ American Academy of Pediatrics
- ☐ American Speech-Language-Hearing Association
- ☐ Directors of Speech and Hearing Programs in State Health and Welfare Agencies

Source: Joint Committee on Infant Hearing. 1994 Position Statement. *Audiology Today* 6(6): 6–9, 1994.

Features of the JCIH 1994 Position Statement

- ☐ Techniques for infant hearing screening must:
  - ✔ detect hearing loss of 30 dB HL
  - ✔ detect hearing loss in the speech frequency region (500 through 4000 Hz)
  - ✔ be feasible in infants within the birth to 3-month age range
- ☐ Screening program personnel
  - ✔ audiologists (should supervise programs)
  - ✔ physicians (otolaryngologists and pediatricians)
  - ✔ nursing personnel
- ☐ Timing of screening and intervention
  - ✔ universal detection of infants with hearing loss as soon as possible
  - ✔ identification by 3 months of age
  - ✔ intervention by 6 months of age
- ☐ Team for diagnostic audiologic assessment and intervention planning for children identified with hearing loss
  - ✔ physician with expertise in pediatric otologic disorders
  - ✔ audiologist with expertise in assessment and management of pediatric hearing loss
  - ✔ specialist in aural habilitation (speech-language pathologist, audiologist, sign language specialist, teacher of children with hearing impairment)
  - ✔ other personnel as appropriate

Source: Joint Committee on Infant Hearing. 1994 Position Statement. *Audiology Today 6*(6): 6–9, 1994.

Development of Auditory Responses

Age	Response(s)
0 to 4 months	✔ eye widening ✔ eye blink ✔ arousal from sleep
4 to 7 months	✔ head turn
Older than 7 months	✔ direct localization of sounds

Source: McConnell and Ward (1967); Northern and Downs (1978)

Development of Hearing

Minimal Response Levels

	Minimal Response Level in dB HL	
Age	Warble Tone Signal	Speech Signal
0 to 6 weeks	75	40–60
6 weeks to 4 months	70	47
4 to 7 months	51	21
7 to 9 months	45	15
9 to 13 months	38	8
13 to 16 months	32	5
16 to 21 months	25	5
21 to 24 months	26	3

Source: McConnell and Ward (1967); Northern and Downs (1978)

Auditory Behavior Index for Infants

Stimulus and Level of Response*

Age	Startle to Noisemakers (approx. dB SPL)	Warbled Pure Tones (dB HL)	Speech (dB HL)	Expected Response
0–6 wk	50–70	75	40–60	Eye widening, eye blink, stirring or arousal from sleep, startle
6 wk–4 mos	50–60	70	45	Eye widening, eye shift, eye-blink quieting; beginning rudimentary head turn by 4 months
4–7 mos	40–50	50	20	Head turn on lateral plane toward sound; listening attitude
7–9 mos	30–40	45	15	Direct localization of sounds to side; indirectly below ear level
9–13 mos	25–35	38	10	Direct localization of sounds to side; directly below ear level, indirectly above ear level
13–16 mos	25–30	30	5	Direct localization of sound on side, above and below
16–21 mos	25	25	5	Direct localization of sound on side, above and below
21–24 mos	25	25	5	Direct localization of sound on side, above and below

*Testing done in a sound room. (Modified with permission from McConnell, F., Ward, PH. *Deafness in childhood*, Nashville, Tennessee, Vanderbilt University Press, 1967.

Source: Adapted from: Northern JL, Downs MP. *Hearing in children* (4th ed.). Baltimore: Williams & Wilkins, 1991.

Piaget Stages of Cognitive Development

Stage	Age range	Main features
Sensorimotor period	birth to 2 years	Development of action patterns. Through them, the child learns that objects in space have permanence. Six substages in this period include: 1) consolidation and perfection of reflexes, 2) formation (primary) of motor habits and perceptions, 3) beginning of intentional acts (first clear differentiation between accomodation and assimilation), 4) more goal directed behavior and application of secondary schemata to new situations, 5) child discovers new approaches to obtain desired goals (assuming maturation of necessary motor-perceptual responses), and 6) integration of sensori-motor schemata and objects take on permanency.
Concrete thinking period *	2 to 12 years	A period of formation and then equilibration. In the former (to age 6 years), the child achieves symbolic thought and can carry out concrete operations. Mental actions are not reversible. Reversibility in thinking occurs after 7 years of age.
Formal operations period	12 years to adulthood	Usually reaches equilibrium by age 14 or 15 years. Child is capable of deductive thinking and is able to solve a number of conceptual problems. With the appropriate environmental conditions, the child is able to perform creative scientific research.

* Early preoperational period = 2 to 4 yrs; Late preoperational period = 4 to 7 yrs; Concrete operations period =7 to 11 or 12 yrs

Sources: Piaget J, Inhelder B. *The psychology of the child*. New York: Basic Books, 1969.

Piaget J. *The language and thought of the child*. New York: Harcourt, Brace & World, Inc., 1926.

Articulation Development in Children

Speech sound	Age in Yearsr* Templin (1957)	Prather et al. (1975)
m	3	2
n	3	2
h	3	2
p	3	2
ŋ	3	2
f	3	2 to 4
j	3 to 6	2 to 4
k	4	2 to 4
d	4	2 to 4
w	3	2 to 8
b	4	2 to 8
t	6	2 to 8
g	4	3
s	4 to 6	3
r	4	3 to 4
l	6	3 to 4
ʃ	4 to 6	3 to 8
ch	4 to 6	3 to 8
ð	7	4
zh	7	4
dʒ	7	4+ **
th	6	4+ **
v	6	4+ **
z	7	4+ **
hw	**	4+ **

*Adapted from Peterson HA, Marquardt TP. *Appraisal and diagnosis of speech and language disorders* (3rd ed.). Englewood Cliffs, NJ: Prentice-Hall, 1994, p. 58.

Sources: Prather EM, Hendrick EL, Kerin CA. Articulation development in children aged two to four years. *J Speech Hear Dis 40:* 179–191, 1975.

Templin MC. *Certain language skills in children*, Institute of Child Welfare Monograph Series, No. 26. Minneapolis: University of Minnesota,1957.

**Sound not produced correctly by 75% of children at the oldest age level tested.

Sensitivity and Specificity of Audioscope

By Signal Frequency and Test Site

	Physicians' Offices/Hearing Center			
Signal Frequency (Hz)	Failure to Hear (%)	*N*	Sensitivity (in %)	Specificity (in %)
Right Ear				
500	13.7	175/172	79/92	76/93
1000	18.3	175/172	91/97	69/85
2000	31.4	175/172	87/79	88/96
4000	63.0	173/172	89/89	78/91
Left Ear				
500	16.1	174/172	79/89	77/94
1000	16.7	174/172	93/97	70/87
2000	32.8	174/171	88/88	89/93
4000	69.0	171/170	83/87	72/87

Source: From Bess, F, Lichtenstein M., Logan S. Audiology assessment of the elderly. In Rintlemann W (ed.). *Hearing assessment* (2nd ed.)., 1991, p. 521.

DIAGNOSTIC AUDIOLOGIC ASSESSMENT OF CHILDREN

General Strategies For Pediatric Hearing Assessment

Three different age groups. The order of the different types of procedures reflects their importance in the age group.

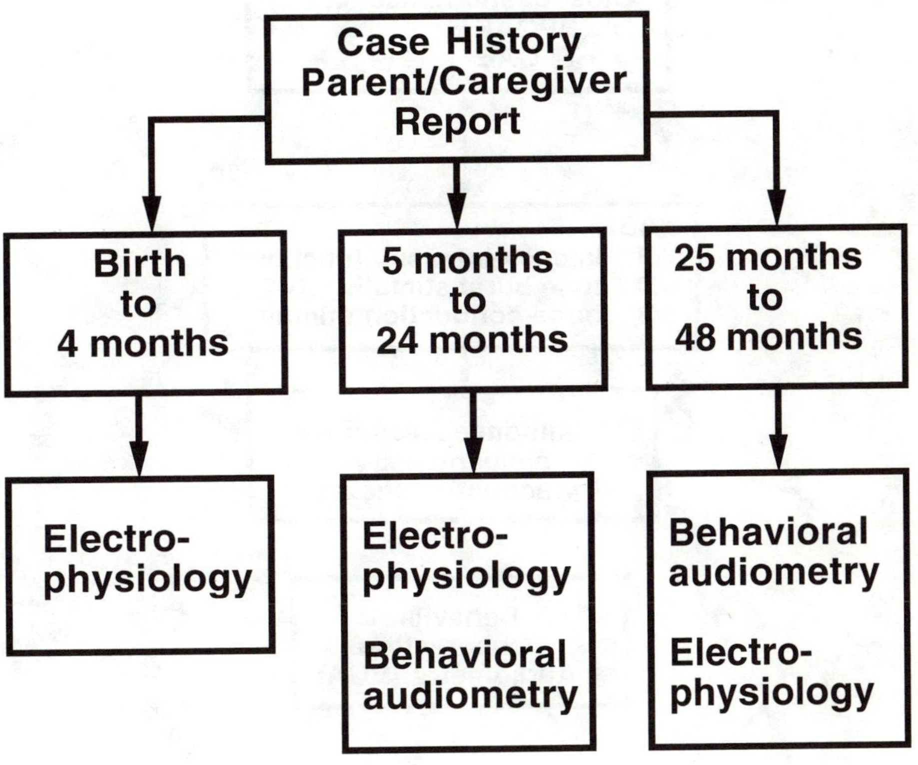

Pediatric Audiology Flowchart

Birth to 4 Months

Sequence of audiologic test procedures performed, or attempted, in the assessment of children in the birth to 4 months age category. For a sizable proportion of children, estimation of hearing status will be dependent mostly or entirely on just ABR and OAE.

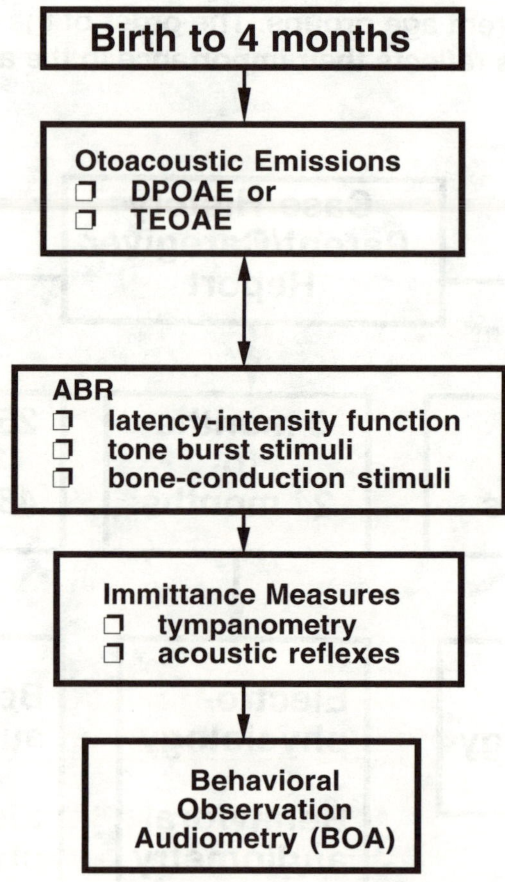

Pediatric Audiology Flowchart

5–24 Months

Sequence of audiologic test procedures performed, or attempted, in the assessment of children in the 5 to 24 months age category. For some children (e.g., developmentally delayed), it might be necessary to rely mostly or exclusively on electrophysiologic measures. In many clinics, OAE are performed as the initial procedure for rapid determination of ear-specific and frequency-specific peripheral (cochlear) auditory status.

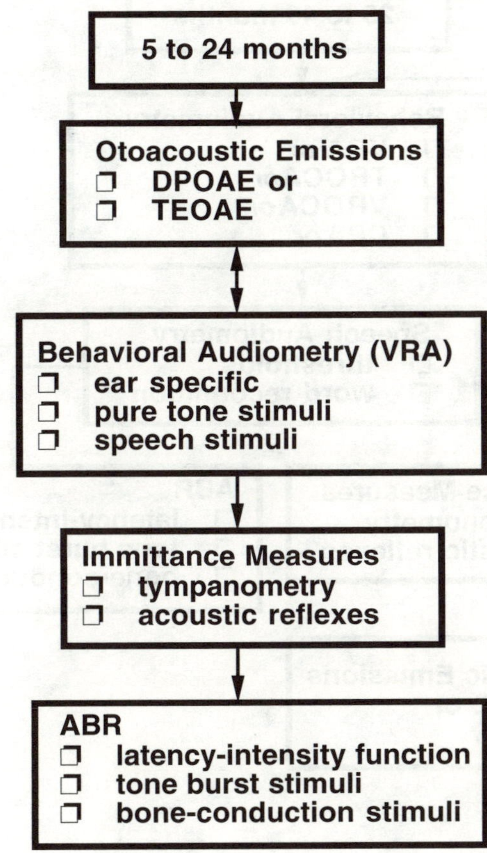

Pediatric Audiology Flowchart

25–48 Months

Sequence of audiologic test procedures performed, or attempted, in the assessment of children in the 25 to 48 months age category. In many clinics, OAE are performed as the initial procedure for rapid determination of ear-specific and frequency-specific peripheral (cochlear) auditory status in almost all children.

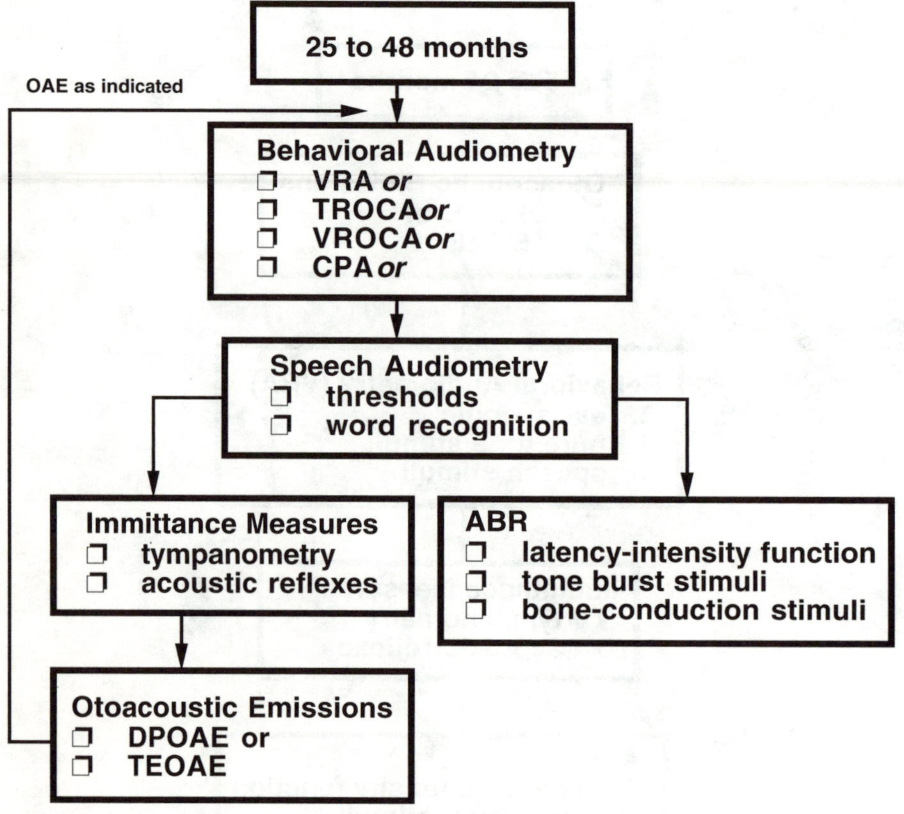

Diagnostic Test Battery Patterns

KEY:
normal ○
maybe abnormal ◍
abnormal ●

PEDIATRIC AUDIOLOGY TEST BATTERY PATTERNS						
	DISORDER / DISEASE					
TEST PROCEDURE	Otitis media	Meningitis	CMV	Hyper-bilirubinemia	Developmental Delay	Degenerative Disease
Aural immittance						
tympanometry	●	○	○	○	○	○
acoustic reflexes	●	◍	●	◍	◍	◍
Pure tone audiometry	●	◍	◍	◍	◍	◍
Word recognition	◍	◍	◍	◍	◍	◍
Otoacoustic emissions	●	◍	◍	◍	○	○
Diagnostic speech audiometry	○	◍	●	●	●	●
Evoked Responses						
ABR	●	◍	●	●	●	●
AMLR	NA	◍	◍	◍	●	●
P300/MMN	NA	◍	◍	◍	●	●

Classic Quote

Jerger and Hayes on the "cross-check principle"

"We have found that simply observing the auditory behavior of children does not always yield an accurate description of hearing loss. In our experience, we have seen too many children at all levels of functioning who have been misdiagnosed and mismanaged on the basis of behavioral test results alone.

"During the past decade two new techniques, uniquely suited to the evaluation of young children, have been made available to clinicians. The first, impedance audiometry, is not only sensitive to middle ear disorders, but in the case of normal middle ear function permits quantification of sensorineural level. The second technique, brain-stem-evoked response (BSER) audiometry, is an electrophysiologic technique that permits the clinician to estimate sensitivity above 500 Hertz by both air and bone conduction.

For the past three years, we have used these two techniques in combination with conventional behavioral audiometry as a pediatric test battery. Our fundamental approach has been to use either impedance audiometry or BSER audiometry as a cross-check of the behavioral test results" (Jerger and Hayes, 1976, p. 59).

"In summary, we believe that the unique limitations of conventional behavioral audiometry dictate the need for a 'test battery' approach. The key concept governing our assessment strategy is the cross-check principle. The basic operation of this principle is that no result be accepted until it is confirmed by an independent measure. . . . We believe that the application of the cross-check principle to our clinical population has had an appreciable effect on the accuracy with which we can identify and quantify hearing loss during the critical years for language-learning." (Jerger and Hayes, 1976, p. 65)

Source: Jerger JF, Hayes D. The cross-check principle in pediatric audiometry. *Archives of Otolaryngology 102:* 614–620, 1976.

ADR NOTE: The pediatric audiometric test battery now includes otoacoustic emissions, in addition to behavioral techniques, auditory brainstem response (ABR), and immittance measures. Details are provided in ADR Chapters 4 (immittance measures), 5 (otoacoustic emissions), and 7 (ABR).

DPOAE in Pediatric Hearing Assessment

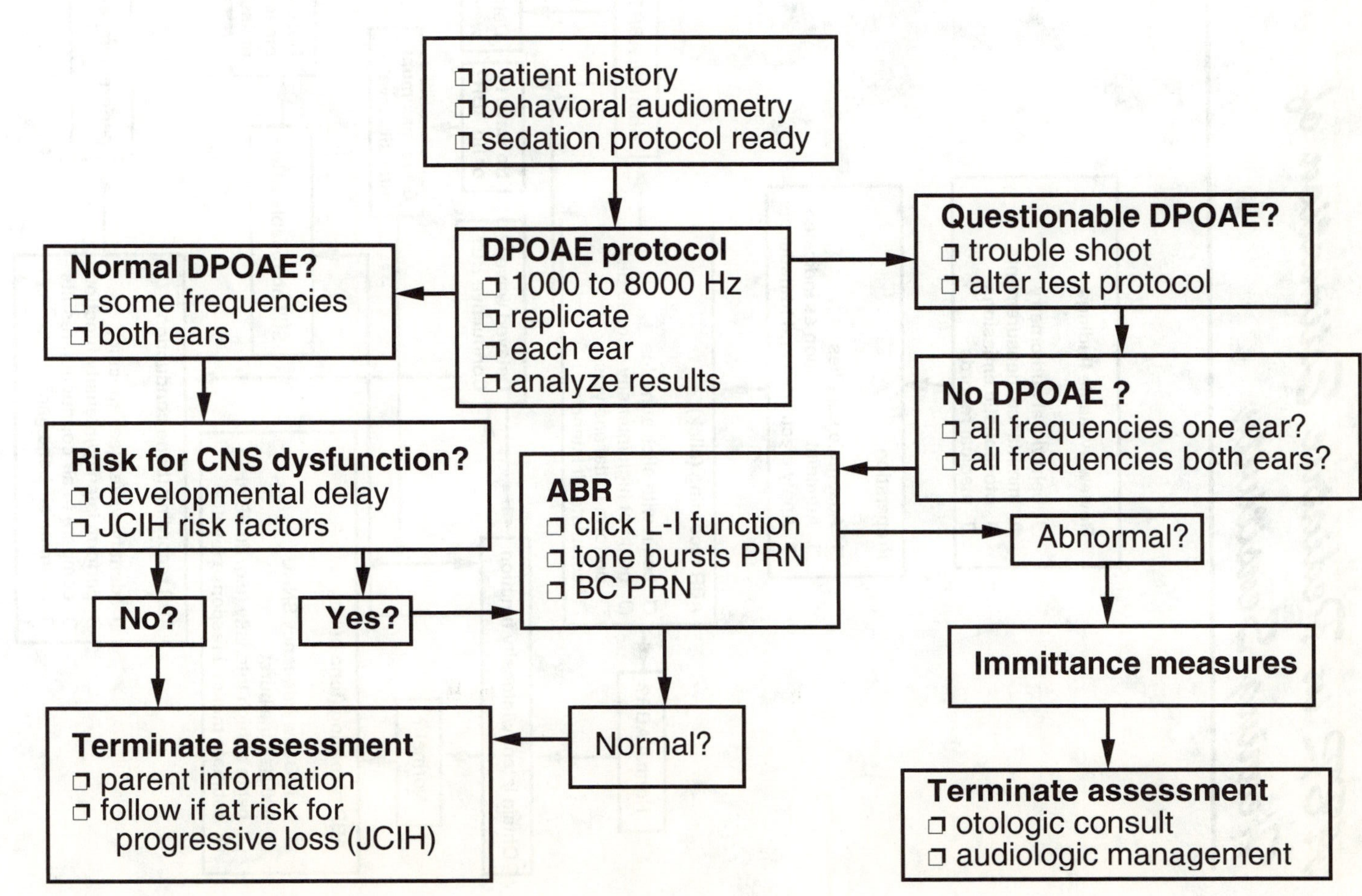

ABR in Pediatric Estimation of Hearing Sensitivity

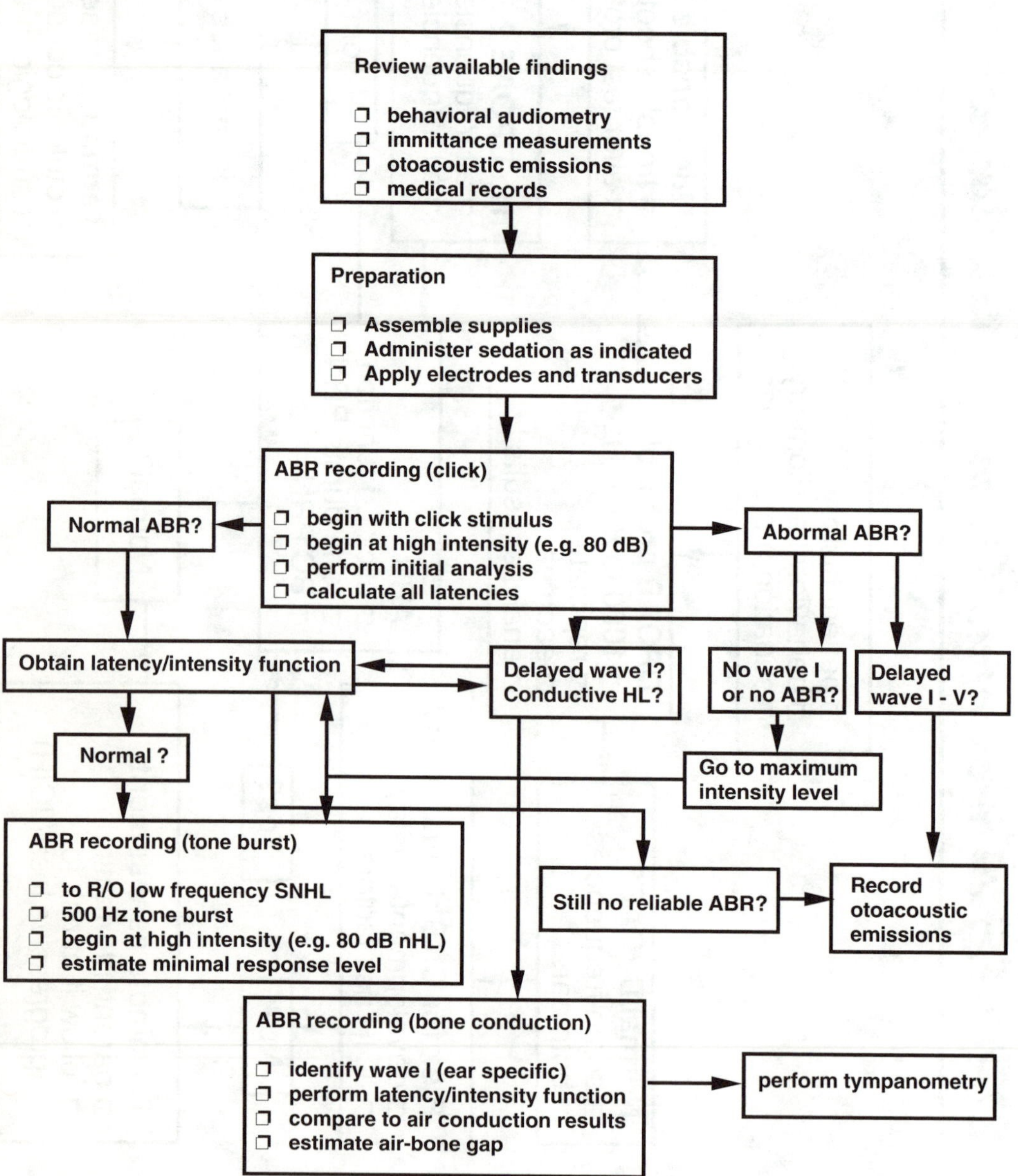

Review available findings
❒ behavioral audiometry
❒ immittance measurements
❒ otoacoustic emissions
❒ medical records
Preparation
❒ Assemble supplies
❒ Administer sedation as indicated
❒ Apply electrodes and transducers
ABR recording (click)
❒ begin with click stimulus
❒ begin at high intensity (e.g. 80 dB)
❒ perform initial analysis
❒ calculate all latencies
Normal ABR?
Abormal ABR?
Obtain latency/intensity function
Delayed wave I? Conductive HL?
No wave I or no ABR?
Delayed wave I - V?
Normal ?
Go to maximum intensity level
ABR recording (tone burst)
❒ to R/O low frequency SNHL
❒ 500 Hz tone burst
❒ begin at high intensity (e.g. 80 dB nHL)
❒ estimate minimal response level
Still no reliable ABR?
Record otoacoustic emissions
ABR recording (bone conduction)
❒ identify wave I (ear specific)
❒ perform latency/intensity function
❒ compare to air conduction results
❒ estimate air-bone gap
perform tympanometry

Guidelines for Speech Threshold Testing of Children

Approximate Level of Function*	Type of Measurement	Test Stimuli	Response Task	Type of Reinforcement
≥ 10 years	Conventional SRT	Spondee	Verbal	Verbal (intermittent)
5 to 10 years	Conventional SRT	Child spondee list	Verbal	Verbal (intermittent)
30 months to 6 years	Modified SRT	Selected child's spondees	Picture or object pointing	Social, visual, or tangible
Less than 3 years	SAT	Repetitive speech utterance	Conditioned	Play, visual, or tangible
Limited	SAT	Repetitive speech utterance	Unconditioned response	None

* Dependent on cognitive, motor, and language development and attending behavior

Source: From Olsen WO, Matkin ND. In WF Rintelmann (Ed.). *Hearing assessment*, 2nd ed., Austin, TX:Pro-Ed, 1991, p. 55. Reprinted with permission.

Clinical Concept

Visual Reinforcement in Pediatric Audiometry

- ☐ Using two visual reinforcers permits more behavioral responses before the child habituates than a single reinforcer
- ☐ After a child habituates to the test signals, taking a 10-minute break during testing will usually lead to at least five more responses, at least in 1-year-old children.
- ☐ Most 2-year-old children habitutate faster than 1-year-old children.

Source: Adapted from Thompson G, Thompson M, McCall A. Strategies for increasing response behavior of 1- and 2-year-old children during visual reinforcement audiometry (VRA). *Ear and Hearing 13:* 236–240, 1992.

CHILDREN WITH UNILATERAL HEARING LOSS

Problems of Children with Unilateral Hearing Loss

- ☐ About 50% of children with unilateral hearing loss will be retained in a grade or will require resource assistance in school
- ☐ Risk of academic failure is 10 times greater for child with unilateral hearing loss than the general school population
- ☐ Seriousness of academic problems is greater for:
  - ✔ early age of onset
  - ✔ right ear impairment
  - ✔ severe-to-profound impairment
- ☐ Most serious auditory problems include:
  - ✔ impaired ability to localize the source of sound
  - ✔ increased difficulty distinguishing sounds, including speech sounds, in the presence of background noise
  - ✔ confusion in social interactions, especially when speaker is on the side of the "bad" ear
  - ✔ apparent disinterest, inattention, and perceived "behavior problem"
  - ✔ may give the impression of being hyperactive and immature

Characteristics of Children with Unilateral Hearing Loss

- ☐ Subjects
  - 60 unilaterally hearing-impaired children
  - age range of 6 to 18 years (mean of 13 years)
  - gender: male = 45%; female = 55%
- ☐ Findings
  - about 50% of the children were experiencing some difficulty in academic progress, including failing at least one grade (35%) or requiring resource assistance (13%)
  - localization scores were significantly poorer for children with unilateral hearing loss than for normal hearing counterparts
  - more localization errors were found for the 3000 Hz than the 500 Hz stimuli
  - localization errors increased with the degree of hearing loss
  - children with unilateral hearing loss had more difficulty in auditory skills and understanding speech in monaural direct and monaural indirect listening conditions in both quiet and in noise (by the nonsense syllable test, or NST)
  - poorer speech understanding scores were noted for children with right ear hearing impairments versus left ear impairments
  - errors were greater for final versus initial consonant identification, and for voiceless versus voiced consonants

Sources: Bess FH, Tharpe AM. Case history data on unilaterally hearing-impaired children. *Ear and Hearing 7:* 14–19, 1986; Bess FH, Tharpe AM, Gilbert AM. Auditory performance of children with unilateral sensorineural hearing loss. *Ear and Hearing 7:* 20–26, 1986.

Management of Children with Unilateral Hearing Loss

- ☐ Teacher in-service training
- ☐ Parent counseling
- ☐ Information for others who interact with the child (coaches, siblings, etc.)
- ☐ Speech-language evaluation
- ☐ Close monitoring of hearing and for middle ear dysfunction
- ☐ Acoustic treatment of the classroom
- ☐ Modification of classroom activities
- ☐ Preferential seating in classroom (only management if child is performing appropriately academically)
- ☐ FM assistive listening device between the teacher and the child

Sources: Bess FH, Tharpe AM. Case history data on unilaterally hearing-impaired children. *Ear and Hearing 7:* 14–19, 1986; Bess FH, Tharpe AM, Gilbert AM. Auditory performance of children with unilateral sensorineural hearing loss. *Ear and Hearing 7:* 20–26, 1986.

Key References

Unilateral Hearing Loss in Children

Bess FH, Klee T, Culbertson JL. Identification, assessment, and management of children with unilateral sensorineural hearing loss. *Ear and Hearing 7:* 43–51, 1986.

Bess FH, Tharpe AM. Unilateral hearing impairment in children. *Pediatrics 74:* 206–216, 1984.

Oyler RF, Oyler, AL, Matkin ND. Unilateral hearing loss: Demographics and educational impact. *Language, Speech & Hearing in the Schools 19:* 201–210, 1988.

Management Stragegies for Children with Unilateral Hearing loss

- ☐ Increase awareness of the child's hearing loss among those who interact with the child
  - ✓ parents and other adult family members
  - ✓ siblings
  - ✓ family physician
  - ✓ classroom teacher
  - ✓ classmates
  - ✓ other school personnel
  - ✓ school bus driver
  - ✓ coaches and team members (e.g., baseball, soccer). Consider preferential positions in baseball (e.g., child with "bad" left ear might play first base, whereas the child with a "bad" right ear would play third base)
  - ✓ other significant persons for child (e.g., at church, day care workers, counselors at summer camps, Santa Claus at the mall)
- ☐ Closely monitor speech-language development, and academic progress, especially in language arts, spelling, and reading
- ☐ Closely monitor hearing in the "good" for early detection and aggressive management of otitis media or other potential causes of hearing impairment
- ☐ Locate child toward the front of and in the quietest area of the classroom, with the "good ear" toward the teacher
- ☐ Have the teacher obtain the child's attention before giving instructions or aural information
- ☐ Rephrase statements that the child doesn't understand the first time
- ☐ Provide visual cues to help the child's understanding of spoken information
- ☐ For older children, supplement aural with written material
- ☐ Consider the use of a no-gain FM or infrared light assistive listening device to improve signal-to-noise conditions for the child in the classroom, or the use of a CROS hearing aid arrangement

IMPACT OF HEARING LOSS IN CHILDREN

Language and Speech

Relationship of Degree of Long-term Hearing Loss to Language and Speech

Degree of Hearing Loss (PTA of (500–4000 Hz)	Possible Effects of Hearing Loss on Understanding of Language and Speech
Normal hearing (–10 to +15 dB HL)	Children have better hearing sensitivity than the accepted normal range for adults. A child with hearing sensitivity in the –10 to +15 dB range will detect the complete speech signal even at soft conversation levels. However, good hearing does not guarantee good ability to discriminate speech in the presence of background noise.
Minimal hearing loss (16 to 25 dB HL)	May have difficulty hearing faint or distant speech. At 15 dB student can miss up to 10% of speech signal when teacher is at a distance greater than 3 feet and when the classroom is noisy, especially in the elementary grades when verbal instruction predominates.
Mild hearing loss (26 to 40 dB HL)	At 30 dB can miss 25–40% of speech signal. The degree of difficulty experienced in school will depend upon the noise level in classroom, distance from teacher, and the configuration of the hearing loss. Without amplification the child with 35–40 dB loss may miss at least 50% of class discussions, especially when voices are faint or speaker is not in line of vision. Will miss consonants, especially when a high-frequency hearing loss is present.
Moderate hearing loss (41 to 55 dB HL)	Understands conversational speech at a distance of 3–5 feet (face-to-face) only if structure and vocabulary controlled. Without amplification the amount of speech signal missed can be 50% to 75% with 40 dB loss and 80% to 100% with 50 dB loss. Is likely to have delayed or defective syntax, limited vocabulary, imperfect speech production, and an atonal voice quality.
Moderate to Severe hearing loss (56 to 70 dB HL)	Without amplification, conversation must be very loud to be understood. A 55 dB loss can cause child to miss up to 100% of speech information. Will have marked difficulty in school situations requiring verbal communication in both one-to-one and group situations. Delayed language, syntax, reduced speech intelligibility, and atonal voice quality likely.
Severe hearing loss (71 to 90 dB HL)	Without amplification may hear loud voices about 1 foot from ear. When amplified optimally, children with hearing ability of 90 dB or better should be able to identify environmental sounds and detect all the sounds of speech. If loss is of prelingual onset, oral language and speech may not develop spontaneously or will be severely delayed. If hearing loss is of recent onset, speech is

	likely to deteriorate with quality becoming atonal.
Profound hearing loss (91 dB HL or more)	Aware of vibrations more than tonal pattern. Many rely on vision rather than hearing as primary avenue for communication and learning. Detection of speech sounds dependent on loss configuration and use of amplification. Speech and language will not develop spontaneously and are likely to deteriorate rapidly if hearing loss is of recent onset.
Unilateral hearing loss (a normal ear and a hearing-impaired ear)	May have difficulty hearing faint or distant speech. Usually has difficulty localizing sounds and voices. Unilateral listener will have greater difficulty understanding speech when environment is noisy and/or reverberant. Difficulty detecting or understanding soft speech from side of bad ear, especially in a group discussion.

Education

Potential Educational Needs and Programs for Children with Long-term Hearing Loss

Degree of Hearing Loss PTA of (500–4000 Hz)	**Potential Educational Needs and Programs**
Normal hearing (–10 to +15 dB HL)	May benefit from mild gain/low MPO hearing aid or personal FM system dependent on loss configuration.
Minimal hearing loss (16 to 25 dB HL)	Would benefit from soundfield amplification if classroom is noisy and/or reverberant. Needs favorable seating. May need attention to vocabulary or speech, especially with recurrent otitis media history. Appropriate medical management necessary for conductive losses. Teacher requires inservice training on impact of hearing loss on language development and learning.
Mild hearing loss (26 to 40 dB HL)	Will benefit from a hearing aid and use of a personal FM or sound-field FM system in the classroom. Needs favorable seating and lighting. Refer to special education for language evaluation and educational follow-up. Needs auditory skill building. May need attention to vocabulary and language development, articulation or speechreading, and/or special support in reading. May need help with self-esteem. Teacher inservice training required.
Moderate hearing loss (41 to 55 dB HL)	Refer to special education for language evaluation and educational follow-up. Amplification is essential (hearing aids and FM system). Special education support may be needed, especially for primary children. Attention to oral language development, reading, and written language. Auditory skill development and speech therapy usually are needed. Teacher inservice training required.
Moderate to severe hearing loss (56 to 70 dB HL)	Full-time use of amplification is essential. Will need resource teacher or special class depending on magnitude of language delay. May require special help in all language skills, language-based academic subjects, vocabulary, grammar, and pragmatics

	as well as reading and writing. Probably needs assistance to expand experiential language base. Inservice training of mainstream teachers required.
Severe hearing loss (71 to 90 dB HL)	May need full-time special aural/oral program with emphasis on all auditory language skills, speech reading, concept development, and speech. As loss approaches 80–90 dB, may benefit from a Total Communication approach, especially in the early language-learning years. Individual hearing aid/personal FM system essential. Need to monitor effectiveness of communication modality. Participation in regular classes as much as beneficial to student. Inservice training of mainstream teachers essential.
Profound hearing loss (≥91 dB HL)	May need special program for deaf children with emphasis on all language skills and academic areas. Program needs specialized supervision and comprehensive support services. Early use of amplification likely to help if part of an intensive training program. May be cochlear implant or vibrotactile aid candidate. Requires continual appraisal of needs in regard to communication and learning mode. Part-time in regular classes as much as beneficial to student.
Unilateral hearing loss (a normal hearing ear and a permanent hearing-impaired ear)	May benefit from personal FM or sound-field FM system in classroom. CROS hearing aid may be of benefit in quiet settings. Needs favorable seating and lighting. Student is at risk for educational difficulties. Educational monitoring warranted with support services provided as soon as difficulties appear. Teacher inservice training is beneficial.

Sources: Developed by Karen L. Anderson and Noel D. Matkin, (1991)

Psychosocial Function

Relationship of Degree of Long-term Hearing Loss to Psychosocial Function

Degree of Hearing Loss (PTA (500–4000 Hz)	**Possible Psychosocial Impact of Hearing Loss**
Normal hearing (–10 to +15 dB HL)	May be unaware of subtle conversational cues which could cause child to be viewed as inappropriate or awkward.
Miminal hearing loss (16 to 25 dB HL)	May miss portions of fast-paced peer interactions which could have an impact on socialization and self-concept. May have immature behavior. Child may be more fatigued than classmates due to listening effort needed.
Mild hearing loss (26 to 40 dB HL)	Barriers beginning to build with negative impact on self-esteem as child is accused of "hearing when he or she wants to," "daydreaming," or "not paying attention." Child begins to lose ability for selective hearing and has increasing difficulty suppressing background noise which makes the learning environment stressful. Child is more fatigued than classmates due to listening effort needed.
Moderate hearing loss (41 to 55 dB HL)	Often with this degree of hearing loss, communication is significantly affected, and socialization with peers with normal hearing becomes increasingly difficult. With full-time use of hearing aids/FM systems child may be judged as a less competent learner. There is an increasing impact on self-esteem.
Moderate-to-severe hearing loss (56 to 70 dB HL)	Full-time use of hearing aids/FM systems may result in child being judged by both peers and adults as a less competent learner, resulting in poorer self-concept, social maturity, and contributing to a sense of rejection. Inservice training to address these attitudes may be helpful.
Severe hearing loss (71 to 90 dB HL)	Child may prefer other children with hearing impairments as friends and playmates. This may further isolate the child from the mainstream; however, these peer relationships may foster improved self-concept and a sense of cultural identity.
Profound hearing loss (≥91 dB HL)	Depending on auditory/oral competence, peer use of sign language, parental attitude, and so on, child may or may not increasingly prefer association with the deaf culture.
Unilateral hearing loss (a normal hearing and permanently hearing-impaired ear)	Child may be accused of selective hearing due to discrepancies in speech understanding in quiet versus noise. Child will be more fatigued in classroom setting due to greater effort needed to listen. May appear inattentive or frustrated. Behavior problems sometimes evident.

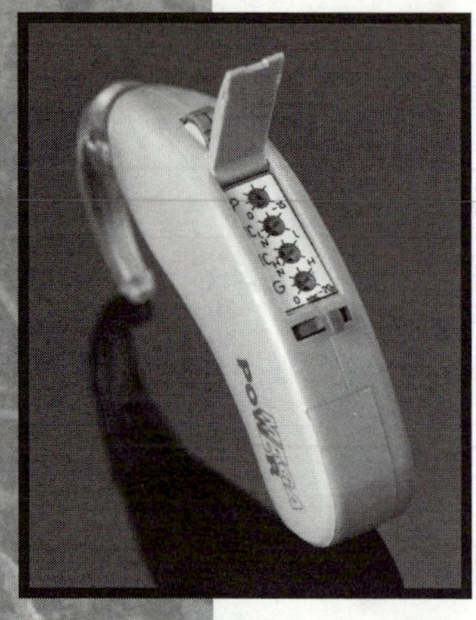

How Does 78dB Gain Sound?

The Answer Is Profoundly Clear.

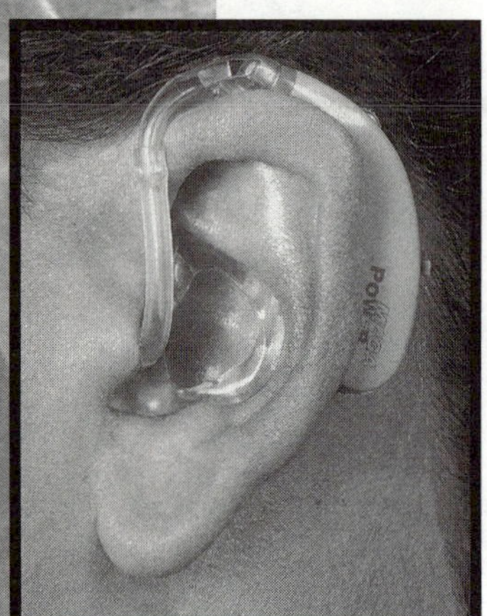

The Mega Power is your advantage for fitting severe to profound hearing losses. Loaded with an amazing 78dB full on gain, maximum 137dB SSPL90 and Class B output compression, this compact unit provides powerful, yet undistorted and clear amplification.

The four adjustable trimmers (power, high & low frequency and gain control) and optional audio input offer additional acoustic flexibility.

RESPONSE CURVE AT REFERENCE TEST GAIN*

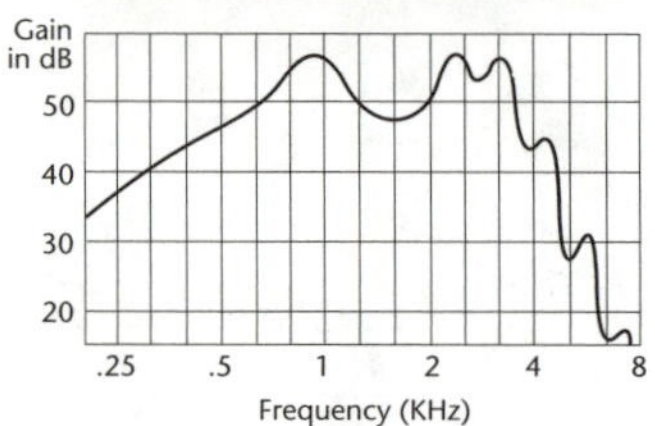

**Volume control set at reference test gain 60dB SPL input.*

ISO PENDING

Other fine Interton models available:

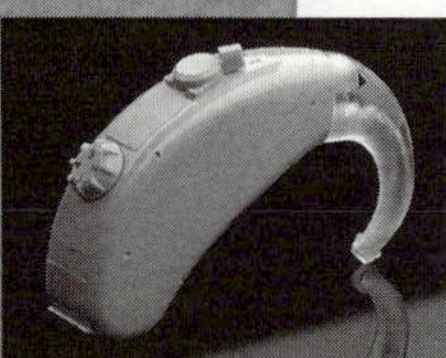
Futura M Series

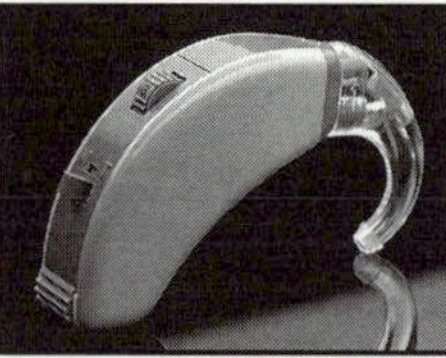
Integra

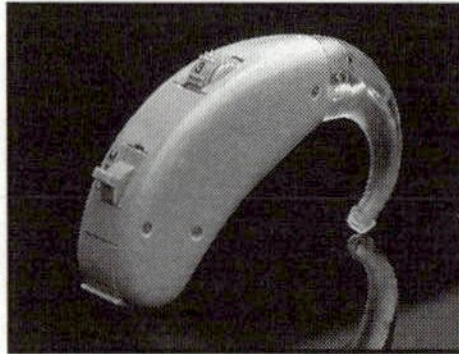
Supra Series

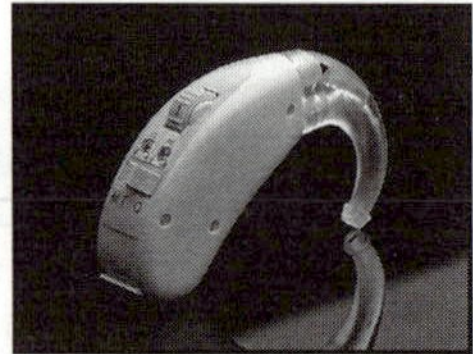
Suprema Series

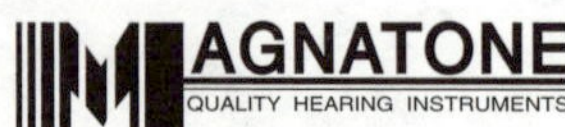

P.O. BOX 180964 • CASSELBERRY, FL 32718-0964 U.S.A.
(800) 327-5159 • (407) 339-2422

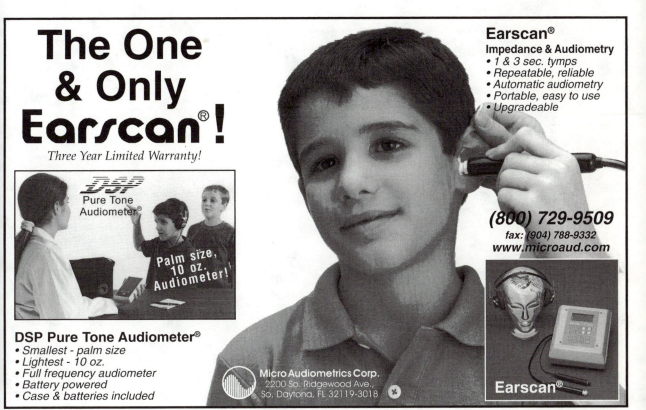

The One
& Only
Earscan®!
Three Year Limited Warranty!
DSP
Pure Tone
Audiometer®
Palm size,
10 oz.
Audiometer!
DSP Pure Tone Audiometer®
• Smallest - palm size
• Lightest - 10 oz.
• Full frequency audiometer
• Battery powered
• Case & batteries included
Earscan®
Impedance & Audiometry
• 1 & 3 sec. tymps
• Repeatable, reliable
• Automatic audiometry
• Portable, easy to use
• Upgradeable
(800) 729-9509
fax: (904) 788-9332
www.microaud.com
Earscan®
Micro Audiometrics Corp.
2200 So. Ridgewood Ave.,
So. Daytona, FL 32119-3018

CHAPTER 10

Infant Hearing Screening

In This ADR Chapter

Perspective

Early identification of hearing impairment is the best strategy for maximizing the benefits of intervention for hearing impairment for persons of all ages, but especially infants and young children. The rationale for this statement is well-appreciated by audiologists. The first 4 to 5 years of life are most important for the development of speech and language skills. Delaying appropriate intervention for hearing impairment in this time period has a more profound and long-term effect than a delay at a later age. For this reason, the information herein is heavily weighted toward hearing screening of infants. Of course, early identification of hearing impairment at any age is the goal of any audiologist.

Since the earliest attempts at infant hearing screening more than 30 years ago by Marion Downs, the "mother of infant hearing screening," there have been remarkable technological advances in hearing screening strategies. Infant hearing screening is conducted in hundreds of hospitals in the United States and around the world. Audiologists at over 150 hospitals in the U.S. have implemented universal newborn hearing screening programs.

Do we have optimal techniques for infant hearing screening? Probably not yet. Should we defer our efforts at early identification of infant hearing loss until someone confirms unquestionably high test performance for a technique? Absolutely not. We must do the best we can with existing techniques, which aren't all that bad, while simultaneously refining them or searching for even better techniques.

FOUNDATIONS OF INFANT HEARING SCREENING

Prevalence of Infant Hearing Loss

Estimated Number of Infants with Hearing Loss in the At-risk versus Healthy Populations Born in the United States Each Year.

Category	Number Born Annually	Prevalence	Total Number of Hearing Impaired
Healthy	3,600,000	3:1000	10,800
At-risk	400,000	30:1000	12,000
Total	4,000,000	5.7:1000	22,800

Source: Northern JL, Hayes, D. Universal screening for infant hearing impairment: Necessary, beneficial and justifiable. *Audiology Today 6:* 1994.

Neo-Classic Quote

Joint Committee on Infant Hearing Rationale for Infant Hearing Screening

"The prevalence of newborn and infant hearing loss is estimated to range from 1.5 to 6.0 per 1000 live births. Risk factor screening identifies only 50% of infants with significant hearing loss. Failure to identify the remaining 50% of children with hearing loss results in diagnosis and intervention at an unacceptably late age."

This 1994 Position Statement:

1. Endorses the goal of universal detection of infants with hearing loss and encourages continuing research and development to improve techniques for detection and intervention of hearing loss as early as possible;
2. Maintains a role for the high-risk factors (hereafter termed indicators) described in the 1990 Position Statement, and modifies the list of indicators associated with sensorineural and/or conductive hearing loss in newborns and infants;
3. Identifies indicators associated with late-onset hearing loss and recommends procedures to monitor infants with these indicators;
4. Recognizes the adverse effects of fluctuating conductive hearing loss from persistent or recurrent otitis media with effusion (OME) and recommends monitoring infants with OME for hearing loss;

5. Endorses provision of intervention services in accordance with Part H of the Individuals with Disabilities Education Act (IDEA); and
6. Identifies additional considerations necessary to enhance early identification of infants with hearing loss." (p. 6)

Source: Joint Committee on Infant Hearing. 1994 Position Statement. *Audiology Today 6*: 6–9, 1994.

Neo-Classic Quote

NIH Consensus Development Conference on Early Identification of Hearing Impairment Panel on Rationale for Infant Hearing Screening

"There is a clear need in the United States for improved methods and models for the early detection of hearing impairment in infants and young children. Approximately 1 of every 1000 children is born deaf. Many more are born with less severe degrees of hearing impairment, while others develop hearing impairment during childhood. Reduced hearing acuity during infancy and early childhood interferes with the development of speech and verbal language skills. Although less well documented, significantly reduced auditory input also adversely affects the developing auditory nervous system and can have harmful effects on social, emotional, cognitive, and academic potential. Moreover, delayed identification and management of severe to profound hearing impairment may impede the child's ability to adapt to life in a hearing world or in the deaf community.

"The most important period for language and speech development is generally regarded as the first 3 years of life and, although there are several methods of identifying hearing impairment during the first year, the average age of identification in the United States remains close to 3 years. Lesser degrees of hearing loss may go undetected even longer. The result is that for many hearing-impaired infants and young children, much of the crucial period for language and speech learning is lost. There is general agreement that hearing impairment should be recognized as early in life as possible, so that the remediation process can take full advantage of the plasticity of the developing sensory systems and so that the child can enjoy normal social development." (p. 3)

Source: NIH Consensus Statement (Volume 11, Number 1, March 1–3, 1993). "Early Identification of Hearing Impairment in Infants and Young Children."
Available from: Office of Medical Applications of Research, National Institutes of Health, Federal Building, Room 618, Bethesda, MD 20892 (TEL: (800) 644-6627)

Summary of Cochlear Development

Developmental Event	Time of Emergence (weeks after conception)
Hair cell differentiation	?
Afferent 8th nerve fibers in cochlear epithelium	10
Inner hair cells histologically distinguished	10 to 12
Outer hair cells histologically distinguished	12 +
Synapses between hair cells and afferent 8th nerve fibers	11 to 12
Development of stereocilia on inner hair cells	12
Development of stereocilia on outer hair cells	12+
Efferent 8th nerve fiber endings below inner hair cells	14
Maturation of inner hair cell—8th nerve synapse	15
Onset of hearing function by structural criteria	20
Efferent synapses with outer hair cells	22
Maturation of outer hair cell—8th nerve synapse	22
Stereocilia maturation (inner and outer hair cells)	22
Outer hair cells and related structures appear mature	30
Normal (mature) auditory sensitivity and frequency resolution	?

Source: Adapted from Pujol R, Lavigne-Rebillard, M. Development of neurosensory structures in the human cochlea. *Acta Otolaryngologica (Stockh) 112*: 259–264, 1992.

Rationale for Hearing Screening Techniques

- ☐ "Hearing loss of 30 dB HL and greater in the frequency region important for speech recognition will interfere with the normal development of speech and language.
- ☐ Techniques used to assess hearing of infants must be capable of detecting hearing loss of this degree in infants by age three months and younger.
- ☐ Of the various approaches to newborn hearing assessment currently available, two physiologic measures . . . Auditory brainstem response (ABR) and otoacoustic emissions (OAE) . . . Show good promise for achieving this goal."

Source: Joint Committee on Infant Hearing. 1994 Position Statement. *Audiology Today 6:* 8.

Effect of Early Identification of Hearing Loss on Development

- ☐ Children identified [with hearing loss] between birth and 6 months of age with immediate intervention (e.g., amplification, family-centered programs) have significantly higher developmental function than those with delayed identification in:
  - ✔ expressive language
  - ✔ expressive vocabulary
  - ✔ receptive vocabulary
  - ✔ communicative gestures
  - ✔ comprehension
  - ✔ number of consonants and vowels

Source: Yoshinaga-Itano, C. University of Colorado. Research study funded by NIH.

Economics of Hearing Impairment

The Cost of Delayed Identification/Intervention of Hearing Loss

- ☐ The estimated cost associated with deafness from birth to adulthood (education, medical/audiologic expenses, special living expenses) is approximately $900,000.
- ☐ Annual earnings for manually communicating persons with deafness are 30% less than the general population.
- ☐ Children with deafness from birth earn, as adults, 5% less than those with onset of deafness after 3 to 6 years of normal hearing.
- ☐ The rate of unemployment is twice as great for high school graduates who are deaf as those who are normal hearing.
- ☐ Profound deafness produces an estimated annual loss of income of approximately $2.5 billion in the United States.

Source: Downs, MP. *Seminars in Hearing 15*: 1994.

Classic and Pseudo-Classic Quotes

Economic Impact of the Early Identification of Hearing Impairment

"Remember that time is money."

Benjamin Franklin
Philadelphia, PA
Advice to a Young Tradesman (1748)

"It is inescapable to conclude that language is money."

Marion Downs
Denver, CO
"The Case for Detection and Intervention of Hearing Impairment at Birth."
Seminars in Hearing 15: 1994

"Don't forget . . . hearing is money too."

Jay Hall
Franklin, TN
Advice to Anyone Who Will Listen (1995)

Effects of Hearing Impairment in Infancy

- ☐ "Reduced hearing acuity during infancy and early childhood interferes with the development of speech and verbal language skills. Although less well documented, significantly reduced auditory input also adversely affects the developing auditory nervous system and can have harmful effects on social, emotional, cognitive, and academic development, as well as on a person's vocational and economic potential.
- ☐ "The most important period for language and speech development is generally regarded as the first 3 years of life . . . . The average age of identification in the United States remains close to 3 years. The result is that, for many hearing-impaired infants and young children, much of the crucial period for language and speech learning is lost.
- ☐ "There is general agreement that hearing impairment should be recognized as early in life as possible, so the remediation process can take full advantage of the plasticity of the developing sensory system and so that the child can enjoy normal social development."

Source: National Institutes of Health Consensus Statement. "Early Identification of Hearing Impairment in Infants and Young Children," March 1–3, 1993.

Rationale for Universal Hearing Screening

- ☐ "The prevalence of newborn and infant hearing loss is estimated to range from 1.5 to 6.0 per 1000 live births.
- ☐ Risk factor screening identifies only 50% of infants with significant hearing loss.
- ☐ Failure to identify the remaining 50% of children with hearing loss results in diagnosis and intervention at any acceptable late age."

Source: Joint Committee on Infant Hearing. 1994 Position Statement.

Apgar Scores

The Apgar score is a rating of the vital signs of newborn infants calculated at 1 minute and 5 minutes after delivery. Virginia Apgar introduced the general scoring system in the early 1950s. A neonate with an Apgar score of 4 to 6 usually requires resuscitation, whereas scores of 0 to 3 reflect acute distress.

	Scores		
Sign	**0**	**1**	**2**
Appearance	Blue or pale	Blue extremities	Pink
Pulse	Absent	Less than 100/min	More than 100/min
Grimace	No response	Grimace	Cough or sneeze
Activity	Limp	Some flexion	Active
Respiration	Absent	Slow, irregular	Good, crying

Criteria for Newborn Screening

Summary of Six General Criteria for Newborn Screening and Their Application to Hearing Screening

	General Criteria	Applied to Hearing Screening
Importance	To warrant screening, a disorder must be serious.	Hearing impairment can cause significant and long-term speech and language deficits.
Prevalence	Screening is efficient only if the disorder is sufficiently prevalent.	Hearing impairment is found in approximately 4–5% of at-risk infants.
(Diagnosis	The disorder can be diagnosed on the basis of clinically established signs and symptoms.	The signs of symptoms of newborn otologic pathology and auditory deficits are well defined and can be evaluated clinically.
Treatment resources	Effective therapies for treatment of the disorder must be available.	Medical, surgical, and audiologic management for auditory impairment is available in most medical and many educational institutions.
Responsiveness to treatment	The disorder responds to appropriate therapy, and its effects on the infant are thereby reduced or eliminated.	Some otologic pathologies are cured with medical or surgical therapies; amplification and education contribute to improved communication skills.
Advantages of early identification	Screening for a disorder in newborns is warranted only if there is an advantage to early intervention.	Speech and language deficits are associated with hearing impairment with the first months of life; delay in identification and intervention usually leads to irreversible loss of communicative potential.

Source: Ruth RA, Dey-Sigman S, Mills JA. Neonatal ABR hearing screening. *The Hearing Journal, 40*: 1985, p. 39.

1994 JCIH Indicators for Sensorineural Hearing Loss

Birth through 28 days (neonate)

1. Family history of congenital or delayed onset childhood hereditary sensorineural hearing loss
2. Congenital infection, such as toxoplasmosis, syphilis, rubella, cytomegalovirus, and herpes
3. Craniofacial anomalies including abnormalities of the pinna and ear canal, absent philtrum, and low hairline
4. Birth weight less than 1,500 grams (3.3 lbs.)
5. Hyperbilirubinemia at level requiring exchange transfusion
6. Ototoxic medications including but not limited to the aminoglycosides (e.g., gentamicin, tobramycin, kanamycin, streptomycin) used in multiple courses or in combination with loop diuretics
7. Bacterial meningitis
8. Apgar scores of 0 to 4 at 1 minute or 0 to 6 at 5 minutes
9. Mechanical ventilation lasting 5 days or longer
10. Stigmata or other findings associated with a syndrome known to include sensorineural and/or a conductive hearing loss (e.g., Waardenburg or Usher's Syndrome)

Age 29 days through 2 years (infant)

1. Parent/caregiver concern regarding hearing, speech, language, and/or developmental delay
2. Bacterial meningitis and other infections associated with sensorineural hearing loss
3. Head trauma associated with loss of consciousness or skull fracture
4. Stigmata or other findings associated with a syndrome known to include sensorineural and/or a conductive hearing loss
5. Ototoxic medications including but not limited to chemotherapeutic agents or aminoglycosides used in multiple courses or in combination with loop diuretics
6. Recurrent or persistent otitis media with effusion for at least 3 months
7. Childhood infectious diseases known to be associated with sensorineural hearing loss (e.g., mumps, measles)

Neo-Classic Quotes

NIH Consensus Development Conference on Early Identification of Hearing Impairment Panel on Techniques for Infant Hearing Screening

- ☐ High-risk criteria: (Joint Committee on Infant Hearing, 1994) ". . . . which identify approximately 9 percent of newborns, encompass half of the children who are subsequently found to have hearing impairment . . . The principal disadvantage is that 50 percent of newborns with congenital hearing deficits are not in the high-risk criteria group." (p. 11)
- ☐ Auditory brainstem response: "Can be used to screen for hearing impairment in newborns, since ABRs do not require a voluntary response and can be done without selection. This screening test is highly sensitive; nearly all children born with significant congenital hearing deficits could be detected in the newborn nursery using ABR and can be referred for further evaluation . . . Newer automated ABR technology and innovative analysis schemes may diminish costs." (pp. 11 and 12)
- ☐ Evoked otoacoustic emissions (EOAE): "Represent a newer type of newborn screening method that offers potential additional benefits. Like the ABR, this technique could be applied to all newborns prior to hospital discharge . . . The sensitivity of EOAE in the detection of congenital hearing impairment is very high, but newborn EOAE testing tends to have more false-positives when compared to ABR, especially during the first 48 hours of life . . . Over-referral may be a major problem." (p. 12)

Source: NIH Consensus Statement (Volume 11, Number 1, March 1–3, 1993). "Early Identification of Hearing Impairment in Infants and Young Children."
Available from: Office of Medical Applications of Research, National Institutes of Health, Federal Building, Room 618, Bethesda, MD 20892 (TEL: (800) 644-6627)

Testing Neonates

Factors Influencing the Effect of Sound on Auditory and General Physiologic Function

- ☐ Intensity level of sound in the nursery
- ☐ Duration of sound exposure in the nursery
- ☐ Maturity of the infant, and the infant's auditory system
- ☐ Health of the infant
  - ✓ asphyxia?
  - ✓ hyperbilirubinemia?
  - ✓ infections?
- ☐ Ototoxic medications
  - ✓ blood levels
  - ✓ duration
  - ✓ synergistic effects
  - ✓ renal status

Recommendations for Caregivers in the Nursery

Minimizing Adverse Effects of Sound on Neonates

- ☐ Regularly monitor and document sound, noise, and vibration in the intensive care unit
- ☐ Assess or screen hearing of preterm infants and other infants at risk for hearing impairment before discharge
- ☐ Establish guidelines for ICU sound levels
- ☐ Carefully evaluate any sound attenuation devices for direct use on infants, including assessment of benefit and potential harm. Utilize devices that contribute to sound attenuation with no unwanted effects
- ☐ Educate ICU personnel, and the parents of infants, on noise reduction

ABR IN INFANT HEARING SCREENING

Characteristics of the ABR

Anatomic generators, electrode sites for detection of the response, components of an evoked response system, and an example of an ABR waveform. Typical absolute and interwave latency values are displayed for major ABR components (recorded with a high stimulus intensity level from a person at least 18 months or older in age). See Chapter 7 for more information on the ABR.

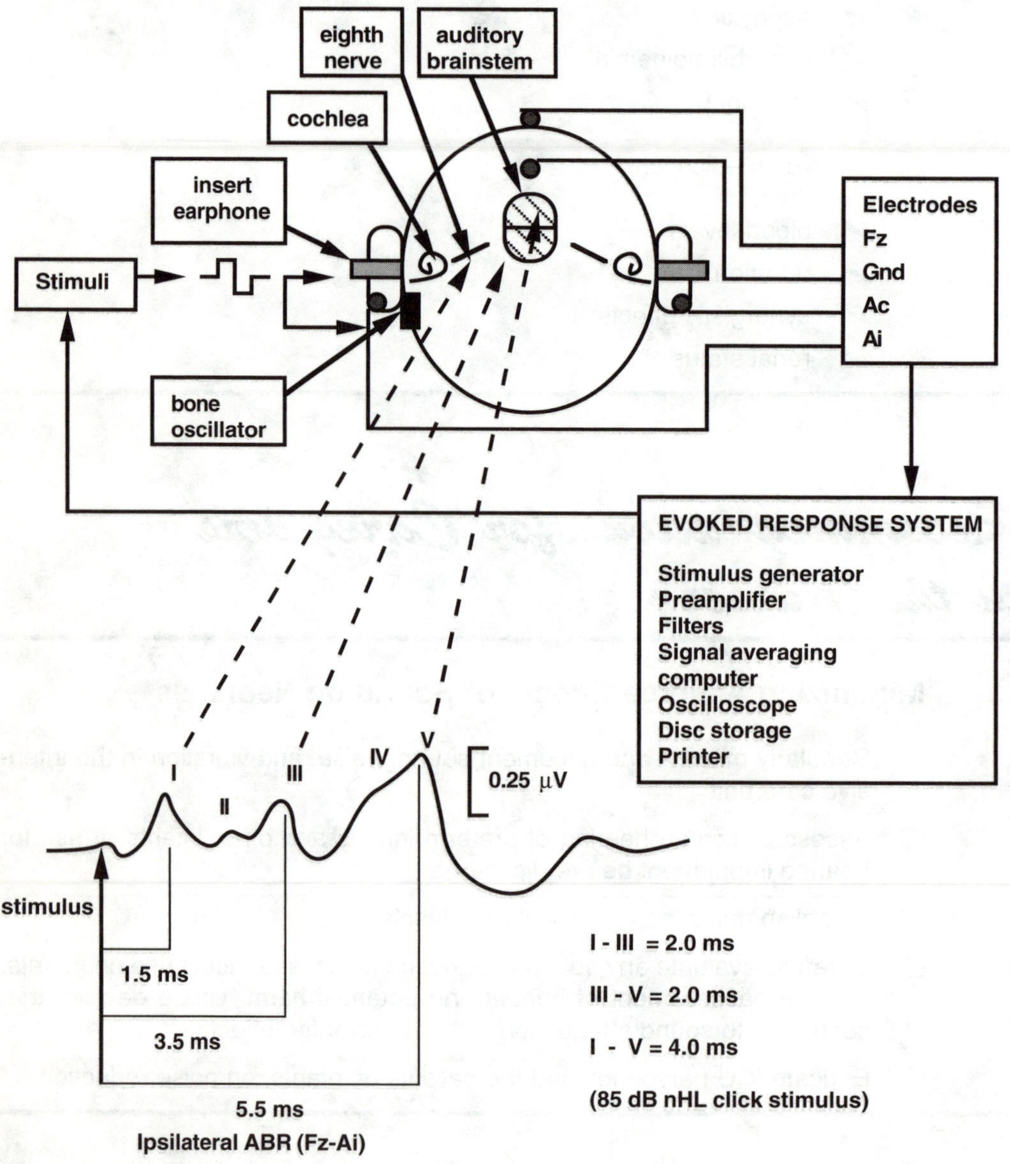

Protocol

Auditory Brainstem Response (ABR) Measurement Parameters for Newborn Auditory Screening Used at the Vanderbilt University Clinics.

	Screening Equipment	
Parameter	**Conventional ABR system**	**Automated ABR (ALGO-1 or -2)**
Stimulus		
transducer	infant Tubephone	special design
type	click	filtered click
duration	0.1 msec	0.1 msec
rate	37.1/sec	37/sec
polarity	rarefaction	alternating
intensity	35 dB HL	35 dB HL
ear	monaural, each	monaural, each
Acquisition		
gain	×100,000	?
artifact reject		
electrical	maybe	yes
myogenic	usually	yes
acoustic	yes	yes
analysis time	15 msec	20 msec
filter settings		
high pass	30 Hz	50 Hz
low pass	1500 Hz	1400 Hz
60 Hz notch	no	yes
number of sweeps	variable*	500 to 15,000
electrode array (s)		
Channel 1		
inverting	Fz	Fz
noninverting	nape	nape
Channel 2**		
inverting	Fz	—
noninverting	(Ai) ipsi earlobe	—
Channel 3**		
inverting	Ac (contra earlobe)	—
noninverting	Ai	—
ground	Fpz	cheek

*Number of sweeps necessary is defined by signal to noise (ratio), and may range from several hundred to 4000 or more

**The second and third channels are optional; one may be used without the other

ABR Interpretation in Newborn Hearing Screening

Two general strategies for analysis of auditory brainstem response (ABR) in neonatal hearing screening. In the top portion of the figure, a "pass" outcome is indicated if there is any reliably recorded wave component, whereas the absence of a response is interpreted as a "fail" outcome. Latency is not analyzed with this strategy. The lower portion of the figure illustrates an analysis strategy that takes into account ABR wave V latency. If a reliable wave V is recorded with a latency within age-corrected normal limits (e.g., normative ABR latency data for 38 week gestational age infants, in this case), the screening outcome is a "pass." If an ABR is present, but the wave V latency value exceeds age-corrected normal limits (or if there's no response of course), the outcome is a "fail."

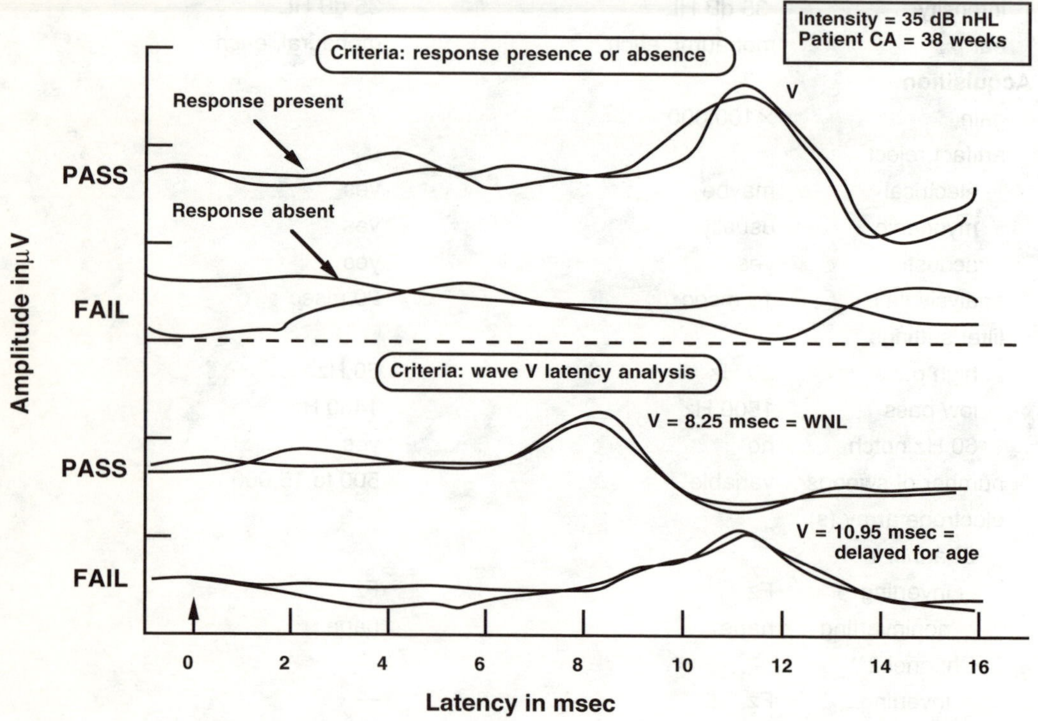

Problems and Solutions

Infant Hearing Screening with ABR*

Problem	Solution
☐ Prematurity	✓ Defer hearing screening until about 40 weeks postconceptional age.
☐ Transient, minor, middle-ear dysfunction	✓ Otologic management ✓ Immittance measurement ✓ Bone-conduction stimulation (in follow up diagnostic ABR assessment)
☐ Neurologic disease involving auditory CNS	✓ Analyze wave I only ✓ Perform otoacoustic emissions screening
☐ Imprecise earphone placement	✓ Insert transducer
☐ Collapsing ear canal	✓ Insert transducer
☐ Inappropriate stimulus rate	✓ Rate consistent with normative data rate
☐ Excessive ambient noise	✓ Insert transducer ✓ Attempt to reduce noise (see other LIST in this ADR chapter) ✓ Test in sound booth (not practical usually)
☐ Excessive movement artifact	✓ Pause or abort recording and wait it out ✓ Increase the number of sweeps averaged ✓ Return to test again after the infant has been fed and is happy
☐ Poor signal to noise ratio (SNR)	✓ Extend averaging to > sweeps to reduce noise ✓ Reduce movement artifact (see above)
☐ Small wave V amplitude	✓ Extend the high-pass filter to 30 Hz ✓ Use a noncephalic "reference" electrode (e.g., nape of neck)
☐ Poor waveform morphology, especially for wave I	✓ Slow the stimulus rate ✓ Rule out neurologic dysfunction by chart review ✓ Increase the number of sweeps ✓ Is the infant premature?

*For most ABR systems; some automated ABR infant hearing screening devices (e.g., the ALGO-1 and ALGO-2) incorporate these or other strategies for solving screening problems.

Step-by-Step

Flowchart illustrating the sequence of steps involved in newborn hearing screening of infants at risk for hearing impairment, according to the Joint Committee on Infant Hearing (JCIH), and screened with an automated auditory brainstem response (ABR) technique. A full listing of the JCIH risk indicators can be found in this ADR chapter.

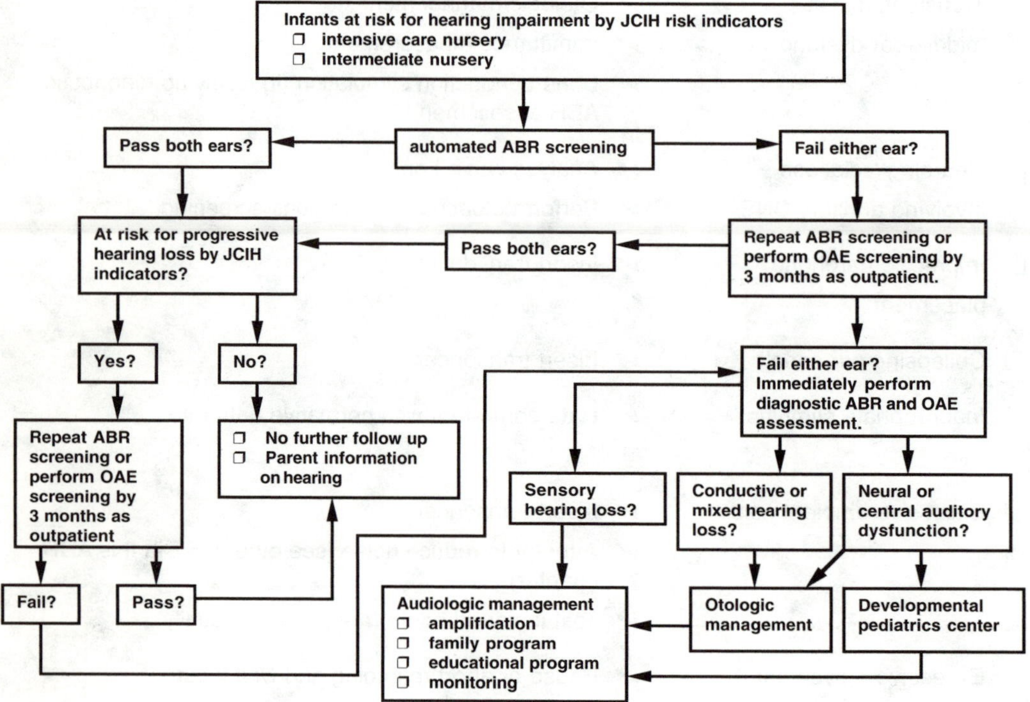

Newborn Hearing Screening

Chart Review Form

Form used for reviewing infant medical charts to determine risk status for hearing impairment at the Vanderbilt University Medical Center. Risk indicators are recommended by the 1994 Joint Committee on Infant Hearing (JCIH). Chart review is performed by either an audiologist or a resident in the Department of Pediatrics.

MC 0003 (1/95)

HEARING RISK CRITERIA CHART REVIEW RECORD

Vanderbilt University Hospital

NEWBORN AUDITORY SCREENING PROGRAM

Name: ____________________ (LAST) , ____________________ (FIRST) Sex: ______ VUH #: __________

DOB: __________ Transported From: L&D / Other: ____________________

Mother / Father Name: ____________________ Telephone #: (_____) __________

Address: ____________________

City: ____________________ State: __________ Zip: __________

Gestational Age: _____ weeks Chart Reviewer ____________________ Date __________

Pediatrician: ____________________ City: __________

RISK INDICATORS	Y	N
1. Low Birth Weight (<1500 grams): Specify		
2. APGAR Scores: 0-4 at 1 min, 0-6 at 5 min Specify: _____ 1 _____ 5 _____ 10		
3. Ototoxic Medications ≥ 5 days (e.g. aminoglycosides, loop diuretics) Specify: __________ (date _____) Recheck: __________ (date _____)		
4. Mechanical Ventilation ≥ 5 days Specify: __________ (date _____) Recheck: __________ (date _____)		
5. Congenital Perinatal Infection: Toxoplasmosis, Other (syphillis, HIV), Rubella, CMV, Herpes		
6. Craniofacial / Syndromal Abnormalities: ____ external ear abnormalities, ____ cleft palate/lip, ____ skull abnormalities, ____ underdeveloped maxillae or mandible, ____ short neck, ____ dwarfism, ____ skeletal and cranial defects, ____ absent clavicles		
7. Bacterial Meningitis		
8. Family History of hereditary childhood SNHL		
9. Hyperbilirubinemia (requiring exchange transfusion) BW — Bili Level 1000-1250 — 10.0 1251-1500 — 13.0 1501-2000 — 15.0 2001-2500 — 17.0 >2500 — 18.0		
10. Syndrome Associated with Hearing Loss (Conductive and/or Sensorineural)		
11. Other (Maternal substance abuse, fetal alcohol syndrome, at risk twin, etc.):		

ALGO: Right ear LR: _____ SWPS: _____ PASS / REFER **OAE:** PASS / REFER
Left ear LR: _____ SWPS: _____ PASS / REFER **OAE:** PASS / REFER

Audiologist: ____________________ Date: __________

Reporting Screening Results

Form used for reporting the results of infant hearing screening with an automated auditory brainstem response (ABR) technique at the Vanderbilt University Medical Center.

MC 0006 (7/91)

NEWBORN AUDITORY SCREENING REPORT

AUDIOLOGY SERVICE/OTOLARYNGOLOGY

The Vanderbilt Clinic

Room 1501
Nashville, TN 37232-5555
(615) 322-6180

Date of screening: ____________________

Name: ______________________________, ______________________________ Sex: __________

Birthdate: __________________ Gestational age: __________________ VUH #: __________

Referring Physician: ____

POTENTIAL RISK FACTOR (S):

_____ Family history of hearing loss
_____ Congenital perinatal infection
_____ Head/neck deformity
_____ Birth weight less than 1500 grams
_____ Hyperbilirubinemia
_____ Bacterial meningitis
_____ Asphyxia
_____ Mechanical Ventilation
_____ Ototoxic medications
_____ Syndrome
_____ Physician order

SCREENING PROTOCOL:

Test: auditory brainstem response (ABR)

Equipment: _____ ALGO-1 _____ Bio-Logic Traveler

Stimulus parameters: type: click rate: 37/.sec;
intensity: 35 dB nHL mode: monaural

Test site: _____ ICU _____ Intermediate Nursery
_____ Normal Nursery _____ Audiology facility

SCREENING RESULTS:

_____ Pass: peripheral hearing sensitivity is within or near normal limits bilaterally in the 1000 to 4000 Hz region

_____ Refer: _____ right ear fail _____ left ear fail

_____ Incomplete: _____ right _____ left

RECOMMENDATIONS:

_____ No further testing is required at this time. Retest only if a change in hearing is suspected.
_____ Follow up audiologic testing in 3 months. Did not pass auditory screening.
_____ Follow up audiologic testing in 3 months. At risk for progressive hearing loss ______________.
_____ Follow up audiologic testing in 6 months. At risk for progressive hearing loss (ototoxic meds).

Audiologist: ______________________________________ Date: ________________

OAE IN INFANT HEARING SCREENING

Step-by-Step

Flowchart illustrating the sequence of steps involved in newborn hearing screening of healthy infants that are not at risk for hearing impairment (according to the Joint Committee on Infant Hearing), and screened with either an automated auditory brainstem response (ABR) or an otoacoustic emission (OAE) technique.

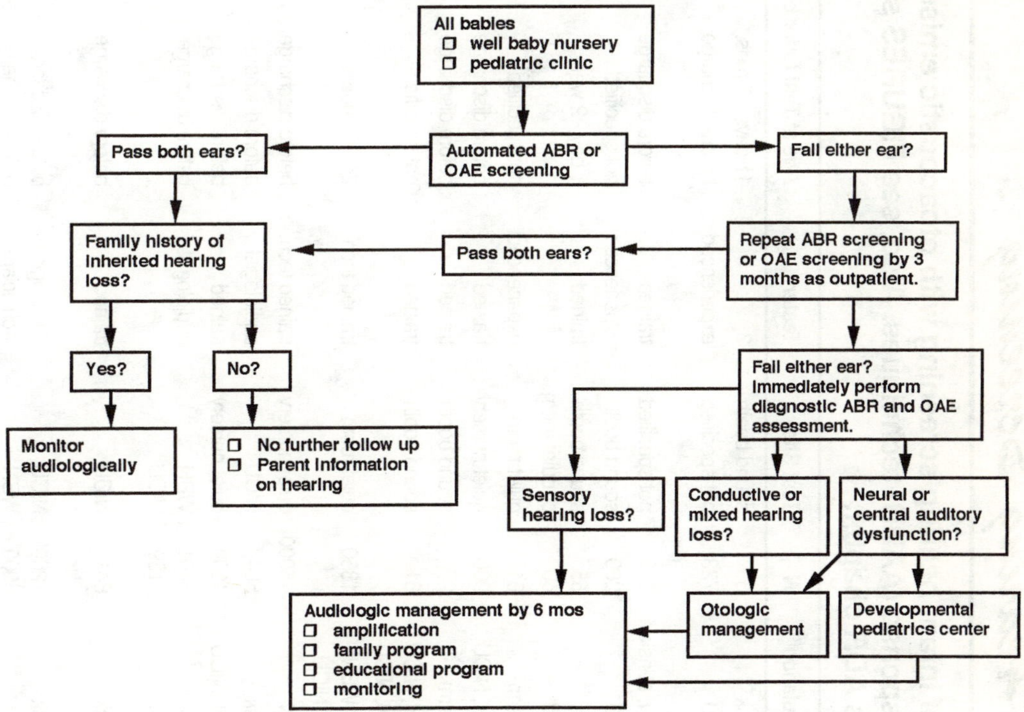

OAE in Infant Hearing Screening

Summary of studies of infant hearing screening with otoacoustic emissions (OAE) or automated auditory brainstem response (AABR) techniques. Also, see FIGURES showing failure rates for OAE and AABR in this ADR chapter.

Study, year	Technique	Population	*N*	Test Site	Tester	Age at Test (after birth)	Pass rate (%)	Fail rate (%)
Plinkert et al, 1990	TEOAE	at-risk	53	sound booth	?	11 days - 7 mos.	70%	30%
Stevens et al, 1990	TEOAE	NICU	723	not specified	experienced	before discharge	80% (inpts) 75% (outpts)	20% (inpts) 25% (outpts)
Kennedy et al, 1991	TEOAE	WBN, at-risk	370	not specified	trained	before discharge	97%**	3%
Webb & Stevens, 1991	TEOAE	NICU*	260	sound booth	experienced	not specified	84%	16%
Uziel and Piron, 1991	TEOAE	WBN NICU	55 40	sound booth or quiet room	trained	1 day - 2 weeks	97% (WBN) 79% (NICU)	3% 21%
Bonfils et al, 1992	TEOAE	preterm	61	quiet room	experienced	not specified	93%	7%
Giebel, 1992	TEOAE	WBN, NICU	900	quiet nursery	trained	before discharge	83%	17%
Bonfils et al, 1992	DPOAE	full term	27	sound booth	trained	before discharge	85%	15% (CNT crying)
Smurzynski et al, 1993	TEOAE DPOAE	WBN, NICU WBN, NICU	61	sound booth	trained	not specified	74%	26% (+7% with middle ear dis.)
White et al, 1993	TEOAE	84% WBN* 16% NICU	1850	quiet room	trained tech.	24 - 60 hours	73%	27
Vohr et al, 1993	TEOAE	WBN	>6000	quiet nursery	trained tech.	before discharge	96%	4%
Hall, Kileny, & Ruth, 1988	AABR*	at-risk	504	NICU	audiologist	before discharge	95%	5%
Giebel, 1992	AABR*	WBN, NICU	1000	quiet nursery	trained	before discharge	98%	2%
Covenant Medical Ctr., 1992	AABR*	WBN NICU	1491 189	WBN NICU	audiologist	before discharge	97% 97%	3% 3%
Stewart et al., 1993	AABR	at-risk	841	NICU	trained	before discharge	87%	12% (+1% CNT)
Hall, Freeman, et al., 1996	AABR**	at-risk WBN	>2000 6000	NICU WBN	audiologists technicians	before discharge before discharge	85% 98.4%	15% 1.6%

*AABR with ALGO-1 Infant Hearing Screener **AABR with ALGO-2 Infant Hearing Screener

Failure Rates

Automated ABR vs. DPOAE and TEDAE

Newborn hearing screening failure rates for transient evoked otoacoustic emissions (TEOAE) and distortion product otoacoustic emissions (DPOAE), as compared to automated auditory brainstem response (AABR) in a sample of infants in the intensive care nursery (ICN) and well baby nursery (WBN) at Vanderbilt University Medical Center, and as reported in the recent literature. All Vanderbilt data were collected in the nursery setting by licensed audiologists with experience in newborn hearing screening. The TEOAE screening procedure was as described by Kemp (1993), and was supervised by a manufacturer representative. DPOAE data in the ICN were collected with a prototype of the Grason Stadler 60 device. DPOAE data in the WBN were collected with the Virtual 330 device. All OAE data analyses were limited to the 1000 to 4000 Hz frequency region for more direct comparison with ABR findings. For enrollment in this study, all infants were required to pass an ABR screening at 35 dB nHL.

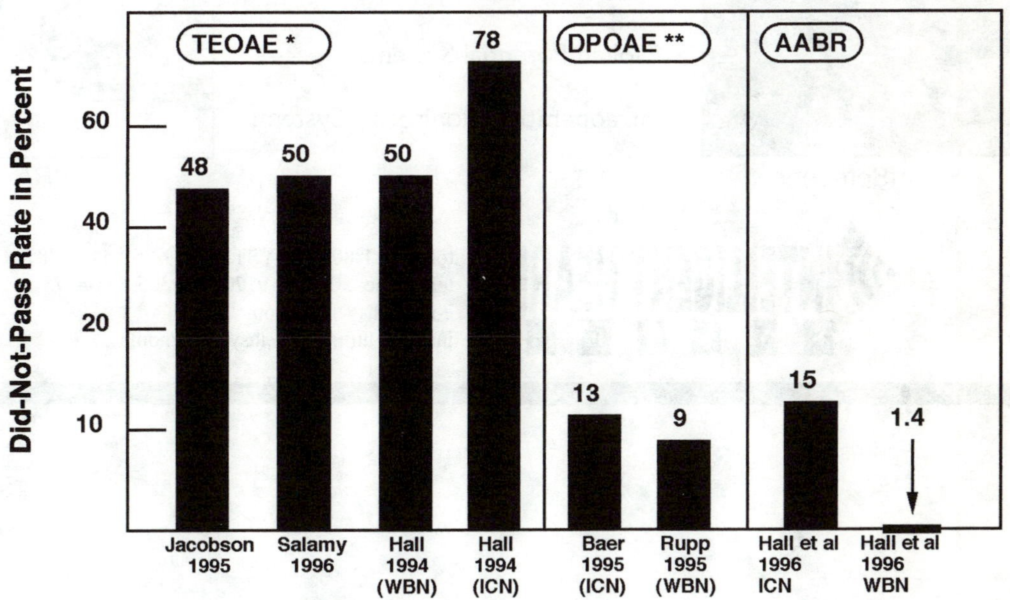

CHAPTER 11

Central Auditory Processing Disorder (CAPD)

In This ADR Chapter

Perspective

Over 40 years ago, Mylkebust (1954) pointed out that "hearing is a receptive sense . . . and essential for normal language behavior" (p. 11), and noted that "the diagnostician of auditory problems in children has traditionally emphasized peripheral damage. It is desirable that he also include considerations of central damage" (p. 54). He also explained that "central deafness [central auditory processing disorder] is a deficiency in transmitting auditory impulses to the higher brain centers while receptive aphasia [language disorder] is a deficiency in the interpretation of these impluses after they have been delivered" (p. 153). During this era, Bocca et al. (1954) reported that surgically confirmed central auditory system pathology could be detected with sufficiently sensitive audiologic procedures. These pioneering observations and studies have since been validated by many clinical investigations. There are now a variety of behavioral and electrophysiologic techniques for the assessment of peripheral and central auditory system function, including central auditory processing disorders (CAPD). The term CAPD is used to describe a deficit in the perception or complete analysis of auditory information due to central auditory nervous system dysfunction, usually at the level of the cerebral cortex (Jerger, Martin, & Jerger, 1987; Jerger et al., 1991; Keith, 1977; Musiek, 1984, 1986; Musiek et al., 1982, 1984, 1990, 1991; Pinheiro & Musiek, 1984). Central auditory processing takes place before language processing or comprehension. The evaluation and management of CAPD is within the scope of audiologic practice and is an accepted clinical activity within the field of communicative disorders (American Academy of Audiology, 1993; American Speech-Language-Hearing Association, 1990).

FOUNDATIONS OF CENTRAL AUDITORY PROCESSING DISORDER

Step-by-Step

CAPD Assessment and Management

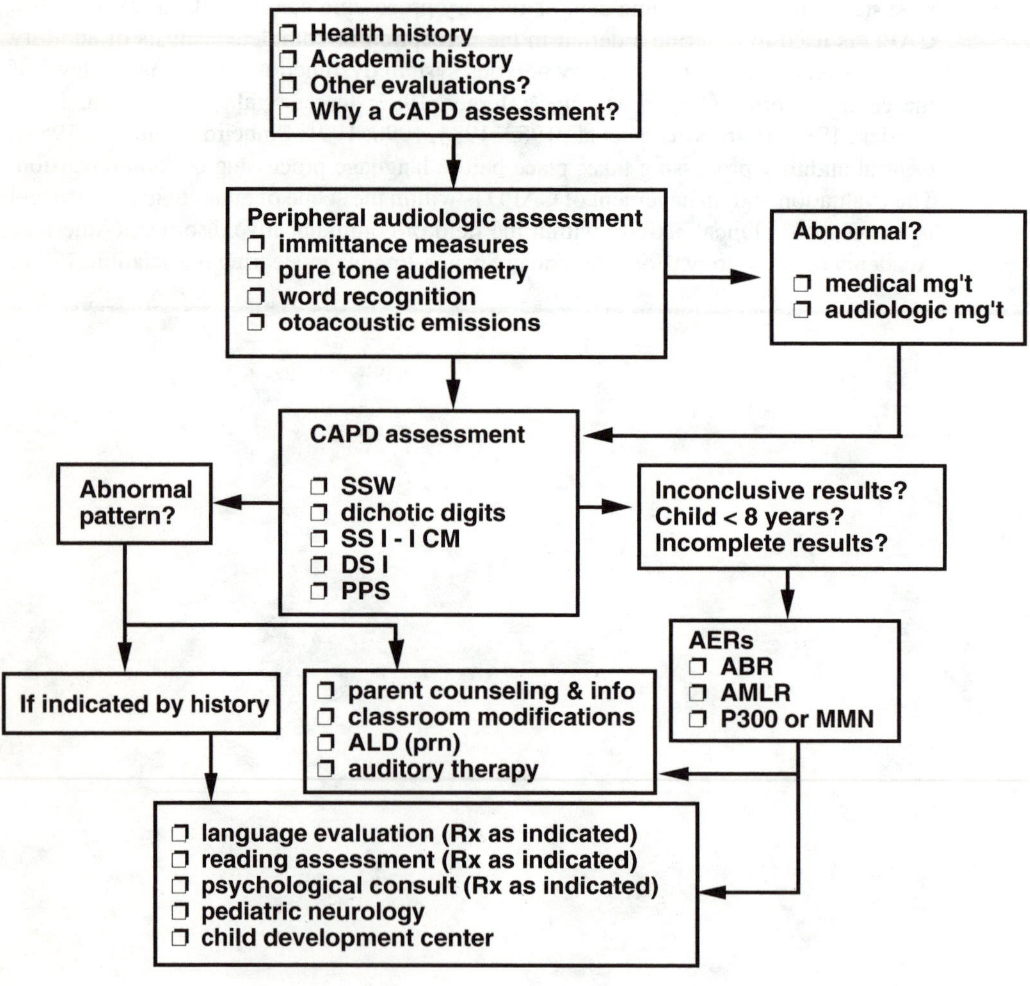

Technical Tip

The Audiologist in CAPD Assessment and Management

The first author's experience confirms that, with an appropriate battery of existing tests, it is possible for audiologists to evaluate, with diagnostic finesse, and to manage, with rehabilitative success, both peripheral *and* central auditory dysfunction. Thorough audiologic assessment of children with suspected or confirmed communication problems contributes to complete diagnosis and appropriate and effective management. Although dealings with this patient population, their parents, and professionals involved in their educational or medical management can be quite time-consuming, and sometimes frustrating, audiologists can make a real difference in the lives and future of children with CAPD.

Components of Auditory Processing

- ☐ **Auditory discrimination:** "The ability to distinguish similarities and differences in sounds." (Gillet, 1993, p. 17)
- ☐ **Auditory memory:** "Involves the ability to retain and recall material presented through the auditory channel . . . general memory refers to global, gross forms of retaining information . . . Sequential memory is involved in remembering things presented in a specified order." (Gillet, 1993, p. 35)
- ☐ **Auditory perception:** "The ability to receive and understand sounds and words . . . Auditory perception has a key role in the development of efficient reading skills, processing incoming verbal information, conceptual development, basic communication, social relationships, and in the ability to respond in an appropriate and safe manner to the environment." (Gillet, 1993, p. 51)
- ☐ **Auditory-vocal association:** "Involves the ability to draw relationships from what is heard, and then to respond verbally in a meaningful way to these spoken words." (Gillet, 1993, p. 63)
- ☐ **Auditory synthesis (closure, sound blending):** "Involves the ability to combine smoothly all the sounds or syllables of words to make them a whole, or the ability to analyze a word into its separate sounds . . . This skill, as well as auditory sequencing, is closely related to the reading and spelling process." (Gillet, 1993, p. 73)
- ☐ **Auditory-vocal automaticity:** "The ability to predict future linguistic events from past experience." (Gillet, 1993, p. 63)
- ☐ **Auditory figure-ground:** "Figure-ground relegates certain sounds into the background while selecting others as the focus of attention. An auditory figure-group problem consists of difficulty perceiving relevant auditory stimuli in the presence of background stimuli or when there is a significant change in intensity of the stimuli." (Gillet, 1993, p. 89)

Source: Gillet P. *Auditory processes.* Novato CA: Academic Therapy Publications, 1993.

Key Members of the CAPD Team

(in addition to audiology)

- ☐ Before an audiologist begins the assessment and management of children with CAPD, he or she should develop a working relationship with a variety of professionals who can provide valuable contributions to both assessment and management of this challenging patient population. Of course, the persons who fulfill these roles should have an interest in, and appreciation of, children with CAPD. Among the team members are representatives of:
  - ✔ **Speech-language pathology.** A properly credentialed person (e.g., master's degree and licensed, as required) with expertise in the evaluation and management of child language disorders is an essential member of the team.
  - ✔ **Neuropsychology.** A properly credentialed clinical neuropsychologist will provide valuable services, such as independent assessment of intelligence.
  - ✔ **Special education.** This person must have expertise in learning disabilities, including assessment and remediation of reading disorders. Special training in reading techniques designed for children with weak auditory processing skills (e.g., Lindamood Bell Learning Process) is particularly important.
  - ✔ **Pediatric neurology.** The population of children suspected of having CAPD will include some who are suspected of having neurologic disorders, including seizure disorders and developmental delay. The pediatric neurologist can evaluate these children and order appropriate diagnostic medical studies (e.g., MRI, lab tests, EEG).
  - ✔ **Otolaryngology.** Optimally, an otologist and/or a pediatric otolaryngologist is available. A substantial proportion of children undergoing CAPD assessment will have peripheral hearing loss. Middle ear disorders are especially common during the winter months. Whenever possible, peripheral auditory dysfunction should be treated medically or surgically before CAPD assessment is carried out.
  - ✔ **Child Development Center.** Children with multiple psychoeducational, communicative, and/or medical problems are often best referred to a center staffed by multiple disciplined professionals.
  - ✔ **Classroom teacher.** Implementation of recommendations for educational modifications begin and end with this important team member.
  - ✔ **Parents.** Implementation of recommendations for home management, and assurance that all recommendations for management are implemented, is usually the responsibility of the parents and other family members. They must understand what CAPD is and what can be done about it.
  - ✔ **Child advocate.** Unfortunately, parents often need the assistance of someone who can serve as an advocate for their child to ensure that an appropriate education plan is developed and carried out fully. This person, who accompanies the parents to M-team (multidisciplinary-team) meetings, may be a professional, or another parent, well-versed in state and federal educational laws, or even a lawyer.

Auditory Processing and Reading

Ways Auditory Processing Problems Can Influence Reading

☐ "Reading is a visual symbol superimposed on previously acquired auditory language. Before a child learns to read, language learning depends almost exclusively on the auditory channel . . ..The three aspects of the auditory processes that are most significant for reading are discrimination of particular phonemes within words, auditory discrimination of words, and auditory synthesis." (Gillet, 1993, p. 95)

- "inability to hear the similarities in the initial and final sounds of words
- cannot perceive the similarities in words (e.g., *fat* and *pat*)
- unable to hear the double consonant sounds in consonant blends
- lack of discrimination of short vowel sounds: *ten*, *tin*, *ton*
- cannot break words into syllables
- cannot break words into individual sounds
- inability to combine parts of words to form a whole
- cannot remember the sounds for the printed symbols or the names for the printed word
- inability to detect rhyming element of words
- difficulty in distinguishing similarities and differences in sounds
- lack of retention of sounds or syllables long enough to make matches or blends
- inability to relate the visual components of words to their auditory counterparts
- does not relate a part of a word to the whole word
- inability to synthesize or analyze unfamiliar words" (Gillet, 1993, pp. 95–96)

Source: From Gillet P. *Auditory processes.* Novato CA: Academic Therapy Publications, 1993. Reprinted with permission.

Clinical Concept

Relation of CAPD to Attention Deficit Disorder (ADD)

Diagnosed or suspected attention deficit disorder (ADD) or attention deficit hyperactivity disorder (ADHD) is often cited as a reason for referral for CAPD (Gascon, Johnson, & Burd, 1986). Parents, and even professionals, seem to be unclear as to the definition of ADHD and its possible relation to language/learning disorders, as well as CAPD. Close examination of the diagnostic criteria for ADHD (American Psychiatric Association, 1987) fails to reveal a direct link between ADHD and CAPD. Although the attention-related criteria of ADHD sometimes involve communication activities (e.g., "often does not seem to listen to what is being said"; "has difficulty following through on instructions from others"), none of the criteria specifically address auditory skills or performance. Our experience clearly suggests that ADHD/ADD and CAPD are independent and unrelated disorders. However, there appears to be a relationship among certain CAPD measures and receptive language and reading skills (Keith & Novak, 1984).

CAPD and ADD/ADHD

Characteristics that may be shared by children with CAPD and children with attention deficit hyperactivity disorder (ADHD). It appears that CAPD and ADD/ADHD are independent disorders.

- ☐ A male-to-female ratio of about 2:1
- ☐ Depressed academic performance
- ☐ "Seems not to listen" (DSM IV)
- ☐ "Easily distracted" (DSM IV)

CAPD Screening Survey History Form

NAME______________________________ AGE_____ GENDER_______

GRADE__________ DATE__________ DOB__________

ADDRESS______________________________

PARENT/GUARDIAN______________________________

BREIFLY DESCRIBE REASON FOR VISIT______________________________

____

REFERRED BY______________________________

*Circle the number that best describes your child's behavior

BEHAVIOR	**DEGREE OF PROBLEM** **1-mild to 5-severe**					
1. Inattentiveness	0	1	2	3	4	5
2. Hearing loss (in light of normal hearing)	0	1	2	3	4	5
3. Hearing in noise	0	1	2	3	4	5
4. Educational/psychological information	0	1	2	3	4	5 (x2)
5. Confuses directions	0	1	2	3	4	5
6. Reverse words, numbers, tones, etc . . .	0	1	2	3	4	5
7. General behavior	0	1	2	3	4	5
8. Asks to repeat	0	1	2	3	4	5
9. Space perception/coordination	0	1	2	3	4	5
10. Music skills	0	1	2	3	4	5
11. Art skills	0	1	2	3	4	5
12. Genetic LD factors	0	1	2	3	4	5
13. Medical findings	0	1	2	3	4	5
14. Handedness		RIGHT			LEFT	
		TOTAL SCORE				

Measures of Child Language

Procedure	Description	Reference
Mean Length of Response (MLR)	A five-stage grading system for estimating approximate language age in the 12 to 46 month age range based on the linguistic complexity of a child's utterances	Templin, 1957
Developmental Sentence Scoring (DSS)	Systematic analysis of 50 consecutive complete (subject + predicate) utterances; for each sentence, scores are given in eight grammatical categories; normative data are available in 6-month intervals for ages 2 to 7 years	Lee, 1974
Length-Complexity Index (LCI)	Analysis of utterances (responses) (e.g., counting types words and sentence components), according to specific rules; normative data not available, but results are useful in planning therapy	Shriner & Sherman, 1967
Peabody Picture Vocabulary Test—Revised (PPVT-R)	Results reported as age equivalent and standard score equivalent values; not an intelligence (cognitive) or receptive language (semantic) test; test consists of 175 plates with 4 pictures per plate (two different versions for repeat administration), with 8 plates for each year of development; normative data are available for ages 2.6 to 40 years	Choong & McMahon, 1983
Vocabular Comprehension Scale (VCS)	A vocabulary test utilizing objects (not pictures); normative data available in 6 month intervals for children aged 2 to 6 years; provides information on the child's understanding of specific pronouns etc, rather than a vocabulary age (versus PPVT for example)	Bangs, 1975
Test of Word Finding (TWF)	Assesses the accuracy and speed of word retrieval for the child's existing vocabulary; test consists of 6 sections (e.g., Picture naming nouns, sentence completion naming); standardized on children aged 6.6 to 12.11 years; reliability and validity have been demonstrated	German, 1986
Test of Adolescent/Adult Word Finding	Follow-up to TWF procedure for older children aged 12 to 19.11, or in grades 7 through 12	German, 1990

(continued)

(continued)

Procedure	Description	Reference
Berko Test of Morphology (Berry-Talbot Exploratory Test of Grammar)	Morphemes are the smallest units of meaning; test employs pictures to evaluate a child's knowledge of plurals, tense, possessives, etc; validity of the original test paradigm has been questioned (Templin, 1966)	Berko, 1958; Newfield & Shlanger, 1968
Northwestern Syntax Screening Test (NSST)	A screening procedure for receptive and expressive language skills that utilizes a variety of syntactic structures represented in increasing difficulty in a series of illustrations; child performs a picture-pointing task; normative data are available for children aged 3 to 7.11 years	Lee, 1969; Lee, 1971 Ratusnick & Koenigsknect, 1975
Carrow Elicited Language Inventory (CELI)	A sentence-repetition test using 51 sentences that vary in length from 2 to 10 words and in grammatical categories and features; assumes that, when a child can repeat an utterance, then he or she has the linguistic structures contained within the utterance within his or her repetoire; normative data are available; takes about 45 minutes to administer	Carrow, 1974
Assessment of Children's Language Comprehension (ACLC)	A four-part test of receptive language requiring about 10 minutes to administer; some parts involve a picture-pointing task; normative data are available separately for boys and girls for ages 3 to 6.5 years	Foster, Giddan, & Stark, 1973
Test for Auditory Comprehension of Language—Revised (TALC-R)	Auditory comprension is assessed with a picture-pointing task; normative data available for ages 3 to 9.11, or for children in grades kindergarden through sixth	Carrow-Woolfolk, 1985
Bankson Language Screening Test (BLST)	153 item test which includes a 38-item screening version that assesses five general areas (including auditory perception and visual perception); normative data are available for ages 4.1 to 8 years	Bankson, 1977
Illinois Test of Psycholinguistic Abilities (ITPA)	A diagnostic measure which involves decoding, encoding, and association concepts of language; ITPA has 12 distinct subtests, which include auditory measures (auditory reception, auditory association, auditory sequential memory, auditory closure, and sound blending); normative data are available for ages 2 to 10 years, and testing yields a psycholinguistic age	McCarthy & Kirk, 1961

(continued)

(continued)

Procedure	Description	Reference
Sequenced Inventory of Communication Development (SICD)	Assesses expressive and receptive language skills with a variety of subtests; normative data are available for children aged 4 to 48 months	Hedrick, Prather, & Tobin, 1975
Preschool Language Scale—3	Consists of four receptive and four expressive language tasks; normative data are available for children aged birth to 4.11 years	Zimmerman, Steiner & Pond, 1992
McCarthy Scales of Children's Abilities (MSCA)	Consists of six scales which assess, in addition to language, numerical concepts, motor abilities, cognition, and memory; normative data are available for children aged 2.5 to 8.5 years	McCarthy, 1972
Language Assessment Tasks (LAT)	A measure for description of language function of, uniquely, older children aged 9 to 14 years; sections of the test measure language expression and reception; utilizes Piaget stages of cognitive development; normative data are not available for all subtests	Kellman, Flood, & Yoder, 1977
Basic Language Concepts Test (BLCT)	Assesses language concepts children should have mastered to succeed in the second grade; normative data are available for children aged 4 to 6.5 years	Engelmann, Ross, & Bingham, 1982
Test of Language Development—Primary (TOLD-P)	Receptive and expressive language measure for children aged 4 to 9 years that assesses vocabulary, syntax, and phonology; normative data are available	Hammill & Newcomer, 1982
and		
Test of Language Development—Intermediate (TOLD-I)	Same as TOLD-P but for older children (aged 8.6 to 12.11 years)	Newcomer & Hammill, 1982
Clinical Evaluation of Language Fundamentals—Revised (CELF-R)	Consists of 11 subtests assessing receptive and expressive language; normative data are available for children aged 5.0 to 16.11 years; a common test of language function used in the public schools with children who are referred for CAPD assessment at Vanderbilt University Medical Center	Semel, Wiig, & Secord, 1987

Source: Peterson HA, Marquardt TP. *Appraisal and diagnosis of speech and language disorders.* (3rd ed). Englewood Cliffs, NJ: Prentice-Hall, 1994.

Patient Perspective

The following poem was written by a 52-year-old female adult with recently diagnosed CAPD.

NOISE CALLED SPEECH

oh, what to say
that might express
the reason why
I do delay
to say anything at all

It's because of the squishy stuff
Masquerading as a mind

the slowness with which it takes things in
the confusion in the turn-around bin
the fear there is no way to win
all caused by this horrendous din
of noise, called speech

The muck leaves me in a bind

And blind.

Blind to the wealth of words
That used to flow both ways quite well
Verbiage now a consummate chore
Sometimes a private hell

Actually, most do not know
That speaking is a strain
For it is the lesser of the losses
From blackouts in the brain

And some, poor sweet fools,
Haven't caught on yet
Are left in first impressions mode
Notions quite set

they rattle on
assuming I
do hear

and then they think
that comprehension
follows

but the masquerading mind
belies

for truly, now
incoming stuff
decries

its lies.

Words coming in seem foreign
I catch them as I can
Most travel on beyond me though
Obeying comprehension's ban

catch a few
hold them tight
watch the rest
continue flight

take the few
turn them 'round
fitting pieces
'til sense they sound

work hard! work fast!
spit out a reply
wondering always
if it will fly

Thus communication
By oral/aural means at least
Is so considerable a task

Not that I would give it up
I just...
Need help; this is what I ask.

Jesse VanVolkenburgh
1995

Handedness and Hemispheric Dominance for Language

Handedness	Dominant Hemisphere (%)		
	Left	Right	Both
Right	96	4	0
Left-or mixed-handed	70	15	15

Key References

Central Auditory Processing Disorders

Blake R, Field B, Foster C, Platt F, Wertz P. (1991). Effect of FM auditory trainers on attending behaviors of learning-disabled children. *Language, Speech, and Hearing Services in Schools 22*: 111–114.

Bocca E, Calearo C, Cassinari V. (1954). A new method for testing hearing in temporal lobe tumors. *Acta Otolaryngologica 44*: 219–221.

Burch-Sims PG, Hall JW III. Auditory mismatch negativity response in adults and normal versus brain injured infants. [Abstract]. *Audiology Today 6*: 1994.

Chermak GD, Musiek FM. Managing central auditory processing disorders in children and youth. *American Journal of Audiology 1*: 61–65, 1992.

Fifer R, Jerger J, Berlin C, Tobey E, Campbell J. (1983). Development of a dichotic sentence identification test for hearing impaired adults. *Ear and Hearing 4*: 300–305.

Flexer C, Savage H. (1992). Using an ALD in speech-language assessment and training. *The Hearing Journal 45*: 26–35.

Gascon G, Johnson R, Burd, L. Central auditory processing and attention deficit disorder. *Journal of Childhood Neurology 1*: 27–33, 1986.

Hall JW III. The acoustic reflex in central auditory dysfunction. In *Assessment of Central Auditory Dysfunction: Foundations and Clinical Correlates*. Pinheiro ML, Musiek FE (eds.). Baltimore: Williams & Wilkins, 1984, pp. 103–130.

Hall JW III, Baer JE, Prentice C, Wilson D, Byrn A. Central auditory processing disorder: A case report. *Seminars in Hearing 14*: 254–264, 1993.

Hawkins DB. Comparisons of speech recognition in noise by mildly-to-moderately hearing-impaired children using hearing aids and FM systems. *Journal of Speech and Hearing Disorders 49:* 409–418, 1984.

Jerger J, Jerger S. Clinical validity of central auditory tests. *Scandinavian Audiology 4*: 147–163, 1975.

Jerger S, Johnson K, Loiselle L. Pediatric central auditory dysfunction: Comparison of children with confirmed lesions versus suspected processing disorders. *American Journal of Otology 9* (Suppl): 63–71, 1988.

Jerger J, Johnson K, Jerger S, Coker N, Pirozzolo F, Gray L. Central auditory processing disorder: A case study. *Journal of the American Academy of Audiology 2*: 36–54, 1991.

Jerger S, Martin RC, Jerger J. Specific auditory perceptual dysfunction in a learning disabled child. *Ear and Hearing 8*: 78–86, 1987.

Jirsa RE, Clontz KB. Long latency auditory event-related potentials from children with auditory processing disorders. *Ear and Hearing 11*: 222–232, 1990.

Jirsa RE. The clinical utility of the P3 AERP in children with auditory processing disorders. *Journal of Speech and Hearing Research 35*: 903–912, 1992.

Kamhi AG, Beasley DA. Central auditory processing disorder: Is it a meaningful construct or a twentieth century unicorn? *Journal of Childhood Communication Disorders 9*: 5–13, 1985.

Keith RW, ed. *Central auditory dysfunction*. New York: Grune & Stratton, 1977.

Keith RW. Interpretation of the staggered spondee word (SSW) test. *Ear and Hearing 4*: 287–292, 1983.

Keith RW. *A screening test for auditory processing disorders*. The Psychological Corporation, Harcourt Brace Jovanovich, 1986.

Keith RW, Novak KK. Relationships between tests of central auditory function and receptive language. *Seminars in Hearing 5*: 243–250, 1984.

Keith RW, Rudy J, Donahue PA, Katbamna B. Comparison of SCAN results with other auditory and language measures in a clinical population. *Ear and Hearing 10*: 382–386, 1989.

Kraus N, McGee TJ. Mismatch negativity in the assessment of central auditory function. *American Journal of Audiology: A Journal of Clinical Practise 3*: 39–51, 1994.

Lindamood P. Auditory discrimination in depth program for phonologic awareness deficits. *Annals of Dyslexia*: 1991.

Musiek FM. (ed). Selected topics in central auditory dysfunction. *Seminars in Hearing 5*: 219–349, 1984.

Musiek FM. Hearing beyond the eighth nerve. *The American Journal of Otology 7*: 1986.

Musiek FM, Baran JA, Pinheiro, ML. P300 results in patients with lesions of the auditory areas of the cerebrum. *Journal of the American Academy of Audiology 3*: 5–15, 1992.

Musiek FM., Geurkink N, Keitel S. Test battery assessment of auditory perceptual dysfunction in children. *Laryngoscope 92*: 251–257, 1982.

Musiek FM, Gollegly KM, Baran JA. Myelination of the corpus callosum and auditory processing problems in children: Theoretical and clinical correlates. *Seminars in Hearing 5*: 231–241, 1984.

Musiek FM, Gollegly KM, Kibbe KS, Verkest-Lenz SB. Proposed screening test for central auditory disorders: Follow-up on the dichotic digits test. *The American Journal of Otology 12*: 109–113, 1991.

Musiek FM, Gollegly KM, Lamb LE, Lamb P. Selected issues in screening for central auditory processing dysfunction. *Seminars in Hearing 11*: 372–384, 1990.

Mylkebust HR. *Auditory disorders in children: A manual for differential diagnosis*. New York: Grune & Stratton, 1954.

Peck DH, Gressard, RP, Hellerman SP. Central auditory processing in the school-aged child: Is it clinically relevant? *Developmental and Behavioral Pediatrics 12*: 324–326, 1991.

Pinheiro ML, Musiek FM, eds. *Assessment of central auditory dysfunction*. Baltimore: Williams and Wilkins, 1984.

Classic Quote

Holy Bible on Ears and Hearing

"They have mouths, but they speak not;
eyes have they, but they see not.
They have ears, but they hear not."

Old Testament of the Holy Bible
Psalms 115:5–6

"Hear now this, O foolish people, and without understanding;
which have eyes, and see not;
which have ears, and hear not."

Old Testament of the Holy Bible
The Book of the Prophet Jeremiah 5:21

CAPD ASSESSMENT AND TEST PROTOCOLS

Selected Tests

Auditory Processing and Central Auditory Nervous System Functioning. List is limited to commercially available behavioral procedures.

General Audiologic

- binaural fusion
- competing sentences test
- compressed speech
- dichotic CVs
- dichotic digits test
- dichotic rhyme test
- dichotic sentence identification (DSI) test
- duration patterns test
- low pass filtered speech (LPFS)
- masking level difference (MLD)
- pediatric speech intelligibility (PSI) test
- pitch pattern sequence (PPS) test
- rapidly alternating speech perception (RASP)
- SCAN
- speech-in-noise
- staggered spondaic word (SSW) test
- synthetic sentence identification-ipsilateral competing message (SSI-ICM)

Auditory Discrimination

- Wepman Auditory Discrimination Test
- Seashore Measures of Musical Talents
  rhyme subtest
- SCAN
- Valett's Developmental Survey of Basic Learning Abilities
  auditory discrimination subtest

- Stanford Diagnostic Reading Test
  auditory discrimination subtest
- Doren Diagnostic Reading Test of Word Recognition Skills
  rhyming subtest
- Goldman, Fristoe, and Woodcock Diagnostic Auditory Discrimination Test
- Robbins Speech Sound Discrimination and Verbal Imagery Type Test
- Test of Nonverbal Auditory Discrimination
- Flowers Auditory Test of Selective Attention
- Accelerated Speech Perception Test
- Test of Awareness of Language Segments (TALS)
- Lindamood Auditory Conceptualization Test (LAC), revised
- Nemner Group Test of Auditory Discrimination
- Kindergarten Auditory Screening Test

Auditory Memory and Sequencing

- Illinois Test of Psycholinguistic Abilities (ITPA), revised
  auditory vocal sequencing subtest
- Goldman, Fristoe, and Woodcock Auditory Memory Tests
- Detroit Tests of Learning Aptitude
  auditory attention span for unrelated words subtest
  auditory attention span for related syllables subtest
  oral commission subtest
- Auditory Pointing Test
- Auditory Sequential Memory Test
- Lindamood Auditory Conceptualization (LAC) test, revised
- Language Structured Auditory Retention Span Test
- Auditory Memory Span Test
- Carrow Auditory-Visual Abilities Test
- Short-Term Auditory Retrieval and Storage Test
- Screening Test for Auditory Perception (STAP)
  remembering rhymes subtest

Auditory Perception

- Test for Auditory Comprehension of Language
- Test of Auditory-Perception Skills (TAPS)
- Detroit Tests of Learning Aptitude
  oral commissions and oral directions subtests
- Test of Auditory Analysis Skills (TASS)
- Katz Auditory Screening Test

- Screening Test for Auditory Perception (STAP)
- Flowers-Costello Test of Central Auditory Abilities
- Illinois Test of Psycholinguistic Abilities (ITPA)
  auditory perception subtest

Auditory Synthesis (closure or blending)

- Kindergarten Auditory Screening Test
- Illinois Test of Psycholinguistic Abilities (ITPA)
  sound blending subtest
- Roswell-Chall Auditory Blending Test
- Readiness Skills
  auditory blending subtest
- Katz Auditory Screening Test
- Flowers Phonics and Blending Test
- Goldman, Fristoe, Woodcock Sound Symbol Tests
- Test of Awareness of Language Segments (TALS)
- Auditory Blending Test

Auditory Figure-Ground

- Auditory Selective Attention Test
- Goldman, Fristoe, Woodcock Auditory Skills Test Battery
- Kindergarten Auditory Screening Test
- Carrow Auditory-Visual Abilities Test
- SCAN
  auditory figure-ground subtest

Source: Gillet P. *Auditory processes.* Novato, CA: Academic Therapy Publications, 1993.

Referral Sources for CAPD Patients

Referral sources for a consecutive series of 257 pediatric CAPD patients assessed by the first ADR author at Vanderbilt University Medical Center. Speech language pathologists, parents, physicians, and neuropsychologists refer the majority of patients to audiology. It is important to note that the center is the sole provider of audiologic CAPD assessment in the region.

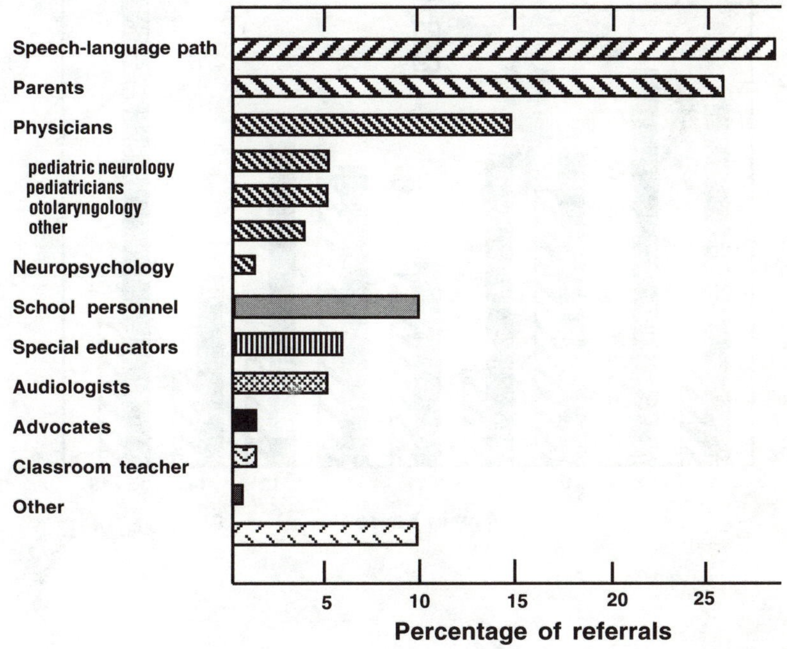

Distribution of CAPD Patients

Age and gender distribution for a consecutive series of 239 pediatric CAPD patients assessed by the first ADR author at Vanderbilt University Medical Center. Male patients exceed females at every age.

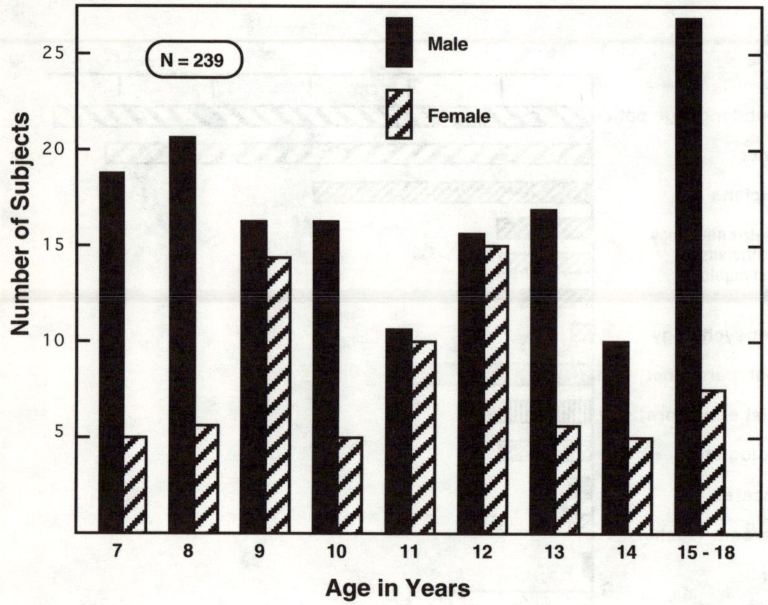

CAPD Test Battery

Assessing Peripheral Auditory Function and Central Auditory Processing Disorders (CAPD) at Vanderbilt University Medical Center

Procedure	Description	Reference
Peripheral auditory function		
pure tone audiometry	Hearing thresholds for octave frequencies of 250 through 8000 Hz	Hall & Mueller, 1995
word recognition	Perception of single syllable words presented in quiet	Hall & Mueller, 1995
aural immittance measures	Tympanometric measurement of middle ear function and acoustic reflex thresholds for ipsilateral and contralateral signals	Hall & Mueller, 1995 Hall, 1984
otoacoustic emissions (OAE)	Electrophysiologic measure of cochlear function	Hall et al., 1984
CAPD: behavioral audiometry*		
Children 8 years and older:		
dichotic digits	Different pairs of numbers presented simultaneously to each ear	Musiek et al., 1982, 1991
Staggered Spondaic Word Test (SSW)	Different two-syllable words presented simultaneously to each ear	Musiek et al., 1982; Jerger & Jerger, 1975 Pinheiro & Musiek, 1984
Dichotic Sentence Identification (DSI)	Different nonmeaningful sentences presented to each ear	Fifer et al., 1893 Hall et al., 1993
Synthetic Sentence Identification with Ipsilateral Competing Message (SSI-ICM)	Nonmeaningful sentences presented to one ear with meaningful story in the same ear at different intensity levels	Jerger & Jerger, 1975 Hall et al., 1993
Competing Sentences Test	Sentences presented to each ear with attention to one ear	Musiek et al., 1982
Pitch Pattern Sequence (PPS) Test	Randomized sequence of three tones of two frequencies	Musiek et al., 1982; Pinheiro & Musiek, 1984

(continued)

(continued)

Procedure	Description	Reference
Children less than 8 years:		
Pediatric Speech Intelligibity (PSI) Test	Single words and sentences presented with a competing message at varying levels of difficulty; performance adjusted for language age	Jerger et al., 1988, 1991
CAPD: auditory evoked responses		
Auditory Brainstem Response (ABR)	Electrophysiologic measure of 8th cranial nerve and auditory brainstem	Hall, 1982
Auditory Middle Latency Response (AMLR)	Electrophysiologic measure of primary auditory cortex function	Hall, 1992
Auditory P_{300} Response	Electrophysiologic measure of hippocampal and auditory cortex function	Hall, 1992
Mismatch Negativity Response (MMN)	Electrophysiologic measure of auditory cortex function (does not require subject attention or participation)	Kraus & McGee, 1994

*All behavioral CAPD test materials are available in analog or digital tape format from: AUDiTEC of St. Louis, 2515 S. Big Bend Blvd., St. Louis, MO 63143-2105 (TEL: (800) 669-9065; FAX: (314) 781-4946)

Rationale for Vanderbilt CAPD Test Battery

Also see tables, lists, and figures in this chapter.

- ☐ Documented sensitivity to surgically or radiologically confirmed central auditory nervous system dysfunction (see CAPD Test Battery).
- ☐ Test battery includes a variety of procedures:
  - ✓ dichotic word tests
  - ✓ dichotic sentence test
  - ✓ speech-in-competition test
  - ✓ auditory sequencing test
- ☐ Adequate age-adjusted normative data are available for children 8 years and older.
- ☐ Relatively brief time (less than 2 hours) is typically needed to administer the entire test battery (peripheral and central auditory procedures).
- ☐ CAPD test results are not significantly influenced by mild peripheral hearing loss.
- ☐ Test materials are available commercially in tape-recorded or CD formats.

Rationale

CAPD Test Battery

CAPD assessment is carried out with a battery of behavioral tests that have proven sensitivity to central auditory dysfunction (refer to CAPD Test Strategy). Our battery of audiologic tests, which is applied annually in over 75 patients referred to the Vanderbilt Balance and Hearing Center for CAPD assessment, is summarized on page 507. If a peripheral hearing loss (unilateral or bilateral) is discovered, we initiate medical or audiologic management and postpone further CAPD assessment. Typically, however, peripheral auditory function is normal and we proceed with the CAPD test battery. Due to age and time constraints, and to avoid a redundancy of information, all of these procedures are not usually applied with each patient. Behavioral CAPD tests are administered first. Our overall goal is to measure reliable performance for each ear on a series of speech audiometry procedures, including a dichotic word test (dichotic digits and often the Staggered Spondaic Word Test), a dichotic sentence test (the Dichotic Sentence Identification Test or, for younger children with poor reading skills, the Competing Sentences Test), a speech-in-competition test (the Synthetic Sentence Identification

Test with an ipsilateral competing message), and reliable performance with binaural stimulation on one or more *non*-speech measures, such as the pitch pattern sequence and duration pattern tests. Auditory evoked responses are recorded if specifically requested by the referring person or if we have any concerns about the reliability or questions about the interpretation of behavioral test performance. CAPD findings for children are analyzed in comparison to age-corrected normative data. Minimal criteria for confirmation of CAPD are scores that are below the age-corrected normal region (2.5 standard deviations below the mean) for one or both ears for at least two different procedures in a child with normal peripheral auditory test findings. Among children referred to our center for evaluation, two-thirds show consistent evidence of CAPD. For the remaining one third, however, CAPD suspected by parents, teachers, speech-language pathologists, or another referral source, was not confirmed and management of CAPD was, therefore, not indicated. For these children, appropriate referrals were initiated.

In constructing a CAPD test battery, it is wise to rely on procedures that are not apt to be influenced by linguistic, cognitive, or attentional disorders. Interpretation of CAPD tests is most straightforward when deficits are unilateral, which confirms that the patient understood the task and that the outcome was not due to a linguistic, cognitive, or attention disorder. A pronounced unilateral abnormality, specifically a marked left ear deficit, is one of the most common patterns of CAPD test battery findings in our experience. Another rather definite CAPD test battery pattern is when reduced performance is apparent only on difficult (vs. easier) portions of a test. This finding also implies an auditory versus linguistic, cognitive, or strictly attentional explanation for the child's poor performance.

Other important features of a clinically feasible CAPD test battery are:

- resistence to the influence of even slight peripheral auditory dysfunction
- the availability of adequate age-matched normative data
- professionally produced tape-recorded or compact disk-recorded test materials.

Earlier concerns about the usefulness of CAPD assessment with rudimentary procedures lacking these criteria were justifiable. Now, however, clinical feasible and commercially available procedures are available for young children, such as the *Pediatric Speech Intelligibility* (PSI) test (Jerger et al., 1987), as well as older children and adults.

Some authors who have questioned the usefulness of CAPD assessment have, unfortunately, not appreciated these criteria, nor taken advantage of a true battery of current, sensitive, and clinically proven procedures (Kamhi & Beasley, 1985). Peck, Gressard, and Hellerman (1991), for example, took issue with the "clinical relevance," "cost-benefit ratio," the over-referral rate, and "resulting management recommendations" of CAPD assessment. Yet, their discouraging conclusions were apparently due to a survey of 26 university clinics and their direct experiences with only three procedures. One was a screening test and not a diagnostic measure (the SCAN). The other two were the Competing Sentences Test and the Staggered Spondaic Word Test. Only the latter measure is a diagnostic procedure for assessment of CAPD that incorporates each of the three features noted above. Furthermore, these authors defined an abnormal CAPD outcome as a score that was only 1 standard deviation below the mean, and the specific normative database used to interpret the test results was not noted.

Diagnostic Codes for CAPD Assessment

Selected Diagnostic Codes Appropriate for Children Undergoing CAPD Assessment. (See appendix for complete listing of diagnosis, and CPT codes, used in audiology.)

Description	Code
Central hearing loss	389.14
Academic underacheivement	313.83
Attention deficit disorder	314.0
Head injury	854.00
Language disorder	315.31
Learning disorder	315.2

Clinical Documentation

The Vanderbilt Balance and Hearing Center CAPD Test Battery

Procedure	Studies
Staggered Spondaic Word (SSW) test	Katz et al., 1983
	Lynn & Gilroy, 1972
	Jerger & Jerger, 1975
	Musiek & Guerkink, 1982
	Hall et al., 1983
	Hall, 1983
	Musiek et al., 1994
	Musiek, 1983
	Musiek et al., 1984
	Musiek et al., 1994
Dichotic Digits Test	Musiek, 1983
	Musiek et al., 1984
	Musiek et al., 1994
	Mueller et al., 1985

Procedure	Studies
Synthetic Sentence Identification-	Jerger & Jerger, 1974
Ipsilateral Competing Message (SSI-ICM)	Jerger & Jerger, 1975
	Hall et al., 1983
	Hall, 1983
	Russolo & Poli, 1983
Dichotic Sentence Identification (DSI)	Jerger et al, 1983
Pitch Pattern Sequence (PPS)	Musiek et al., 1980
	Musiek et al., 1984
	Musiek et al, 1994

Normal Distribution

Bell-shaped curve, with corresponding regions representing mean (average) and variability (standard deviations), standard score equivalents, and stanines.

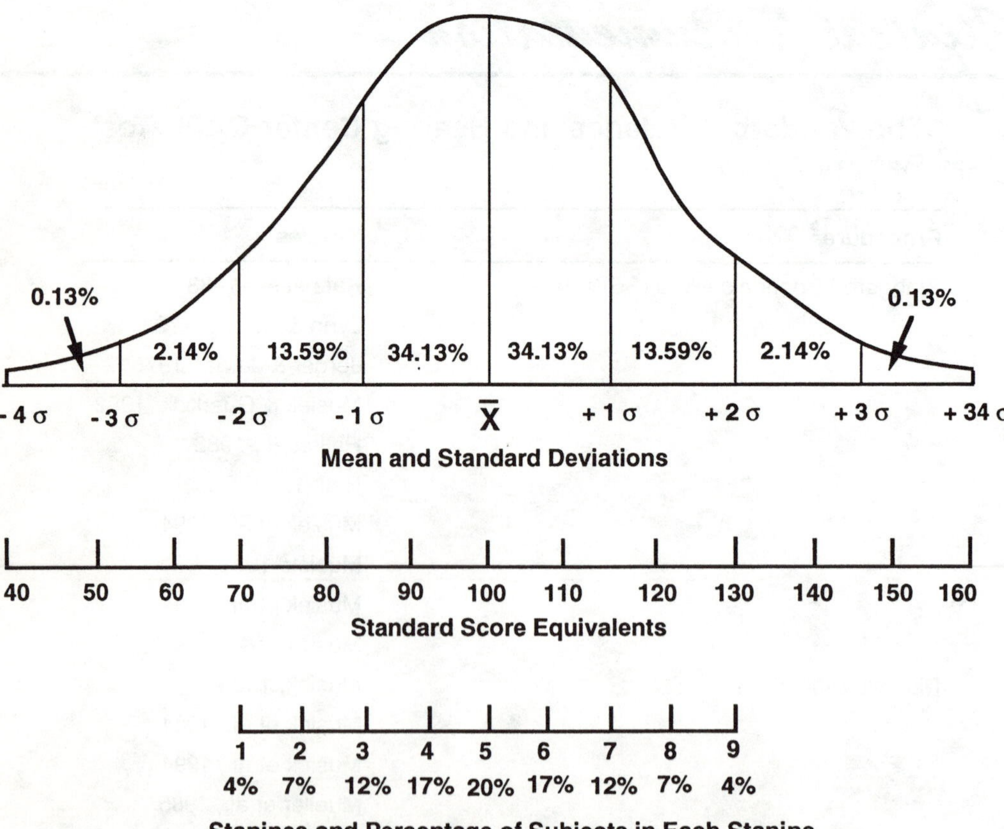

Strategies for Assessment and Management

Peripheral Versus Central Auditory Dysfunction. Note that there isn't really a heck of a big difference.

Strategies	Peripheral	Central
Assessment		
Test battery available	yes	yes
Behavioral measures used	yes	yes
Electrophysiologic measures used	yes	yes
General site-of-lesion information	yes	yes
Specific site-of-lesion information	no	no
Clinical experience reported	> 50 years	> 40 years
Test performance in diagnosis	unknown	unknown
Management		
Medical referrals based on tests	yes	yes
Counseling patient and family members	yes	yes
Classroom modifications	yes	yes
Hearing instruments fitted	yes	yes
Referral to speech-language pathology	sometimes	sometimes
Psychoeducational recommendations	sometimes	sometimes
Auditory rehabilitation/training	sometimes	sometimes
Outcome of management predictable	no	no

Staggered Spondaic Word (SSW) Test Paradigm

A dichotic procedure using spondee word materials. The four conditions shown include: right ear noncompeting ("up"), the competing condition (right ear lead with the word "stairs" and left ear lag with the word "down"), and a left ear noncompeting condition ("town"). The lead vs. lag words (e.g., right then left) are reversed after the first 20 sets of words. The primarily decussating (crossing) auditory pathways are represented by the dashed arrows. LH = left hemisphere auditory cortex and RH = right hemisphere auditory cortex.

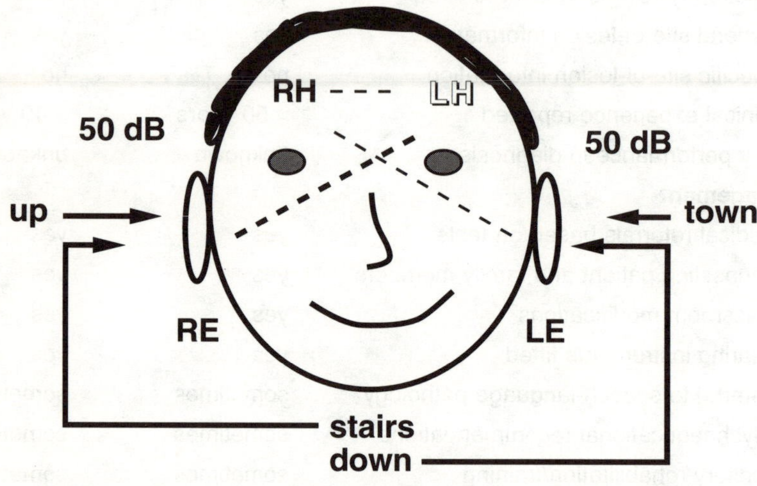

Stimuli: *40 pairs of spondee words presented dichotically to each ear*

Response: *repeat in any order*

Protocol

Staggered Spondaic Word (SSW) Test (see related figure)

☐ General Information

- First reported by Katz (1962, 1968). The use of spondaic words was expected to provide a high degree of test-retest reliability.
- Probably most widely used central auditory procedure.

☐ Clinical Validity

- Clinically proven value in detecting cortex temporal lobe lesions.
- Performance deficit is for ear contralateral to side of cortical dysfunction.
- May observe ipsilateral performance deficit in brainstem dysfunction.
- Retrocochlear (eighth cranial nerve) dysfunction produces an ipsilateral pattern of findings.
- Lower performance accuracy noted among the Alzheimer population.
- Especially useful in evaluating children and adults with relatively good hearing sensitivity.

☐ Test Administration

- Presentation Level = 50 dBSL (re: SRT)
- Composed of two spondees with a staggered onset.
- The second syllable of the first spondee and the first syllable of the second spondee are presented dichotically (time difference of milliseconds) in a "competing" condition, whereas the remaining syllables are presented in isolation to opposite ears.
- Example: Right ear leading = hot; Right ear competing = dog; Left ear competing = air; Left ear lagging = plane.
- There are 40 total test items. Twenty pairs of words are presented with the right ear leading and then another 20 are presented with the left ear leading.
- Patient is instructed to repeat both words as soon as both are heard.

☐ Scoring and Interpretation

- Percent correct scores are computed for each of the four conditions.
- Each syllable is worth 5%.
- Different scoring strategies have been described (see Katz, 1994, p. 239 for details).

- With simple method, competing scores for right and left ears are compared for asymmetry (>20% is abnormal) and compared to age-corrected normative data.
- Account for peripheral hearing loss by subtracting the percent error for speech discrimination from the SSW raw score in each condition.

☐ Advantages

- Widely used.
- Scoring takes into account peripheral hearing loss.
- Sensitive to retrocochlear, brainstem, and temporal lobe dysfunction.
- Good noncompeting syllable scores or significant asymmetry in scores with good performance for one ear argues strongly against the influence of cognition, attention, and intelligence on test performance.

☐ Disadvantages

- May not differentiate brainstem vs. cerebral auditory dysfunction.
- Some scoring procedures are complex.

Available from: AUDiTEC of St. Louis (800-669-9065).

Form

VANDERBILT UNIVERSITY MEDICAL CENTER
Division of Audiology

STAGGERED SPONDEE WORD TEST (SSW)*

Name:______________________ Age:____ Sex:____ Date:______________

Ear Leading______ Ear Trailing______ HL:______ Tester:______________________

1.	up	stairs		11.	meat	sauce	
		down	town			base	ball
2.	out	side		12.	king	pin	
		in	law			cod	fish
3.	cow	boy		13.	black	board	
		raw	hide			air	mail
4.	day	light		14.	sauce	pan	
		lunch	time			birth	day
5.	rain	bow		15.	house	fly	
		cough	drop			wood	work
6.	wash	tub		16.	oil	cloth	
		black	board			mail	man
7.	corn	bread		17.	green	bean	
		oat	meal			home	land
8.	bed	spread		18.	sun	day	
		mush	room			shoe	shine
9.	flood	gate		19.	air	port	
		flash	light			jet	plane
10.	sea	shore		20.	white	walls	
		cut	side			dog	house

*Only first 20 of 40 test items are shown.

Dichotic Digits Test Paradigm

A dichotic procedure using numbers from one to 10 (except the two-syllable number seven). A different number is presented to each ear at the same time (e.g., 1 and 5), then a second different number follows immediately to each ear. The primarily decussating (crossing) auditory pathways are represented by the dashed arrows. LH = left hemisphere auditory cortex and RH = right hemisphere auditory cortex.

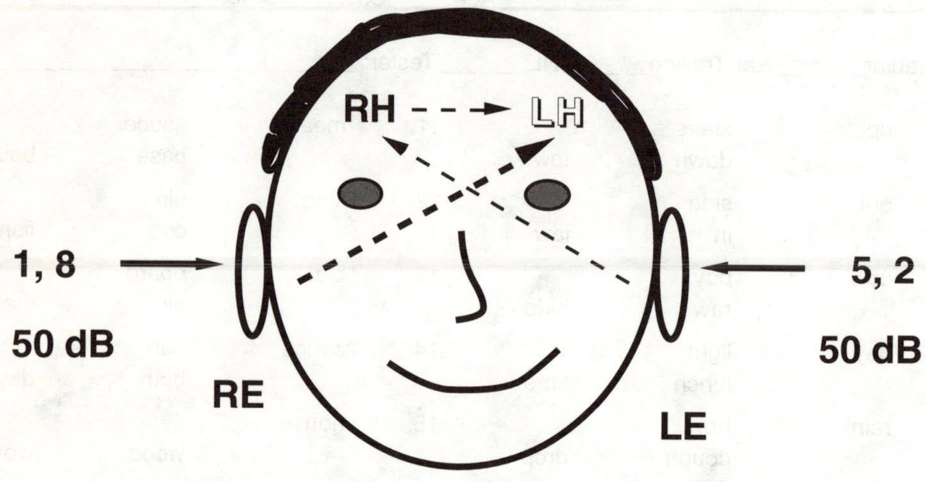

Stimuli: ***20 pairs of numbers to each ear***

Response: ***repeat in any order***

Protocol

Dichotic Digits Test (DDT) (see figure above.)

☐ General Information:

- First reported by Kimura in 1961 using three stimuli (digits) to each ear.
- Modified by Musiek in 1983 using two stimuli (digits) to each ear.

☐ Clinical Validity

- Used mostly in cortical/hemispheric and interhemispheric disorders.
- Reduced performance for the ear contralateral to lesion.
- May be of value in detecting brainstem lesions.

☐ Test Administration

- Presentation Level = 50 dB SL (re: SRT).
- Twenty digit pairs are presented simultaneously to each ear; numbers include 1 through 10, excluding 7 (because of two syllables).
- Example: 8, 1 presented to left ear while 2, 9 are presented to right ear.
- Subject instructed to repeat back all digits heard in any order.

☐ Scoring and Interpretation

- Percent correct scores are derived for each ear.
- Each number in pair is worth 2.5%
- Normal subjects yield a right ear advantage (REA) of 2–6%.
- Normative data are available from 8 years of age to adulthood.

  NOTE: see normative data in this chapter.

☐ Advantages

- Relatively resistant to cochlear loss.
- Simple stimuli vocabulary and closed set response allows use with a wide range of patients.
- Time efficient.
- Sensitive to brainstem and cortical lesions.
- Easy to score.

☐ Test-retest Reliability

- Good noncompeting syllable scores or significant asymmetry with good performance for one ear argues strongly against the influence of cognition, attention, and intelligence on test performance.

☐ Disadvantages

- Two-digit version is not currently available in CD format.
- Normative data not available for children younger than 8 years.

Available from: Auditec of St. Louis (800-669-9065).

Form

Dichotic Digits Test

Name:______________________ Age:____ Sex:____ Date:______________

Practice Items

Channel #1	Channel #2	Channel #1	Channel #2
___ 5	___ 2	5 , 4	2 , 1
___ 1	___ 8	8 , 3	6 , 4
___ 3	___ 10	2 , 8	3 , 5

Test Items

Channel #1	Channel #2	Channel #1	Channel #2
___ 1	___ 7	6 , 1	8 , 2
___ 8	___ 3	2 , 5	10 , 4
___ 2	___ 6	4 , 3	9 , 5
___ 3	___ 4	8 , 6	3 , 1
___ 1	___ 3	9 , 2	4 , 6
___ 7	___ 5	3 , 10	2 , 4
___ 5	___ 3	5 , 8	1 , 10
___ 1	___ 2	2 , 9	5 , 3
___ 3	___ 10	10 , 5	4 , 9
___ 10	___ 7	1 , 9	6 , 4
___ 6	___ 2	3 , 1	8 , 6
___ 4	___ 9	5 , 3	2 , 9
___ 8	___ 1	2 , 4	3 , 10
___ 3	___ 5	8 , 2	6 , 1
___ 8	___ 10	10 , 4	2 , 5
___ 6	___ 2	9 , 5	4 , 3
___ 9	___ 4	4 , 9	10 , 5
___ 1	___ 9	6 , 4	1 , 9
___ 2	___ 8	1 , 10	5 , 8
___ 10	___ 3	4 , 6	9 , 2
		SCORES: ______	______

Courtesy of Frank E. Musiek, Ph.D.

SSI-ICM Paradigm

Synthetic Sentence Identification (SSI) with Ipsilateral Competing Message (ICM) Test

A synthetic sentence is presented at a comfortable level (e.g., 50 dB HL) to one ear while a meaningful competing message (story about Davy Crockett) is presented to the same ear. The intensity level of the competing message is varied after each presentation of a list of 10 randomly ordered sentences. The primarily decussating (crossing) auditory pathways are represented by the dashed arrows. LH = left hemisphere auditory cortex and RH = right hemisphere auditory cortex.

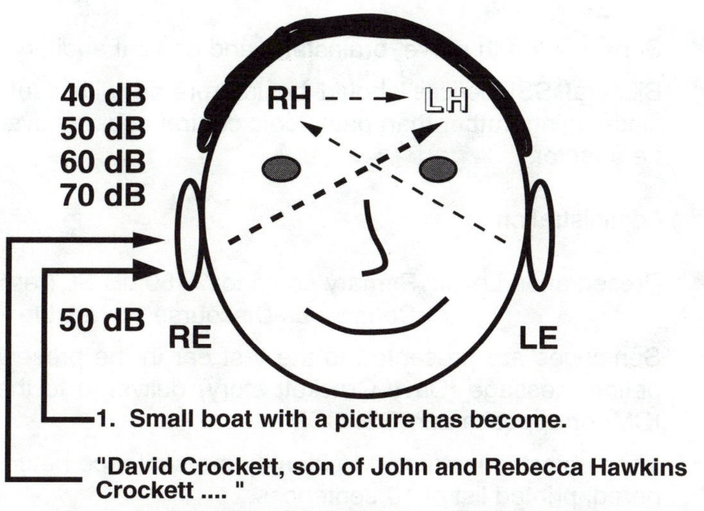

Stimuli: ***closed set of nonsense sentences presented in presence of ongoing story about Davy Crockett***

Response: ***identify number of sentence heard from printed list of 10 sentences***

Protocol

Synthetic Sentence Identification with Ipsilateral or Contralateral Competing Message (SSI-ICM/SSI-CCM) (see related figure on page 521)

☐ General Information

- First reported in 1965 by Speaks and Jerger.
- Was designed to minimize the subject's reliance on linguistic skills by utilizing third order approximations of English sentences.

☐ Clinical Validity

- Sensitive to 8th nerve, brainstem, and cortical auditory dysfunction.
- Bilateral SSI deficits should be interpreted with caution in elderly since aging, rather than pathologic central auditory dysfunction, may be a factor.

☐ Test Administration

- Presentation Level: Primary sentence = 50 dB SL (re: SRT)
Continuous Discourse = variable
- Sentences are presented to the test ear in the presence of a competing message (Davy Crockett story) delivered to the same (SSI-ICM) or opposite ear (SSI-CCM).
- The subject is instructed to identify the sentence heard from a numbered, printed list of 10 sentences.
- For the SSI-ICM, the primary message remains fixed at the same intensity level (e.g., 50 dB HL), whereas the continuous discourse is varied from +10 to −20 dB in the same ear.
- For the SSI-CCM, the primary message remains fixed at the same intensity level, whereas the continuous discourse is typically set at −40 MCR.

☐ Scoring and Interpretation

- Scores are plotted as a function of MCR.

  NOTE: see score sheet and figure in this chapter.
- Norms are available.

  NOTE: see figure in this chapter.
- Retrocochlear findings are ipsilateral for both ICM and CCM.

- With brainstem lesions, performance on the SSI-CCM generally will be good, whereas performance on the SSI-ICM shows deficit in the ear contralateral to the site of lesion.
- With temporal lobe pathology, performance on the SSI-CCM is poor in the contralateral ear. One or both ears show a deficit on the SSI-ICM.

☐ Advantages

- Widely used.
- Available in tape-recorded or CD recorded format.
- Available in English, Spanish, French, Arabic, and other languages.
- Independent of degree of hearing loss and cognitive function.
- Closed message set minimizes dependence on linguistic skill.
- Easily scored.
- Can be performed with pointing versus oral response.
- Sensitive to 8th nerve, brainstem & cortical auditory dysfunction.

☐ Disadvantages

- More variable results in elderly population.
- Requires rudimentary reading skills and visual acuity.

Available from: Auditec of St. Louis (800-669-9065).

Materials

Synthetic Sentence Identification (SSI) Test Materials

1. Small boat with a picture has become
2. Built the government with the force almost
3. Go change your car color is red
4. Forward march said the had a
5. March around without a care in your
6. That neighbor who said business is better
7. Battle cry and be better than ever
8. Down by the time is real enough
9. Agree with him only to find out
10. Women view men with green paper should

Graph For Plotting SSI-ICM and SSI-CCM

Percent correct performance (%) is plotted as a function of the difference between the sentences and the competing, the message-to-competition ratio (MCR), in dB. The hatched region on the SSI-ICM graph represents the adult (10 years and older) region.

Vanderbilt Balance and Hearing Center

Synthetic Sentence Identification (SSI)

NAME: AGE: SEX: DATE: SPL OF PRIMARY MESSAGE:
TESTER:

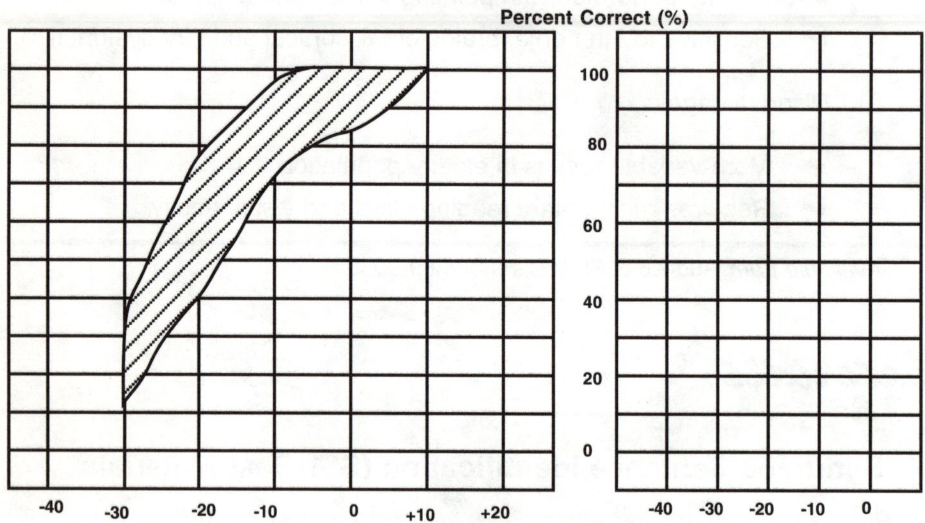

Dichotic Sentence Identification (DSI) Test Paradigm

A Dichotic Procedure Using the Synthetic Sentences from the SSI Procedure.

One synthetic sentence is presented at a comfortable level (e.g., 50 dB HL) to one ear while another synthetic sentence is presented at the same intensity level to the opposite ear. The primarily decussating (crossing) auditory pathways are represented by the dashed arrows. LH = left hemisphere auditory cortex and RH = right hemisphere auditory cortex.

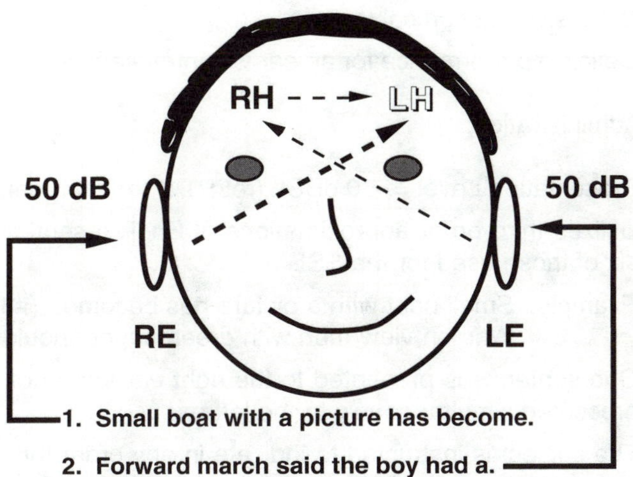

Stimuli: ***closed set of nonsense sentences presented in pairs dichotically***

Response: ***identify number of sentence heard from printed list***

Protocol

Dichotic Sentence Identification (DSI) Test (see related figure)

☐ General Information

- First reported by Fifer et al. (1983).
- Goal was to develop a dichotic test that could be administered to individuals with hearing loss.

☐ Clinical Validity

- Persons with PTAs up to 50 dB HL can be tested.
- Is sensitive to cortical lesions.
- Deficit in performance for an ear is contralateral to site of dysfunction.

☐ Test Administration:

- Presentation Level = 50 dBSL (re: PTA) for each ear.
- Utilizes third order approximations of English sentences identical to six of those used for the SSI.
- Example: Small boat with a picture has become. (#3)
Women view men with green paper should. (#6)
- One sentence is presented to the right ear and another sentence is presented simultaneously to the left ear.
- The subject is instructed to indicate in any order the numbers of the two sentences heard from a numbered, printed list.

☐ Scoring and Interpretation

- A percent correct score is calculated separately for right and left ears.
- Scores are evaluated for each ear in symmetry and relative to normative data.
- If the subject's PTA ranges from 5 to 25 dB, the normal DSI scores range from 75% to 100%.
- If the subject's PTA is greater than 35 dB, results become more variable, but norms are available.
- If the PTA of poorer ear is <39 dB HL, the asymmetry should be no greater than 16%.
- If the PTA of the poorer ear is from 40–59 dB, the asymmetry should be no greater than 39%.

☐ Advantages

- ✓ Not affected by peripheral hearing loss.
- ✓ Time efficient.
- ✓ Easily scored.
- ✓ Can be performed with pointing versus oral response.
- ✓ Sensitive to cortical lesions with scoring of ear differences.

☐ Disadvantages

- ✓ Insensitive to brainstem lesions.
- ✓ Rudimentary reading skills and visual acuity ability are required.

Materials

Dichotic Sentence Identification (DSI) Test

1. Small boat with a picture has become.
2. Built the government with the force almost.
3. Go change your car color is red.
4. Down by the time is real enough.
5. Agree with him only to find out.
6. Women view men with green paper should.

Available From: Auditec of St. Louis (800-669-9065).

Pitch Pattern Sequence (PPS) Test Paradigm

An Auditory Sequencing Procedure.

Three tones (some combination of high or low frequency, as illustrated by the bars) are presented either monaurally or binaurally. The patient response may be verbal (identification of the frequencies as high or low) or humming the pattern. The primarily decussating (crossing) auditory pathways are represented by the dashed arrows. LH = left hemisphere auditory cortex and RH = right hemisphere auditory cortex.

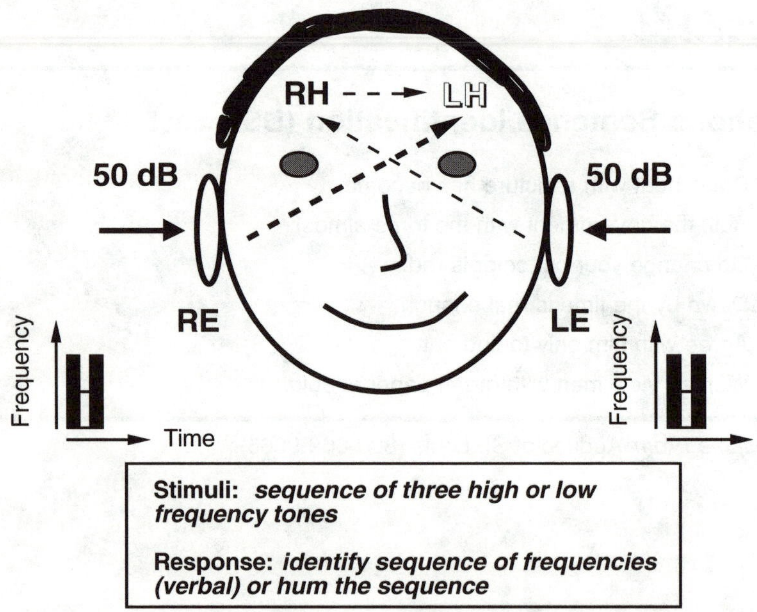

Protocol

Pitch Pattern Sequence Test (PPS) (see related figure)

- ☐ General Information
  - First reported by Pinheiro and Ptacek in 1971.
  - Utilizes nonverbal stimulus.
- ☐ Clinical Validity
  - Yields bilateral deficits for lesions limited to one hemisphere, thus does not provide clear laterality information. This is related to the interaction of both hemispheres in decoding the pattern for verbal response.
  - Split-brain patients and other patients with corpus collosum lesions can hum sequences but fail at verbal report.
  - Sensitive to cerebral lesions, but less sensitive to brainstem lesions.
  - Patients with lesions of either hemisphere or of interhemispheric pathways experience difficulty.
- ☐ Test Administration
  - Three tones are presented in succession, one of which is a different frequency than the other two, thus six patterns are possible.
  - Two test frequencies (pitches): high (H) = 1122 Hz
low (L) = 880 Hz
  - Examples: HHL LLH HLH LHL HLL LHH
  - 30 to 50 pitch pattern sequences are presented.
  - Five to 10 practice items precede actual scored patterns.
  - A verbal subject response is usually requested initially. Then, if scores are abnormal a humming response is requested.
- ☐ Scoring and Interpretation
  - Percent correct score are derived for the binaural presentation.
  - Normal limits vary depending on source of test material. Scores less than 75% are considered abnormal with adults suspected of auditory central nervous system lesions, although pediatric normative data are also available.

- Advantages
  - Relatively resistant to cochlear loss.
  - Sensitive to cortical and interhemispheric lesions based on large and varied published clinical database.
  - Does not use speech as a stimulus, and thus can be used to assess individuals with limited or impaired language skills.
- Disadvantages
  - Not sensitive to brainstem lesions.
  - Yields bilateral deficits for lesions limited to one hemisphere, and thus cannot provide definitive laterality information.

Available from: Auditec of St. Louis (800-669-9065).

Competing Sentences Test (CST) Paradigm

A Dichotic Procedure Using Actual Sentences.

One sentence is presented to one ear at 35 dB HL, while the other sentence is presented to the other ear at 50 dB HL. The patient listens only for the sentences presented to the target (35 dB HL) ear, and attempts to repeat them correctly. The primarily decussating (crossing) auditory pathways are represented by the dashed arrows. LH = left hemisphere auditory cortex and RH = right hemisphere auditory cortex.

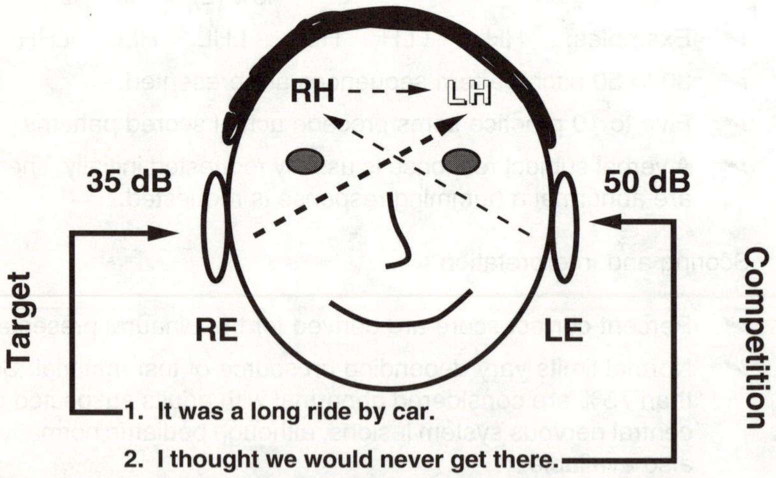
RH
LH
35 dB
50 dB
Target
Competition
RE
LE
1. It was a long ride by car.
2. I thought we would never get there.

Stimuli: ***pairs of real sentences presented dichotically***

Response: ***repeat sentence heard in target ear only***

Protocol

Competing Sentences Test (CST) (see related figure)

☐ General Information

- First reported by Willeford in 1968.
- Rationale in design was to avoid dependence on identification of highly transient single words and to simulate language constructions that one might encounter in everyday life.

☐ Clinical Validity

- Sensitive to temporal lobe lesions.
- Contralateral ear deficits in individuals with posterior temporal lobe lesions.
- Brainstem auditory dysfunction (unilateral) produces ipsilateral ear effects.
- Difficult to differentiate between hemispheric and brainstem lesions.

☐ Test Administration

- Composed of 30 pairs of simple sentences that are six to seven words in length.
- Sentences are presented dichotically but at different intensity levels in each ear.
- Target sentence is presented at 35 dB SL (RE: SRT) and the competing sentence at 50 dB SL.
- Example: I think we'll have rain today. (TARGET)
There was frost on the ground. (COMPETING)
- Subject is instructed to repeat the target sentence while ignoring the competing sentence.
- Five target sentences are presented to one ear as practice, and the next 10 as the test. Then the process is repeated for the other ear.

☐ Scoring and Interpretation

- Scoring guidelines are somewhat vague and not well-defined.
- Each correctly repeated target sentence is worth 10%.
- A sentence does not have to be repeated verbatim to be considered correct, although the content/meaning of the sentence cannot be compromised.

- Incorrect repetitions are assigned a value of 0, 2.5, 5, or 7.5% depending on how much meaning is lost.
- Scores for normal adults and children above age 10 should be 90–100%.
- Maturation effects are observed with children. Scores improve with age, especially for the nondominant (usually left) ear.
- Temporal lobe lesions are associated with poorer performance in the contralateral ear, especially for posterior temporal lobe lesions. Lesions in the anterior temporal lobe usually do not affect performance.

  Note: See normative data in this chapter.

☐ Advantages

- Sensitive to temporal lobe lesions.
- Somewhat sensitive to brainstem lesions.

☐ Disadvantages

- Guidelines for scoring not well-defined.
- Variability of results.
- Open set paradigm maximizes dependence on language skills.
- Difficult to differentiate hemispheric vs. brainstem lesions.

Available from: Auditec of St. Louis (800-669-9065).

Form

Competing Sentences Test

Name________________________________ Age_____ Date__________________

1. It was a long ride by car.
   I thought we would never get there.
2. He went to the South on his vacation.
   I get two weeks off in the summer.
3. He read the whole book in one week.
   I think they made the book into a movie.
4. I put the letter in the mail box.
   You must write to her more often.
5. He drank all of the milk.
   I like my coffee black.
6. He watched the cartoon on TV.
   I like the Bugs Bunny cartoon.
7. He was very late to class yesterday.
   I went to the cafeteria at noon.
8. The airplane flew very low.
   The jet took off smoothly.
9. I have the best teacher in school.
   He was a student here before me.
10. I saw the funny clown.
    The circus was very good.
11. This is a long freight train.
    The caboose is always last.
12. I don't like to go to school either.
    Recess is my favorite time.
13. My car is very fast.
    Put gas in the tank.
14. They say candy is bad for your teeth.
    I do not like to eat dinner alone.
15. Put a clean bandage on that cut.
    That scratch may get infected.
16. That movie was on TV.
    I saw it when it was a play.
17. I saw lots of different kinds of animals.
    There are lions and tigers in the zoo.
18. It is dangerous to swim there.
    He likes to swim the backstroke.
19. He is only resting.
    I had to take a nap.
20. I had a wonderful Christmas.
    He's off for Easter week.
21. I think hide and seek is a lot of fun.
    The children played tag for a long time.
22. They went to the zoo Sunday.
    I was able to go to the park.
23. My sister is older than I am.
    Your uncle is not over there.
24. There is a color television over there.
    I think I hear a radio playing.
25. He's too old to play with toys.
    I like to run my model train.
26. There was fried chicken for dinner.
    I had a sandwich for lunch.
27. Dessert was a chocolate sundae.
    I put strawberries on my ice cream.
28. Mother made pancakes for breakfast.
    I like maple syrup on my waffles.
29. Nobody is at home.
    They won't answer the phone.
30. It's raining very hard.
    There's a lot of snow on the ground.

NOTE: Target sentence = 35 dB HL
Competing sentence = 50 dB HL
5 practice and 10 test sentences in each ear.
Patient attends to target sentence in test ear.

Duration Pattern Test

DURATION PATTERN TEST

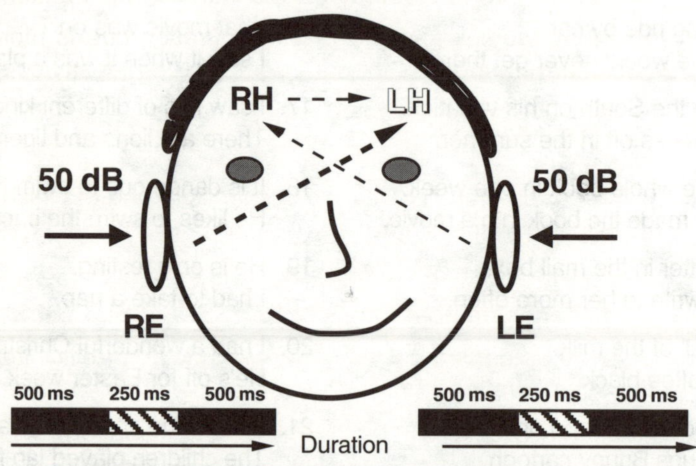

Stimuli: ***sequence of three short or long duration tones***

Response: ***identify sequence of durations (verbal, pointing, or humming response)***

Protocol

Duration Pattern Test (DPT) (see figure above)

- ☐ General information:
  - First reported by Musiek and colleagues in 1990.
  - Rationale in development was that the DPT does not require good frequency discrimination as only one frequency is used. Thus the effects of frequency distortion that could be caused by cochlear hearing loss are minimized.

☐ Clinical Validity

- Yields bilateral deficits for lesions limited to one hemisphere, and thus cannot provide definitive laterality information. This is related to the interaction of both hemispheres in decoding the pattern for verbal report.
- More sensitive to cerebral lesions than the pitch pattern test.
- Previous studies showed that the duration cue is more resistant to cochlear hearing loss than a frequency or intensity cue.

☐ Test Administration

- Three tones are presented in succession, one of which is different in duration than the other two.
- Long (L) = 500 msec; short (S) = 250 msec
- Six patterns are possible: LLS SSL LSL SLS LSS SLL
- 30 to 50 patterns are presented, with 5 to 10 practice items preceding the actual testing.
- Subject response can be verbal, manual (pointing), and/or humming.

☐ Scoring

- Percent correct score are derived for binaural presentation.
- Scores less than 70% are considered abnormal by some investigators, although normative data are limited especially for children.

☐ Advantages

- Relatively resistant to cochlear loss.
- Flexibility (any frequency can be used).
- Sensitive to cortical and interhemispheric lesions.
- Does not use speech as a stimulus thus can by used to assess individuals with limited or impaired language skills.

☐ Disadvantages

- Not sensitive to brainstem auditory dysfunction.
- Yields bilateral deficits for dysfunction that is limited to one hemisphere, and thus cannot provide definitive laterality information.
- Lack of published investigations in literature describing clinical applications.

Available from: Auditec of St. Louis (800-669-9065).

PATTERNS OF CAPD FINDINGS

Abnormal CAPD Test Findings

Proportion of abnormal behavioral CAPD test findings for a consecutive series of 239 pediatric CAPD patients assessed by the first ADR author at Vanderbilt University Medical Center. Abbreviations in the figure are as follows: DD = dichotic digits; SSW = staggered spondaic word test; SSI = synthetic sentence identification; DSI = dichotic sentence identification; PPS = pitch pattern sequence test; CST = competing sentences test. Abnormalities were significantly more common for the left vs. right ear, and most likely for the dichotic digits test.

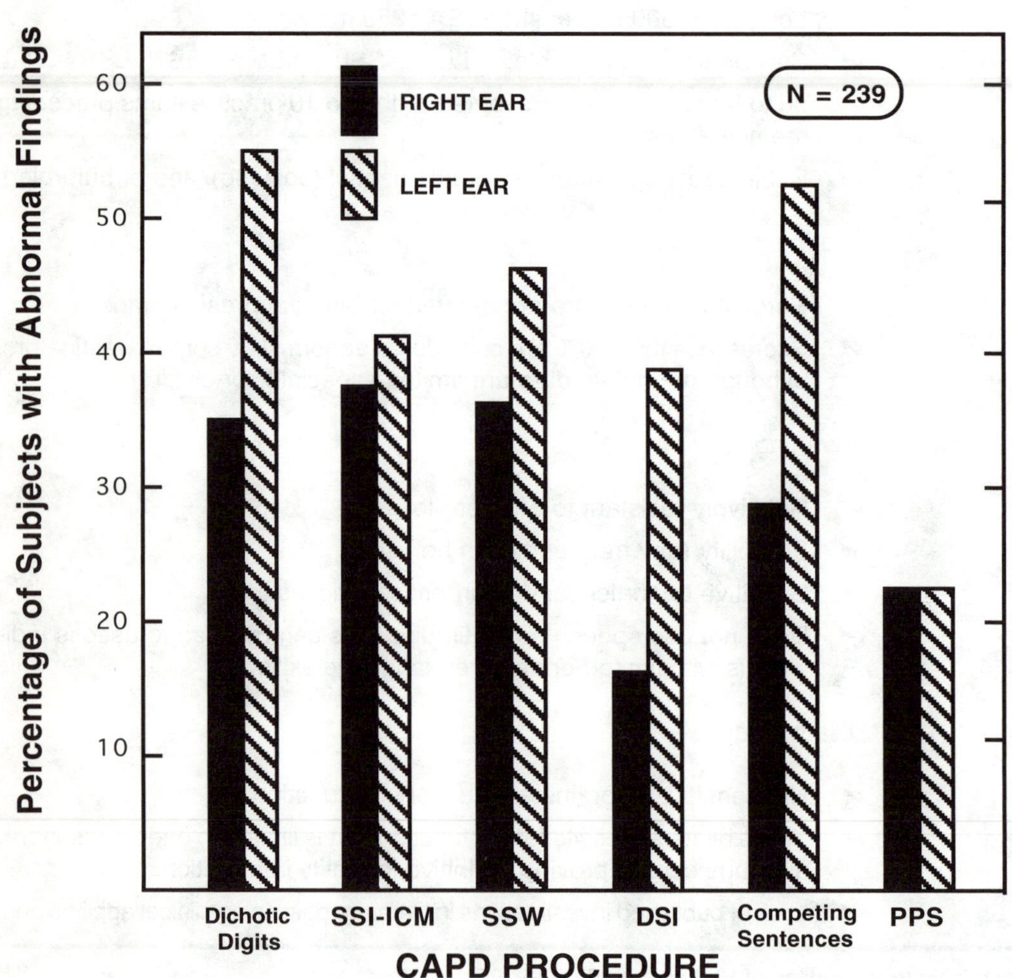

Comparison of Test Specificity

Number of Patients with Normal (N) vs. Abnormal (A) Findings

SSW (*N* = 188)	DD* (*N* = 190)		SSI-ICM* (*N* = 183)		DSI* (*N* = 99)		PPS* (*N* = 188)	
	N	**A**	**N**	**A**	**N**	**A**	**N**	**A**
Right ear								
N	101	24	90	37	66	5	102	26
A	23	42	25	31	20	8	42	18
Left ear								
N	73	32	83	30	46	16	96	15
A	17	68	24	46	18	20	47	30

*SSI-ICM = Synthetic Sentence Identification-Ipsilateral Competing Message
DSI = Dichotic Sentence Identification
PPS = Pitch Pattern Sequence Test

Electrophysiologic Test Findings in CAPD

Proportion of abnormal electrophysiologic CAPD test findings for a consecutive series of 196 pediatric CAPD patients assessed by the first ADR author at Vanderbilt University Medical Center. Abbreviations in the figure are as follows: Ipsi ART = ipsilateral (uncrossed) acoustic reflex threshold; Contra ART = contralateral (crossed) ART; ABR = auditory brainstem response; AMLR = auditory middle latency response; ALR = auditory late response. Abnormalities were significantly more equivalent for the left vs. right ear, but more likely for contra vs. ipsilateral ARTs and for two cortical auditory evoked responses (AMLR and P300).

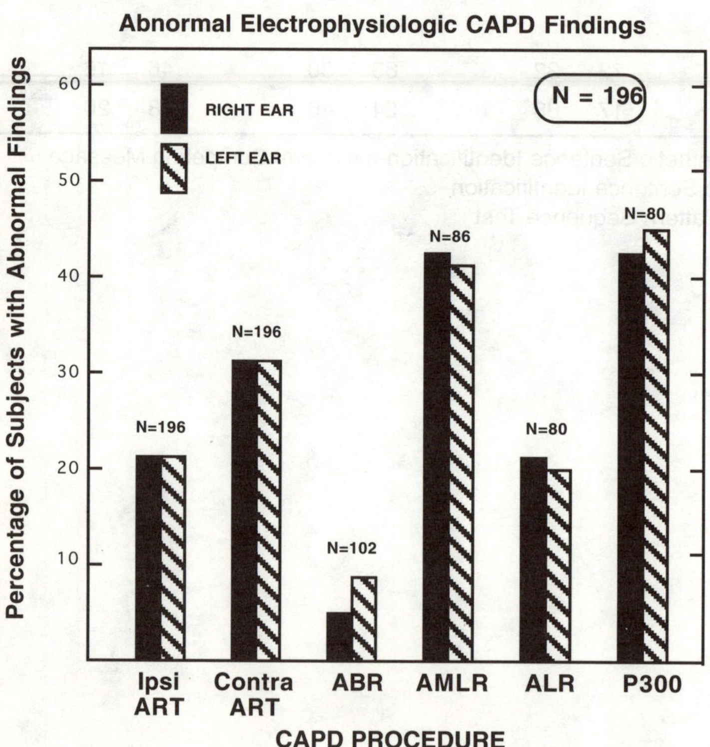

Case Example

Abnormal Findings for an 8-Year-Old Boy

Form used for plotting right and left ear results of CAPD test battery. Shaded region represents abnormal region. Typical findings are plotted for an 8-year-old boy with CAPD. Note that scores are consistently lower for the left vs. right ear. SSI and DSI procedures could not be administered because of the child's young age.

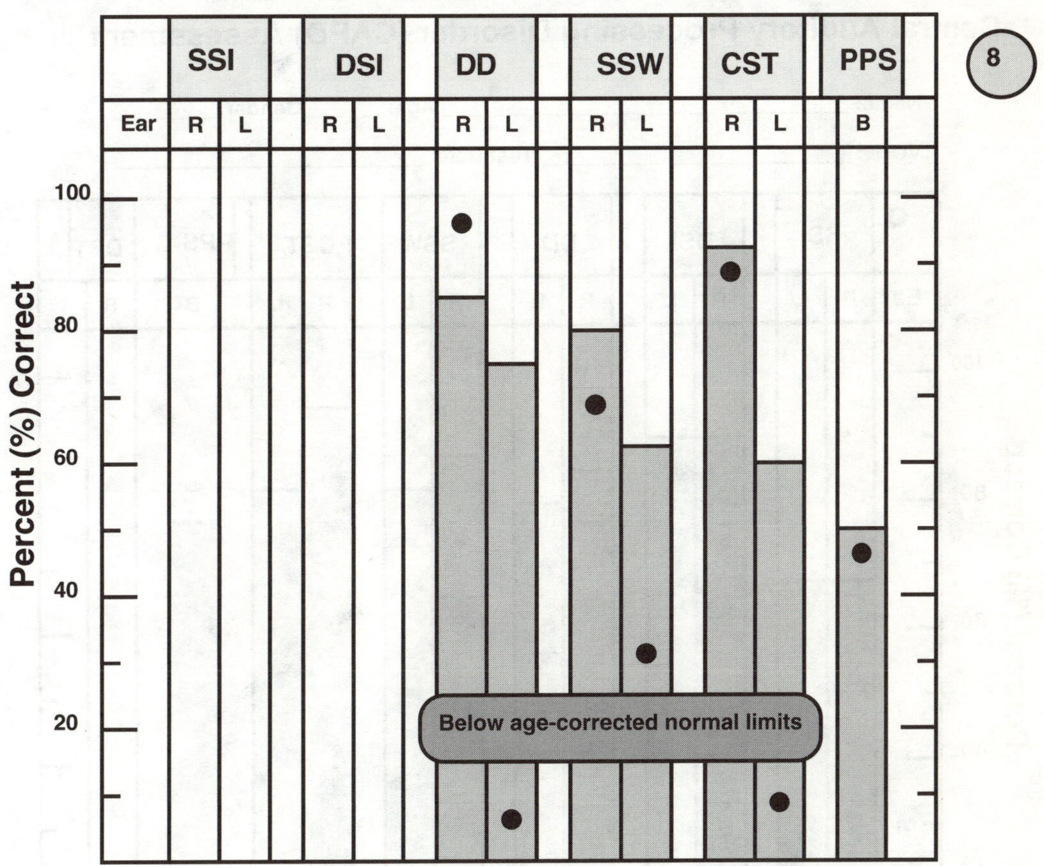

Form

Graph for Plotting CAPD Findings for 9-Year-Old Children

Form used for plotting right and left ear results of CAPD test battery. Shaded region represents abnormal region for 9-year-old child.

VANDERBILT BALANCE & HEARING CENTER
1500 21st Avenue South, Suite 2600
Nashville, TN 37212-3102
TEL: 625-322-HEAR FAX: 615-343-0872

Central Auditory Processing Disorder (CAPD) Assessment

Name: ____________________ Age: ______ Gender: ________

VUH#: ____________________ Test Date: ____________________

O	SSI		DSI		DD		SSW		CST		PPS	DPT
Ear	R	L	R	L	R	L	R	L	R	L	B	B

Percent (%) Correct: 100, 80, 60, 40, 20

Below age-corrected normal limits

SSI-ICM = synthetic sentence identification-ipsilateral competing message;
DSI = dichotic sentence identification; DD = dichotic digits; SSW = staggered spondaic words;
CST = competing sentence test; PPS = pitch pattern sequence; DPT = duration pattern test

Case Example

Abnormal Findings for a 9-Year-Old Boy with CAPD

Form used for plotting right and left ear results of CAPD test battery. Shaded region represents abnormal region for a 9-year-old child. Typical findings are plotted for an 9-year-old boy with CAPD. Note that scores are consistently lower for the left vs. right ear.

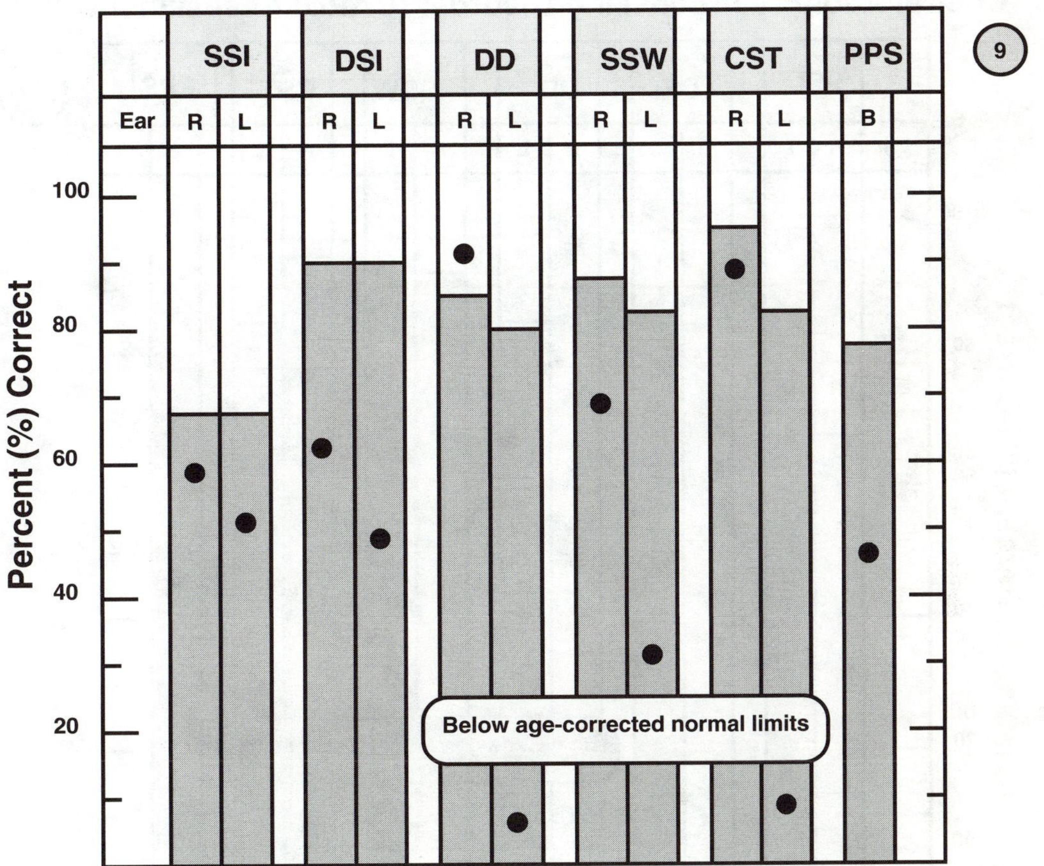

Form

Graph for Plotting CAPD Findings for 10-Year-Old Children

Form used for plotting right and left ear results of CAPD test battery. Shaded region represents abnormal region for 10-year-old child.

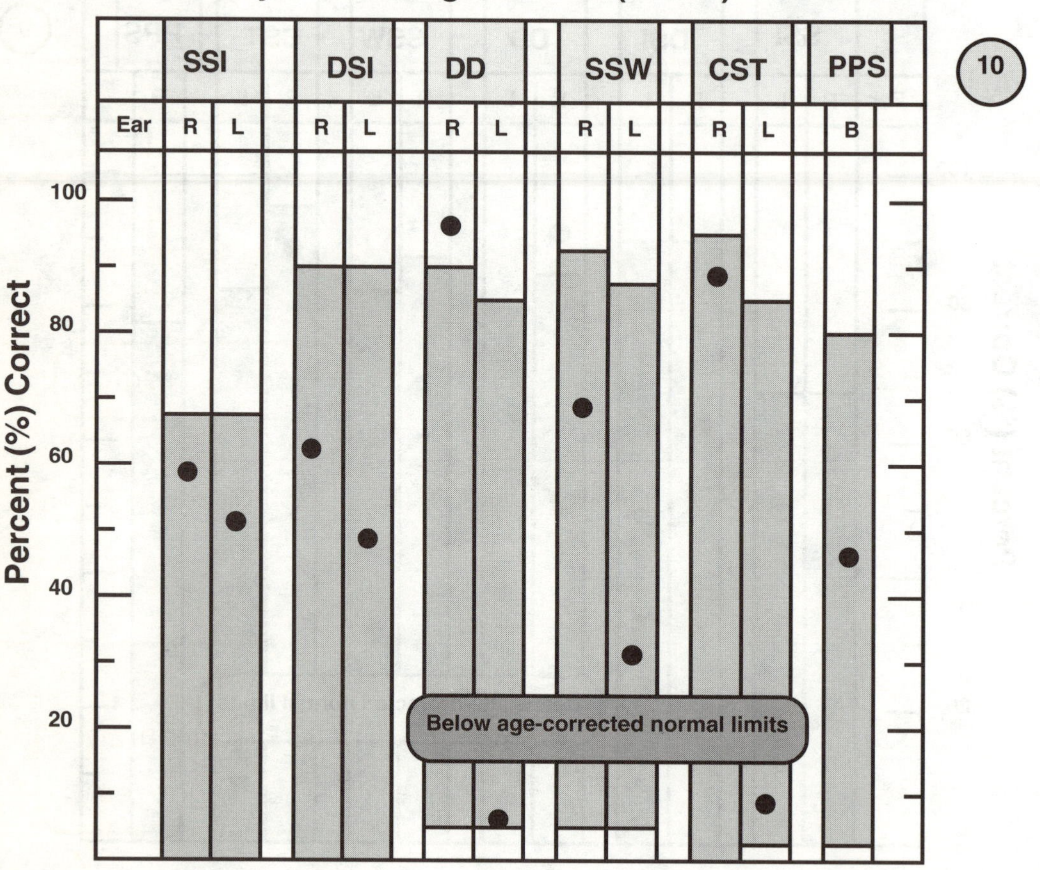

Evaluation of Assistive Listening Device

Plotting results for Synthetic Sentence Identification with Ipsilateral Competing Message (SSI-ICM) in the assessment of performance with an assistive listening device (ALD). Percent correct performance (%) is plotted as a function of the difference between the sentences and the competing, the message-to-competition ratio (MCR), in dB. The hatched region on the SSI-ICM graph represents the normal adult (10 years and older) region.

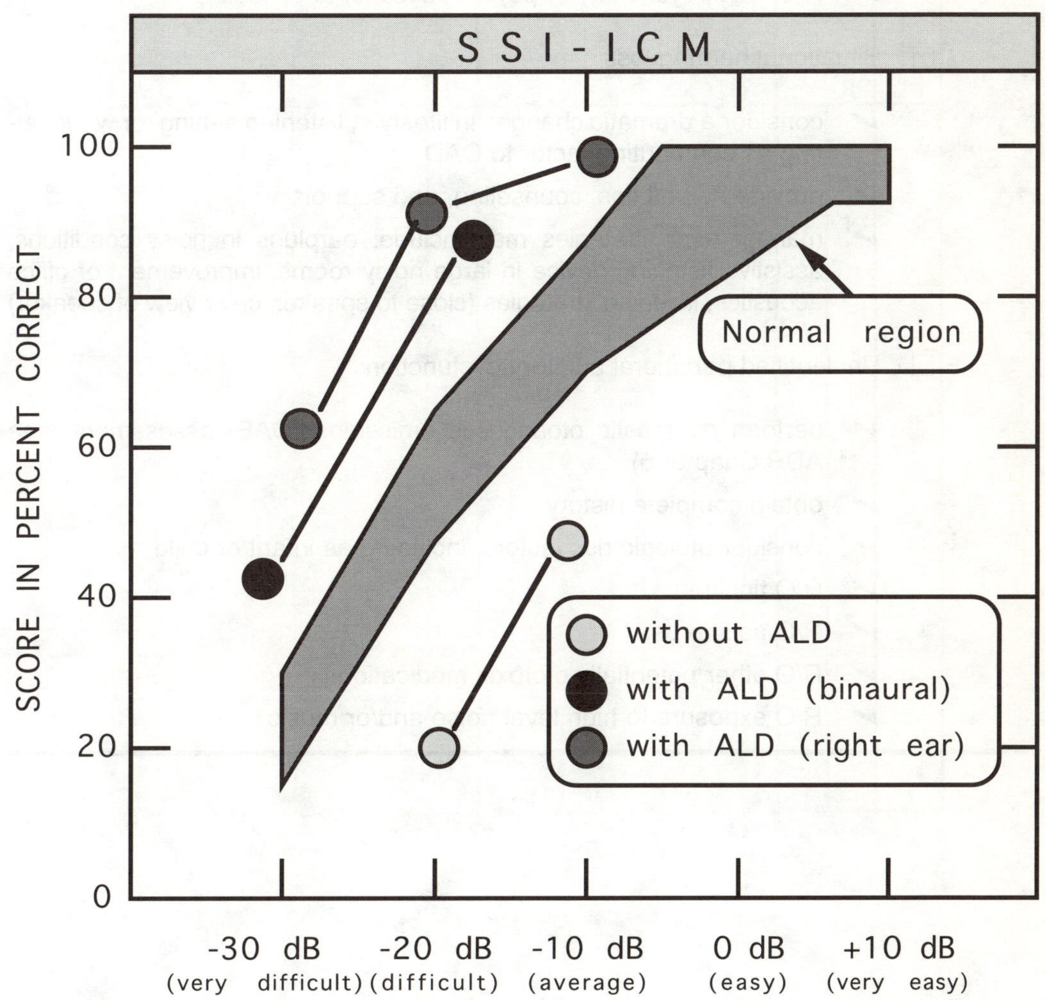

Obscure Auditory Dysfunction (OAD)

Four Possible Underlying Explanations

- ☐ Central auditory processing disorders (CAPD) and possible associated learning disabilities
  - ✓ R/O (rule out) with comprehensive CAPD assessment.
- ☐ Psychological or anxiety problems
  - ✓ R/O with psychology or psychoeducational consult
- ☐ Situational hearing loss
  - ✓ consider a dramatic changes in lifestyle, listening setting, or work setting as contributing factor to OAD
  - ✓ provide helpful tips, counseling, and support
  - ✓ management strategies may include: earplugs in noisy conditions, assistive listening device in large noisy rooms, improvement of office acoustics, listening strategies (close to speaker, clear view of speaker)
- ☐ Unidentified peripheral auditory dysfunction
  - ✓ perform diagnostic otoacoustic emissions (OAE) assessment (see ADR Chapter 5)
  - ✓ obtain complete history
  - ✓ consider otologic risk factors, including as infant or child
  - ✓ R/O tinnitus
  - ✓ R/O aspirin use
  - ✓ R/O other potentially ototoxic medications
  - ✓ R/O exposure to high level noise and/or music

MANAGEMENT OF CAPD

Checklist

Audiologic Management of CAPD

- Parent and teacher counseling and detailed information regarding characteristics and management of children with CAPD
- Modification of teaching strategies at school and at home the use of earplugs during deskwork and homework to attenuate background sounds
- Aural rehabilitation designed to develop auditory and listening skills (Gillette, 1992)
- The use of an assistive listening device (ALD) by teacher and child to enhance the signal-to-noise relationship in the classroom. The ALD consists of a directional microphone and FM transmitter worn by the speaker, and a receiver coupled to some type of earphone which is worn by the listener. There is mounting evidence that the latter management strategy is beneficial in the classroom setting for certain students (Blake et al., 1991; Flexer & Savage, 1992; Hawkins, 1984).
- Appropriate referrals for nonaudiologic assessments and management (see LIST: CAPD. Team of professionals involved in management)
- Advocacy for children and parents
- Expert legal opinion and testimony in depositions, due process hearings, and court litigation

Technical Tip

Guidelines for Recommending an FM Assistive Listening Device

☐ **Age**

Most children who comply with ALD use are younger than 13 years or older than 18 years. Children in the middle school and high school grades are generally less likely to readily use an ALD, probably because they are conscious of the reaction of their peers. This problem also applies to hearing aid use for children with peripheral hearing loss.

☐ Test findings

An ALD is most appropriate for management of persons meeting clear and well-defined criteria for CAPD. These criteria include depressed performance in comparison to age-corrected normative data (e.g., outside of the normal region as defined by the 10th percentile or 2.5 standard deviations below average performance) for one or both ears on at least two different CAPD test procedures. The strongest recommendation is made when performance is abnormally depressed for a procedure involving a signal-to-noise, figure-ground, or speech-in-competition task (e.g., the SSI-ICM).

☐ Educational setting

The need for an ALD is greater for children who are typically in classrooms with many other students (20 or more), rather than children who are taught with only a few other students (e.g., home schooled children or those in self-contained special classes). The noisier the typical classroom setting, the more an ALD is likely to help the child.

☐ Other educational, communicative, and medical needs

As a rule, a recommendation for classroom use of an ALD is one component of a comprehensive and multidisciplinary management strategy. In some cases, it is advisable to delay initiation of ALD use until other evaluations (e.g., speech-language, psychoeducational, neurologic, otologic) are completed and the results known or other management recommendations are implemented. There is a tendency by some educational personnel to rely on the ALD to solve all of the child's academic and communicative problems. The ALD is, however, really a tool which should enhance the effectiveness of other management strategies. Consider the analogy of a hearing aid. A child identified with a peripheral hearing impairment who is a candidate for a hearing aid will benefit maximally from amplification when it is used as part of an aural rehabilitation program and speech-language remediation.

☐ Features of the ALD

Usually, a no-gain personal ALD is indicated. Many children prefer to use an ear-bud type earphone rather than the head-set style because it is less conspicuous. If more than one child requires an ALD in a classroom, a classroom FM system should be considered. A variety of personal and classroom FM ALD systems are commercially available. A directional microphone typically is coupled to the transmitter.

☐ Trial period versus extended use?

Sometimes school personnel may recommend a relatively brief (e.g., 4 to 6 weeks) trial period of ALD use. The assumption is that clear signs of benefit will be evident within this period if the ALD is educationally indicated. If these signs are not observed, ALD use is discontinued. This strategy is used quite freely, even with children who appear to have some characteristics of children with CAPD, but who have not undergone diagnostic assessment.

In the author's experience, the trial period approach to ALD use is, with many children, counterproductive. Because ALD are used by children without an adequate diagnostic assessment, those who do not have CAPD undergo the trial period. Naturally, this population does not benefit from ALD use. The child, and most everyone involved with the child, may become frustrated and confused. School personnel may form the opinion that ALDs are of little value. The cost-to-benefit ratio of ALD use is very high. Limited school system resources (time and money) are not well spent. The child, parents, and classroom teacher are apt to approach ALD use half-heartedly, without full commitment. Even the child with definite CAPD may not obtain maximum benefit from ALD use is such a short time period. As with hearing aids, there is an adjustment period with ALD use which may extend well beyond the trial period. Relatively long-term academic and communicative benefits, and personal benefits (e.g., improved self-esteem) by definition do not occur within a span of just a few weeks.

A more effective approach is to limit recommendations for ALD use to children with clear and consistent audiologic evidence of ALD. The child, parents, teachers, approach ALD use with total commitment and a positive attitude. ALD use is introduced with care and the understanding that benefits will occur over time. The likelihood of benefit from ALD use is much higher with careful selection of the appropriate users. ALDs are viewed as a necessary and potentially very beneficial treatment strategy for CAPD, rather than a hit-or-miss effort that is tried without much hope that it will produce any benefit.

Misconceptions of School Personnel about CAPD

(Gleaned and in some cases quoted from tape recordings of M-team meetings and transcriptions of due process hearings.)

- ☐ "One of the reasons that we've [school personnel] been more cautious about that [implementing ALD use with CAPD children] is that it's kind of like doing drug trials in that to the extent to which you don't want to prescribe something that has been limitly (sic) researched. And the ALDs have not been widely researched."
- ☐ "Audiologists say that ALDs just simply make their job easier. But again, that's something that they say intuitively and not from a research base."

- ☐ "If he were to go [for CAPD assessment] he's probably going to come back as positive for central auditory processing because, number one, he has attention deficit disorder and the research shows us that kids who have ADDs typically come back as positive for auditory processing as well."
- ☐ "I don't really agree with [the parents request for a CAPD assessment] . . . I have recommended those for other kids and I'm so sure that this kid has characteristics of CAPD that it would be superfluous information. We already have indicators for CAPD . . . I'm convinced that [the CAPD assessment] will come back positive."
- ☐ "One of the things that he [the audiologist] recommends for every kid is an ALD."
- ☐ The cost for a CAPD assessment ranges from $500 to as high as $3000.
- ☐ ALDs are very expensive. We can't afford to fit 10 to 30% of the children in any given class with an ALD.
- ☐ "No matter how the CAPD assessment comes out, it won't affect the kind of program that is going to be provided."
- ☐ "An audiologist is not an educator. An audiologist hasn't had the training or classroom experience which would qualify him or her to make recommendations about the educational management of a child with CAPD."
- ☐ "All of the tests used in assessment of CAPD are quite new, and experimental. This is really a controversial issue among audiologists."
- ☐ "We could go ahead and complete the CAPD assessment, but what do you do if the child is shown to have CAPD?"

Handy Handout

Cover Letter

This letter accompanies the "Handy Handouts" in this chapter. All of these materials can be organized in a folder with several pockets to give to parents of children with diagnosed CAPD with the report of CAPD findings. We use a colorful and classy Vanderbilt University folder which has a small slot for a business card.

TO PARENTS:

There are three sets of information in this folder.

1. The first section (white paper) summarizes characteristics of children with auditory processing disorders (CAPDs). It was prepared for parents of children with CAPD, but not all of the information in this section may apply to your child. This section includes guidelines on how you might modify the home environment, and how you might interact with your child, in order to help your child improve listening skills and better acheive his or her academic and communicative potential. Keep in mind that as your child progresses in school, more and more learning will (or should) take place out of the classroom. These guidelines can be followed by the entire family, along with anyone else who comes into contact with your child.

2. The next section (yellow paper) is for your child's classroom teacher and other appropriate school personnel. It includes a summary of characteristics of children with CAPD, and lists suggestions for dealing with children with central auditory processing disorders at school. These include how the learning environment can be modified to help your child.

3. The final section consists of General Directions for Selective Listening Exercises with Background Noise (green paper). This information was provided by Dr. Frank Musiek of Dartmouth-Hitchcock Medical Center in Hanover, New Hampshire. Dr. Musiek has written and lectured widely on the topic of CAPD.

James W. Hall III, Ph.D.
Director
Vanderbilt Balance and Hearing Center

Handy Handout

Information for Parents, Teachers, and Other Important Persons in the Life of the Child with CAPD

CHARACTERISTICS OF CHILDREN WITH AUDITORY PROCESSING PROBLEMS

Definition: A person with auditory processing problems has difficulty in the reception and interpretation of auditory information in the absence of a hearing loss.

When one begins to look at a list of the symptoms of an auditory processing problem, often the results look very similar to the symptoms of peripheral hearing loss (a loss of hearing caused by a problem in the ear itself). The list will be very similar because in both cases the person with the problem can not make sense out of what he or she is hearing. The person with the auditory processing problem may hear the sounds loud enough, but not understand the message, and therefore act like he or she cannot hear. The following list gives some things to look for in these children, but understand that children with these symptoms need a regular hearing test to determine if their hearing is normal. It is possible that a child with a central auditory processing problem will demonstrate only some of these symptoms or perhaps none of these symptoms. These are areas that a teacher or parent could begin to look at to obtain some information about the child's listening behavior.

1. Does the child have difficulty in the areas of reading and spelling?
2. Does the child "pay attention only when he or she wants to," or have difficulty responding to part of the message?
3. Does the child appear puzzled by some auditory information and say "huh" or "what" often?
4. Does the child have difficulty staying on task and completing an assignment or project?
5. Does the child look around for visual cues from other children before beginning an assignment?
6. Does the child appear to tune out what is in the environment and become lost in "his or her own little world"?
7. Does the child have upper respiratory problems such as allergies, sinus, colds, adenoid problems, or mouth breathing?
8. Does the child have a history of fluctuating hearing loss or ear infections?
9. Has the child had earaches, feelings of pressure in the ears, discharge from the ears, or complained of noises in the ears?
10. Does the child ever seem confused about where sounds are coming from and have trouble locating them quickly?
11. Does the child have difficulty telling the difference between words that sound similar, such as cone/comb, and lath/laugh?
12. Does the child demonstrate unusual expressions or body postures while listening, such as facial expressions, turning or tilting of the head, or turning the body?

13. Does the child respond fairly well in quiet situations, but have great difficulty listening in noisy situations such as with the T.V. on or in a noisy crowd or classroom?
14. Does the child have difficulty remembering what is heard such as names, stories, numbers, multiple directions?
15. Does the child have trouble saying certain sounds correctly or have reduced language abilities or know the meaning of words as well as other children of his or her age group?
16. Can the child learn children's songs and T.V. jingles easily?
17. Does the child pay attention to sounds in the environment? Is there curiosity about sound and attempts to imitate sounds?
18. Can the child associate certain sounds correctly with the source, such as a moo sound with a picture of a cow?
19. Does the child often confuse directions or words and think something else was said?
20. Does the child have difficulty keeping information heard in the correct sequence?
21. Does the child respond to very simple instructions, but not to more complex instructions?
22. Does the child tend to use the same words or phrases over and over instead of responding appropriately to changing verbal information?
23. Is the child very visually alert, as demonstrated by watching the speakers faces very closely or by watching what others are doing?
24. Does the child have difficulty associating letters of the alphabet with the sounds being made?
25. Does the child show behaviors that are inappropriate (i.e., aggression, withdrawal, or impulsiveness)?
26. Is the child slow to respond to auditory information, as if it takes longer to think through the information?
27. Is the child easily distracted and appear to have a short attention span?
28. Does the child do poorer on tests that require verbal language understanding than on tests where something is actually done with the hands?
29. Does the child have trouble working independently?
30. Does the child perform very inconsistently, well at times, and very poorly on the same task at other times?

The list could go on and on, but these suggested areas to look for can give you a place to start. Many of these symptoms are seen at times in a lot of children without central auditory processing problems. If, however, your child or student is having some or many of these symptoms much of the time and is not progressing as you expect, a closer look at the problem is warranted.

Handy Handout

Common-sense Suggestions for Parents of Children with CAPD

May be limited to a single sheet, and laminated for posting on the refrigerator, and other handy places. Parents often report that simply knowing what their child's problem is, and the increased appreciation of their child's problems, has made a big difference to the entire family, including of course their child.

VANDERBILT BALANCE and HEARING CENTER
1500 21st Avenue South, Suite 2600
Nashville, TN 37212-3102
TEL: 615-322-HEAR (4327) FAX: 615-343-0872

Director: James W. Hall III, Ph.D., CCC/SP, CCC/AUD

CHILDREN WITH CENTRAL AUDITORY PROCESSING PROBLEMS

SUGGESTIONS FOR PARENTS

1. A child with auditory processing problems seems to hear inconsistently. If your child seems to hear some things, but not others, do not assume he or she is purposely ignoring you.
2. You will have greater success in communicating with your child if there are no other activities (other children or adults laughing or talking, television or radio playing, dishwasher or vacuum cleaner running, etc.) competing with you.
3. During communication, learn to control your child's environment by providing a quiet setting. Take the child to a quiet room, shut off the TV, ask others to be quiet for a moment, etc.
4. Delay important conversation until a quiet time can be found.
5. Make a point of finding "quiet conversation periods" on a regular basis during the course of each day.
6. Simplify your language level if your child does not seem to understand.
7. Try slowing down your rate of speech if your child continues to have trouble understanding. One way to accomplish this is to pause between utterances, especially after your child has finished talking and before you respond.
8. If you have to repeat something for your child, try saying it in a different way (different words, different type sentence).
9. Do not try to have discussions when you and your child are in separate rooms.
10. When conversing, allow the child adequate time to respond.
11. Your child may need time to rest and recuperate after school. Allow time for relaxation before asking him or her to do chores, homework, and so on.
12. Read aloud to your child and discuss what you have read.
13. Praise any accomplishment (academic or otherwise) that represents even small improvements over previous levels. It is not helpful to compare his or her performance to other children.

Handy Handout

Suggestions for Teachers

Students with central auditory processing problems will respond to changes their environment and teaching program in a variety of ways. Some of these suggestions will help some students but of no benefit to others. Some students will appear to be helped by most suggestions; others will be very difficult to help, no matter what is tried. The best suggestion is to try these ideas and carefully observe the student to see what works. The goal is to help the student become more comfortable and learn better in his or her educational environment. Parents, administrators, and educational staff can work together as a team in determining what appears to be in the best interest of a particular student.

1. **Reduce Distractions:** Avoid extraneous noises and visual distractions, especially when giving instructions and teaching new concepts. Before giving instructions, stand close to the student and call the student's name or touch his or her shoulder to make sure you have his or her attention. Use of the student's name during teaching time will also help hold his or her attention. Traditional classrooms are generally less distracting than open-style classrooms. Reduce motor activities during verbal presentations (i.e., in P.E., avoid giving complicated directions during calisthenics; avoid explanations while student is drawing or coloring).
2. **Preferential Seating:** Provide seating away from known auditory and visual distractions such as open windows, pencil sharpeners, doorways, air conditioners, computers, and learning centers. You may have to experiment to find the best location for each student.
3. **Delivery Style:** Avoid multiple commands. Presenting instructions in the simplest form possible. Gestures that enhance the message may be helpful, but extraneous gestures and excessive movement while delivering the message may be distracting. Speaking at a slower than normal rate will improve auditory comprehension skills. Speak clearly and at a comfortably loud level, using words within the student's vocabulary. Research has shown that background noise is often equal to or louder than the teacher's voice.
4. **Instructional Transitions:** By reviewing past material before beginning new lessons, the teacher will give the student a feeling of success. In addition, the student will be better prepared to assimilate new information. Preassigned readings and home assignments will also help when introducing new concepts and topics. Try to use "pretuning" techniques to focus the student's attention on the subject coming up. Words such as "Listen," "Ready," and "Remember this one" seem to be effective for signaling an important message.
5. **Attenuate Distractions:** Sound-attenuating ear muffs and earplugs may help the student tune out distractions during seatwork. If several pairs of ear muffs are made available to the class, the student with auditory processing difficulties will not feel singled out.
6. **Visual Aids:** Visual aids, including overheads, opaque projectors, and computers may be utilized to supplement the teacher's oral presentations as well as to provide an alternative mode to the auditory channel. Combining the visual and auditory modes of learning may benefit all students in the classroom. Written instructions

may be provided in conjunction with verbal instructions to aid the student in following directions.

7. **Auditory Exhaustion:** Students with auditory processing problems tend to fatigue or exhaust more easily due to the external distractions of the classroom. Teachers may want to consider special adaptations to allow for this fatigue. These might include avoiding demanding auditory tasks when the student is already fatigued. This might be accomplished by presenting auditory tasks early in the day or by alternating lessons requiring a higher amount of auditory processing with less demanding study periods. Physical activity can be used for reduction of the stress. Keeping such a child in from recess should be used with caution.
8. **Check Comprehension:** The teacher should watch for signs of inattention, decreased concentration or understanding. Instructions may need to be repeated and/or simplified for the student. To check for understanding, the student should be asked to repeat the instructions in his or her own words. Besides being a good check, this will also improve his/her listening habits since the student knows he or she will be expected to do this occasionally. To help with reading comprehension, the student may be allowed to subvocalize while reading until such time as this is unnecessary.
9. **Be Supportive:** Many students with auditory processing problems experience a lack of self-confidence or diminished self-worth due to comparisons made by self or others concerning their performance versus classmates. Demanding performance that is comparable to other students is not recommended. Professionals working with the student should reinforce all work performed successfully to help alleviate this problem.
10. **Buddy System:** A buddy system can be started by having one student, who appears to be strong in auditory processing, help the student who is having difficulty. Various methods may be tried to find what seems to be the most beneficial. Assistance may include note-taking, assistance with instructions, small group projects, and tutoring.
11. **Classroom Adaptations:** Class lessons or instructions can be recorded so the child can hear the material again at a later time. Mild amplification might be used to assist the student in attending to the teacher. This should be done with caution, and only with the assistance and supervision of an audiologist. The classroom may be sound treated to reduce background noise by adding drapes, carpets, and sound-absorbing materials. The teacher may wish to structure the classroom in a more traditional format to reduce background distractions. Written directions and assignments should be given, along with verbal instructions. The student should be encouraged to ask for repetition of instructions, if needed. When repeating instructions, rephrase and reword the instructions. Verbal information should be presented in a brief, concise, and clear fashion. Another compensatory practice would be teaching the student good note-taking skills. Small group and individual instruction is very helpful whenever possible.

Handy Handout

Behavior Characteristics of the Child with CAPD

General information for parents and other family members, teachers, coaches, and any one else coming into contact with a child who is diagnosed with CAPD. It is important for all to recognize that the child has a real "hearing problem" and needs their help and support.

BEHAVIOR CHARACTERISTICS OF THE CHILD WITH CENTRAL AUDITORY PROCESSING DISORDERS (CAPD)

Children with central auditory processing disorders often have the following hearing difficulties and behavior characteristics.

HEARING DIFFICULTIES

1. Inability to follow verbal commands of instructions, particularly if they are long and complex.
2. Gives inappropriate response to questions.
3. Inconsistent response to auditory stimulation (sometimes responds appropriately, sometimes not) or inconsistent auditory awareness (one-to-one conversation is better than in a group).
4. Repeatedly asks for repetition. Poor auditory discrimination skills—misunderstands what is said.
5. Poor listener: Ignores sound totally (ignoring because he or she cannot process)—difficulty attending to class work.
6. Difficulty with auditory localization skills.
7. Says what/huh: Is buying time to process or figure out what is being said.
8. Sometimes responds too quickly (before instructions are completely given) to avoid fear of failure, although this impulsive behavior actually may increase his or her failure. By this over-hasty responding, child is not aware of the rest of the incoming message.
9. Discrepancy in performance on verbal versus written instruction.
10. Frightened or upset by loud noise.
11. Uses a loud voice.
12. Withdraws in a group or when there is excessive noise. May have poor "social skills" and be immature for age.

BEHAVIOR CHARACTERISTICS

Academic Performance

1. Having academic problems (especially in reading, spelling and writing) nonachievers, academic failures, performing below expected academic levels.
2. No correlation between I.Q. and CAPD, but there is often a discrepancy between I.Q. and achievement.
3. Difficulty completing class assignments.

4. Short attention span, fatigued easily by a long or complex activity.
5. Easily distracted by auditory or visual stimuli.
6. Not able to remember long or short term information. (Is the difficulty in storing or did he get the information auditorally in the first place?)

Behavior

1. Hyperactive—high activity levels. Acting out in class with classroom behavior problems.
2. Hypoactive—passive, reserved, lethargic. Trouble beginning task, seldom completes a task. Very fatigued after school (goes home and goes to sleep).
3. Loners—may play with younger children or adults rather than with peers (can better control conversation with younger children or adults).
4. Poor self-concept (in older group there is a high drop-out rate).
5. Reluctance to try new tasks for fear of failure—"I can't do it."
6. "Don't care" attitude.
7. Emotional and social overlays—inadequacy, rejection, unacceptability, depression in the older child (may result in delinquency).

Other

1. Uncoordinated.
2. Difficulty with time concepts.
3. Speech and language problems (obvious or subtle).

Handy Handout

Strategies for Dealing with the CAPD Child at Home

SUGGESTIONS FOR THE HOME

1. Limit extraneous noise.
   a. During homework: provide a quiet place, ear muffs, turn TV and/or radio off, limit visual distractions.
   b. Your child will have greater success communicating if there are no other activities going on (children/adults talking, T.V., radio, vacuum cleaner, dishwasher). This kind of noise seriously interferes with your message regardless of how hard your child attempts to listen. Listening under these conditions is simply more difficult for a child with CAPD compared to others.
   c. Control your child's environment by making it quiet by any means available. (Take child to quiet room, shut off T.V., ask others to be quiet.) If you cannot control the auditory environment, it is better to delay conversation.
   d. Members of the family should make a point of finding quiet conversation periods on a regular basis during the day.
   e. Don't attempt to talk from another room or when your child is preoccupied with other thoughts or activities.
   f. Using ear plugs in car often settles children.

2. Put structure in your child's life. With knowledge of what to expect, your child will be better able to anticipate speech content.
   a. Set controls on daily activities. Structure all activities so that your child has fewer opportunities to be confused.
   b. Have daily routines, a schedule. Your child will perform better if he or she knows what to expect.
   c. In disciplining your child, be sure to indicate what specific behavior is being punished and why.
   d. Be certain you avoid punishing a behavior which your child could not help. It is important to set enforceable and realistic rules.
   e. When reprimanding, choose a time when you have your child's attention. Make sure your child knows exactly why he or she is being reprimanded. Also, do this in private so you don't embarrass your child and damage your child's self-esteem and self-image.

3. Other
   a. Use simple language, shorter words and short sentences, and state one idea at a time. Get your child's attention first, either by saying his or her name or by touching him or her. Children may also attend better if from time to time they repeat back the instructions. In this way, the adult can also monitor where the message may have broken down and then repeat the parts the child missed. Do not ask, "Did you hear me?" Rather, ask specific questions about the instructions.
   b. Move on to areas of new learning gradually so that your child knows what is expected of him or her and what is coming next. Review the areas that your child knows.

c. Multiple-part directions instructions should be given one part at a time with a slight pause (long enough for the adult to mentally repeat each part back to him- or herself) in between the parts to allow your child time to receive the message and comprehend each part.
d. Put the person speaking on the side of your child's "strong ear."
e. Conversations at the dinner table may be difficult for your child. Make sure that your child is a part of the conversation.
f. You may wish to write important chores or instructions on a blackboard.
g. For now, settle for limited success by praising often any accomplishment that represents an improvement over your child's previous levels.
h. Visual tasks may be your child's strongest ability and visual cues should be used whenever possible to supplement auditory understanding.

Handy Handout

General Directions for Selective Listening Exercises

Simple activities and excercises for children with CAPD. These are usually completed by parents or speech-language pathologists. For more detailed and extensive activities, see citations in Key References in this chapter, especially Gillet (1993).

GENERAL DIRECTIONS FOR SELECTIVE LISTENING EXERCISES WITH BACKGROUND NOISE

The purpose of these exercises is to improve your child's ability to understand what is said when there are distracting background noises. The louder the background noise and the more similar it is to what your child is listening for, the harder it will be for your child to understand.

Materials

Cassette tape-recording of background sounds containing approximately 3 minutes of each of the following kinds of sounds:

Level I: *Nonverbal constant noise*
Examples: kitchen fan, vacuum cleaner, hair dryer

Level II: *Nonverbal variable noises*
Examples: washing dishes, crowd noise, recess

Level III: *Verbal and Nonverbal music*
Examples: classical, folk songs, rock or country music

Level IV: *Verbal, nonmeaningful conversation*
Examples: foreign language, reading philosophy

Level V: *Verbal, meaningful conversation*
Examples: reading a story, TV show

Note: If this tape is not available, a similar one can be made at home. The tape should have a variety of nonverbal and verbal sounds and should roughly follow the above sequence. If a tape recorder is not available, use a sound source found at home such as a hair dryer, record player, TV, or a second person reading a story in the background.

Directions

Place the tape recorder or other sound source so that the sounds reach your child's ears equally—either directly behind the child, between you and your child, or directly behind you. Mark the volume dial (low, medium, high) so that you can return to the same volume or can increase the volume in some measurable way. The High volume should not be louder than your speaking voice. Your child should not be able to *see* your mouth, so have your child turn his back toward you or place a piece of paper in front of your mouth to block his view.

For each exercise, first be sure that your child can perform the required task with at least 80% accuracy *without* the background noise. **Any exercise from other parts of this booklet which the child has mastered can now be done again with background noise.** Begin with a low volume of Level I sounds. Once your child can complete an exercise with 80% accuracy, increase the volume. The volume should be increased until your child can understand the desired verbal task when the background noise is as loud as your voice, but not louder.

Once your child has mastered an exercise with Level I sounds, proceed to Level II and repeat the above procedures. Some children may move quickly to Levels IV and V; others may have to work hard to understand what is said when there are Level I sounds.

Record your child's accuracy on each exercise using a score sheet. Indicate the date, the name of the exercise, which Level of sounds was used, and the volume. If your child asks you to repeat what you said, mark it as an error, as you are trying to encourage good listening skills the first time something is said.

SELECTIVE LISTENING WITH BACKGROUND NOISE

Purpose

The purpose of this exercise is to improve your child's ability to understand what is said when there are distracting background sounds.

Description

Following Directions: Simple one-step directions (for younger children)

The parent gives the child a direction to follow when there are increasingly louder background sounds.

Materials

Tape-recording of background sounds and tape recorder or other sound source such as radio, hair dryer. (See General Directions at the beginning of this section.)

Directions

The parent says, "I am going to tell you some things to do. You will hear some other sounds at the same time. Listen to my voice and do what I say." Any simple commands may be substituted for the following directions. Be sure your child is able to follow the directions without the background sounds before you turn on the tape.

Examples

List 1

1. Raise your hand
2. Point to the floor
3. Touch your nose
4. Point to the ceiling
5. Touch your ear
6. Hold up three fingers
7. Close your eyes
8. Clap two times
9. Touch your hair
10. Point at me

List 2

1. Shake your head "yes"
2. Point to the door
3. Hold up 5 fingers
4. Open your mouth
5. Point to the floor
6. Touch your teeth
7. Point to the window
8. Clap 3 times
9. Touch your neck
10. Point to your eyes

SELECTIVE LISTENING WITH BACKGROUND NOISE

Purpose

The purpose of this exercise is to improve your child's ability to understand what is said when there are distracting background sounds.

Description

Following Directions: Simpler Drawing Task (for younger children)

The parent gives the child a direction to follow when there are increasingly louder background sounds. (See General Directions at the beginning of this section.)

Materials

Tape-recording of background sounds and tape recorder or other source of background sound; paper, crayons or pens (red, green, blue, yellow)

Directions

The parent says, "I am going to tell you some things to draw. You will hear some other sounds at the same time. Listen to my voice and draw what I tell you to." Any simple directions may be substituted for the following drawing tasks. Be sure your child is able to follow the directions without the background sounds before you turn on the tape.

Examples

1. Draw a red circle
2. Color it red
3. Draw a blue square
4. Draw two green triangles
5. Make 2 blue lines
6. Make 3 red lines
7. Draw 2 green squares
8. Color the squares red
9. Draw 2 blue circles
10. Color them yellow

SELECTIVE LISTENING WITH BACKGROUND NOISE

Purpose

The purpose of this exercise is to improve your child's ability to understand what is said when there are distracting background sounds.

Description

Following Directions: Harder drawing task (for older children)

The parent gives the child a direction to follow when there are increasingly louder background sounds. (See General Directions at the beginning of this section.)

Materials

Tape recording of background sounds and tape recorder or other source of background sound; paper, crayons or pens (red, green, blue, yellow)

Directions

The parent says, "I am going to tell you some things to draw. You will hear some other sounds at the same time. Listen to my voice and draw what I tell you to." Any similar directions may be substituted for the drawing tasks given below. Be sure your child is able to follow the directions without the background sounds before you turn on the tape.

Examples

1. Draw a small blue square.
2. Draw a red circle *around* it.
3. Make a green line *under* the red circle.
4. Make 2 blue lines *beside* the red circle.
5. Make 3 yellow lines *over* the red circle.

6. Draw 3 small green triangles.
7. Color them yellow.
8. Make a blue square around one triangle.
9. Make a green square around one triangle.
10. Make a red circle around one triangle.

SELECTIVE LISTENING WITH BACKGROUND NOISE

Purpose

The purpose of this activity is to improve the child's ability to understand what is said when there are distracting background noises.

Description

Following Directions: Harder drawing task

The parent gives the child a direction when there are increasingly louder background sounds. (See General Directions at the beginning of this section.)

Materials

Tape-recording of background sounds and tape recorder; paper, crayons, pens.

Directions

The parent says, "I am going to tell you some things to draw. You will hear some other sounds at the same time. Listen to my voice and draw what I tell you to draw." Be sure the child is able to follow the directions without the background sounds before you turn on the tape.

Examples

1. Draw a small green circle.
2. Draw a blue square on the right side of the circle.
3. Draw a yellow wavy line on the left side of the circle.
4. Draw a straight line below the circle.
5. Draw a green circle over the blue square.
6. Draw 4 blue triangles in a row.
7. Draw 4 red circles around the triangles.
8. Draw a yellow line below the first triangle.
9. Draw a blue line above the second triangle.
10. Draw a green square around the third and fourth triangles.

Source: Materials supplied by Dr. Frank E. Musiek, Professor and Director of Audiology, Dartmouth-Hitchcock Medical Center, Hanover, NH.

CHAPTER 12

Diagnostic Audiometry

In This ADR Chapter

Perspective

Every time a patient undergoes a hearing assessment, some measure of diagnostic audiometry comes into play. The clinical challenge is to know when more than the basic hearing test battery is required and what procedures will best define the patient's auditory status. The audiologist must, of course, be able to carry out sophisticated audiology procedures and analyze the results. Then, the pattern of diagnostic audiometry findings must be properly interpreted. In this era of health care cost containment, this entire process is a balancing act in which the consequences of not enough diagnostic assessment (e.g., the audiologist fails to identify serious auditory dysfunction) are weighed against the consequence of performing unecessary procedures (i.e. additional cost to the patient or the third party payer). Of course, the same dilemma arises in the decision regarding the need for referral of the patient to other health care providers for even more financially costly neurodiagnostic evaluation.

The diagnostic audiometry test battery has evolved considerably since the traditional site-of-lesion test battery of the 1960s. Then we performed, analyzed, and interpreted tests such as the SISI, ABLB, tone decay tests, and Bekesy audiometry in an attempt to differentiate cochlear (sensory) versus retrocochlear (usually neural) auditory dysfunction accurately. Today, these tests are obsolete. Instead, we apply a variety of other procedures, such as ABR and other evoked responses, OAE, and behavioral measures of central auditory function, in both adult and pediatric patient populations. The goal remains essentially the same—description of the type, degree, and, whenever possible, the site of auditory dysfunction.

FOUNDATIONS OF DIAGNOSTIC AUDIOLOGY

Seven Signs of Serious Ear Disease

Primary care providers are asked to evaluate and treat an ever-increasing number of both routine and complex medical problems. It is critical that the primary care provider be knowledgeable in a broad spectrum of routine medical problems, yet also recognize when the consultation of a specialist is indicated.

Seven signs of serious otologic (ear) disease that indicate the need for an evaluation by a specialist are:

1. Ear pain or fullness
2. Discharge or bleeding from the ear
3. Sudden or progressive hearing loss, even with recovery
4. Unequal hearing between ears or noise in the ear
5. Hearing loss after an injury, loud sound, or air travel
6. Slow or abnormal speech development in children
7. Balance disturbance or dizziness

1. Ear pain or fullness

Ear pain (otalgia) may arise as a result of ear diseases or as a result of an illness elsewhere in the head and neck. Otitis externa, or swimmer's ear, is often a benign infection that responds well to topical therapy; but in cases of immunocompromise or diabetes, otitis externa may be the first sign of and eventually lead to skull base osteomyelitis. Acute otitis media is a frequent cause of otalgia and is usually effectively treated with antibiotics, but a middle ear infection can become complicated and lead to facial paralysis, intracranial abscess, or meningitis. Referred otalgia, or pain referred to the ear from another source, may be due to temporomandibular joint dysfunction (TMJ) as well as cancers of the upper aerodigestive tract. Tumors in the pharynx and base of tongue have a particular tendency to cause referred otalgia through a neural network that innervates both the source of the cancer and the ear.

2. Discharge or bleeding from the ear

Discharge or bleeding from the ear commonly results from infection or tumor. Otitis externa may lead to purulent discharge (otorrhea) or bleeding and is accompanied by severe otalgia. More diffuse disorders of the temporal bone include chronic otitis media and cholesteatoma. These are often associated with multiple episodes of ear drainage. Cholesteatoma is a slow-growing lesion that erodes bone so that critical anatomy becomes vulnerable to erosion and infection over time. Complications of cholesteatoma include facial paralysis, labyrinthitis, meningitis, and brain abscess. Tumors of the external auditory canal, middle ear, and other regions of the temporal bone may present with bleeding from the ear. Bleeding from the ear may also be a result of trauma and can be a harbinger of more serious medical problems.

3. **Sudden or progressive hearing loss: even with recovery**
Sudden sensorineural hearing loss is often ascribed to a viral infection or an ischemic event but may be a symptom of a far more ominous pathology. Up to one third of patients with acoustic neuromas experience a hearing loss at some point during their illness. These tumors most commonly present as a unilateral or asymmetric sensorineural hearing loss, often with tinnitus. Hearing loss with recovery or fluctuating sensorineural hearing loss is also frequently noted in patients with Ménière's disease along with whirling vertigo, aural fullness, and tinnitus. Progressive losses may also be caused by immune disorders, syphillis, or infections at other sites in the body. Conductive hearing losses should be evaluated medically because of the risks of cholesteatoma and because most causes of conductive hearing loss can be readily treated.

4. **Unequal hearing between ears or noise in the ear**
Progressive asymmetric hearing loss or unilateral noise in the ear may be associated with acoustic neuroma or other tumors.

5. **Hearing loss after injury, loud sound, or air travel**
Hearing loss after an injury may be conductive or sensorineural. Conductive hearing losses are due to a disruption of the free movement of the vibrating tympanic membrane and ossicular unit. Both blunt and penetrating trauma may lead to tympanic membrane perforation or ossicular discontinuity. Noise-induced sensorineural hearing loss may occur after a single extremely loud noise or after repeated exposures to loud sounds. Air travel is one cause of otologic barotrauma and scuba diving is another. Hearing loss again may be either conductive, as in the case of hemorrhage behind an intact tympanic membrane (hemotympanum), or sensorineural, as in the case of an inner ear membrane tear. The membranes that are most vulnerable to this type of injury are the oval and round window membranes.

6. **Slow or abnormal speech development in children**
Abnormal speech development in children very frequently is a result of the child's inability to hear speech, recognize it, mimic it, and learn to use it appropriately. A common reason for hearing loss in young children may be otitis media with effusion that does not clear with treatment and leads to a significant conductive hearing loss. However, significant delays in speech acquisition are usually due to more serious, permanent sensorineural losses. Abnormal speech development in children requires immediate action because speech and language are most efficiently acquired in early years of life.

7. **Balance disturbance or vertigo**
Balance disturbance or vertigo may originate from an otologic or a neurological source. A variety of specific otologic etiologies for vertigo are amenable to either medical or surgical treatment, as in Ménière's disease or perilymphatic fistula. It is particularly important to exclude some specific potentially dangerous etiologies for vertigo including acoustic neuroma and other intracranial tumors, stroke, or demyelinating disease.

Conclusion

Primary care providers must be familiar with many types of diseases and decide which are to be treated in the primary care environment and which are to be referred to a specialist. The seven warning signs of serious ear disease were created to help in making that decision. Each warning sign should be a "red flag" and could indicate a potentially serious condition. When these warning signs appear, the patient should be referred to an otolaryngologist—head and neck surgeon to rule out serious disease of the ear, nose, or throat. The American Academy of Otolaryngology—Head and Neck Surgery is a resource that can be contacted and can supply a list of Academy members in a given region who may be of help.

Source: From American Academy of Otolaryngology-Head and Neck Surgery, Inc., *Seven signs of serious ear disease* (leaflet), 1995. Reprinted with permission of the American Academy of otolaryngology. Head and Neck Surgery, Inc. Alexandria, VA.

Indicators for Diagnostic Audiology

Retrocochlear Signs in the Basic Audiometric Test Battery

- ☐ Asymmetry in hearing sensitivity
- ☐ Rollover in PI-PB functions
- ☐ Acoustic reflex abnormalities in normal middle ear function
- ☐ Unilateral vestibular findings
- ☐ Unilateral tinnitus with any of the above

Reasons to Pursue a Central Auditory Assessment in Adults (See ADR Chapter 1 for more information on CAPD in children.)

- ☐ The patient complains of a hearing problem, but the results of basic audiologic assessment (aural immittance, pure tone audiometry, word recognition) are normal.
- ☐ Patient is 65 years or older and complains of difficulty hearing in the presence of background sounds, yet hearing is reasonably good for higher frequencies.
- ☐ History of neurologic disease or dysfunction, including but not limited to:
  - stroke
  - head injury
  - meningitis
  - anoxic/ischemic event
  - hydrocephalus
  - Alzheimer's disease
  - chronic alcoholism
  - demyelinating disease

External Ear Pathologies and Disorders

See Chapter 15 for more information on diseases.

External ear (benign tumors)

- ☐ Angiomas
  - ✔ capillary hemangioma
  - ✔ cavernous hemangioma
  - ✔ lymphangioma
- ☐ Cysts
  - ✔ sebaceous cysts
  - ✔ preauricular cysts (and fistulas)
- ☐ Fibroma
  - ✔ fibroma
  - ✔ keloids
- ☐ Papilloma
  - ✔ cutaneous horn
  - ✔ keratoacanthama
  - ✔ senile kertoses

External auditory canal

- ☐ Cerumen
- ☐ Foreign bodies
- ☐ External otitis (inflammatory)
  - ✔ acute localized external otitis
  - ✔ acute diffuse external otitis (swimmer's ear)
  - ✔ chronic diffuse external otitis
  - ✔ eczematoid external otitis
  - ✔ seborrheic external otitis
- ☐ External otitis (malignant)
- ☐ Chronic stenosing external otitis

- ☐ Keratosis obliterans
- ☐ Tumors (benign)
  - exostosis
  - adenoma
- ☐ Tumors (malignant)
  - carcinoma
  - ceruminoma
  - cystic adenoid carcinoma (Brooke's tumor)
  - malignant melanoma

Source: Adapted from Austin DF. Diseases of the external ear. *Otorhinolaryngology: Head and Neck Surgery*, 15th ed. (JJ Ballenger, JB Snow, Jr, Eds). Baltimore: Williams & Wilkins, 1996, pp. 974–988.

Cochlear Pathologies and Disorders Associated with Sensorineural Hearing Loss

See ADR Chapter 15 for more information on diseases.

Sudden sensorineural hearing loss

- ☐ Viral etiologies
  - ✔ mumps
  - ✔ measles
  - ✔ rubella
  - ✔ influenza
  - ✔ adenoviruses
  - ✔ cytomegalovirus (CMV)
  - ✔ human immunodeficiency virus (HIV)
- ☐ Infection
  - ✔ Lyme disease
  - ✔ syphilis
  - ✔ bacterial meningitis
- ☐ Vascular
- ☐ Rupture of the labyrinthine membranes
- ☐ Congenital
- ☐ Neoplasm
- ☐ Trauma
- ☐ Ototoxicity
- ☐ Neurologic disorders
  - ✔ multiple sclerosis
  - ✔ lateral pontomedullary syndrome (AICA stroke)

Autoimmune inner ear diseases and disorders

- ☐ Cogan's syndrome
- ☐ Rheumatoid arthritis
- ☐ Wegener's granulomatosis
- ☐ System lupus erythematosus (SLE)
- ☐ Vasculitides
- ☐ Ulcerative colitis

Source: Adapted from Harris JP, Ruckenstein MJ. Sudden sensorineural hearing loss, periplymph fistula, and autoimmune inner ear disease. *Otorhinolaryngology: Head and Neck Surgery*, 15th ed. (JJ Ballenger, JB Snow, Jr, Eds). Baltimore: Williams & Wilkins, 1996, pp. 1109–1117.

Clinical Entities Associated with Dynamic or Treatable SNHL

Entity	Characteristics	Medical treatment	Surgical treatment	Audiologists' role
Autoimmune disease	rapid, progressive SNHL	steroids, cyclophosamide, plasmaphoresis	none	detection, audiologic monitoring, amplification
Ménière's disease	fluctuating SNHL, episodic vertigo, ear fullness, tinnitus	salt and caffeine restriction, diuretics, vestibular suppressants, aminoglycosides	endolymphatic sac decompression/shunt, vestibular neurectomy	neurodiagnosis (ABR, OAE, ECochG, vestibular assessment, intraoperative, vestibular and audiologic monitoring
Meningitis	progressive or reversible SNHL	antibiotics	none	early detection, audiologic assessment, monitoring, & management
Syphilis	variable SNHL, some symptoms as in Ménière's disease	steroids, antibiotics	none	detection, neurodiagnosis, amplification
Otosclerosis	conductive or apparently mixed hearing loss	fluoride	stapedectomy	pre- and postoperative audiologic assessment
Otosclerosis (cochlear)	flat SNHL; usual family history	fluoride, calcium, Vitamin B	none	detection, amplification
Sudden deafness	rapid (<72 hrs) SNHL; possible vertigo	steroids, carbogen, I.V contrast media	none	detection and audiologic monitoring
Perilymph fistula	SNHL, dizziness	bedrest, stool softeners, cough suppressants	tympanotomy with fistular grafting	neurodiagnosis
Ototoxic drugs	SNHL which may progress or reverse	cessation or reduction of drugs	none	early detection, audiological assessment, monitoring, and management
Head injury	flat, reversible SNHL	bedrest, ?	none	audiologic assessment and monitoring

Semi-Classic Quote

Medical Referral Guidelines

You've completed the basic audiologic assessment for your patient. There are some questionably suspicious findings. Is a referral to a physician in order? Follow this simple policy:

"When in doubt . . . refer your patient out"

Historical Perspective

Then and Now (1948* versus 1995)

Baseball (ML)

- ☐ 1948: Cleveland Indians beat Boston Braves in the World Series
- ☐ 1995: Atlanta Braves beat Cleveland Indians in the World Series

Football (college)

- ☐ 1948: Northwestern University goes to the Rose Bowl
- ☐ 1995: Northwestern University has very successful season and goes to the Rose Bowl as representative from Big Ten Conference when Michigan upsets Ohio State

Audiology

- ☐ 1948: Diagnostic test battery consists of:
  - ✓ pure tone audiometry (air and bone conduction)
  - ✓ spondee reception threshold
  - ✓ word recognition (PAL PB word lists)
- ☐ 1995: Diagnostic test battery consists of:
  - ✓ pure tone audiometry (air and bone conduction)
  - ✓ spondee reception threshold
  - ✓ word recognition (variety of materials)
  - ✓ CAPD procedures
  - ✓ auditory brainstem response (ABR)
  - ✓ otoacoustic emissions (OAE)

* One of first ADR author's favorite years.

Classic Quote

Harold Schuknecht on Pathophysiology of Loudness Recruitment and Outer Hair Cells

"The phenomenon of loudness recruitment appears to be the psycho-acoustic expression of the loss of a large component of outer hair cells and the concurrent preservation of a large component of inner hair cells and type I cochlear neurons.

"It is well established that the outer hair cells are more susceptable than inner hair cells to almost all types of injury (e.g., inflammatory disease, trauma, ototoxic drugs) and that nerve fibers undergo degeneration only as a retrograde effect following injury to the sustenacular cells, particularly the inner pillar cells and the inner phalangeal cells."

Source: From Schuknecht HF. *Pathology of the Ear* (2nd ed). Philadelphia: Williams & Wilkins, 1993, p. 91.

Classic Quote

Benjamin Franklin on Writing and Doing (Words of wisdom to doctoral students embarking on a clinical scholar career track)

"If you would not be forgotten,
As soon as you are dead and rotten,
Either write things worthy of reading,
Or do things worth the writing."

Benjamin Franklin (1706–1790)
Poor Richard's Almanac (May)

Test Performance

Sensitivity and Specificity

	Disorder (Disease) Is Present	No Disorder (Disease) Is Not Present	
Test is positive for disorder	True Positive (hit rate)	False Positive (false alarm)	**Total Positive**
Test is negative for disorder	False Negative (miss rate)	True Negative (correct negative)	**Total Negative**
Total Number:	**with disorder (disease)**	**without disorder (disease)**	

Terminology of test performance:

Sensitivity = True Positive/total number with the disease
Specificity = True Negative/total number without the disease
Predictive value = True Positive/total number positive
Predictive value = True Negative/total number negative
Efficiency = True positive + true negative

Mover & Oscillator

James F. Jerger, the "Father of Diagnostic Audiology"

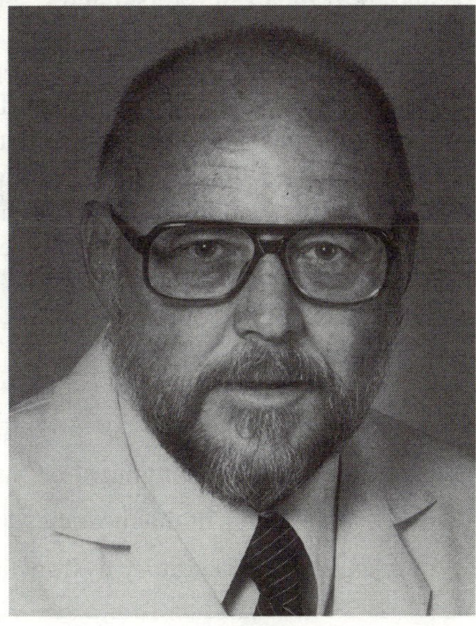

James Jerger

A synopsis of his work in his own words.

"My first exposure to clinical research was a study of the diagnostic value of the intensity difference limen (DL) in identifying cochlear hearing loss. That led eventually to my doctoral dissertation, a study of the DL in cochlear loss using the quantal psychophysical method. Interestingly, Ray Carhart was one of the experimental subjects.

He had sustained a modest high-frequency loss from aspirin toxicity. This research led ultimately to the SISI test, a clinical measure of intensity sensitivity. Here at Baylor College of Medicine, we stopped doing SISI tests about 25 years ago, as better diagnostic techniques based on the acoustic reflex and ABR became available, but the test is still very much alive in other parts of the world and, I note, is still included on some commercial diagnostic audiometers. My interest in differential sensitivity, in the late 1950s, coincided with the introduction of the Bekesy-type audiometer by the Grason Stadler Company. I used the Model E-800 to study the relation between thresholds for interrupted and continuous tones, leading to the classification of Bekesy-audiograms as types I, II, III, IV, or V.

In the early 1960s, Charles Speaks, Susan Jerger, and I developed the Synthetic Sentence Identification (SSI) procedure for speech audiometry, and I have used it fairly consistently ever since. It has furthered in important ways our understanding of the speech processing difficulties of persons with both cognitive and specifically auditory processing deficits.

The 1970s were devoted largely to impedance (now called "immittance") audiometry. My main thrust was to provide the framework for including the immittance battery as a part of routine audiologic evaluation. During the 1980s I was chiefly occupied with the auditory brain stem response (ABR) and the other auditory evoked potentials. Throughout the 1970s and the 1980s I developed and evaluated diagnostic test protocols based on the combination of speech, immittance, and evoked response measures. Another landmark event, during the 1980s, was the development of the Dichotic Sentence Identification (DSI) test based on the SSI materials. This was the result of a suggestion by Chuck Berlin and our subsequent collaboration to develop the DSI test protocol. More recently, I have initiated topographic brain mapping of auditory evoked potentials, chiefly the P-300 event-related potential, and have brought this new technology to bear on the auditory processing problems of elderly persons.

Looking back over all this, I can identify four contributions that I hope will have a sustained effect:

1) The concept of the diagnostic test battery for identifying site of auditory disorder.

2) The immittance battery as an essential component of basic audiologic evaluation.

3) The importance of speech audiometry in diagnostic evaluation.

4) Understanding the complex nature of auditory dysfunction in elderly persons."

Prepared by James Jerger in March 1996.

THE RISE AND FALL OF THE TRADITIONAL SITE-OF-LESION DIAGNOSTIC TEST BATTERY

Classic Quote

James Jerger and Deborah Hayes on the value of diagnostic speech audiometry

"The diagnostic value of traditional speech audiometry is extremely limited. If measurement is confined to the usual combination of spondee threshold and 'PB max' at a single suprathreshold level, the performance variation within distinct diagnostic categories is so great that there is a real problem of overlapping ranges. The difficulty is further compounded by the extreme dependence of monosyllabic word intelligibility on high-frequency sensitivity loss, a factor which places the PB score at the mercy of audiometric configuration to an undesirable extent. For very thorough and insightful treatment of the general problem of diagnostic speech audiometry the interested reader is urged to obtain a copy of the report entitled 'A Feasibility Study of Diagnostic Speech Audiometry,' by P. Lyregaard, D. Robinson, and R. Hinchcliffe.

During the past several years, we have experimented with a combination of speech tests designed to produce more useful diagnostic information. The test battery includes performance vs intensity (PI) functions for both conventional phonemically balanced (PB) monosyllables and for the synthetic sentence identification (SSI) task. In actual test-battery administration, blocks of 25 PB words are presented at four to six speech levels in order to define the PI-PB function, and blocks of ten sentences are presented, usually at the same levels, to define the PI-SSI function.

The importance of defining a reasonably complete PI function for each set of speech materials cannot be overemphasized. Presentation of a single block of either PB words or sentences at a single level, assumed to be at the plateau or maximum of the PI function, is almost never satisfactory for two reasons. First, in the cases of greatest interest, eighth nerve and central disorders, the exact shape of the PI function is so unpredictable that the speech level producing maximum performance can seldom be accurately estimated a priori. Second, the consistency of the relationship between the two complete functions, over their entire range, often reveals subtle effects not as evident or discernible from a comparison of single scores."

Source: Jerger J, Hayes, D. Diagnostic speech audiometry. *Archives of Otolaryngology 103*: 216–222, 1977.

Classic Quote

James Jerger, while he was at Northwestern University, on the detection of extremely small changes in sound intensity (SISI)

"A unique method for the clinical assessment of differential intensity discrimination is described. Short (200 msec.) 1-dB intensity increments are superimposed, at 5-second intervals, on a pure tone of constant amplitude at a sensation level of 20 dB. The patient responds to the momentary changes in loudness. The procedure is called SISI (short increment sensitivity index), and results are expressed in terms of the percentage of 20 increments to which a response is made.

Findings on selected individual cases are reported in order to illustrate the manner in which the SISI score varies with different kinds of hearing loss.

Results obtained in 75 patients with various types of hearing loss are reviewed. Conductive and retrocochlear losses showed very low SISI scores, never exceeding 15%. Ménière and noise-induced losses, on the other hand, yielded relatively high percentages, the lowest score obtained in any of these patients being 70%."

Source: Jerger, J, Lassman, S, Harford E. On the detection of extremely small changes in sound intensity. *A. M. A. Archives of Otolaryngology 69:* 200–211, 1959.

Major Advances in Classic Diagnostic Audiology

Procedures for Site-of-Lesion Assessment

Year	Procedure	Principle Investigator(s)
1930	audiometer	Western Electric
1935	monaural loudness balance	Reger
1937	alternate binaural loudness balance (ABLB)	Fowler
1946	impedance audiometry	Metz
1947	Bekesy audiometer	Bekesy
1948	ABLB in site-of-lesion evaluation	Dix, Hallpike, & Hood
1948	difference limen for intensity	Luscher & Zwislocki
1957	tone decay	Carhart
1959	short increment sensitivity index	Jerger, Shedd, & Harford
1960	Bekesy threshold types	Jerger
1969	acoustic reflex decay	Anderson, Barr & Wedenberg
1970–71	auditory brain stem response	Jewett & Williston
1971	performance-intensity functions for PB words	Jerger J & Jerger S
1972	Bekesy forward-backward	Jerger J, Jerger S, Mauldin
1974	tone decay	Olsen & Noffsinger
1974	Bekesy comfortable loudness (BCL)	Jerger J & Jerger S
1975	suprathreshold adaptation test (STAT)	Jerger J & Jerger S
1975	discovery of computerized tomography (CT)	Sir Hounsfield
1977–79	ABR in eighth nerve pathology	Selters & Brackmann; Clemis & McGee; Thomsen, Terkildsen, & Osterhammel, 1978 Terkildsen et al., 1977 Rosenhamer, 1977

Procedures and Principles

Alternate Binaural Loudness Balance (ABLB)

General Principles

- ☐ Test is performed to determine whether recruitment is present or absent, or whether decruitment is present.
- ☐ Compares loudness growth in an impaired ear versus a normal ear.
- ☐ Applicable only with patient having unilateral hearing loss.
- ☐ *Basic Principle:* intensity increases above threshold required to produce the sensation of equal loudness are much less for the impaired ear than the normal ear.

Background Information

- ☐ Concept first discovered in the mid-1930s:
  - ✔ Scott Reger (1935): Monaural loudness balance (MLB). Loudness growth compared between two frequencies in the same ear when there is impaired hearing at one frequency and normal hearing sensitivity at the other.
  - ✔ Edward Fowler (1936 & 1937): ABLB. Compares loudness growth between the two ears for the same frequency.
  - ✔ Began to be utilized as a site-of-lesion test in 1948 by Dix, Hallpike, and Hood.
- ☐ Physiological Bases (probable):
  - ✔ General consensus that the anatomic site responsible for abnormal loudness recruitment is at the hair cell level of the cochlea. However, the reason for its occurrence is a bit more controversial
  - ✔ Hair cell loss/dysfunction
  - ✔ Decoupling of stereocilia from tectorial membrane
  - ✔ 8th nerve function
  - ✔ Physiologic difference between OHC and IHC
  - ✔ CNS mechanisms

Test Administration

- ☐ Test is performed by alternating a pure tone between two ears, keeping the intensity in one ear (usually the good ear) fixed and varying the intensity in the other until the two tones are judged to be equally loud.
- ☐ The patient is told that he or she will hear two tones, one constant in loudness and one variable. Judgments in loudness are to be made only from the

variable tone to the reference. Patient's task is to state whether the variable tone is softer than, louder than or equal in loudness to the reference ear.

- ☐ Test begins at 20 dB SL in the fixed (normal hearing) ear.
- ☐ After equal loudness is judged, the intensity is increased in 20 dB increments until either the patient's tolerance level or the maximum output of the audiometer is reached.

Test Interpretation

- ☐ Findings plotted graphically using laddergrams.
  - ✔ *No Recruitment.* The decibel level between the two ears remains constant (i.e., intensity is raised by an equal amount above threshold for each ear).
  - ✔ *Complete Recruitment.* When equal loudness occurs at equal intensities (i.e. the patient perceives the stimuli to each ear as equally loud when the tones are at the same level-equal levels).
  - ✔ *Partial Recruitment.* When there is a decrease in the stimulus intensity difference between the two ears, but equal loudness for equal intensities is not reached.
  - ✔ *Decruitment/Derecruitment.* When an increase in intensity to the impaired ear is necessary to achieve equal loudness; thus, there is an increase in decibel difference between the two ears to achieve equal loudness.

- ☐ Significance of test results:
  - ✔ *Cochlear Pathology.* An abnormally rapid growth in loudness as the intensity of a pure tone is increased above threshold in the impaired ear. Typical findings are complete recruitment or partial recruitment.
  - ✔ *Retrocochlear Pathology.* An abnormally slow growth in loudness. This is a very rare finding, but it is positive for retrocochlear pathology. It is referred to as decruitment.

ABLB

- ☐ Advantages
  - ✔ Effective test of recruitment
  - ✔ Effective in detecting cochlear disorder
  - ✔ Easy and quick to administer

- ☐ Disadvantages
  - ✔ Cannot be administered in cases of bilateral hearing loss
  - ✔ Less effective in detecting retrocochlear pathology

Classic References

ABLB (Alternate Binaural Loudness Balance)

Dix M. Hallpike C, and Hood J. Observations upon the loudness recruitment phenomenon with especial reference to the differential diagnosis of disorders of the internal ear and the VIIIth nerve. *Journal of Laryngology and Otology 62:* 671-686, 1948.

Fowler EP. The diagnosis of diseases of the neural mechanism by the aid of sounds well above threshold. *Transactions of the American Otological Society 70:* 27-219, 1937.

Reger S. Loudness level contours and intensity discrimination of ears with raised auditory threshold. *Journal of the Acoustical Society of America 7:* 73 (Abstract), 1935.

Procedures and Principles

Short Increment Sensitivity Index (SISI)

General Principles

☐ Based on Difference Limen for Intensity (DLI). Defined as the increment in intensity of a sound in which the subject perceives a change in loudness 50% of the time.

☐ Designed to test the ear's ability to detect very small changes in intensity.

☐ Screening test to identify site of lesion as cochlear versus noncochlear.

Basic Principles

☐ *Normal auditory system.* Not as sensitive to changes in intensity when listening to low-level signals. Very sensitive to intensity changes when listening to high-level signals (can detect changes as small as 1 dB!).

☐ *Cochlear loss.* Individuals with cochlear loss are able to detect small increments in intensity (as small as 1 dB) at low sensation levels (dB SL).

Background Information

☐ Evolved indirectly from Fowler's description of "loudness recruitment" in 1936 and 1937.

☐ Evolved directly from work on differential sensitivity to intensity changes in the late 1940s and early 1950s (difference limens). Early work focused on difference limens as an indirect test of recruitment because a strong relationship was found between the ability to detect small changes in intensity and the presence of recruitment associated with cochlear hearing loss.

☐ Named SISI by Jerger et al. in 1952. Instead of studying the relationship between DLI and recruitment, they looked at whether sensitivity to small-changes in intensity was related to site of lesion within the auditory system. This type of work led to the more current forms of the test.

☐ Not trying to find the patient's difference limen, just trying to find the proportion of 1-dB increments (out of 20) the person can detect.

Test Administration

☐ Patient is instructed to indicate that he has heard a brief "jump" in the loudness of the tone.

☐ A continuous carrier tone is presented at 20 dB SL and the patient listens for brief presentations of an increment of the same pure tone frequency that is 1 dB greater in intensity, superimposed on the carrier tone.

- ☐ Before testing begins, increments of 5 dB and then 2 dB are presented to acquaint the patient with the task. Do not just begin testing at 1 dB increments.
- ☐ Increments are presented periodically (every 5 seconds) for a total of 20 increments of 1 dB at each frequency, for each ear.
- ☐ The percentage of 1 dB increments detected by the patient is calculated (Number of jumps detected multiplied by 5 = score).

Test Interpretation

- ☐ Scores:
  - 70% or greater = positive for cochlear pathology
  - 30% or less = negative for cochlear pathology
  - 30% to 70% = not strongly diagnostic/Inconclusive
- ☐ Patients with cochlear loss of less than 50 to 60 dB do not achieve high SISI scores, so a number of investigators used 75 to 90 dB SL instead of 20 dB SL. At this higher intensity level, patients with mild-to-moderate impairment were more likely to show a positive test outcome.
- ☐ Thompson (1963) first reported a high-intensity SISI technique. Found that when SISI was administered at 75 dB on two patients with surgically confirmed tumors and normal-hearing sensitivity bilaterally. Each patient achieved low scores whereas normal ears yielded high scores.
  - high scores (>70%) = normal cochlear function or cochlear pathology
  - low scores (<30%) = retrocochlear lesions

Advantages and Disadvantages

- ☐ Advantages
  - Easy and quick to administer. Shortened versions are available.
  - Fairly sensitive to cochlear pathology.
- ☐ Disadvantages
  - Conflicting reports on effectiveness. Predictive accuracy in 8th nerve pathology has traditionally been low, often at the level of chance, whereas normal-hearing persons can detect small intensity increments at high intensity levels, and patients with cochlea loss do not necessarily detect small increments at low intensity levels.
  - Best used as part of a test battery.
  - Limited understanding of physiological basis.
  - OHC (low threshold) vs. IHC (high threshold of excitability).

Classic References

SISI (Short Increment Sensitivity Index)

Jerger J, Shedd J, and Harford E. On the detection of extremely small changes in sound intensity. *Archives of Otolaryngology 69*: 200–211, 1959.

Luscher E, and Zwislocki J. A simple method for indirect monaural determination of the recruitment phenomenon (difference limen in intensity in different types of deafness). *Acta Oto-laryngologica (Stockholm) 78(Suppl.)*: 156–168, 1949.

Thompson GA. A modified SISI technique for selected cases with suspected acoustic neuroma. *J Speech Hear Dis 28*: 299–302, 1963.

Procedures and Principles

Tone decay tests

General Principles

- ☐ Based on auditory adaptation.
- ☐ Normal phenomenon in the auditory system.
- ☐ A perceived decrease in the loudness of a steady-state signal.
- ☐ Excessive tone decay. Observed by presenting a continuous tone in the ear and attempting to quantify the ability of the patient to sustain it over time.
- ☐ Quantified in two ways:
  - ✓ Measure amount of tone decay in dB (subtract beginning presentation level from ending level).
  - ✓ Measure "time to inaudibility" as a function of signal level. It may be due to neural degeneration or to space occupying lesions (such as tumor pressing against the 8th nerve). Other sites suggested include chemical synapse between hair cell and afferent 8th nerve fibers.

Background Information

- ☐ Gradenigo and Allen successfully distinguished cochlear from 8th nerve pathology using a rudimentary tone decay test in 1893.
- ☐ Tests were originally concerned only with measuring tone decay at or near threshold levels.

- ☐ Carhart (1957) developed the first widely used clinical test of tone decay.
- ☐ Several modifications of Carhart's classic tone decay test now exist.

Carhart Threshold Tone Decay Test

- ☐ Test Administration
  - Patient is instructed to raise hand when the tone is perceived and keep hand raised as long as the tone is heard.
  - Tone is initially presented below threshold and increased slowly in 5 dB steps until patient first responds.
  - As soon as patient responds, timing begins.
  - If the tone is heard for a full minute the test is terminated.
  - If the signal becomes inaudible and patient stops responding before the 1-minute period is over, the intensity is increased by 5 dB without interruption and timing is restarted.
  - Procedure continues until the patient is able to sustain the tone for 1 full minute or until the signal reaches 30 dBSL.
- ☐ Test Interpretation
  - Slow tone decay is associated with cochlear pathology (Carhart, 1957)
  - Marked or rapid decay is associated with retrocochlear pathology.
  - Tone decay in excess of 30 dB is very likely associated with retrocochlear pathology, regardless of its rapidity (Green, 1978).
  - The greater the number of frequencies involved, the greater the likelihood of retrocochlear involvement.
- ☐ Advantages
  - Several modifications exist to shorten test time.
  - Effective in identification of retrocochlear lesions.
  - Low cost and general accessibility.
- ☐ Disadvantages
  - Can be time consuming, possibly requiring as much as 4 to 4.5 minutes for each frequency tested.
  - No universal classification system for test findings.

Modifications of Carhart's Tone Decay Test

- ☐ Rosenberg (1958). Measures decay over a single 60-second time period. If the patient stops responding, the signal is increased without interruption. The amount of tone decay (in dB) occurring in 60 seconds is measured.

- ☐ Green (1963). Same as Rosenberg's 60 second test, but patients are instructed to raise hand at 90 degree angle to stimuli having tonal quality. If tone is still perceived, but has lost its tonality, the patient is to lower hand to 45 degree angle.

  - ✓ *Advantage:* Increases sensitivity of the test, especially in differentiating patients with abnormal decay due to retrocochlear lesions from those with cochlear lesions. Patients who have abnormal decay and lose tonality and audibility are more likely to have retrocochlear pathology than those who only lose tonality.

- ☐ Olsen-Noffsinger (1974). Same as Carhart test, but test begins at 20 dB SL rather than at threshold. This saves test time.

  - ✓ *Advantage:* Makes test easier for the patient because the tone is less difficult to perceive.

Owens Threshold Tone Decay Test

- ☐ Test Administration

  - ✓ Tone presentation begins at 5 dB SL.
  - ✓ If tone decays before the 60–second period, the stimulus is discontinued for 20 seconds before introduction of the tone at a 5 dB increment.
  - ✓ Procedure continues until the stimulus is perceived for 60 seconds or a level of 20 dB SL is reached.
  - ✓ Measures amount of tone decay in dB and time to inaudibility.

- ☐ Test Outcomes

  - ✓ TYPE I = Normal ears show little or no tone decay.
  - ✓ TYPE II = Cochlear pattern. Time to inaudibility increases when signal level increases.
  - ✓ TYPE III = Retrocochlear. Time to inaudibility is not affected by increases in signal level.

- ☐ Test Interpretation

  - ✓ Patients with retrocochlear disorders characteristically show decay at all frequencies and the rapidity of the decay does not change substantially with increases in intensity.
  - ✓ Patients with cochlear pathology show decay at one or two frequencies, but the decay is slower as intensity is increased.

- ☐ Advantages
  - Possible to differentiate between decay occurring with cochlear versus retrocochlear site of lesion.
  - Has specific classification system for results.
- ☐ Disadvantages
  - Less sensitive than Carhart and Olsen-Noffsinger for detection of retrocochlear pathology.

Classic References

Tone Decay

Carhart R. Clinical determination of abnormal auditory adaptation. *Archives of Otolaryngology, 65:* 32–39, 1957.

Gradenigo G, Allen SE. On the clinical signs of affections of the auditory nerve (German). *Archives of Otorhinolaryngology 22:* 213–215, 1893.

Green DS, The modified tone decay test (MTDT) as a screening procedure for eighth nerve lesions. *J Speech Hearing Disord 28:* 31–36, 1963.

Jerger J, Jerger S. A simplified tone decay test. *Archives Otolaryngolgy 101:* 403–407, 1975.

Olsen W, Noffsinger D. Comparison of one new and three old tests of auditory adaptation. *Archives Otolaryngolgy 99:* 94–99, 1974.

Rosenberg P. Abnormal auditory adaptation. *Archives Otolaryngolgy 94:* 89, 1971.

Procedures and Principles

Békèsy Audiometry

General Principles

- ☐ Based on auditory adaptation *and* difference limen for intensity.
- ☐ Used for determination of auditory thresholds and site of lesion testing.

Background Information

- ☐ Békèsy (1947) developed an audiometer that allowed threshold assessment by having patients record their own thresholds.
- ☐ Jerger (1960) delineated four distinct Bekesy tracings; a fifth was added later.

General Test Administration

- ☐ Patient is instructed to activate the intensity switch when the test tone is just heard and release the switch immediately when the test signal becomes inaudible.
- ☐ The audiometer automatically increases intensity 2.5 dB/sec—when the patient activates the switch, the intensity of the signal gradually decreases.
- ☐ The audiometer makes a graphic record of the patient's responses.
- ☐ Signal can be presented continuously or intermittently (pulsed) and the frequency of the signal can be swept across frequencies (sweep frequency) or remain at a constant frequency (fixed frequency).
- ☐ Threshold testing can be performed, although use of Békèsy tracings for site of lesion testing is the focus here.

Diagnostic Békèsy Audiometry

- ☐ Thresholds for continuous tone are compared to pulsed tone thresholds.
- ☐ ADAPTATION: The difference in threshold between pulsed and continuous tones is an index of tone decay.
- ☐ DLI: The difference in tracing width between pulsed and continuous tones. A narrower tracing for continuous tone is indicative of cochlear pathology.

Test Interpretation

☐ Five classical patterns:

- TYPE I. Continuous and pulsed tones are superimposed and the amplitudes (widths) are constant throughout the frequencies tested. This pattern is consistent with normal, conductive, or SNHL of unknown etiology.
- TYPE II. Continuous and pulsed tones are superimposed up to 1000 Hz; above this frequency the tracings for the continuous tone drop below the pulsed tracing by 20 dB or less and the amplitude of the continuous tracing becomes noticeable smaller. This pattern is consistent with SNHL due to cochlear pathology.
- TYPE III. Continuous tone tracing drops immediately and dramatically from that of the pulsed tone and sometimes falls to the limits of the audiometer. This pattern is consistent with retrocochlear auditory dysfunction, often due to acoustic neuroma or CPA tumor.
- TYPE IV. Early drop of the continuous tracing before 500 Hz; separation typically continues across frequency range but may interweave in the middle and high frequencies. Amplitude may or may not be reduced. This pattern is consistent with cochlear or retrocochlear auditory dysfunction.
- TYPE V. Thresholds for pulsed tracing are obtained at a higher intensity than the continuous tone tracing. The intensity level of the continuous tracing is suggestive of non-organic hearing loss.

Modifications of Békèsy Audiometry

☐ Reverse-sweep Békèsy

- Tones presented from high to low frequencies.
- With retrocochlear auditory dysfunction, more hearing loss is present in reverse-sweep mode than in the forward-sweep mode for continuous tone tracing. This pattern does not occur in all retrocochlear lesions.
- Also, in retrocochlear there is a discrepancy in low-high versus high-low tracings. Not all retrocochlear lesions will show this.
- Discrepancies are found more frequently with continuous tracings.
- Jerger also found discrepancies in cases of nonorganic loss.

Békèsy Comfortable Loudness (BCL)

- ☐ Developed in an effort to increase sensitivity for retrocochlear disorders.
- ☐ Békèsy audiograms are traced at suprathreshold levels rather than threshold levels.
- ☐ Patients respond when the signal is "uncomfortably loud" and stop responding when signal is less than "comfortably loud."
- ☐ Six types of tracings:
  - ✔ N1, N2, N3 patterns show no unusual adaptation for continuous vs. pulsed tones. This outcome is consistent with normal, conductive, mixed, and cochlear auditory dysfunction.
  - ✔ P1, P2, P3 patterns show an unusual adaptation for the continuous tone compared to the pulsed tone. This outcome is consistent with retrocochlear auditory dysfunction.
- ☐ Advantages
  - ✔ Documents patient's responses during the test.
  - ✔ Very effective in detecting cochlear disorders.
  - ✔ Several modifications available.
- ☐ Disadvantages
  - ✔ Cost of initial equipment purchase.
  - ✔ More involved calibration procedures required.
  - ✔ Some patients have difficulty responding appropriately due, for example, to tinnitus.
  - ✔ Value in identifying retrocochlear disorders is questionable.
  - ✔ Békèsy audiometers are not readily available in most audiology clinics today.

Classic Quote

James Jerger on the application of Békèsy audiometry in the analysis of auditory disorders

"Less than 14 years has elapsed since Bekesy's original description of a self-recording audiometer. Within this period, however, the technique of 'Bekesy audiometry' has rapidly gained the stature of a major clinical and research tool in audiology.

Bekesy audiometry refers to a method in which the subject traces his own auditory threshold by means of a suitable self-recording audiometer. The threshold tracing signal may be either a fixed-frequency or a gradually changing frequency, and the signal may be either continuous or periodically interrupted in time, but the essence of Bekesy's method is, first, that the signal intensity is always changing at a constant rate, and second, that the subject determines the direction of this change by alternately pressing and releasing a key that reverses the direction of a motor-driven attenuator. He is instructed to press this key when he just hears the tone and to release it when he just-no-longer hears it. By connecting a pen-writing system to the attenuator a graphic representation, or tracing, of the subject's successive threshold crossings may be obtained.

The Bekesy technique is particularly useful in psychoacoustics. It lends itself admirably, for example, to the measurement of temporary threshold shift following acoustic stimulation and has been so employed by several investigators. It finds use in the measurement of pure-tone masking.

Type I. The type I relationship is characterized by an interweaving or superposition of continuous and interrupted tracings, and by a tracing width which is constant over frequency and averages about 10 dB. There is, however, considerable variation about this mean value. Tracing widths as small as 3 dB and as large as 20 dB are not uncommon.

In the case of fixed-frequency tracings, the type I relationship is reflected in two interweaving, horizontal tracings.

Type II. Type II tracings differ from type I in two respects. First, the continuous tracing drops below the interrupted at high frequencies, but never to a substantial extent. The gap seldom exceeds 20 dB and ordinarily does not appear at frequencies below 1000 cps. Second, the width or amplitude of the continuous tracing is often quite small (3 to 5 dB) in these higher frequencies. This narrowing of the width or amplitude of the continuous tracing is, of course, the classical Bekesy sign thought by many to indicate the presence of loudness recruitment.

In fixed-frequency tracing the type II result is quite clear-cut. The interrupted tracing is, again, horizontal and of normal width, but the continuous trace drops from 5 to 20 dB below the interrupted, **within the first minute;** *thereafter, it maintains a fairly stable level. There is a reliable difference between interrupted and continuous tracings but the difference is relatively small and remains quite constant after the first 60 seconds of tracing. Furthermore, the difference appears only at mid- and high frequencies (that is, above 500 to 1000 cps).*

Type III. Type III tracings are quite dramatic. The continuous tracing drops below the interrupted to a remarkable degree. Furthermore, the two curves may diverge at relatively low frequencies (100 to 500 cps). It is not uncommon to observe the continuous tracing break away at a frequency as low as 150 cps and drop to a level as much as 40 to 50 dB below the interrupted tracing. The width of the continuous tracing ordinarily remains, however, quite normal.

In type III fixed-frequency tracings the interrupted tracing is horizontal but the continuous drops very rapidly and ordinarily does not stabilize at all. Typically, the continuous tracing begins at the same level as the interrupted but describes a rapidly descending trace to the limit of the equipment. A 40-to-50-dB drop within as little as 60 seconds is not unusual.

Type IV. Type IV tracings more closely resemble type II than type III but differ in one important respect. The continuous tracing falls consistently below the interrupted at frequencies below 500 cps. At higher frequencies the continuous may fall a constant distance below the interrupted, resembling a type II in this respect. The tracing width may or may not become abnormally small, further adding to possible confusion with type II. At mid- and high frequencies there may even be some overlap between C and I. The distinguishing feature, however, occurring in both conventional and fixed-frequency tracings, is the gap between C and I at relatively low frequencies (100 to 500 cps). Type IV tracings differ from type III tracings in that C ordinarily does not show a precipitous drop over time.

The vast majority of Bekesy tracings can be fitted into one of these four categories quite reliably. There are, however, a small number that, for one reason or another, do not appear to fit any of the four classic patterns. They may be designated by the label 'questionable.'"

Source: Jerger, J. Bekesy audiometry in analysis of auditory disorders. *Journal of Speech and Hearing Research 3*(3): 45–51, 1960. Reprinted by permission of the American Speech-Language-Hearing Association.

Traditional Diagnostic Audiometry

Accuracy of diagnostic audiometry procedures in correct identification of eighth nerve and cochlear pathology.

	Eighth Nerve		Cochlear	
Procedure	***N***	**%**	***N***	**%**
Short increment sensitivity index (SISI)	720	64	696	92
Tone decay *	737	64	2069	91
Alternate binaural loudness balance (ABLB)	620	68	1067	90
Phonetically balanced word recognition	737	69	250	60
Suprathreshold adaptation test (STAT)	20	70	75	83
Bekesy threshold tracing	44	84	327	96
Bekesy comfortable loudness (BCL)	16	80	101	97
Acoustic reflex**	126	85	218	84
Auditory brainstem response (ABR)	292	96	793	88

*Data for Carhart, Rosenberg, and Olsen/Noffsinger procedures were combined.
**Acoustic reflex threshold or decay.

ADR NOTE: Data for the number of subjects indicated were compiled in 1980 by JW Hall III from studies published up to that year.

The Demise of the Traditional Site-of-Lesion Diagnostic Audiology Test Battery

See Quasi-Classic Quote by Jay Hall in this chapter.

Four factors, occurring by chance in combination over a 2- or 3-year period in the mid-1970s, probably sank the good ship *Traditional Diagnostic Audiology.* They are:

- ☐ **Acoustic reflex measurement:** Clinical application of acoustic reflex measurement in differentiation of cochlear versus retrocochlear auditory dysfunction, including estimation of acoustic reflex threshold and assessment of acoustic reflex decay, became commonplace during the 1970s. Acoustic reflexes very quickly yielded information acquired much more slowly by most of the traditional diagnostic procedures, and were more accurate to boot. (See Traditional Site-of-Lesion Tests in this chapter.)

- ☐ **Auditory brainstem response:** By 1978, an international group of investigators had independently and conclusively shown that the ABR was far more sensitive to retrocochlear auditory dysfunction than the entire traditional site-of-lesion test battery combined. (See Traditional Site-of-Lesion Tests in this chapter.)
- ☐ **CT:** The emergence of computerized tomography (CT) in most major medical centers toward the end of the 1970s and beginning of the 1980s provided a radiologic technique for detection and localization of relatively small neoplasms within posterior fossa and auditory brainstem. By the mid-1980s, magnetic resonance imaging (MRI) began to replace CT scans as the "gold standard" for neuroradiology. These radiologic procedures, especially when applied with techniques for enhancement of small tumors, have even posed a threat to the diagnostic value of the ABR. (See Chapter 16 for more information on CT and MRI.)
- ☐ **Inadequate test performance:** The end of the 1970s saw increased appreciation of the important of test performance characteristics (disease prevalence, sensitivity, specificity, positive and negative predictive value) in the selection of diagnostic procedures in audiology, and medicine in general. Unfortunately, the traditional diagnostic audiology test battery appeared rather shabby when viewed from this nonsentimental perspective. (See Test Performance in this chapter for details on the test performance.)

Quasi-Classic Quote

Jay Hall on the demise of the traditional site-of-lesion diagnostic audiology test battery

"It is tempting to valiantly argue, as have others (Brunt, 1985; Green, 1985; Martin, 1985) that the classic site-of-lesion test battery, or at least one or two procedures, still has a role in diagnostic audiometry, albeit a more limited and less glorious role than in years past. Few audiologists would suggest that we regress to a state-of-the-art that is 20 or 30 years outdated, but there is nevertheless a tendency to look back longingly on the good old days of diagnostic audiology. Nostalgia, however, has no place in modern auditory or otologic neurodiagnosis. Current technology and procedures, including acoustic reflexes and auditory evoked responses, are by no means perfect, but improved neurodiagnosis will be found only in the future and not in the past."

Source: Hall JW III. Classic site-of-lesion tests. In WF Rintelmann (Ed.), *Hearing assessment* (2nd ed.). Needham Heights, MD: Allyn & Bacon, 1991, p. 669.

DIAGNOSTIC AUDIOLOGY TODAY

Diagnostic Audiology Strategy

The Major Steps in Diagnostic Assessment

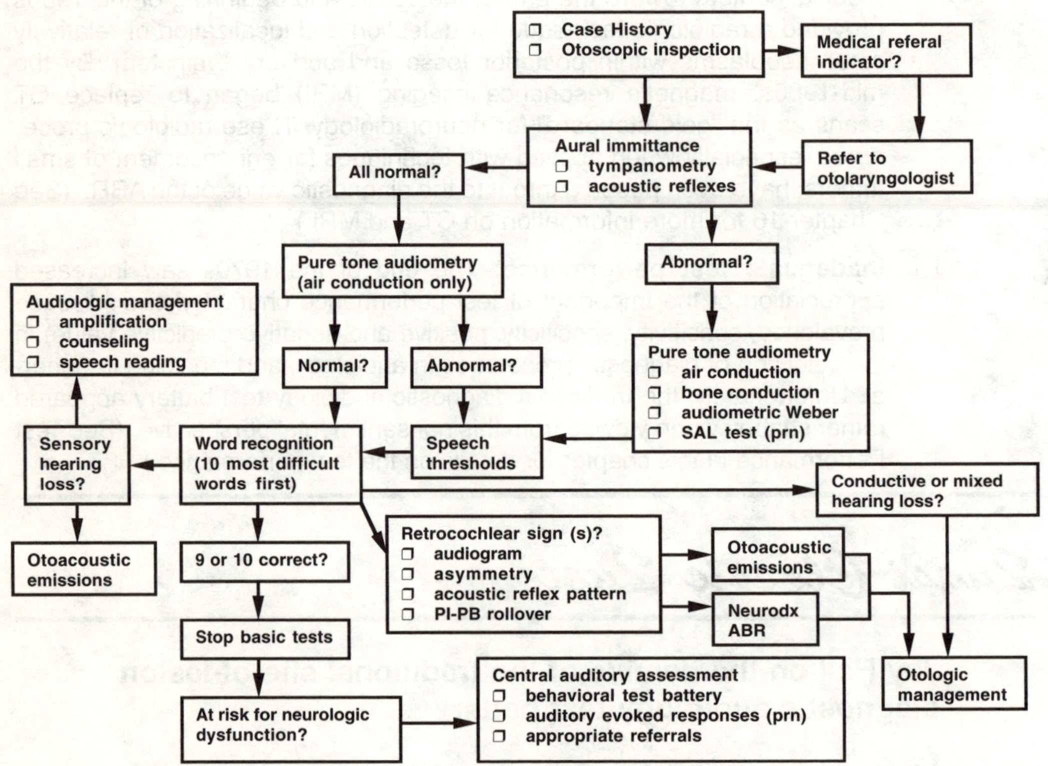

Test Battery Patterns

Contribution of state-of-the art test procedures to the diagnostic audiology test battery in various sites of lesions. Note the unique findings for certain procedures relative to others.

KEY: normal ○; maybe abnormal ⊘; abnormal ●

DIAGNOSTIC AUDIOLOGY TEST BATTERY PATTERNS

TEST PROCEDURE	SITE OF LESION					
	Middle ear	Cochlea	Eighth nerve	Brainstem Caudal	Brainstem Rostral	Cerebrum
Aural Immittance						
tympanometry	●	○	○	○	○	○
acoustic reflexes	●	⊘	●	⊘	○	○
Pure tone audiometry	⊘	●	⊘	○	○	○
Word recognition	○	⊘	⊘	○	○	○
Otoacoustic emissions	●	●	○	○	○	○
Diagnostic speech audiometry	○	○	●	●	●	●
Evoked Responses						
ECochG	⊘	⊘	○	○	○	○
ABR	●	⊘	●	●	●	○
AMLR	○	○	○	○	○	●
P300/MMN	○	○	○	○	○	●

Pediatric Audiology Test Battery Patterns

Contribution of test procedures to the pediatric diagnostic audiology test battery in different diseases. Note the unique findings for certain procedures relative to others. For example, otoacoustic emissions (OAE) may confirm normal cochlear function in patients with retrocochlear dysfunction (e.g. developmental delay) and abnormal ABR findings.

KEY: normal ○ maybe abnormal ⊘ abnormal ●	PEDIATRIC AUDIOLOGY TEST BATTERY PATTERNS					
	DISORDER / DISEASE					
TEST PROCEDURE	Otitis media	Meningitis	CMV	Hyper-bilirubinemia	Developmental Delay	Degenerative Disease
Aural Immittance						
tympanometry	●	○	○	○	○	○
acoustic reflexes	●	⊘	●	⊘	⊘	⊘
Pure tone audiometry	●	⊘	⊘	⊘	⊘	⊘
Word recognition	⊘	⊘	⊘	⊘	⊘	⊘
Otoacoustic emissions	●	⊘	⊘	⊘	○	○
Diagnostic speech audiometry	○	⊘	●	●	●	●
Evoked Responses						
ABR	●	⊘	●	●	●	●
AMLR	NA	⊘	⊘	⊘	●	●
P300/MMN	NA	⊘	⊘	⊘	●	●

Tests for Pseudohypacusis

Tests developed for use with patients suspected of pseudohypacusis (this group of patients is also sometimes referred by other terms, including malingerers, fakers, crocks, and patients with non-organic hearing loss)

Tests	Appropriate Laterality of Suspected Hearing Loss
Basic audiometry	
☐ Test-retest reliability of pure tone thresholds	Unilateral or bilateral
☐ Speech reception threshold vs. PTA agreement	Unilateral or bilateral
☐ Failure to demonstrate shadow curve	Unilateral
Immittance measures	
☐ Acoustic reflex threshold	Unilateral or bilateral
☐ Sensitivity prediction by the acoustic reflex (SPAR)	Unilateral or bilateral
Otoacoustic emissions (OAE)	
☐ Transient evoked OAE	Unilateral or bilateral
☐ Distortion product OAE	Unilateral or bilateral
Bekesy Audiometry	
☐ Type V pattern	Unilateral or bilateral
☐ Lengthened off-time (LOT) Bekesy	Unilateral or bilateral
☐ Bekesy Ascending-Descending Gap Evaluation (BADGE)	Unilateral or bilateral
Tests specifically for pseudohypacusis	
☐ Speech or pure-tone Stenger	Unilateral
☐ Doerfler-Stewart	Unilateral or bilateral
☐ Lombard reflex	Unilateral or bilateral
☐ Delayed auditory feedback with speech	Unilateral or bilateral
☐ Delayed auditory feedback with pure tones	Unilateral or bilateral
☐ Swinging story	Unilateral

Psuedo-Classic Quote

Motto of the Vanderbilt Audiology Clinics.

"We can, and will, evaluate the hearing of any patient, of any age, at any time, and in any place!"

ACOUSTIC TUMORS AND OTHER DISORDERS

Facts and Figures

Acoustic tumors

☐ The average rate of tumor growth for a group of 51 patients with confirmed, untreated, unilateral acoustic tumors was 0.11 cm per year. The range of growth rate was 0 to 1.1 cm per year.

Source: Strasnick B, Glasscock ME, Haynes D, McMenomey SO, Minor LB. The natural history of untreated acoustic neuromas. *Laryngoscope 104:* 1115–1119, 1994.

☐ "In this study, the overall sensitivity in 40 consecutive acoustic neuromas was 85%. While the ABR was abnormal in 96% of our patients with extracanalicular tumors, it detected only 67% of those with intracanalicular tumors.* However, most patients with intracanalicular acoustic neuromas exhibited significantly reduced caloric responses on the affected side on ENG, indicating superior vestibular nerve tumor origin . . . .When the ABR is abnormal, suggesting retrocochlear pathology, and the EMRI is normal, it is advisable to follow the patient at regular intervals for signs of continued or progressive symptoms."

Source: Wilson DF, Hodgson RS, Gustafson MF, Hogue S, Mills L. The sensitivity of auditory brainstem response testing in small acoustic neuromas. *Laryngoscope 102:* 961–964, 1992.

***ADR note:** tumor size in these patients ranged from 3.0 to 13.0 mm*

☐ "Although most patients with acoustic neuromas will present with a sensorineural hearing loss in the affected ear and an abnormal ABR, approximately 5% of patients will have a normal pure tone audiogram, and at least 2% of patients will have a normal ABR."

Source: Telian SA, Kileny PR, Niparko JK, Kemink JL, Graham MD. Normal auditory brainstem response in patients with acoustic neuroma. *Laryngoscope 99:* 10–14, 1989, p. 13.

***ADR note:** data for 93 patients with confirmed acoustic neuromas for whom ABR data were available.*

Anatomy of the Internal Auditory Canal (IAC)

Note the relation of the cochlear (auditory) portion of the eighth cranial nerve to other structures within the IAC.

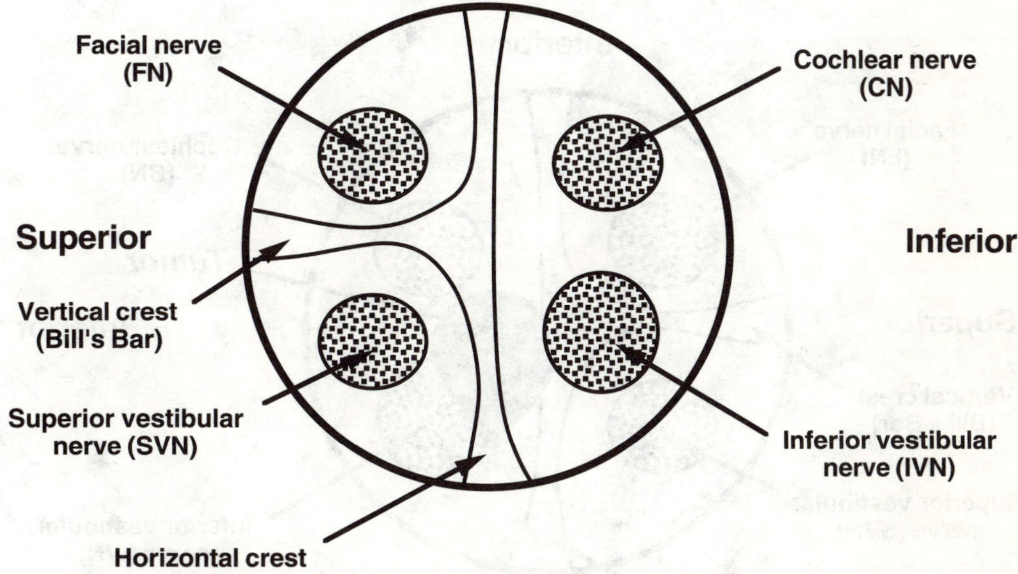

Acoustic Neuroma

An acoustic tumor (neuroma) within the internal auditory canal (IAC) in relation to the cochlear (auditory) nerve. An acoustic tumor is in most cases a vestibular schwannoma (arising from the Schwann cells or sheath of a vestibular nerve).

Right Side

ACOUSTIC NEUROMA ORIGINATING FROM THE INFERIOR VESTIBULAR NERVE

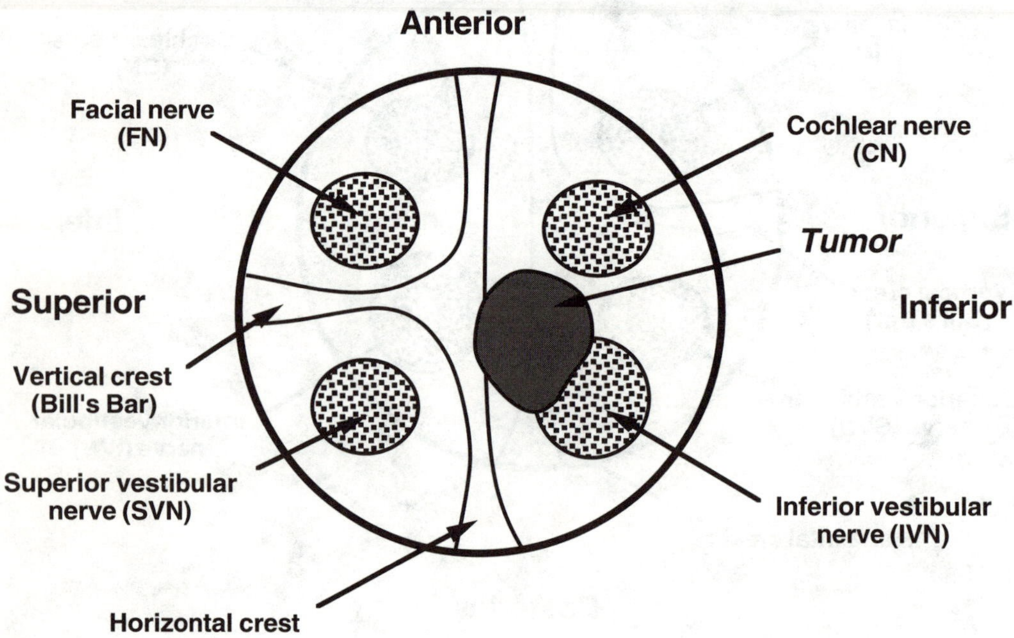

Acoustic Neuroma

Source of most acoustic tumors (neuromas) within the internal auditory canal (IAC), relative to the cochlear (auditory) nerve. The commonest acoustic tumor is really a vestibular schwannoma arising from the superior vestibular nerve.

Right Side

ACOUSTIC NEUROMA ORIGINATING FROM THE SUPERIOR VESTIBULAR NERVE

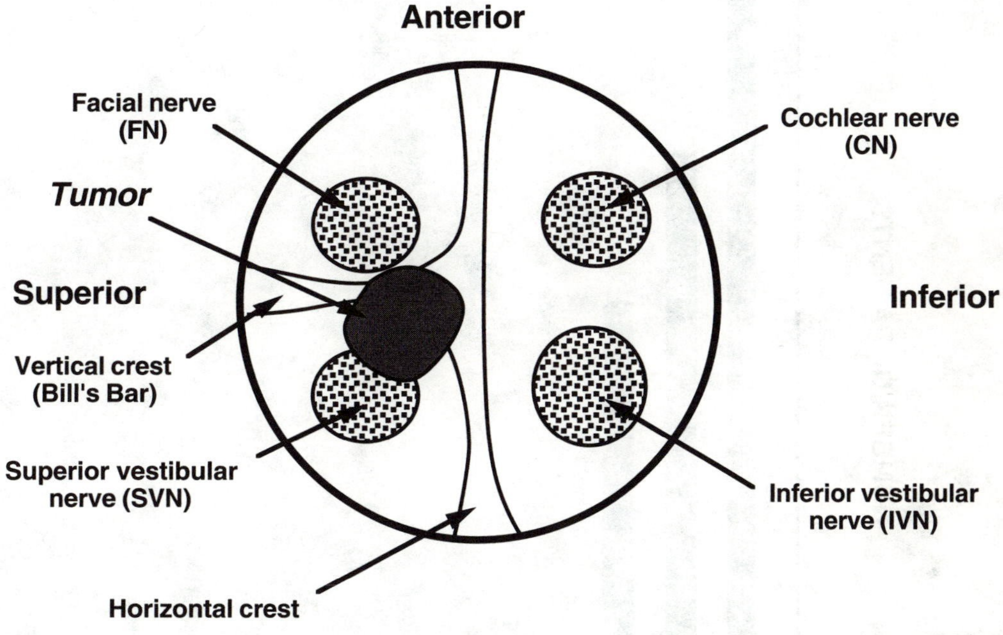

Growth Rates of Acoustic Neuromas

Most acoustic neuromas are very slow growing tumors, growing less than 0.2 cm (2 mm) per year. This graph shows the distribution of 50 patients over a 1-year period. (Adapted from Strasnick B, Glasscock ME, Haynes D, McMenomey SO, Minor LB. The natural history of untreated acoustic neuromas. *Laryngoscope 104:* 1115–1119, 1994.)

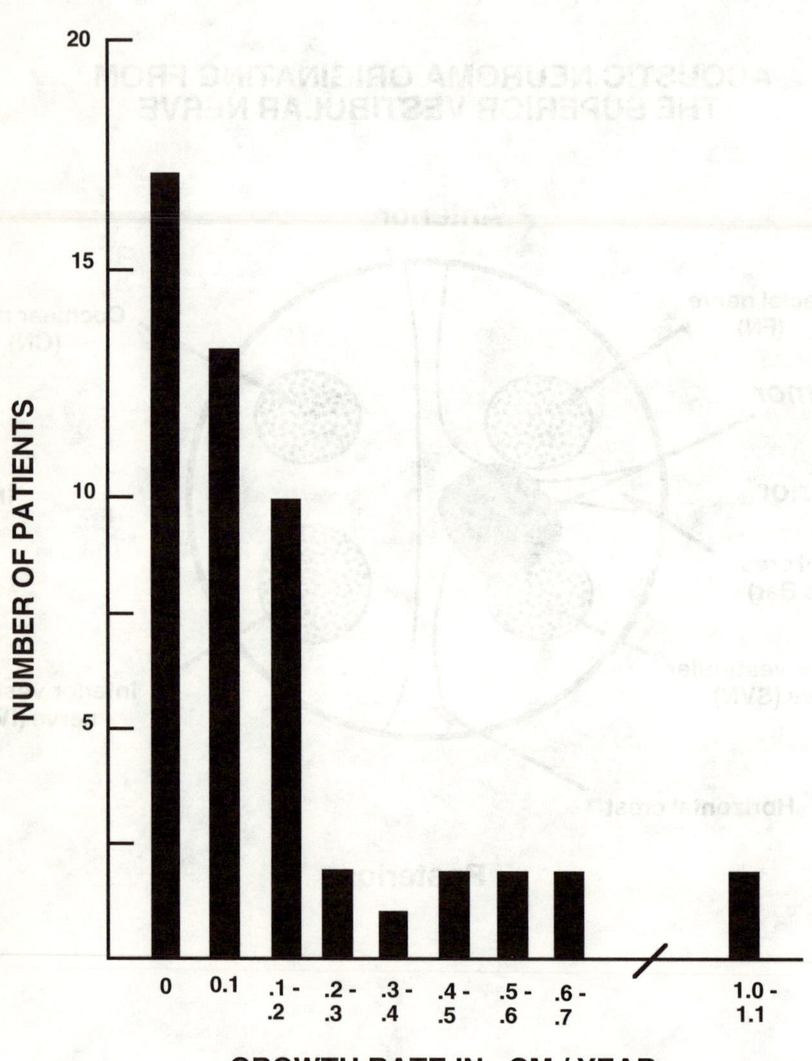

False-Positive MRI in Suspected Retrocochlear Pathology

Data are limited to published reports. These are patients diagnosed with tumors by MRI who did not actually have tumors.The extent of unreported data on false-positive "gold standards" can only be conjectured.

Study, Year	No. of patients	Radiology	Actual Pathology
von Glass et al., 1991	2	Gd-MRI	arachnoiditis
Haberman & Kramer, 1989	case report	CT, MRI	vascular loop compression
Prasher & Gibson, 1983	case report	CT	?
Crain & Dolan, 1990	case report	CT	Paget's disease
Loftus & Wazen, 1990	case report	Gd-MRI	chronic inflammation between flocculus and eighth nerve

ABR in Retrocochlear Pathology

Optimal Criteria

Criteria that most efficiently differentiate patients at low risk for retrocochlear pathology (normal audiometry and radiology) versus those with confirmed retrocochlear pathology.

ABR Variable	Criterion (in msec)	95% Confidence Limit* (in msec)
I–III	2.65	2.52
I–V (female)	4.69	4.34
I–V (male)	4.68	4.46
Interaural latency difference (ILD) for wave V	0.43	0.37
Rate latency shift for wave V (11/sec to 44/sec)	0.45	0.44
Rate latency shift for wave V (11/sec to 88/sec)	0.75	0.81

*Derived from the group without confirmed retrocochlear pathology.
Source: Lightfoot GR. ABR screening for acoustic neuromata: The role of rate-induced latency shift measurements. *British Journal of Audiology 26*: 217–227, 1992.

False-Negative ABR Findings in Retrocochlear Pathology

Recent Studies Utilizing Current Radiologic Techniques. Also see False-Positive MRI in this chapter.

Study, Year	No. of Patients	False-Negative Rate
Bockenheimer et al., 1984	19*	26%
Legatt et al., 1988	39	10%
Grabel et al., 1991	56	11%
Gillen et al., 1991	49	0%
Telian et al., 1992	93	2%

*Small tumors.
Source: Adapted from Jacobson & Reams, 1986.

ADR NOTE: False negative findings for ABR are dependent on at least five variables: (1) Size of tumor, (2) Site of tumor (e.g., Intra- versus extracanalicular), (3) Origin of tumor (e.g., Superior versus inferior vestibular nerve versus meninges), (4) "Gold standard" for confirmation of pathology (e.g., CT, enhanced CT, MRI, gadolinium-enhanced MRI), and (5) ABR measurement strategy and analysis criteria (e.g., slow versus fast stimulus rate, ILD V versus I–V latency interval).

Clinical Concept

ABR Findings in Patients with Confirmed Acoustic Neuromas (*N* = 93)

"Although most patients with acoustic neuromas will present with a sensorineural hearing loss in the affected ear and an abnormal ABR, approximately 5% of patients will have a normal pure tone audiogram, and at least 2% of patients will have a normal ABR."

Source: Telian SA, Kileny PR, Niparko JK, Kemink JL, Graham MD. Normal auditory brainstem response in patients with acoustic neuroma. *Laryngoscope 99*: 10–14, 1989, p. 13.

ABR Findings

Patients with Confirmed Acoustic Neuromas (*N* = 93)

ABR Finding	No. of Patients	% Percent of Sample
Normal (e.g., false-positive)	2	2
Wave I–V latency abnormally delayed	36	39
Abnormal wave V interaural latency difference (only wave V present; no wave I)	17	18
Absent waves II–V with adequate hearing sensitivity	12	13
Wave V absent	1	1
No ABR observed (profound SNHL)	25	27

Source: Data from Telian SA, Kileny PR, Niparko JK, Kemink JL, Graham MD. Normal auditory brainstem response in patients with acoustic neuroma. *Laryngoscope 99*: 10–14, 1989.

Key References

Radiologic vs. ABR Findings in Retrocochlear Auditory Pathology

Loftus B, Wazen JJ. A false-positive gadolinium-enhanced MRI: Acoustic neuroma versus cochleovestibular neuritis. *Otolaryngology—Head and Neck Surgery 103:* 299, 1990.

Crain MR, Dolan KD. Internal auditory canal enlargement in Paget's disease apearing as bilateral acoustic neuromas. *Annals of Otology Rhinology and Laryngology 99*: 833–834, 1990.

Haberman RS, Kramer MB. False-positive MRI and CT findings of an acoustic neuroma. *American Journal of Otology 10*: 301–303, 1989.

Legatt AD, Pedley TA, Emerson RG, Stein BM, Abramson M. Normal brain-stem auditory evoked potentials with abnormal latency-intensity studies in patients with acoustic neuromas. *Archives of Neurology 45*: 1326–1330, 1988.

Strasnick B, Glasscock ME, Haynes D, McMenomey SO, Minor LB. The natural history of untreated acoustic neuromas. *Laryngoscope 104*: 1115–1119, 1994.

Telian SA, Kileny PR, Niparko JK, Kemink JL, Graham MD. Normal auditory brainstem response in patients with acoustic neuroma. *Laryngoscope 99*: 10–14, 1989.

Wilson DF, Hodgson RS, Gustafson MF, Hogue S, Mills L. The sensitivity of auditory brainstem response testing in small acoustic neuromas. *Laryngoscope 102*: 961–964, 1992.

Clinical Concept

MRI Findings and Small Acoustic Tumors

Gadolinium-enhanced magnetic resonance imaging (MRI) will identify acoustic neuromas which are not likely to become symptomatic. Most are very small (e.g., just a few millimeters) tumors that may grow slowly (e.g., 1 mm per year). Tumor regression may actually occur in a small percentage of cases.

Presenting Symptoms

Patients with Confirmed Acoustic Tumors (N = 51)

Hearing loss	85%
Tinnitus	66%
Vertigo	63%
Ear fullness	47%

Source: Strasnick B, Glasscock ME, Haynes D, McMenomey SO, Minor LB. The natural history of untreated acoustic neuromas. *Laryngoscope 104:* 1115–1119, 1994.

Patterns of Auditory Abnormalities in Multiple Sclerosis

Complete references are listed in Key References: Multiple sclerosis on the following page

Investigator(s)	Year	No. of Subjects	Percent Abnormal *			
			ABR	AR	SA	MLD
Jerger et al.	1986	62	52	71	55	45*
Gollegly et al.	1985	33	63	27	41	52
Kofler	1985	119	74	—	—	—
Oberascher	1985	72	—	64	—	—
Grenman et al.	1984	53	40	32	0	—
Kofler et al.	1984	47	72	64	—	—
Russolo and Poli	1983	20	80	65	55	—
Hannley et al.	1983	20	75	44	25	75
Kjaer	1983	58	78	—	—	—
Parving et al.	1981	13	0	—	—	—
Purves et al.	1981	33	45	—	—	—
Chiappa et al.	1980	81	47	—	—	—
Hausler and Levine	1980	29	62	—	3	—
Maurer et al.	1980	27	89	—	—	—
Tackmann et al.	1980	23	26	—	—	—
Hess	1979	20	—	33	—	—
Lacquaniti et al.	1979	25	64	—	—	—
Robinson and Rudge	1977	51	63	—	—	—
Stockard et al.	1977	30	93	—	—	—
Olsen et al.	1976	100	—	—	—	47
Coletti	1975	13	—	69	0	—
Olsen et al.	1975	31	—	—	19	—
Noffsinger et al.	1972	61	—	—	24	49
Dayal and Swisher	1967	14	—	—	36	—
Average**			61	50	23	56

*ABR = auditory brainstem response; AR = acoustic reflex; SA = speech audiometry; MLD = masking level difference

**Jerger et al. study excluded.

Source: Jerger J, Oliver TA, Chmiel RA, Rivera VM. Patterns of auditory abnormality in multiple sclerosis. *Audiology, 25*, 193–209, 1986. Reprinted with permission.

Key References

Auditory Findings in Multiple Sclerosis

Chiappa KH, Harrison JL, Brooks EB, & Young RR. Brainstem auditory evoked responses in 200 patients with multiple sclerosis. *Annals of Neurology 7:* 135–143, 1980.

Coletti V. Stapedius reflex abnormalities in multiple sclerosis. *Audiology 14:* 63–71, 1975.

Gollegly KM, Kibbe-Michal K, Reeves AG, & Musiek, FE. Auditory behavioral and electrophysiological results in multiple sclerosis. Paper presented at the ASHA Convention, Washington, DC, 1985.

Grenman R, Lang H, Panelius M, Salmivally A, Laine H, & Rintamaki, J. Stapedius reflex and brainstem auditory evoked responses in multiple sclerosis patients. *Scandinavian Audiology 1*3: 109–113, 1984.

Hannley M, Jerger JF, & Rivera VM. Relationships among auditory brain stem responses, masking level differences and the acoustic reflex in multiple sclerosis. *Audiology 22:* 20–33, 1983.

Hausler R, & Levine, RA. Brain stem auditory potentials are related to interaural time discrimination in patients with multiple sclerosis. *Brain Research 191:* 589–594, 1980.

Hess K. Stapedius reflex in multiple sclerosis. *Journal of Neurology, Neurosurgery Psychiatry 42:* 331–337, 1979.

Kjaer M. Evoked potentials. With special reference to the diagnostic value in multiple sclerosis. *Acta Neurologica Scandinavia 67:* 67–89, 1983.

Kofler, B. (1985). Visuell und akustisch evozierte Potentiale bei der multiplen Sklerose. *Wien. Med. Wschr. 135:* 35-38.

Kofler F, Oberascher G, & Pommer B. Brain-stem involvement in multiple sclerosis: A comparison between brain-stem auditory evoked potentials and the acoustic stapedius reflex. *Journal of Neurology 231:* 145–147, 1984.

Lacquaniti F, Benna P, Gilli M, Troni W, & Bergamasco B. Brain stem auditory evoked potentials and blink reflex in quiescent multiple sclerosis. *Electroenceph. Clin. Neurophysiol. 47:* 607–610, 1979.

Maurer K, Schafer E, Hopf HC, & Leitner H. The location by early auditory evoked potentials (EAEP) of acoustic nerve and brainstem demyelination in multiple sclerosis (MS). *Journal of Neurology 223:* 43–58, 1980.

Oberascher G. Otoneurologische Untersuchungsmoglichkeiten bei der multiplen Sklerose. *Wien. Med. Wschr. 135:* 31–33, 1985.

Olsen WO, Noffsinger D, & Carhart R. Masking level differences encountered in clinical populations. *Audiology 15:* 287–301, 1976.

Parving A, Elberling C, & Smith T. Auditory electrophysiology: Findings in multiple sclerosis. *Audiology 20:* 123–142, 1981.

Purves SJ, Low MD, Galloway J, & Reeves B. A comparison of visual, brainstem auditory, and somatosensory evoked potential in multiple sclerosis. *Can J. Neurol. Sci. 8:* 15–19, 1981.

Robinson K, & Rudge P. The early components of the auditory evoked potential in multiple sclerosis. *Prog. Clin. Neurophysiol. 2:* 58–67, 1977.

Russolo M, & Poli P. Lateralization, impedance, auditory brainstem response, and synthetic sentence audiometry in brainstem disorders. *Audiology 22*: 50–62, 1983.

Stockard JJ, Stackard JE, & Sharbrough FW. Detection and localization of occult lesions with brainstem auditory lesions. *Mayo Clin Proc 52:* 761–769, 1977.

Tackmann W, Strenge H, Barth R, & Sojka-Raytscheff A. Auditory brain stem evoked potentials in patients with multiple sclerosis. *Eur. Neurol. 19:* 396–401, 1980.

OBSCURE AUDITORY DYSFUNCTION (OAD)

Clinical Concept

Obscure Auditory Dysfunction (OAD)

See Key References: OAD later in this chapter for sources of more information, and tables for details on assessment.

Some patients who seek professional (e.g., audiologic or otolaryngologic) help for self-reported auditory disability and handicap have pure tone audiograms that are within clinically defined normal limits. In 1989, Englishwoman Gabrielle Saunders and colleagues coined the term "Obscure Auditory Dysfunction" (OAD) to describe this syndrome. Dr. Saunders developed a special test battery for audiologic assessment of persons suspected of OAD. Several investigations yielded group data confirming *"sensory and cognitive underlying genuine performance deficit for understanding speech-in-noise, but that personality-related factors also played an important role in explaining OAD"* (Saunders & Haggard, 1993, p. 242).

Source: Saunders GH. Determinants of objective and subjective auditory disability in patients with normal hearing. Ph.D. Thesis. Nottingham, England: University of Nottingham, 1989; Saunders GH, Haggard MP. The assessment of "Obscure Auditory Dysfunction": Auditory and psychological factors. *Ear and Hearing 10:* 200–208, 1989. Saunders GH, Haggard MP. The influence of personality-related factors upon consultation for two different "marginal" organic pathologies with and without reports of auditory symptomatology. *Ear and Hearing 14:* 242–248, 1993.

Assessment of OAD

Audiologic Test Battery

See Key References: OAD later in this ADR chapter for sources of more information.

Procedure	Description
Pure tone audiogram	Air conduction thresholds from 125 to 8000 Hz
Otoacoustic emissions (OAE)	Transient or distortion product OAE. Note: According to Saunders, OAE do not consistently provide diagnostic information in OAD assessment.
Auditory frequency selectivity at 2000 Hz	Measurement of frequency resolution by comparing a masked threshold within a broad band noise (1) versus a masked threshold within notched noise (2). Frequency resolution = masked threshold (1) − 2 masked threshold (2).
Binaural masking level difference (BMLD)	Measurement of binaural processing that takes into account the peripheral and (BMLD) central mechanisms of localization
Gap detection	Measurement of temporal resolution ability at 500 Hz
Audiovisual adaptive sentences test	Measurement of lipreading ability
Word monitoring in sentences (WMIS)	A measure of a person's reaction time in using context during linguistic processing
Pseudo-free-field speech-in-noise test (PFFIN)	Measurement of adaptive speech reception thresholds in noise (SRTN) in two conditions: (1) Performance condition = measurement of 50% SRTN to test actual speech discrimination ability = PFFIN (I) (2) Self-assessed condition = determination of subject's estimate of his/her own hearing ability = PPFIN (ii) (3) A third derived variable = The difference between (1) and (2) = an esimate of the degree to which the subject misjudges his/her hearing ability = PFFIN (iii)

Source: Saunders GH, Haggard MP. The assessment of "Obscure Auditory Dysfunction": Auditory and psychological factors. *Ear and Hearing 10:* 200–208, 1989; Sanders GH, Haggard MP. The Assessment of "Obscure Auditory Dysfunction" (OAD): Case-control analysis of determining factors. *Ear and Hearing 13:* 241–254, 1992.

Four Possible Underlying Explanations

Obscure Auditory Dysfunction (OAD)

- ☐ Central auditory processing disorders (CAPD) and possible associated learning disabilities
  - ✔ R/O (rule out) with comprehensive CAPD assessment (see Chapter 11)
- ☐ Psychological or anxiety problems
  - ✔ R/O with psychology or psychoeducational consult
- ☐ Situational hearing loss
  - ✔ consider a dramatic changes in lifestyle, listening setting, or work setting as contributing factor to OAD
  - ✔ provide helpful tips, counseling, and support
  - ✔ management strategies may include: earplugs in noisy conditions, assistive listening device in large noisy rooms, improvement of office acoustics, listening strategies (close to speaker, clear view of speaker)
- ☐ Unidentified peripheral auditory dysfunction
  - ✔ perform diagnostic otoacoustic emissions (OAE) assessment (see Chapter 5)
  - ✔ obtain complete history
  - ✔ consider otologic risk factors, including as infant or child
  - ✔ R/O tinnitus
  - ✔ R/O aspirin use
  - ✔ R/O other potentially ototoxic medications
  - ✔ R/O exposure to high level noise and/or music

Key References

Obscure Auditory Dysfunction (OAD)

Saunders GH. Determinants of objective and subjective auditory disability in patients with normal hearing. Doctoral thesis. Nottingham, England: University of Nottingham, 1989.

Saunders GH, Haggard MP. The assessment of "Obscure Auditory Dysfunction". Auditory and psychological factors. *Ear and Hearing 10:* 200–208, 1989.

Saunders GH, Field DS, Haggard MP. A clinical test battery for Obscure Auditory Dysfunction (OAD): Development, selection and use of the tests. *British Journal of Audiology 26:* 33–47, 1992.

Saunders GH, Haggard MP. The assessment of "Obscure Auditory Dysfunction" (OAD). Case-control analysis of determining factors. *Ear and Hearing 13:* 241–254, 1992.

Saunders GH, Haggard MP. The influence of personality-related factors upon consultation for two different "marginal" organic pathologies with and without reports of auditory symptomatology. *Ear and Hearing 14:* 242–248, 1993.

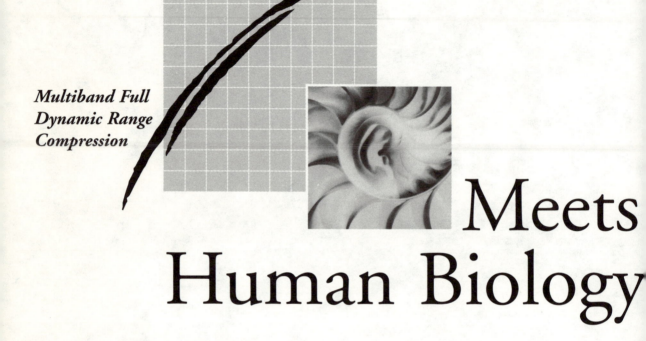

CHAPTER 13

Electroneuronography (ENoG)

In This ADR Chapter

Perspective

Electroneuronography (ENoG)

Some audiologists, particularly those in medical settings, perform electroneuronography (ENoG) as a clinical service. This clinical activity is within the current scope of practice for audiology (the American Academy of Audiology and the American Speech-Language-Hearing Association statements on Scope of Practice are republished in an appendix of the ADR).

Audiologist involvement in the measurement of facial nerve function, and neurodiagnostic application of facial nerve findings, is certainly not new, or unprecedented. In the early 1970s, the diagnostic value of acoustic reflex pattern analysis was confirmed by an international collection of investigators. Erik Borg's careful investigations of the acoustic reflex arc clearly identified the facial nerve, and corresponding nuclei in the pons of the brain stem, as crucial components for recording the acoustic stapedial reflex. Within a few years, there were clinical papers documenting the expected abnormal acoustic reflex pattern in patients with Bell's palsy, and other pathologies affecting the facial nerve (e.g., large acoustic tumors). Current application of ENoG in facial nerve assessment by audiologists is really an extension of these early efforts to expand the diagnostic capabilities of audiologists.

Another factor contributing to the involvement of audiologists in ENoG is the similarity in the instrumentation required for measurement of ENoG and the auditory brainstem response (ABR). Although it is in some respects a case of technological overkill, sophisticated evoked response systems are typically used to record ENoG. With the addition of a somatosensory-evoked response option, which includes an electrical stimulus package, a conventional evoked response system available from a number of manufacturers is adequately equipped for recording ENoG.

In 1982, the first author had access to such an evoked response system, purchased to record somatosensory-evoked responses from severely head-injured patients in the intensive care unit setting. A neurotology colleague and co-worker came back from a scientific meeting where ENoG studies had been reported and expressed interest in introducing this service in our clinic. A quick review of the literature revealed several articles by Dr. Fisch (described briefly in this chapter). Within weeks, we were recording ENoG on the occasional patient with severe facial nerve dysfunction who met the criteria, as detailed Brackmann (defined in a table in this chapter).

The first impression of many clinicians (e.g., me) is that ENoG recording is like taking candy from a baby. Using a hand-held set of stimulus electrodes (in Texas we called it the "cattle prod," away from the ears of anxious patients, of course), stimulation of the stylomastoid foramen region seemed easy enough. And the response was enormous. After analyzing ABR amplitudes on the order of 0.5 microvolt, a healthy ENoG of over 1000 microvolts was almost surreal. As it turned out, ignorance was bliss. The more we learned about ENoG, and facial nerve anatomy and pathophysiology, the more sobering clinical ENoG recordings became.

Before you first attempt to apply ENoG in clinical assessment of facial nerve function, take the time to read the information this chapter, consult an otology text for more details on facial nerve anatomy and the various types of pathology that can compromise facial nerve function, develop a good understanding of the surgical and nonsurgical management strategies used in patients with facial nerve paresis and paralysis. And, by all means, practice your ENoG technique on family, colleagues, and friends (they'd better be good friends) before you see your first patient. Always remember that your ENoG results may contribute to potentially life-threatening surgical treatment for facial nerve dysfunction or, conversely, may lead to a decision for more conservative treatment that conceivably might result in permanent facial nerve dysfunction. Finally, a patient's whole self-concept and personality is largely related to what they see in the mirror each morning—their faces.

FOUNDATIONS OF ELECTRONEURONOGRAPHY

Historical Reverberation

Sir Charles Bell

Sir Charles Bell (1774–1842) was a Scottish physiologist and surgeon. In 1833, Bell discovered that the muscles of the face were innervated by one cranial nerve, the 7th (facial) cranial nerve, whereas the sensation of the face was served by another cranial nerve, the 5th (trigeminal). He is also credited with Bell's law, which posits that anterior spinal nerve roots contain motor fibers only, whereas posterior roots have only motor fibers.

Clinical Concept

Anatomy of the Facial Nerve

The facial nerve consists of about 10,000 fibers, and includes motor fibers (approximately two-thirds) and sensory fibers (approximately one-third). The sensory portion of the facial nerve is known as the *nervous intermedius*.

Facial Nerve Anatomy

Temporal Bone Segments of the Facial Nerve

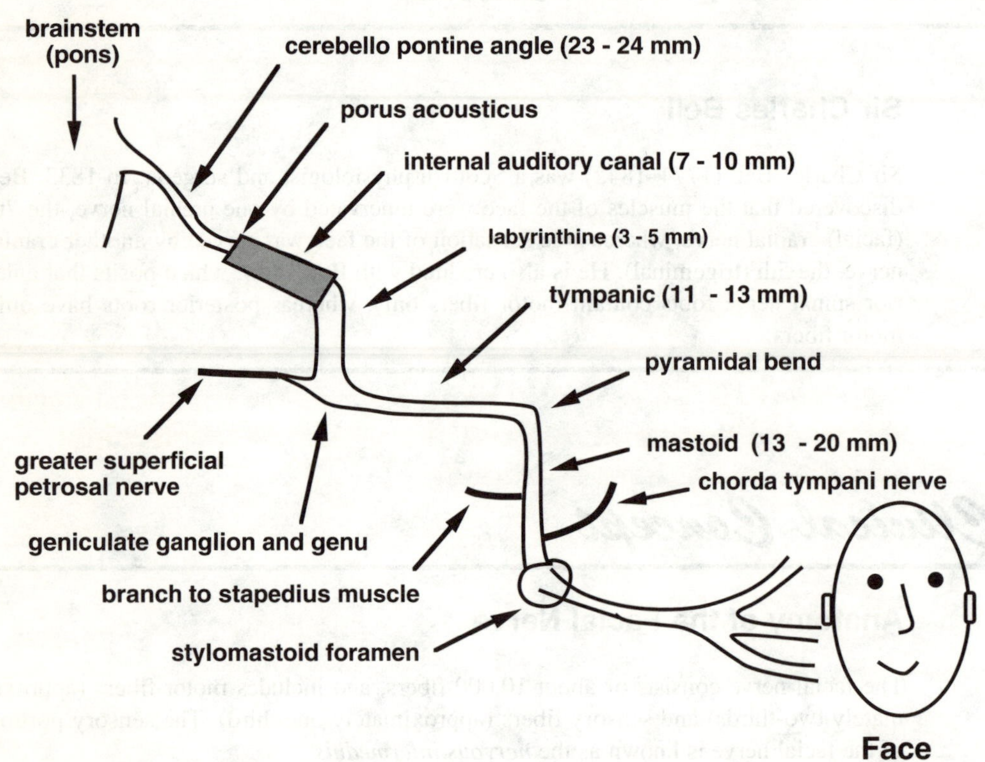

Differential Diagnosis of Facial Nerve Paralysis

Pathologies

- idiopathic Bell's palsy
- head injury
- Herpes zoster oticus (Ramsay-Hunt syndrome)
- otitis media with or without cholesteatoma
- acute and chronic tympanomastoiditis

- neoplasia (tumor), such as Schwannomas or metastatic neoplasms
- congenital facial paralysis (e.g. Treacher Collins syndrome)
- central nervous system disorder (e.g. stroke)
- Guillain-Barré syndrome
- Melkersson-Rosenthal syndrome
- multiple sclerosis

Localization of Traumatic Facial Nerve Lesions

Schematic of the temporal bone segment of the facial nerve illustrating the distribution of injury sites in longitudinal fractures of the temporal bone.

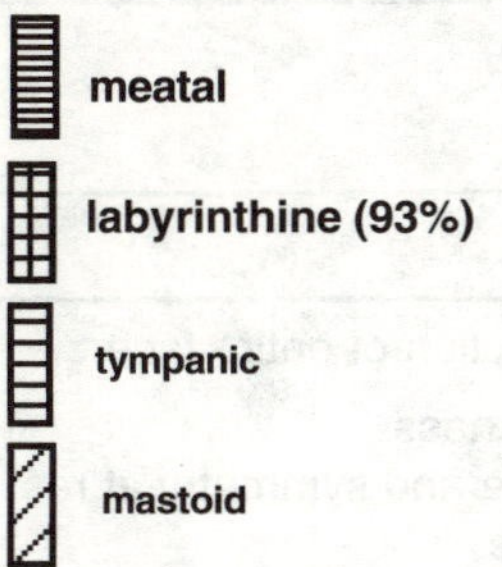

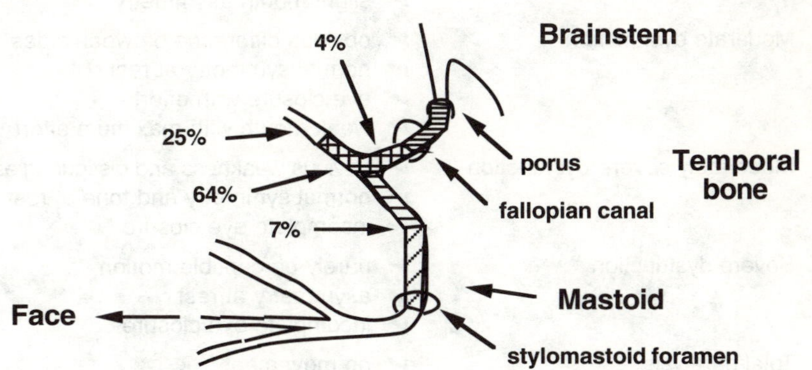

Features of Bell's Palsy

- incidence of 13 to 18 per 100,000 depending on geographic location
- there is a familial tendency for onset of Bell's palsy
- site of lesion most often is at narrowest region of fallopian canal ("meatal foramen"), as shown in a diagram in this chapter
- onset of unilateral paralysis develops within 24 to 48 hours
- Wallerian degeneration occurs within the 48- to 72-hour period after onset
- recovery is complete for about 75 to 80% of patients, beginning within 3 weeks after onset of paralysis
- approximately 15% of patients have some residual weakness and 5% have severe or total paralysis
- Bell's palsy may recur in about 7 to10% of patients

Clinical Grading System

Facial Nerve Function

Grade	Description	Features
I	Normal	normal function of entire face
II	Mild dysfunction	slight weakness normal tone and symmetry at rest eye closure slight mouth asymmetry
III	Moderate dysfunction	obvious difference between sides normal symmetry at rest eye closure with effort weak mouth with maximum effort
IV	Moderately severe dysfunction	obvious weakness and disfiguring asymmetry normal symmetry and tone at rest incomplete eye closure
V	Severe dysfunction	barely perceptible motion asymmetry at rest incomplete eye closure
VI	Total paralysis	no movement

NOTE: ENoG is indicated for patients with grade VI paralysis
Source: House JW, Brackmann DE. Facial nerve grading system. *Otolaryngol Head Neck Surg 93:* 146–147, 1985. Reprinted with permission.

Procedures

Diagnosis of Facial Nerve Disorders

- House-Brackmann grading scale
- Hilger testing
- electromyography
- acoustic stapedial reflex measurement
- evoked accelerometry
- antidromic nerve potentials
- ENoG
- magnetic resonance imaging (MRI)
- high resolution computed tomography scanning

Treatment Options

Facial Nerve Paralysis (dependent on diagnosis)

- observation
- eye care
- medical therapy includes steroids (e.g., Prednisone) and antiviral drugs (e.g., acyclovir)
- surgical decompression of temporal bone (middle fossa approach)
- surgical removal of tumor
- surgical anastomosis of facial nerve with another cranial nerve (hypoglossal)
- physical therapy
- blethraroplasty and insertion of gold weights in eyelids

Clinical Concept

Anatomy

The region around the mouth (the orbicularis oris muscle) is richly innervated by the facial nerve.

Movers and Oscillators

Ugo Fisch

Ugo Fisch is a Swiss neurotologist who, along with Esslen, introduced electroneurography (ENoG) as a clinical procedure for quantifying facial nerve paralysis and degeneration. A number of neurotologists from the United States have traveled to Switzerland to study facial nerve pathophysiology and management with Dr. Fisch.

Key References

Electroneuronography (ENoG)

Esslen E. Electrodiagnosis of facial palsy. In Miehlke, A. *Surgery of the facial nerve* (2nd ed). Urban and Schwarzenberg, 1973.

Fisch U. Facial paralysis in fractures of the petrous bone. *Laryngoscope 84*: 2141–2154, 1974.

Fisch U. Maximal nerve excitability testing versus electroneuronography. *Arch of Otolaryngol 106*: 352–357, 1980.

May M, et al. The prognostic accuracy of the maximal stimulation test compared with that of the nerve excitability test in Bell's Palsy. *Laryngoscope 81*: 931-938, 1971.

Schuknecht HF. *Pathology of the ear* (2nd ed). Philadelphia: Lea & Febiger, 1993.

ENoG RECORDING

Stimulating and Recording Electrode Sites for ENoG

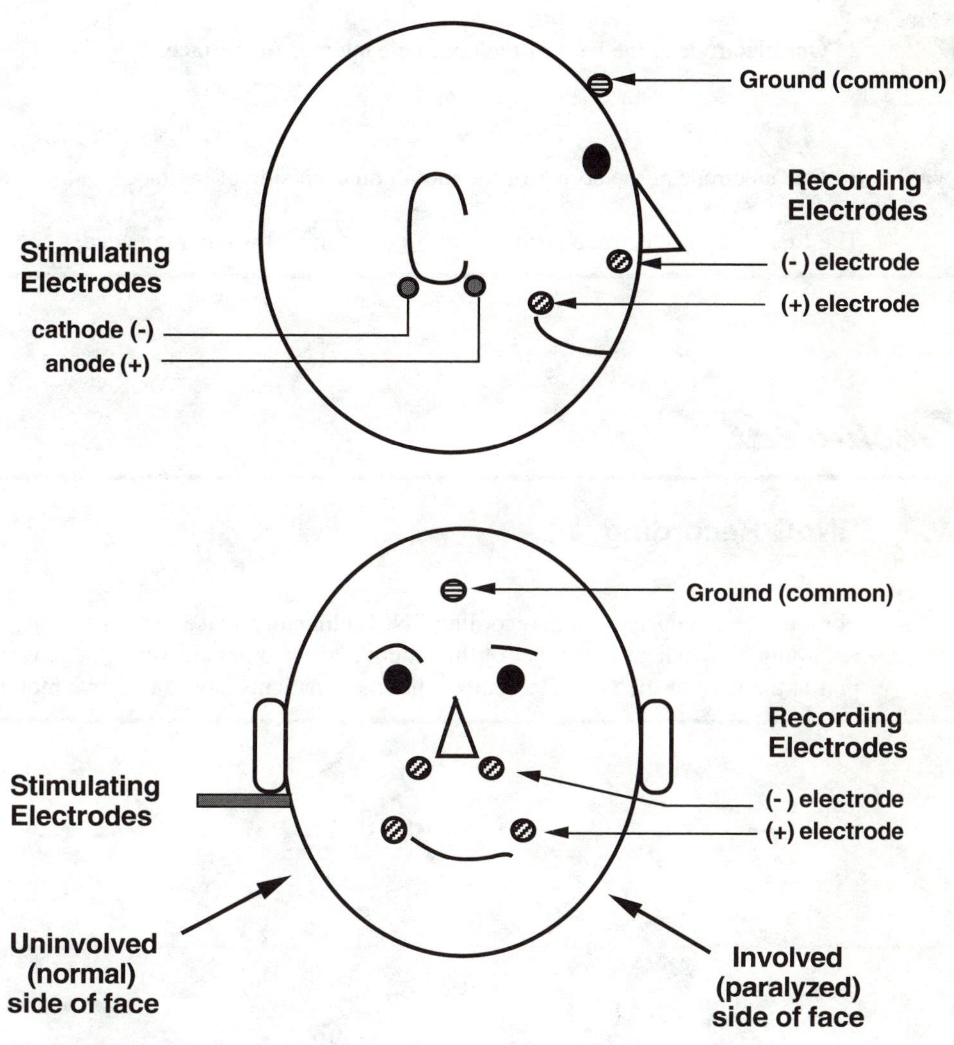

TIP: test this side first and use ENoG values as a reference

Clinical Concept

ENoG Recording

At least three different recording electrode arrays may be used in ENoG:

1. One electrode at the base of the nose and the other electrode of the pair at the corner of the mouth on the side of stimulation (along the nasolabial fold),

   or

2. One electrode at the base of the nose on each side of the face,

   or

3. One electrode at the corner of the mouth on each side of the face.

The first of these electrode arrays is most common and is recommended.

Technical Tip

ENoG Recording

For the sake of consistency in recording ENoG clinically, place the positive or "active" recording electrode at the corner of the mouth and the other electrode (negative) in the pair at the base of the nose. Remember that most patients have an "active mouth."

Protocol

ENoG Measurement Parameters

Stimulus

- ☐ Transducer — pair of electrodes
- ☐ Site — stylomastoid foramen region
- ☐ Orientation — horizontal with cathode (negative) posterior
- ☐ Type — electrical pulse (shock) of constant current or voltage
- ☐ Mode — continuous
- ☐ Duration — 0.2 msec (200 μsec)
- ☐ Rate — 1.1/sec
- ☐ Laterality — unilateral, assess uninvolved side first
- ☐ Intensity — milliamperes (μA) sufficient to produce a supramaximal response (usually 15 to 25 mA)

Acquisition

- ☐ Amplification — X 5000 (or less if response exceeds 1000 μV)
- ☐ Filter setting — 3 to 5000 Hz
- ☐ Notch filter — none
- ☐ Analysis time — 20 msec
- ☐ Prestimulus time — 1 msec
- ☐ Number of sweeps — 1 to 20
- ☐ Electrodes
  - Channel 1 — nasolabial fold (corner of mouth to base of nose) on side ipsilateral to stimulation
  - Ground (common) — forehead
- ☐ Interelectrode impedance — less than 5000 ohms

Step-by-Step

ENoG Measurement

- assemble necessary supplies and equipment (electrodes, paste, tape)
- verify correct instrumentation protocol
- explain the procedure to the patient
- seat patient in swivel chair within reach of examiner's chair
- prepare skin at electrode sites (recording and stimulation)
- attach recording and ground electrodes
- verify interelectrode impedance
- plug in recording electrodes on normal (uninvolved) side of face
- verify adequate distance between stimulus and recording electrode wires
- verify normal versus involved side (chart review, patient history, patient observation)
- verify lowest possible stimulus intensity level
- verify correct stimulus electrode polarity (cathode posterior)
- place recording electrodes and begin to increase stimulus intensity
- examine face for twitch, ask patient about sensation, inspect EEG for response
- increase stimulus intensity to supramaximal level
- move recording electrodes to verify optimal site
- record and store optimal response to supramaximal stimulation from normal side
- plug in recording electrodes on involved (paralyzed) side of face
- verify correct stimulus electrode polarity (cathode posterior)
- repeat recording process for involved side
- calculate degeneration in percent
- remove electrodes and clean electrode sites
- verify patient comfort and status
- determine time of ENoG postonset
- report ENoG findings
- make appropriate recommendations for follow-up ENoG assessments

Clinical Concept

ENoG Stimulation

Supramaximal stimulation is an essential component in ENoG recording. That is, the largest possible response should be elicited from the uninvolved (normal) and involved (paralyzed) side of the face. Supramaximal stimulation implies that all functioning nerve fibers are contributing to the measured response, including those with the highest threshold of firing. ENoG outcome and interpretation may be invalid if submaximal stimulation is used. This point is illustrated by diagrams in this chapter.

Advantages of ENoG versus Clinical Observation

- specifically assesses distal (end of the nerve from mastoid out to face) degeneration, whereas paralysis with voluntary attempts to move facial muscles involves entire length of the facial nerve and central nervous system pathways and nuclei.
- objectivity
- quantified results (in microvolts) permit more accurate monitoring of facial nerve status over time
- storage of data for later analysis
- data can be printed for medical record

Supramaximal Response in ENoG Recovery

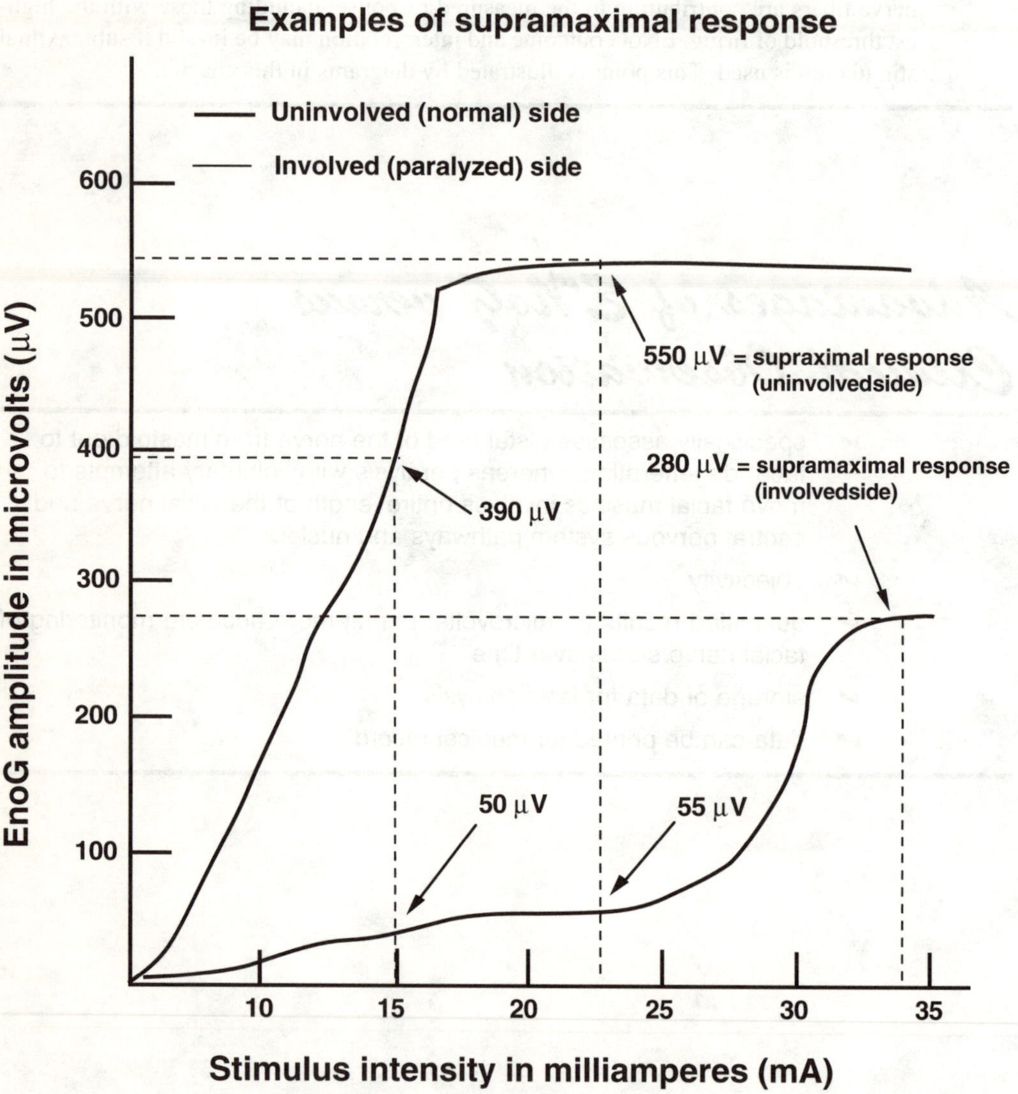

Percent degeneration of involved versus uninvolved side:

87 % @ stimulus intensity of 15 mA on each side = not significant
90 % @ stimulus intensity of 23 mA on each side = significant
49 % @ stimulus intensity producing supramaximal response on each side = not significant

Trouble-Shooting

ENoG Recording Problems and Solutions

Symptom	Problems	Solutions
Poor response bilaterally	✓ ineffective stimulus ✓ obesity ✓ bilateral dysfunction	✓ use needle electrodes ✓ compare patient results to normative database
	✓ edema at stimulus site; ✓ tenderness precludes adequate stimulus electrode pressure	✓ relieve pain ✓ defer testing
No response bilaterally	✓ chemical paralysis (in ICU or O.R.) ✓ improper electrode placement	✓ reverse neuromuscular blocking agent medically ✓ verify correct electrode placement and usage
Poor response unilaterally	✓ inappropriate stimulus site	✓ relocate stimulating electrodes ✓ increase stimulus intensity to supramaximal level
Short latency response	✓ masseter muscle response	✓ move stimulating electrodes posteriorly
Excessive artifact rejection	✓ stimulus artifact	✓ increase distance between stimulus and recording electrodes ✓ avoid crossing stimulus and electrode wires ✓ use post-stimulus time
delay		
	✓ very large response	✓ decrease amplification (gain) and/or increase sensitivity limits

Measurement Parameters

Recording ENoG in the Clinic versus Recording Facial Nerve Integrity in the Operating Room

Parameter	Clinical ENoG	Intraoperative Monitoring
Electrodes	disc type	subdermal needles
Electrode sites	nasolabial fold	corner of mouth and corner of eyes
Stimulation	electrical	facial muscle activity monitored continuously to detect unintentional activation of nerve intraoperatively by surgical manipulations
Stimulus site	stylomastoid foramen	direct stimulation of facial nerve in internal auditory canal or posterior fossa
Stimulus intensity	15 to 40 mA	0.05 to 1 mA
Response analysis	side-to-side amplitude comparison	acoustic events related to facial nerve activation; amplitude of response
Anesthesia	not relevant	no neuromuscular blocker (no muscle paralyzing agent)

Classic Quote

Ugo Fisch on ENoG

"In the case of ENoG, the investigator does not rely on visual observation but takes a graphic record of the compound action potentials originated by the synchronous discharge of the supramaximally stimulated facial nerve in a respresentative number of facial muscles."

Source: Fisch U. Maximal nerve excitability testing versus electroneuronography. *Arch Otolaryngol 106*: 52, 1980.

Important Terminology

ENoG

anode: The positive (+) electrode in the stimulating electrode pair. Placed anteriorly.

axonotmesis: Nerve fibers within the nerve bundle are damaged, but the outer sheath (epineurium) remains intact.

cathode: The negative (−) electrode in the stimulating electrode pair. Placed posteriorly.

dyskinesis: An inappropriate facial movement. For example, the eyes close when the patient attempts to smile.

fixed versus variable recording electrode techniques: With the fixed technique, the skin is prepared and two electrodes (positive and negative) are attached to the face at each end of the nasolabial fold and secured with tape. Usually conventional disc electrodes are used. The same recording electrode array is maintained during all stimulation of this side of the face as different stimulating electrode locations are used in an attempt to obtain the maximal response. With the variable technique, both stimulating and recording electrodes are moved repeatedly in an attempt to record the maximum response amplitude. A specially-designed hand-held electrode bar is typically used for the recording electrodes.

mA: Abbreviation for milliamperes. The unit of electrical stimulation used in ENoG.

neuropraxia: The facial nerve distal (peripheral) to the lesion is intact but not capable of conducting a neural signal. See diagram in this chapter.

neurotmesis: The facial nerve is totally severed. There is no anatomic connection of the fibers or of the epineurium between the two segments.

supramaximal stimulation: The magnitude of electrical stimulation (in mA) that produces the largest facial nerve response. No increase in response amplitude is recorded with further increases in stimulus intensity. In theory, all intact nerve fibers are contributing to the compound action potential with supramaximal stimulation.

synkinesis: Mass movement of facial muscles. For example, the eye on the involved side of the face closes whenever the patient's mouth closes (as during eating).

Wallerian degeneration: The proximal to distal (central to peripheral) progression of facial nerve dennervation or loss of the nerve's capacity to conduct a neural signal. The term honors Augustus Volney Waller (1816-1870), an English physician. Approximately 72 hours (3 days) are required for complete Wallerian degeneration.

ENoG ANALYSIS AND INTERPRETATION

Clinical Concept

ENoG Analysis

ENoG analysis typically is based on a comparison of the amplitude of the facial nerve response for the uninvolved ("good") side of the face versus the involved (paralyzed) side of the face (shown in a diagram in this chapter). This analysis strategy is inappropriate, however, in patients with, or at at risk for, bilateral facial palsy, including those with Guillain-Barré syndrome, herpes zoster oticus, Stevens-Johns syndrome, polyneuritis, neurofibromatosis II, and bilateral temporal bone fractures.

ENoG Waveform Analysis

No Significant Degeneration

Electroneuronography (ENoG) analysis technique with an example of asymmetry in the amplitude of facial nerve response that is within normal variation. That is, there is no significant degeneration on the involved (paralyzed) side of the face.

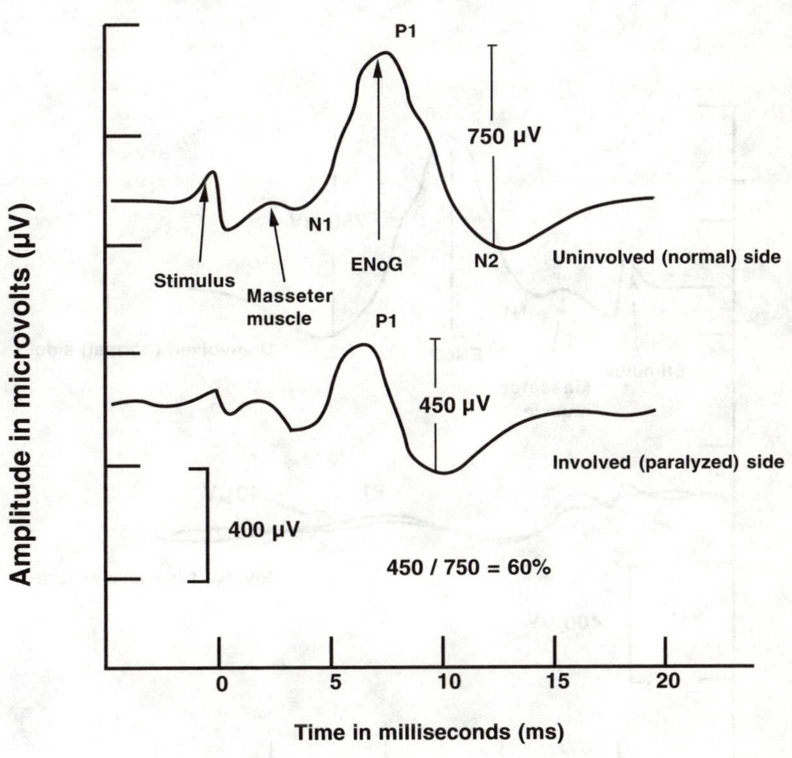

$$\text{Percent degeneration} = 100 - \frac{\text{amplitude on involved side of face } (\mu V)}{\text{amplitude on uninvolved side of face } (\mu V)} \times 100$$

$$\text{Percent degeneration} = 100 - \frac{450\ \mu V}{750\ \mu V} \times 100 = 40\ \%$$

ENoG Waveform Analysis

Significant Degeneration

Electroneurography (ENoG) analysis technique with an example of asymmetry in the amplitude of facial nerve response that reflects significant degeneration in facial nerve function. That is, there is significant degeneration on the involved (paralyzed) side of the face compared to the opposite (normal) side of the face.

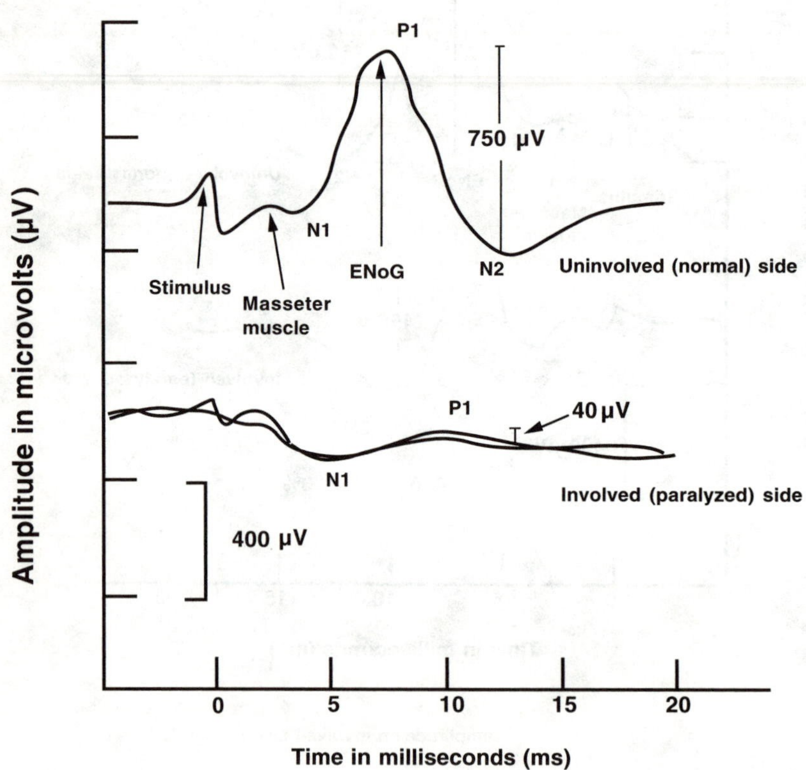

$$\text{Percent degeneration} = 100 - \frac{\text{amplitude on involved side of face } (\mu V)}{\text{amplitude on uninvolved side of face } (\mu V)} \times 100$$

$$\text{Percent degeneration} = 100 - \frac{40\ \mu V}{750\ \mu V} \times 100 = 95\%$$

Timing of ENoG Assessments

- defer initial test until 72 hours (3 days) after injury for completion of Wallerian degeneration
- within 72 hours patient will show paralysis but will still have intact nerve fibers
- repeat ENoG every 4 to 5 days after injury to document improvement or further degeneration
- decrease of ENoG to less than 10% of uninvolved ("good") side (i.e., 90% degeneration) is considered significant
- significant degeneration may warrant aggressive (surgical) therapy
- stable ENoG findings or increase in response suggests good prognosis

Time Course of Degeneration in Bell's Palsy

Degeneration post-onset as described by Fisch for Bell's palsy. More serious injury, poorer prognosis, and the need for aggressive management is usually indicated by degeneration exceeding 90% over a short time period.

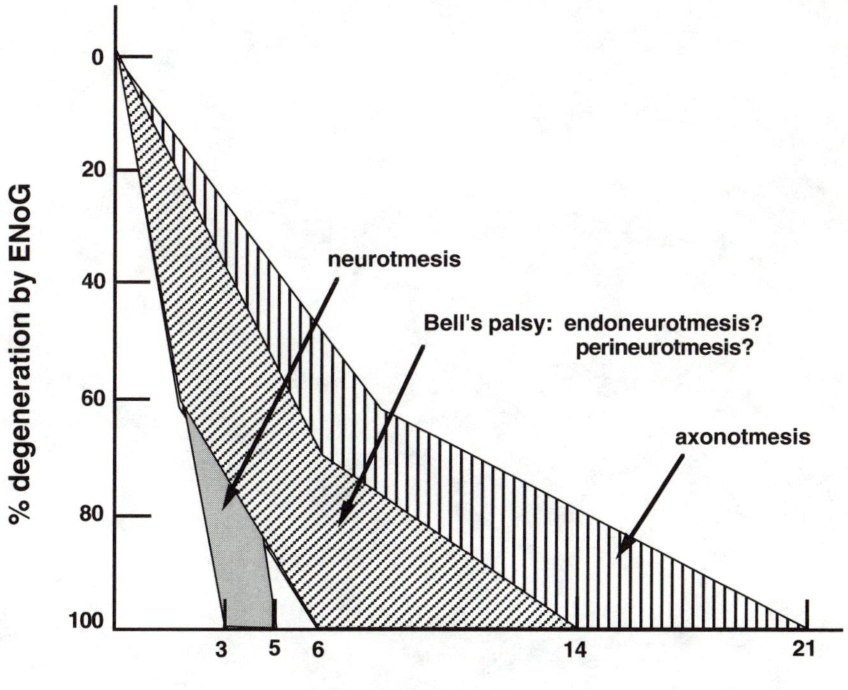

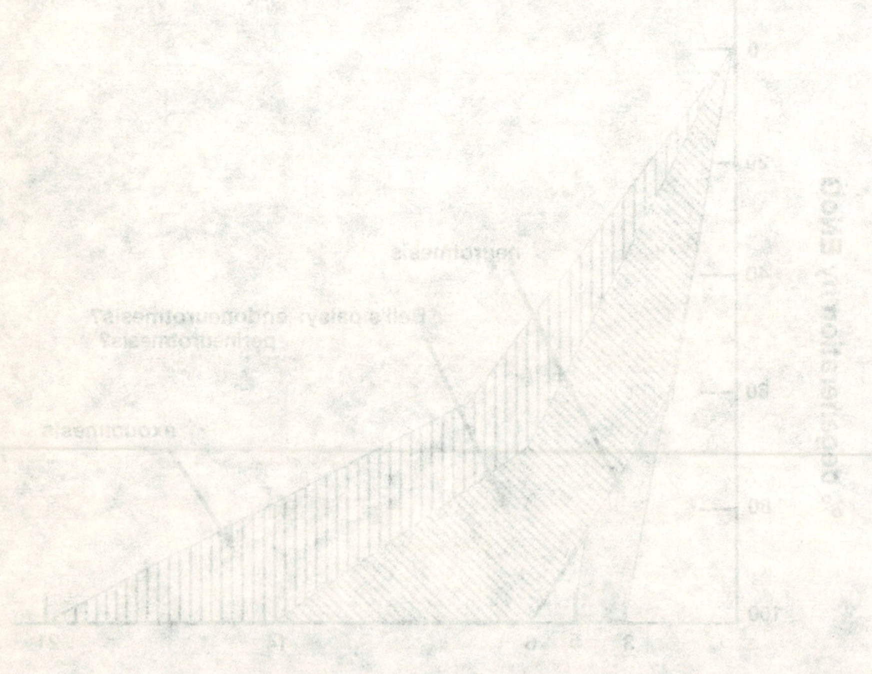

CHAPTER 14

Vestibular Assessment and Rehabilitation

In This ADR Chapter

Perspective

Assessment of, and some forms of rehabilitation for, vestibular disorders is within the official scope of audiology. Audiologists have long appreciated that basic hearing science is the foundation of clinical assessment and audiologic management of persons with hearing impairment. An understanding of vestibular system anatomy and physiology is equally important for the audiologist assessing and managing this patient population.

Indeed, the anatomic link between the auditory and vestibular systems has no doubt contributed to the development of the audiology's clinical role in assessment and management of the patient with vestibular disorders. Many germinal clinical vestibular papers, and several textbooks, have been written by audiologists, often in close collaboration with their otolaryngology colleagues. And, in clinical practice, many of the patients on any audiologist's daily schedule have both auditory and vestibular complaints. The audiologist then has primary responsibility for performing appropriate measures of vestibular function, and interpreting the results in the context of the patient's history and auditory findings. This clinical activity requires a general understanding of clinical pharmacology, along with knowledge of the structure and function of the peripheral and central vestibular system and related systems (e.g., somatosensory and visual). For selected patient etiologies, such as benign paroxysmal positioning vertigo (BPPV), the audiologist may also provide the primary management of the patient. The vestibular subspecialty of audiology is certain to increase in years to come.

FOUNDATIONS OF VESTIBULAR AND BALANCE ASSESSMENT

Clinical Concept

Vertigo

- ☐ Objective = environment is turning
- ☐ Subjective = patient is turning

Clinical Concept

Ewald's Laws

- ☐ Eyes and head move in the direction of the endolymph
- ☐ Ampulopetal flow (toward ampulla) in the lateral canal produces greater stimulus
- ☐ Ampulofugal flow (away from ampulla) in the superior and posterior canal produces greater stimulus

Clinical Concept

Vertigo versus Disequilibrium

- ☐ Vertigo
  - ✓ true sensation of disturbed motion
  - ✓ nystagmus
  - ✓ peripheral or CNS vestibular disorders
- ☐ Disequilibrium
  - ✓ spatial disorientation or ataxia
  - ✓ no nystagmus
  - ✓ systemic disorder or nonvestibular CNS disease

Components of Patient History on Dizziness

- ☐ Chronology
  - ✔ onset
  - ✔ duration
  - ✔ frequency
  - ✔ aura
- ☐ General pattern
  - ✔ falling sensation
  - ✔ nausea
  - ✔ provocation
  - ✔ sensation (objective vs. subjective)
  - ✔ improves and worsens
- ☐ Hearing loss, tinnitus, and ear disease
  - ✔ drainage
  - ✔ surgery
  - ✔ fullness/fluctuation
  - ✔ tinnitus
- ☐ Ocular problems
  - ✔ double vision
  - ✔ difficulty in the dark
  - ✔ new glasses
- ☐ Central nervous system—ataxia
  - ✔ numbness
  - ✔ clumsiness
  - ✔ difficulty speaking or swallowing
- ☐ Disequilibrium
  - ✔ when you're dizzy, are you lightheaded?
  - ✔ swimming in head?

- syncope
- headache
- hunger
- stress

Source: Mitchell K, Schwaber MD, Vanderbilt Vestibular Workshop. Nashville, Tennessee, November 1995

Clinical Concept

Alexander's Law

- ☐ Nystagmus beats most intensely when the eyes are deviated toward the side of the fast phase of the nystagmus. For example, left beating nystagmus is stronger with left lateral gaze compared to right lateral gaze.
- ☐ Spontaneous ocular square waves, observed during a gaze test, are often caused by lesions of the brainstem/cerebellum. They may also be seen with tense or nervous patients.

Causes for Dizziness

- head injury
- neck injury
- vestibular neuronitis
- syphilis
- tuberculosis
- Ramsay Hunt syndrome
- anemia
- hyperviscosity
- valvular disease
- heart failure
- hypoglycemia
- hyperventilation
- posterior fossa tumors
- degenerative neurologic disorder
- skull base abnormalities
- Paget's disease
- medications
- toxins
- Ménière's disease
- fistula
- stroke
- multiple sclerosis
- cholesteatoma

Synonyms for Dizziness

- reeling
- whirling
- faint
- giddy
- heady
- lightheaded
- woozy
- shaky
- unstable
- wobbly
- bewildered
- confused
- dazed
- disequilibrated
- swimmy-head
- clumsy
- off balance
- vertiginous
- floating
- drifting
- falling
- swaying
- weak
- fuzzy-headed
- spinning
- listing
- leaning

Reeling in the Ears

History of Vestibular Testing

1830 Flourens observed connection between the vestibular system and eye movements. When SCC was destroyed in pigeons and rabbits, he noticed uncontrollable eye movement and a change in the animal's body posture.

1849 Du Bois-Reymond discovered electrical potential difference between the cornea and retina which formed the basis for monitoring eye movements. Series of invasive techniques were tried with needle electrodes and contact lenses to record corneal-retinal potential (CRP).

1939 Jung applied surface electrodes around the periphery of the eyes and used CRP for recording nystagmus and other eye movements. This led to development of modern-day ENG.

1950s Although Barany first described a rotatory stimulus to test the vestibular system in the early 1900s, by the 1950s caloric stimulation had proven to be more cinically useful.

1960s ENG under rapid development and clinical acceptance.

1970 Reasonable standardization of caloric tests and ENG techniques led to widespread clinical acceptance.

1980s Computers result in feasability of analysis of rotary testing.

Key References

Vestibular and Balance Assessment and Function

Barber HO, Stockwell CW. *Manual of electronystagmography* (2nd ed). St. Louis: C.V. Mosby Co., 1990.

Brookler K, Rubin W. Objective confirmation of symptoms. In *Dizziness: Etiologic approach to management.* New York: Thieme Medical Publishers, 1991.

Coats A. ENG examination technique. *Ear and Hearing 7:* 143–150, 1986.

Cyr, DG. Vestibular system assessment. In W Rintelmann (ed). *Hearing assessment* (2nd ed). Austin: Pro-Ed, pp. 739-803, 1991.

Hirsch BE. Computed sinusoidal harmonic acceleration. *Ear and Hearing 7:* 198–203, 1986.

Jacobson GP and Newman CW. The development of the dizziness handicap inventory. *Arch Otolaryngol Head Neck Surg* 116: 424–427, 1990.

Jacobson GP, Newman CW, Kartush J (eds). *Handbook of balance function testing.* St. Louis: Mosby/Yearbook, 1993.

Kavanagh KT and Babin RW. Definitions and types of nystagmus and calculations. *Ear and Hearing 7:* 157–166, 1986.

Kileny P, Kemink JL. Artifacts and errors in the electronystagmographic (ENG) evaluation of the vestibular system. *Ear and Hearing 7:* 151–156, 1986.

Lambert PR. Nonlocalizing vestibular findings on electronystagmography. *Ear and Hearing 7:* 182–185, 1986.

McGee ML. Electronystagmography in peripheral lesions. *Ear and Hearing 7:* 167–175, 1986.

Steenerson RL, Van de Water SM, Sytsma WH, Fox EJ. Central vestibular findings on electronystagmography. *Ear and Hearing 7:* 176–181, 1986.

Jacobson GP, Newman CW. Rotational testing. *Seminars in Hearing 12:* 199–224, 1991.

Shephard NT, Telian SA. Balance disorders ("The Dizzy Patient"). In Jacobson J, Northern J. (eds) *Diagnostic audiology,* Boston: Little, Brown, 1990.

Hamid AM. Determining side of vestibular dysfunction with rotatory chair testing. *Otolaryngol-Head Neck Surgery 105:* 40–43, 1991.

O'Leary DP, Davis LL. High-frequency autorotational testing of the vestibulo-ocular reflex. *Neurologic Clinics 8:* 297–312, 1990.

Fineberg R, O'Leary DP, Davis LL. Use of active head movements for computerized vestibular testing. *Arch Otolaryngol Head Neck Surg 113:* 1063–1065, 1987.

ANATOMY AND PHYSIOLOGY

Location of Vestibular Apparatus Within the Temporal Bone

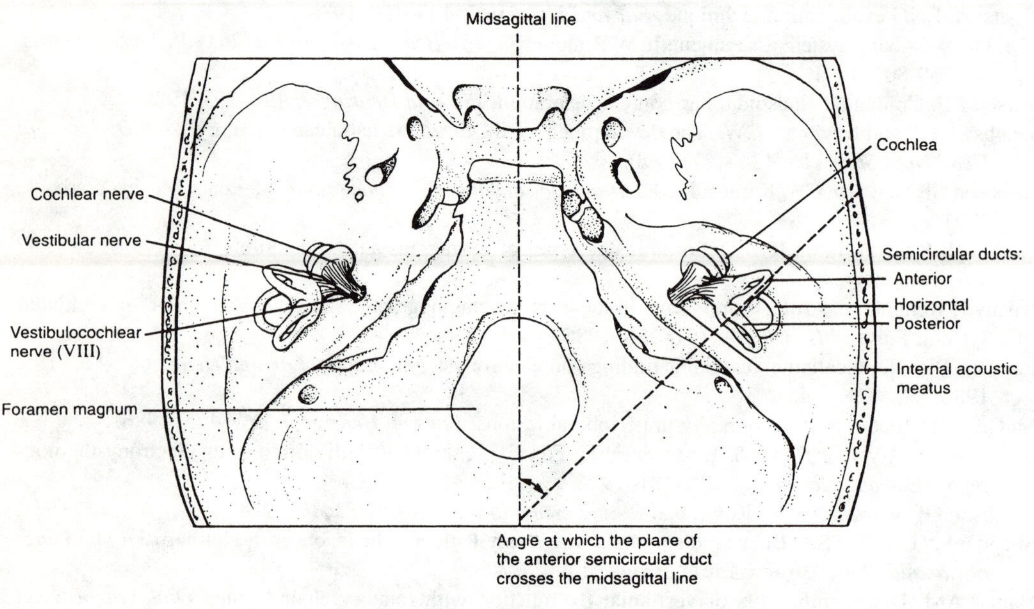

From Kandel ER, Schwartz JH, Jessell TM (eds). (1991). *Principles of neural science* (3rd ed). Norwalk, CT: Appleton & Lange. Reprinted with permission.

Cochlea and Vestibular Structures Within the Temporal Bone

Viewed from the left side of the head (top portion of the figure labeled "**A**") showing their relationship to the auditory and vestibular portions of the eighth cranial nerve. Lower portion (**B**) shows internal view of these structures (i.e., the bony and membranous labyrinths, in relation to the middle ear space)

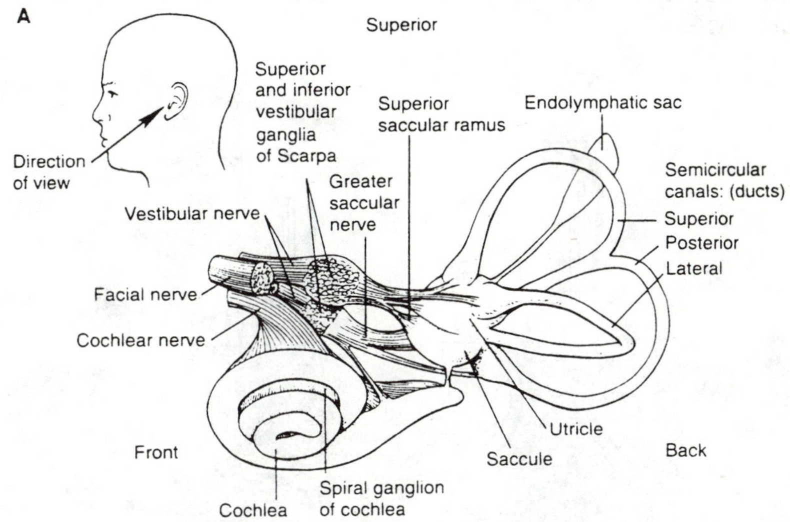

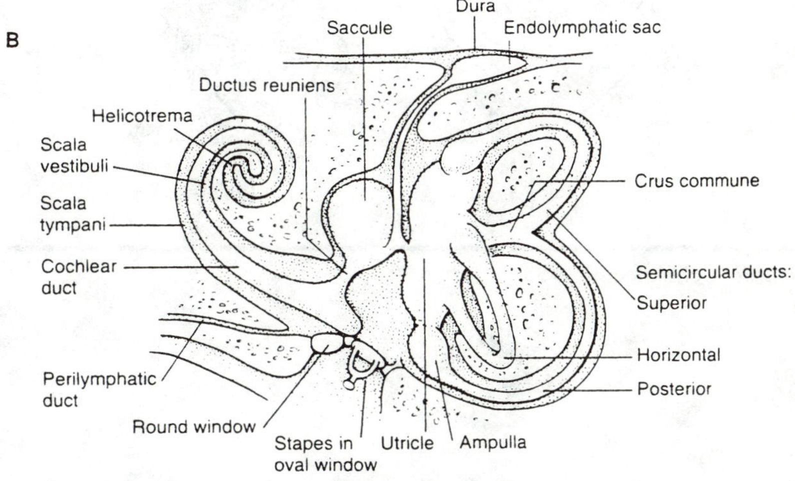

Source: from Kandel ER, Schwartz JH, Jessell TM (eds). *Principles of neural science* (3rd ed). Norwalk, CT: Appleton & Lange, 1991, p. 502. Reprinted with permission.

The Two Types of Hair Cells in the Vestibular Labyrinth

In addition to the obvious difference in shape between the two types, there are functional differences. Type I hair cells are innervated by large afferent vestibular nerve fibers, whereas Type II hair cells are innervated by small afferent fibers (and some small efferent fibers too). The large fibers terminate on the larger neurons in the center of the superior vestibular nucleus. Small fibers terminate on small neurons in a region located between the center of the superior vestibular nucleus and the restiform body. The two different types of vestibular hair cells parallel the two types of cochlear hair cells.

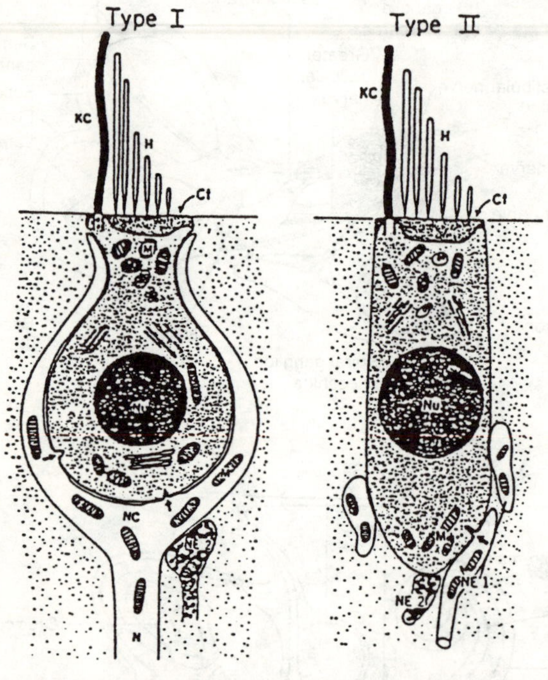

Source: Schuknecht, 1993

Orientation of the Stereocilia and Kinocilium

Vestibular hair cells and the functional state of the hair cells (i.e., resting potential, excitation, or inhibition).

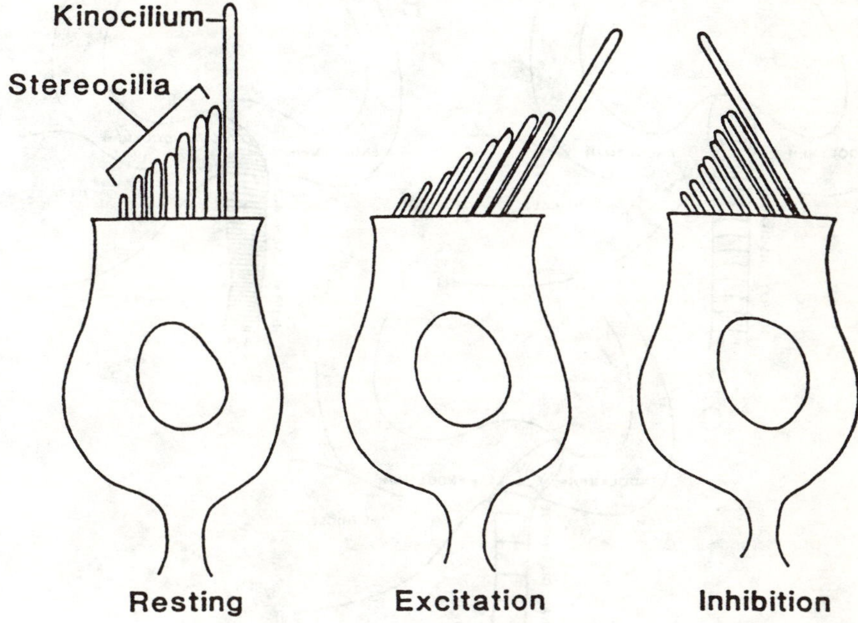

Three Functional States of the Crista

(**A**) The system at rest with a resting vestibular neural discharge or potential, (**B**) The crista is bent toward the utricle (utriculopetal) and the vestibular neural discharge rate is increased, (**C**) The crista is bent away from the utricle (utriculofugal) and the vestibular neural discharge rate is decreased.

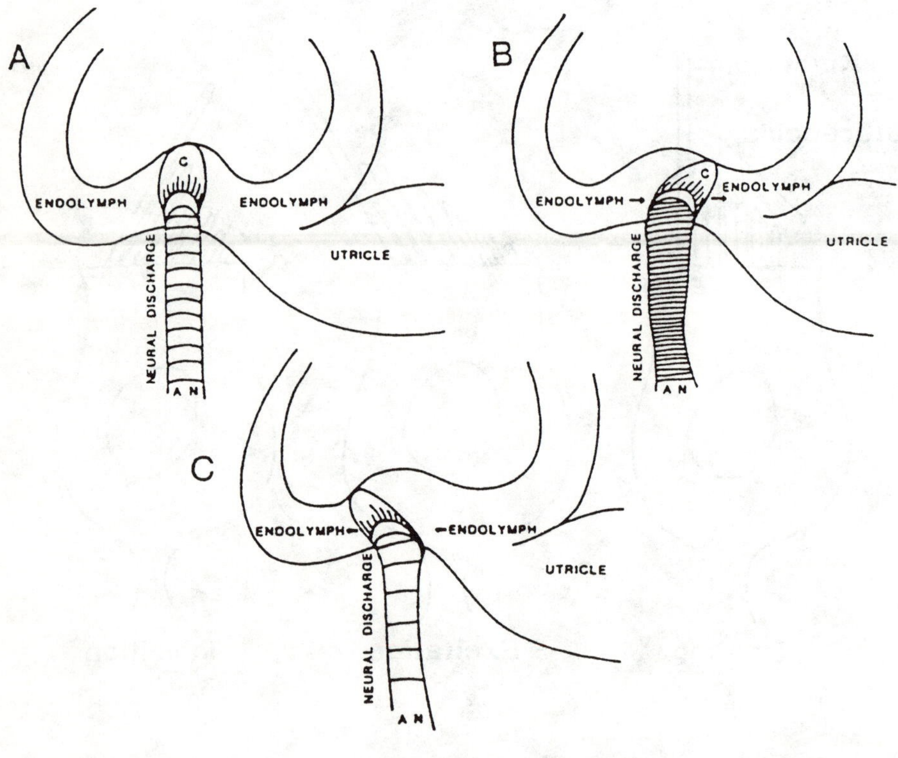

From Cyr D. (1991). Vestibular system assessment. (p. 745). In W. F. Rintelman (Ed.), *Hearing Assessment Second Edition*. Allyn & Bacon: Needham Heights, MA. Reprinted with Permission.

Vestibulo-Oculomotor Reflex Pathways

Highly schematic illustration of the initial portion of the vestibulo-oculomotor (VOR) reflex pathways. Head turning motion in one direction (noted at the top of the figure and at the bottom) is associated with motion of fluid in the ampulla of the semicircular canal that is in the opposite direction. This triggers a sequence of excitations and inhibitations within the central vestibular pathways and centers. As a result of the unique innervation of the ocular muscles for each eye, eyeball movement is in the opposite direction of head turning motion.

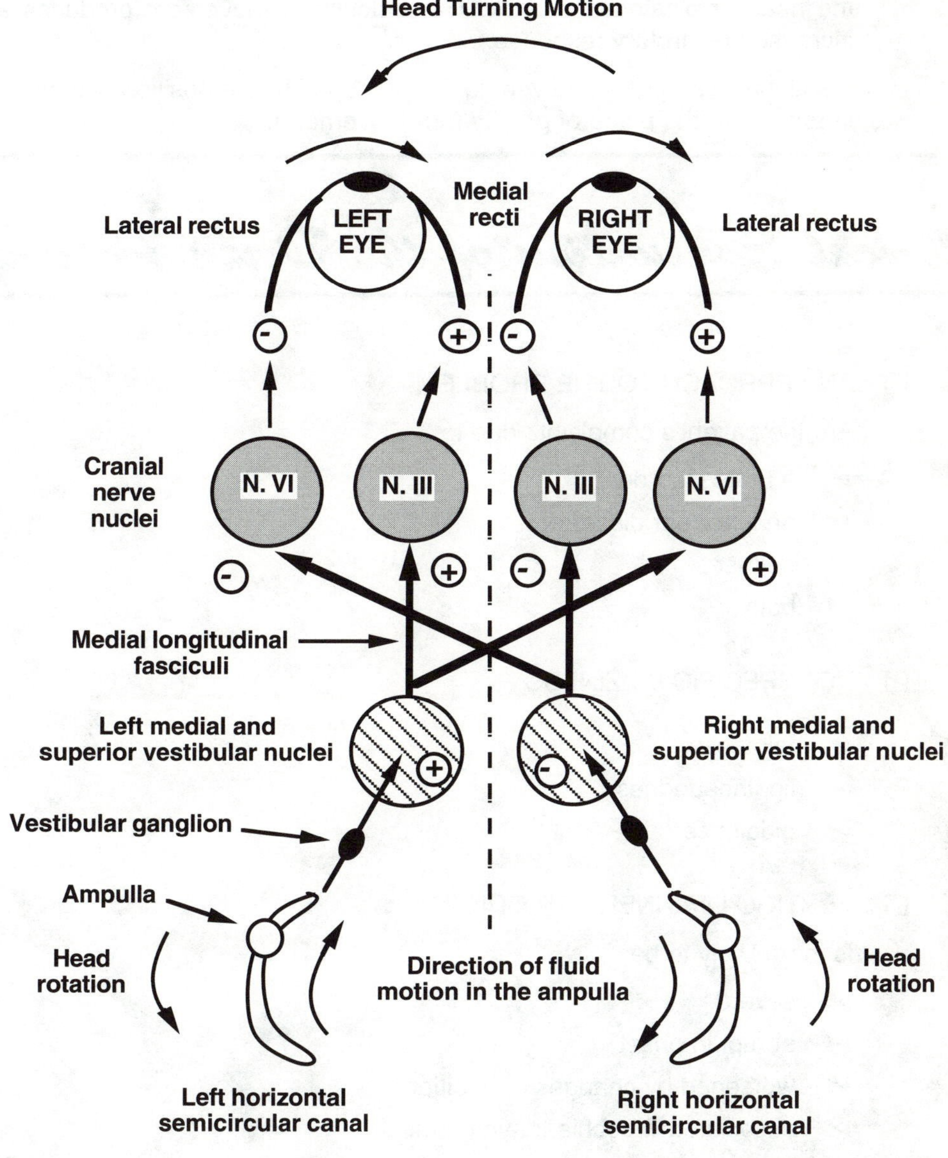

CONCEPTS IN VESTIBULAR ASSESSMENT

Clinical Concept

Positional versus Positioning Nystagmus and Vertigo

- ☐ Positioning nystagmus and vertigo are brought on by quick extension of the head or a lateral head tilt. This velocity of movement produces an increased postrotary response.
- ☐ Positional nystagmus and vertigo are produced by the position of the head in relation to the plane of gravity (not movement).

Clinical Evaluation of the Dizzy Patient

☐ AN APPROACH TO THE PROBLEM

Are the patient's complaints due to:

- ✓ a brain disorder
- ✓ an inner ear disorder
- ✓ neither
- ✓ both

☐ NONSPECIFIC DIZZINESS

- ✓ faintness
- ✓ lightheadedness
- ✓ giddiness

☐ VERTIGO OF INNER EAR ORIGIN

Is more likely to be:

- ✓ severe
- ✓ abrupt in onset
- ✓ worsened by changes of position
- ✓ associated w/cochlear symptoms

☐ CLUES TO VERTIGO OF CNS ORIGIN

- focal neurological symptoms and signs
- alterations in mental status
- "fellow travellers"

☐ QUALITY OF SYMPTOMS

- vertigo or not
- "subjective" vertigo
- "objective" vertigo
- oscillopsia

☐ TEMPORAL COURSE OF SYMPTOMS

- sudden onset versus gradual onset
- intermittent versus continuous symptoms
- duration

☐ CIRCUMSTANCES OF ONSET

- antecedent illness
- head or neck injury
- unusual activity
- significant life stress

☐ EXACERBATING/RELIEVING FACTORS

- change of position
- certain positions
- eyes open versus eyes closed
- worsened by loud noise (Tulio phenomenon)
- worsened by Valsalva
- rapid shifts of attention or of vision
- exercise
- situational stress
- eating

☐ ASSOCIATED SYMPTOMS

- nausea, vomiting, and autonomic symptoms
- shortness of breath, palpitations
- hiccups
- dysarthria and dysphagia
- visual loss and diplopia
- “blurry” vision
- hearing loss, aural fullness-pressure-or-pain, tinnitus
- recruitment
- diplacusis
- headache
- pain
- falling
- alterations or losses of consciousness
- focal numbness or weakness

☐ CLUES FROM THE PAST: THE MEDICAL HISTORY

- previous similar illnesses
- previous otologic problems
- history of hearing problems or motion sickness
- visual problems
- previous syncope, seizures, stroke or TIA
- psychological problems
- migraine
- medications
- family history

Nonvestibular Factors in General Medical Examination of the Dizzy Patient

- ☐ Postural hypotension
- ☐ Hyperventilation
- ☐ Arteriosclerosis
- ☐ Hypertension
- ☐ Hematologic disorders
- ☐ Metabolic disorder
- ☐ Ataxia

Source: Mitchell K. Schwaber MD, Vanderbilt Vestibular Workshop. Nashville, Tennessee, November 1995

Cochleovestibular Disorders Causing Vertigo

- ☐ Intralabyrinthine
  - Ménière's disease
  - Labyrinthitis and labyrintine fistula
  - Otosclerosis
  - Trauma
  - Viral/syphilis
  - Ototoxic drugs
  - Tumors
  - Hereditary or acquired syndromes
  - Motion sickness
  - Congenital vestibular asymmetry
  - Benign paroxysmal positional vertigo (BPPV)
- ☐ Extralabyrinthine
  - Intracanalicular tumor
  - Cerebellopontine angle tumor
  - Anomalous blood vessel
  - Herpes Zoster Oticus
  - Toxic vestibular neuronitis
  - Viral neuronitis

Source: Mitchell K. Schwaber MD, Vanderbilt Vestibular Workshop. Nashville, Tennessee, November 1995

Dizziness Handicap Inventory (DHI)

VANDERBILT BALANCE & HEARING CENTER
THE VILLAGE AT VANDERBILT
1500 21ST AVENUE, SOUTH SUITE 2600
NASHVILLE, TN 37212-3102
TELEPHONE (615) 322-HEAR FAX (615) 343-0872

NAME______________________________ DATE ____________

DIZZINESS HANDICAP INVENTORY

Instructions: The purpose of this scale is to identify difficulties that you may be experiencing because of your dizziness or unsteadiness. Please answer "yes," "no," or "sometimes" to each question by checking the appropriate box. *Answer each question as it pertains to your dizziness or unsteadiness problem only.*

ITEM	YES	NO	SOMETIMES
1. Does looking up increase your problem?	☐	☐	☐
2. Because of your problem, do you feel frustrated?	☐	☐	☐
3. Because of your problem, do you restrict your travel for business or recreation?	☐	☐	☐
4. Does walking down the aisle of a supermarket increase your problem?	☐	☐	☐
5. Because of your problem, do you have difficulty getting into or out of bed?	☐	☐	☐
6. Does your problem significantly restrict your participation in social activities such as going out to dinner, going to movies, dancing, or parties?	☐	☐	☐
7. Because of your problem, do you have difficulty reading?	☐	☐	☐
8. Does performing more ambitious activities like sports, dancing, household chores such as sweeping or putting dishes away increase your problem?	☐	☐	☐
9. Because of your problem, are you afraid to leave your home without having someone accompany you?	☐	☐	☐

ITEM	YES	NO	SOMETIMES
10. Because of your problem, have you been embarrassed in front of others?	☐	☐	☐
11. Do quick movements of your head increase your problem?	☐	☐	☐
12. Because of your problem, do you avoid heights?	☐	☐	☐
13. Does turning over in bed increase your problem?	☐	☐	☐
14. Because of your problem, is it difficult for you to do strenuous housework or yardwork?	☐	☐	☐
15. Because of your problem, are you afraid people may think you are intoxicated?	☐	☐	☐
16. Because of your problem, is it difficult for you to go for a walk by yourself?	☐	☐	☐
17. Does walking down a sidewalk increase your problem?	☐	☐	☐
18. Because of your problem, is it difficult for you to concentrate?	☐	☐	☐
19. Because of your problem, is it difficult for you to walk around your house in the dark?	☐	☐	☐
20. Because of your problem, are you afraid to stay home alone?	☐	☐	☐
21. Because of your problem, do you feel handicapped?	☐	☐	☐
22. Has your problem placed stress on your relationships with members of your family or friends?	☐	☐	☐
23. Because of your problem, are you depressed?	☐	☐	☐
24. Does your problem interfere with your job or household responsibilities?	☐	☐	☐
25. Does bending over increase your problem?	☐	☐	☐

Patient Instructions

Pre-test instructions for balance testing (used at Vanderbilt Balance and Hearing Center)

For all balance testing, electrodes will be taped on your face to measure eye movement. You may be scheduled for one or more of the following tests:

Electronystagmyography (ENG): This test consists of three parts. First, you will be asked to watch a series of lights on the wall. Next, you will be asked to turn your head in several different positions. Finally, your ears will be irrigated with warm and cool water to measure back and forth eye movements called nystagmus.
Test time is 1 1/2 hours.

Rotary Chair: Eye movement is measured while you are seated in a slowly rotating chair in a darkened booth. A speaker system allows communication with the audiologist outside of the booth.
Test time is 45 minutes.

Vestibular Auto-Rotational Test (VAT): Eye movement is measured while you are asked to shake your head in back and forth and up and down motions.
Test time is 20 minutes.

These tests are not painful. However, you may feel dizzy for some time after the test, so we suggest that you arrange for someone to drive you home after the testing is completed.

PLEASE NOTE

Certain medications may change the finding of the ENG exam. We ask that you NOT take any nonessential medications for a period of 48 hours before your appointment time, and that you especially avoid the following:

- ✔ Alcoholic beverages
- ✔ Sleeping pills
- ✔ Tranquilizers
- ✔ Antihistamines
- ✔ Anti-dizzy pills
- ✔ Narcotics of any kind
- ✔ Over-the-counter cold or allergy medications
- ✔ Medications which contain any of the above

If you have any questions about medications or concerning testing, please call the Vanderbilt Balance and Hearing Center at 322-HEAR (4327).

ALSO

- ✔ Do not eat or drink anything for a period of three (3) hours before the time of the test.
- ✔ Do not drink any caffeinated beverages or use any tobacco on the day of the test.
- ✔ Do not wear make-up foundation or face cream the day of the test.

Drugs Associated with Vestibular Disorders

Drugs	Eye Movement Abnormalities
Alcohol (Ethanol)	vestibular dysfunction: positional nystagmus brainstem-cerebellar dysfunction pattern
Aminoglycoside Antibiotics ☐ Streptomycin ☐ Gentamicin	vestibular dysfunction: permanent labyrinthine hypofunction
Antidepressants:	central sedation pattern
☐ Tricyclics (e.g., Elavil)	internuclear ophthalmoplegia
☐ Phenothiazines (e.g., Pamelor)	opsoclonus
☐ Others (e.g., Prozac)	partial or total gaze paresis
☐ Lithium	brainstem-cerebellar pattern opsoclonus
Chemotherapeutic	vestibular dysfunction: permanent labyrinthine hypofunction
Anti-cancer Agents (e.g., cisplatin)	
Diuretics ☐ Lasix ☐ Ethacrynic Acid	vestibular dysfunction: permanent labyrinthine hypofunction
Haldol (Haloperidol)	opsoclonus
Industrial Solvents:	brainstem-cerebellar dysfunction pattern
☐ Xylene	vestibular dysfunction: central positional nystagmus
☐ Trichlorethylene	exaggerated VOR
Marijuana	brainstem-cerebellar dysfunction pattern
Methadone	brainstem-cerebellar dysfunction pattern
Quinine	vestibular dysfunction: positional nystagmus
Salicilates: ☐ Aspirin (acetylsalicylic acid)	vestibular dysfunction: transient labyrinthine hypofunction
Stimulants: ☐ Amphetamine	impaired accommodation/convergence; reduced saccadic latency

Sedatives:	brainstem-cerebellar dysfunction pattern
☐ Barbiturates (e.g., phenobarbital, Seconal)	vestibular dysfunction: central positional nystagmus central sedation pattern
☐ Chloral hydrate	
Tobacco	upbeat nystagmus
☐ Smoking or chewing	square wave jerks
☐ Nicotine gum	
Tranquilizers;	central sedation pattern
☐ Benzodiazepines (e.g., Valium, Ativan, Xanax)	brainstem-cerebellar pattern
Vestibular Suppressants:	central sedation pattern
☐ Meclizine	vestibular dysfunction: transient labyrinthine hypofunction
☐ Benadryl	
☐ Scopolamine	
☐ Phenergan	
☐ Flunarize	

Terms in Vestibular Assessment

Electro-oculography (EOG): A method of monitoring eye movements which provides a permanent record, either with the eyes open or closed, in light or in darkness.

Electronystagmography (ENG): A method of using EOG for clinical study of dizziness and balance disturbance. The term ENG is used because it is primarily used to measure nystagmus.

Corneo-retinal potential (CRP): The eye acts as battery with the cornea the positive pole and the retina the negative pole. The potential difference between poles is normally at least 1 mv. This electrical potential is called the corneo-retinal potential and creates in the front of the head an electrical field that changes its orientation as the eyeballs rotate.

These polarity changes are detected by electrodes placed on the skin, amplified, and transmitted to a computer or to a strip-chart recorder. The tracing shows a displacement that corresponds to the degree and direction of eye displacement.

Questions (sometimes) Answered by ENG

- Does a lesion exist? Especially if the question is whether the lesion is vestibular or oculomotor.
- If a lesion exists, what is the site (location)? Sometimes ENG answers this question in general terms. Information from ENG often is nonlocalizing (no specific site-of-lesion is indicated), but the pattern of abnormalities points toward a peripheral (labyrinth or 8th cranial nerve) or central nervous system lesion.
- If a lesion exists, what is its cause? ENG rarely answers this question.

ENG Abnormalities and Suspected Site-of-Lesion

Test	Type of Abnormality	Suspected Site-of-Lesion
Saccade	ipsilateral dysmetria	cerebellopontine angle
	bilateral dysmetria	cerebellum
	decreased velocity	throughout the CNS, muscle weakness or peripheral nerve palsy
	internuclear ophthalmoplegia	medial longitudinal fasciculus
Pursuit	break-up	brainstem or cerebrum
	saccadic	cerebellum
Gaze	direction-fixed and horizontal	peripheral vestibular
	direction-changing and vertical	brainstem
	up-beating	brainstem or cerebellum
	down-beating	cervico-medullary junction or cerebellum
	rotary	vestibular nuclei/brainstem
FFS	less than 40% decrease	brainstem or cerebellum
Positional	direction-fixed	nonlocalizing or peripheral
	direction-changing	nonlocalizing or central
Dix Hallpike	classic	peripheral vestibular—undermost ear
	nonclassic	nonlocalizing
Caloric	unilateral or bilateral weakness	peripheral vestibular
	directional	nonlocalizing
		preponderance

VESTIBULAR TEST PROCEDURES AND PROTOCOLS

Preparation for ENG Assessment

☐ **The patient**

Does the patient have:

- An intracardiac catheter or pacemaker with exposed leads?
- Alcohol "on board" (i.e., in the blood)?
- Drugs in the system that could affect the test results?
- A hearing loss?
- A severe visual problem (e.g., blind)?
- Seizure disorder?
- A history of back or neck problems?

☐ **Otoscopic examination**

- Check for excessive cerumen which must be removed prior to caloric testing.
- With a tympanic membrane perforation must use air or closed loop calorics.
- Orientation of EAC. For accurate irrigation, it's important for the tester to be familiar with bends in the EAC.

☐ **Electrodes**

- Five electrodes are typically used with a two-channel recording technique (one channel is for horizontal movement and one for vertical). See figure in this chapter.
- Apply the electrodes as soon as possible before actual ENG recording begins. Over the course of minutes after electrodes are applied, interelectrode impedance tends to decrease.
- Prepare the skin with an appropriate abrasive substance.
- Check impedance. Inter-electrode should be lower than 10,000 ohms.
- Darken the test room. A change in darkness will affect the CRP.

CALIBRATION

☐ Calibration verifies the relationship between recorder or pen deflection and the amount of eye movement (in degrees). The patient looks at two fixation points separated by a known horizontal distance, usually a 20° visual angle. The patient alternately looks at one and then the other during the calibration task. As the patient performs this task, the gain is adjusted so that 1 mm of pen movement equals 1 mm of eye displacement. The vertical channel is calibrated similarly with the light points arranged vertically. When horizontal eye movements are recorded, a deflection upward represents eye movement to the right and deflection downward represents eye movement to the left. With vertical eye movements, a deflection upward represents upward movement and a deflection downward represents downward movement.

ENG TEST BATTERY

☐ Tests comprising the basic ENG battery:

- Calibration
- Saccade test
- Gaze tests
- Sinusoidal tracking test
- Optokinetic test
- Dix-Hallpike maneuver
- Positional tests
- Caloric test

Source: Courtesy of Faith Wurm, Ph.D.

Equipment Used in Vestibular Assessment

- ☐ **Room:** The room dimensions are at least 10 × 14 feet. The patient is placed in center of room with the light bar in front and major ENG equipment behind. A sink and cabinet space are also needed.

  Special features of room include:

  - not near X-ray machines which emit electromagnetic energy that interferes with ENG recording
  - air conditioning to keep room cool and dry
  - no windows or very good window coverings to keep the room lightproof.
  - It's important that equipment be grounded.

- ☐ **Eye movement recording system**:

  The system must be able to detect minute voltage changes produced by eye displacement, amplify them by about 20,000 times without distortion, and display them. Equipment needed to measure eye movements are electrodes and computer or nystagmograph.

- ☐ **Electrodes:** Ag/AgCl electrodes are widely used because they do not polarize as other metal electrodes do. They display highest stability and lowest impedance of any readily available electrode.

  Disposable electrodes are used in many clinics.

- ☐ **Nystagmograph:** Amplifies and displays the minute voltage changes detected by the recording electrodes. Also referred to as ENG recorder. May be strip-chart recorders or computer-controlled ENGs.

  From 1 to 4 channels may be used. At least 2 channels are preferrable, one for horizontal nystagmus and one for vertical nystagmus.

- ☐ **Vestibular Stimulators:** Caloric irrigators are stimuli used in ENG. Several types include water, air, closed loop, monothermal, and bithermal.

- ☐ **Water calorics:** have been used successfully for many years and are considered the most reliable stimulus. Fairly well standardized: 250 cc of water delivered to the EAC within 30 seconds. Each ear is irrigated twice, once with 30° and once with 44°. This is referred to as a bithermal stimulus (i.e., one temperature is above and one below body temperature). Each temperature produces a different direction of nystagmus with each stimulus.

  Irrigation system itself consists of three components:

  - a pair of water reservoirs to hold the water at the proper temperatures
  - a calibrated delivery system to deliver the proper amount of water to the ear
  - a timing system to control duration of water flow.

Disadvantages of water calorics include:

- messy
- greater potential for electric shock
- contraindicated in some middle ear pathologies such as tympanic membrane perforation.

- **Air calorics:** eliminate disadvantages of water calorics.

  A greater quantity of air is needed to generate the same caloric stimulus obtained with water stimulation because the transfer of thermal energy between the air and tissue is much less efficient than between water and tissue. The standard is 8 liters of air at either 24° or 50° delivered into EAC within 60 seconds.

  Disadvantage of air calorics:

  - Coats found air responses had significantly greater test-retest variability than water calorics.
  - Ford and Stockwell, however, found no significant difference in responses if care was taken in irrigator placement so that tip was directly aimed at the tympanic membrane. Placement may be more critical with air calorics than water calorics.

- **Closed loop system:** This is also a form of water caloric. Water is circulated in a balloon inserted in the EAC and continuously exchanges the water in the balloon with fresh temperature-controlled water. Cyr has shown that closed loop system yields response intensities and reliabilities that are comparable to those produced by the traditional water caloric system.
- **Visual stimulators**: An array of points is needed for the patient to fixate on for calibration, gaze, and saccade tests. To calibrate, a pair of points must be separated by a desired distance. This instrument is usually called a light bar.
- **Other equipment:** Also needed are an electrode impedance tester and examining table. The examining table allows the patient to be positioned in sitting and supine positions. The table should also have the capability of elevating the head by 30° for caloric testing.

Location of Electrodes in ENG

ENG tracings (bottom portion) are display for horizontal and vertical movement of the eyeballs. A rightward eyeball movement (nystagmus) is reflected by an upward deflection on the tracing, whereas leftward nystagmus is reflected as a downward deflection in the tracing. For vertical movement, up is up and down is down.

ELECTRONYSTAGMOGRAPHY (ENG) ELECTRODE SITES and ENG TRACINGS

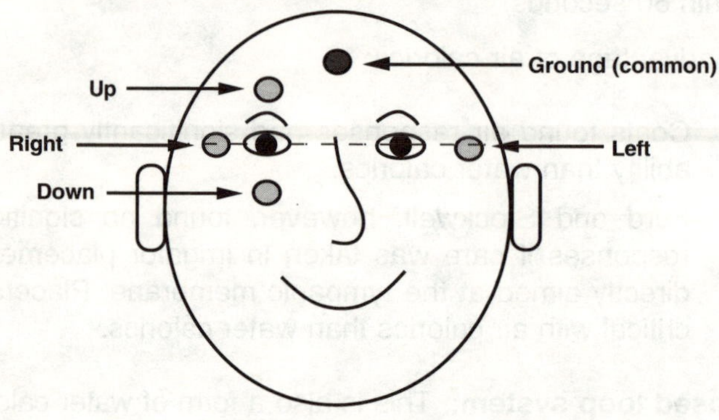

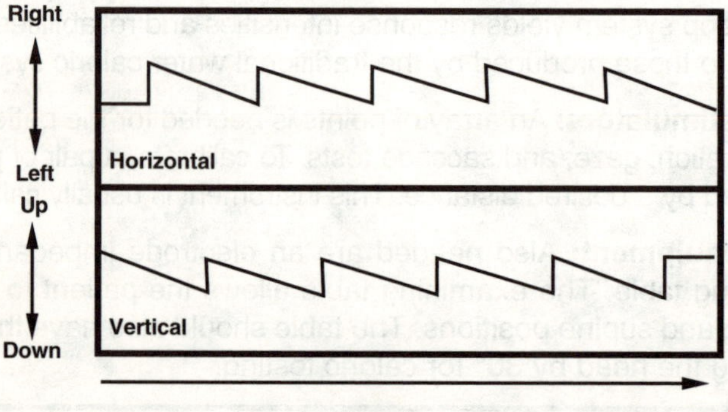

Technical Tip

ENG tracings, or which way is up versus down and right versus left?

Horizontal

- ☐ When horizontal eye movements are recorded, a deflection *upward* represents eye movement to the *right* and deflection *downward* represents eye movement to the *left*.

Vertical

- ☐ With vertical eye movements, a deflection *upward* represents *upward* movement and a deflection *downward* represents *downward* movement.

Protocol

Optokinetic Test

- ☐ Eye movements are recorded while the patient watches an optokinetic stimulus that is moving horizontally, first to the left then to the right. Consider using several velocities.
- ☐ The stimulus is a produced with a light bar, optokinetic drums, and/or vertical moving stripes
- ☐ The function of the optokinetic system is to maintain visual fixation when the head is in motion. The OPK test creates a nystagmus similar to that recorded during head rotation or caloric irrigation.
- ☐ Abnormalities may include
  - ✔ asymmetric nystagmic response
  - ✔ low-amplitude response
  - ✔ poor nystagmic waveform morphology.
- ☐ Most abnormalities are due to brainstem lesions, although some may be cortical.
- ☐ The problem with the OPK test is that its not specific and there may be many interpretation problems, such as:
  - ✔ Type of stimulus used in most clinical settings does not elicit a true OPK response.
  - ✔ Probably evaluates the pursuit system instead of OPK system unless the stimulus fills the visual field.

Protocol

Gaze Test

☐ **Technique**

- The patient's eyes are fixed on a point at a known angle from midline for a period of 20 to 30 seconds.
- Eye movements are recorded at 0°, 20° right, 20° left, 30° right, 30° left, 20° up, 20° down, 30° up, 30° down.
- The purpose of the gaze test is to identify the presence of spontaneous eye motion (usually nystagmus) during visual fixation.
- A patient with normal gaze ability should be able to maintain a steady ocular fixation when looking at fixed targets in the visual field.
- The gaze test is also repeated with eyes closed, but this test is often classified as a positional test.
- Gaze nystagmus with eyes open is a hard central finding while gaze nystagmus with eyes closed is a peripheral finding (called spontaneous nystagmus).

☐ **Types of gaze nystagmus**

- Bilateral horizontal gaze nystagmus
- Unilateral horizontal gaze nystagmus
- Rebound nystagmus
- Rotary gaze, usually consistent with brainstem lesion, often involving vestibular nuclei. Also seen with cerebellar disease
- Periodic alternating nystagmus (PAN), usually present in the primary center gaze position.
- Vertical gaze nystagmus
- Upbeating nystagmus, found on gaze upward or downward. This pattern suggests drug intoxication or posterior fossa disease. It looks like rightbeating nystagmus on the vertical channel.
- Down-beating nystagmus, usually on lateral gaze. This pattern suggests a lesion in the medullary or medullocervical region. It looks like left-beating nystagmus on the vertical channel.
- Direction changing nystagmus, which is gaze nystagmus that changes its direction when the patient changes the direction of the gaze. Usually implies a brainstem/cerebellum lesion.
- Congenital nystagmus, which describes nystagmus that appears at birth or soon after in an otherwise healthy individual. This pattern may occur in a patient with normal or impaired vision, and may be pendular or jerk-type.

Clinical Concept

Differentiating Congenital vs. Gaze Nystagmus

☐ Characteristics of congenital nystagmus

- Nystagmus that appears at birth or soon after in an otherwise healthy individual.
- May be pendular or jerk-type.
- Nystagmus markedly declines or stops at null point.
- Nearly always is horizontal or rotatory, rarely vertical. Nystagmus on gaze upward is virtually always horizontal, not vertical. Remember, vertical nystagmus on upward gaze denotes a pathologic or drug-induced condition.
- Reduction or abolition of the nystagmus on convergence.

Protocol

Tracking Test

☐ **General**

- Patient's eye movements are recorded while he or she follows a visual target moving in the horizontal plane.
- The total excursion should be approximately 30° visual angle and the maximum target speed should not exceed 40 to 50°/sec, because normal persons begin to have difficulty following targets at higher speeds.

☐ **Abnormalities**

- **Saccadic pursuit.** When brainstem disease involves the pursuit system, a patient may substitute saccadic movements for the smooth tracking capacity. This is called "cogwheeling."
- **Disorganized and disconjugate pursuit.** This is reduced horizontal gaze capacity and disconjugate eye movement, and may indicate a brainstem lesion.

☐ **Reasons for variations in persons with normal function**

- Inattentive patient
- Head movement
- Superimposed gaze or congenital nystagmus

Protocol

Saccade Test

☐ **General points**

- Done during calibration.
- Patient looks back and forth between the two dots on the wall.
- If the saccades are normal, the patient's eyes move rapidly and usually stop precisely on each target.
- Some patients with normal findings overshoot or undershoot and then make corrective saccades.

☐ **Abnormalities**

- **Ocular dysmetria:** Ocular counterpart to dysdiadochokinesia. Caused by diseases of the cerebellar system, defect of limb movement.
- **Overshoot or hypermetric saccades:** Eyes remain at a point a few degrees beyond the target of 150 to 200 msec, then return to fixate on the target. Unidirectional is most common.
- **Undershoot or hypometric saccades:** Eyes do not initially reach the target.
- **Saccadic slowing:** saccades are visibly slowed, velocity is abnormal. Can be seen in certain basal ganglia diseases.
- **Internuclear ophthalmoplegia:** rounding one side of plateau on saccades. When attempt is made to fixate, one eye lags behind.

☐ **Normal variations on the saccade test**

- Superimposed gaze nystagmus or congenital nystagmus
- Inattentive patient
- Eye blinks
- Head movements during calibration

MANAGEMENT OF VESTIBULAR DISORDERS

Medical Management

☐ **Vestibular suppressants**

- Antihistimines
- Benzodiazepines
- Anticholinergics

☐ **Anti-inflammatory agents**

- Dosepaks
- Prednisone
- Decadron

☐ **Diets**

- Low salt
- Low caffeine
- Low solute

☐ **Diuretics/calcium channel blockers**

- Thiazides
- Carbonic anhydrase inhibitors
- Furosemide
- Osmotics

☐ **Antinauseants**

- Phenergan
- Reglan
- IV Droperidol
- Bucladin

- ☐ **Vestibular rehabilitation**
  - Cawthorne-Cooksey exercises
  - Modified Epley maneuver
  - Posturography with training
- ☐ **Transtympanic gentamicin infusion**

Source: Courtesy of Mitchell K. Schumberg, M.D.

Features and Factors

Chemical Labyrinthectomy

- ☐ Gentamicin and streptomycin at low to moderate doses are mostly vestibulotoxic, whereas other aminoglycosides, such as amikacin and kanamycin, are cochleotoxic.
- ☐ Drugs cause deterioration of hair cells of the cristae and the ampullae in the vestibular apparatus and in the cochlea.
- ☐ Therapeutic gentamicin and streptomycin administration may be intramuscular, directly to lateral semicircular canal, or intratympanic.
- ☐ Intratympanic aminoglycoside therapy is performed as an outpatient nonsurgical procedure, and has the advantages of reduced risk to the patient and reduced cost.
- ☐ Indications for intratympanic aminoglycoside therapy.
  - patient has symptoms of Ménière's disease
  - clinical results of intratympanic aminoglycoside therapy
  - surgical and anesthetic risk factors
- ☐ Clinical results of intratympanic aminoglycoside therapy
  - control of vertigo in up to 90% of patients
  - hearing preservation in from 55 to 85% of patients

Essentials of Benign Paroxysmal Positioning Vertigo (BPPV)

Introduction

- ☐ First described by Barany in 1921
- ☐ Further defined by Dix and Hallpike in 1952
  - ✓ developed Dix-Hallpike maneuver
  - ✓ localized source of BPPV to undermost ear
- ☐ Incidence: accounts for 20% of vertigo cases presenting to ENT office
- ☐ Age: most common at 40+ years
- ☐ Gender: more women vs. men
- ☐ Other test findings, including calorics, rotary chair, and posturography, typically WNL

Definition

- ☐ Benign (i.e., it is not malignant nor is it life-threatening)
- ☐ Paroxysmal (i.e., response [nystagmus] gradually build, peaks, and fades in its intensity)
- ☐ Positioning (i.e., response is provoked by change in head or body position)
- ☐ Vertigo (i.e., a sensation of movement, usually described as a sensation of spinning or turning)

Classic characteristics

- ☐ Latency: 10 to 30 seconds
- ☐ Paroxysmal
- ☐ Rotary nystagmus
- ☐ Duration <1 minute
- ☐ Fatigues with repetition
- ☐ Dix-Hallpike duplicates patient's symptoms
- ☐ Nystagmus may reverse in upright position
- ☐ Positioning provoked vertigo
- ☐ Periods of exacerbation and remission
- ☐ Onset may follow head trauma or inactivity, although usually idiopathic in origin
- ☐ Usually unilateral
- ☐ Little benefit from medication (Antivert, Meclizine)

Diagnosis

☐ Diagnosis based on a positive Dix-Hallpike

- head hanging right → counter clockwise nystagmus
- head hanging left → clockwise nystagmus

Dix-Hallpike maneuver

☐ Completion of Dix-Hallpike maneuver:

- patient sitting upright
- turn head 45° to right
- eyes remain open
- assist patient into supine, head hanging position; maintain 45° head turn to right
- patient focuses on target; observe for nystagmus
- maintain head hanging position for 30 seconds; if response occurs, wait for nystagmus to fatigue
- patient centers head and returns to upright position
- when seated, patient focuses on target; if response was demonstrated previously, may see nystagmus reversal
- repeat with head hanging left

☐ Variations of the Dix-Hallpike maneuver

- record vs. observe nystagmus
- use Frenzel lenses
- turn head 45° to right (or left) after head hanging position is obtained
- for patients with complaints of back/neck pain, place pillow under middle/lower back; patient hangs head off pillow vs. table edge

Etiology

☐ Cupulolithiasis

- otoconia in utricle break loose and adhere to cupula in posterior semicircular canal (PSC)
- the increased density of the cupula relative to the endolymph causes inappropriate deflection of the cupula.

☐ Canalithiasis

- otoconia are free floating in PSC
- when the head is moved into a provoking position, the otoconia sink

into the most dependent position in the canal, causing the endolymph to move away from the ampulla

- movement of the endolymph overcomes the inertia of the cupula, resulting in inappropriate excitation.

Management

☐ Nothing

- not a life-threatening disorder
- 90% experience a spontaneous resolution of symptoms after a period of weeks to months

☐ Medication (Antivert, Meclizine)

☐ Adaptation exercises

☐ Surgery: intended to restrict fluid movement in the PSC

- PSC fenestration and occlusion
- singular neurectomy—sever nerve that innervates ampulla of PSC

☐ Epley or Semont maneuvers (see Epley Maneuver in this chapter)

- use should follow demonstration of a classic or positive Dix-Hallpike maneuver

Source: Information provided by Mary Beth Trine, M.S., CCC-A, Vanderbilt University

Modified Semont Maneuver

- Developed by A. Semont M.D., a French physician
- Also called the Liberatory Maneuver
- Appropriate for BPPV secondary to cupulolithiasis or canalithiasis
- Completion of modified Semont (Cyr et al., 1994)
    - patient seated on side of bed; turn head 45° to better ear
    - eyes remain open
    - Position #1: assist patient into lateral position on side with BPPV; maintain 45° head position in opposite direction. *Otoconia drift to top of PSC, away from cupula.*
    - observe rotary nystagmus
    - maintain position #1 for 10 minutes
    - Position #2: maintaining 45° head position, assist patient to opposite shoulder. *Otoconia move toward common crus.*
    - observe for reversal of rotary nystagmus
    - if no nystagmus is seen after 15 to 30 seconds, turn patient's head 90° upward and down
    - if absence persists, START OVER
    - maintain position #2 for 10 to15 minutes postnystagmus
    - Position #3: maintaining 45° head position, assist patient to upright position over 15-second period
    - patient slowly centers head. Otoconia move from common crus to utricle.
    - REPEAT maneuver if nystagmus seen in position #3
- Follow-up instructions
    - keep head vertical for remainder of today only; wear neck collar
    - tonight only, do not lie flat in bed
    - for next 3 to 4 days, do not sleep on treated side
- Differences from original Semont maneuver
    - speed of position change
    - duration per position
- Advantages of Semont vs. Epley maneuver
    - less back strain
    - increased time between position changes allows recovery from nausea
    - appropriate for cupulolithiasis or canalithiasis

- Efficacy of modified Semont maneuver (Cyr et al., 1994)
  - Subjects:

N:	115
age:	18–90 y (mean 59.6)
gender:	31 males, 84 females
ear:	43 left, 72 right
symptom duration:	6 days to 24 years (mean = 28 months)
Results:	89% clear after initial maneuver 96% clear after initial or second maneuver Dix-Hallpike was repeated the next day

- Efficacy as reported by Semont (1988)
  - 84% clear after initial maneuver
  - 93% clear after second maneuver
- Conclusion: Semont and Epley maneuvers:
  - have an 80 to 90% success rate or better
  - are noninvasive
  - can be performed in an office setting for a reasonable cost

Source: Information provided by Mary Beth Trine, M.S., CCC-A, Vanderbilt University

Step-by-Step

The Canalith Repositioning Procedure

An illustration of the steps in the canalith repositioning procedure (CRP), also known as the Epley maneuver, for treatment of benign paroxysmal positioning vertigo (BPPV).

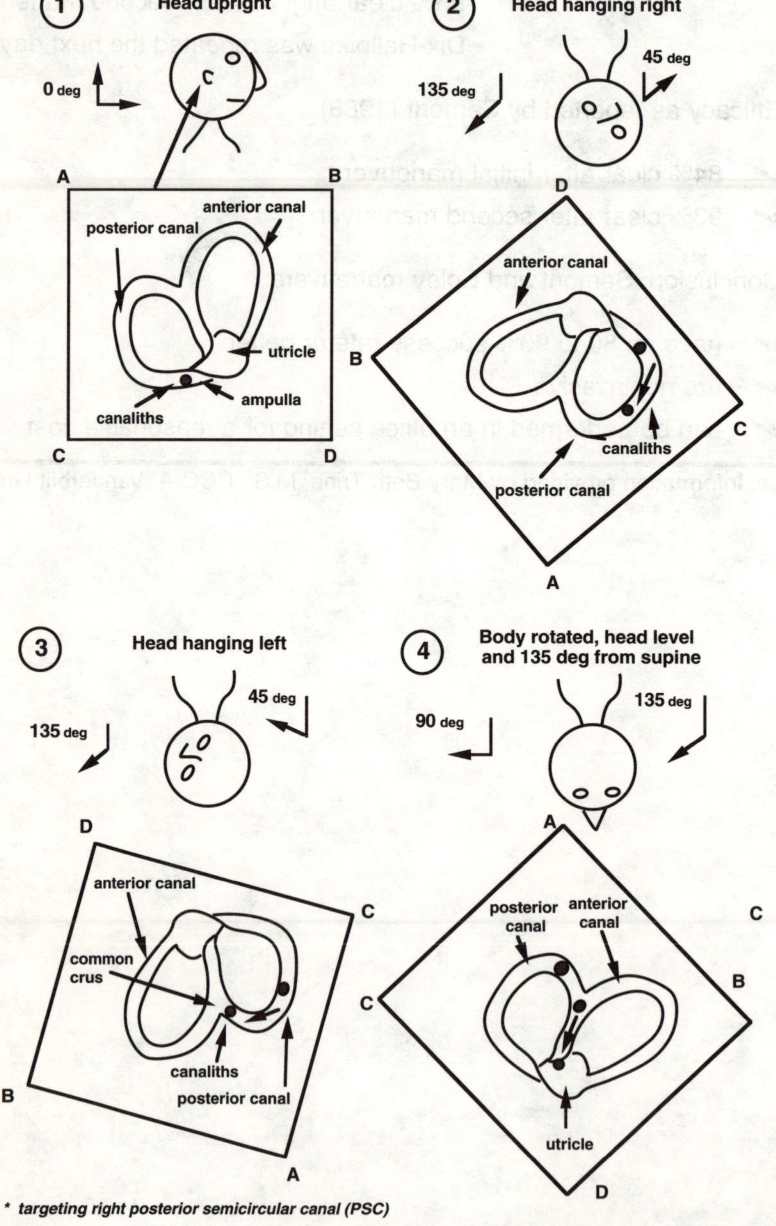

* *targeting right posterior semicircular canal (PSC)*

Key References

BPPV, Epley Manuever, and Semont Maneuver

Cyr DG, Brookhouser PE, Harker LA, Gossman MA. Modified Semont procedure for patients with unilateral BPPV. Presented to the Middle Section Meeting of the Triological Society, January 22, 1994, Rochester, Minnesota.

Epley JM. The canalith repositioning procedure: For treatment of benign paroxysmal positional vertigo. *Otolaryngol Head Neck Surg. 107:* 399–404, 1992.

Gossman MA, Cyr D, White V, Brookhouser PE. Treating patients with BPPV: Nonmedical/surgical approaches. Presented at American Academy of Audiology, April 29, 1994, Richmond, Virginia.

Jacobson GP, Newman CW, Kartush JM. *Handbook of balance function testing*. St. Louis: Mosby-Year Book, 1993.

Lynn S, Pool A, Rose D, Brey R, Suman V. A randomized trial of the Canalith Repositioning Procedure. *Otolaryngol Head Neck Surg,* in press.

Semont A, Freyss G, Vitte E. Curing the BPPV with a liberatory maneuver. *Adv Oto-Rhino-Laryngol. 42*: 290–293, 1988.

BALANCE

Sensory Organization Test

Components Assessed by Computerized Dynamic (platform) Posturography

☐ Subtest #1

- eyes are open
- platform and visual surround are fixed

☐ Subtest #2

- eyes are closed
- platform and visual surround are fixed

☐ Subtest #3

- eyes are open
- the visual surround is sway referenced
- platform is fixed

☐ Subtest #4

- eyes are open
- visual surround is fixed
- platform is sway referenced

☐ Subtest #5

- eyes are closed
- visual surround is fixed
- platform is sway referenced

☐ Subtest #6

- eyes are open
- visual surround is sway referenced
- platform is sway referenced

☐ Balance strategies

- ankle
- hip
- step

Sensory Organization Patterns

- ☐ Vestibular deficit pattern
  - subtests 1 through 4 are normal with appropriate visual and/or proprioceptive information
  - with vestibular input alone, performance is abnormal
  - subtests 5 and 6 or 6 only are abnormal in patients with bilateral vestibular weakness, an acute, unilateral peripheral vestibular weakness (e.g., not compensated yet), or a central vestibular lesion
- ☐ Surface dependency pattern
  - subtests 4, 5, and 6 are abnormal
  - patient can't make appropriate use of visual and/or vestibular cues to maintain balance
  - the patient is unsteady when standing on an uneven, compliant, or moving surface
- ☐ Visual preference pattern
  - subtests 3 and 6 or 6 only are abnormal
  - the patient can't suppress visually inaccurate information
  - balance is normal when eyes are closed
  - example: when you're sitting at a stop light in your car, the car next to you moves, and you hit the brakes
  - this pattern may reflect a central (cerebellar) deficit
- ☐ Vestibular dysfunction with visual preference
  - subtests 3, 5, and 6 are abnormal
- ☐ Vestibular/somatosensory deficit pattern
  - subtests 2, 3, 5, and 6 are abnormal
  - the patient can't make use of proprioceptive and/or vestibular cues to maintain balance
- ☐ Functional (physiologically inconsistent) pattern
  - normal or relatively better performance on the most difficult subtests (4, 5, and 6)
  - poor performance on the easier subtests (1, 2, and 3)

Sensory Organization Test

Six Conditions

The three senses that are integrated are: (1) vision, (2) vestibular, and (3) somatosensory. Each condition differs from the next by elimination of one or more of these sensory systems from the patient's balance system.

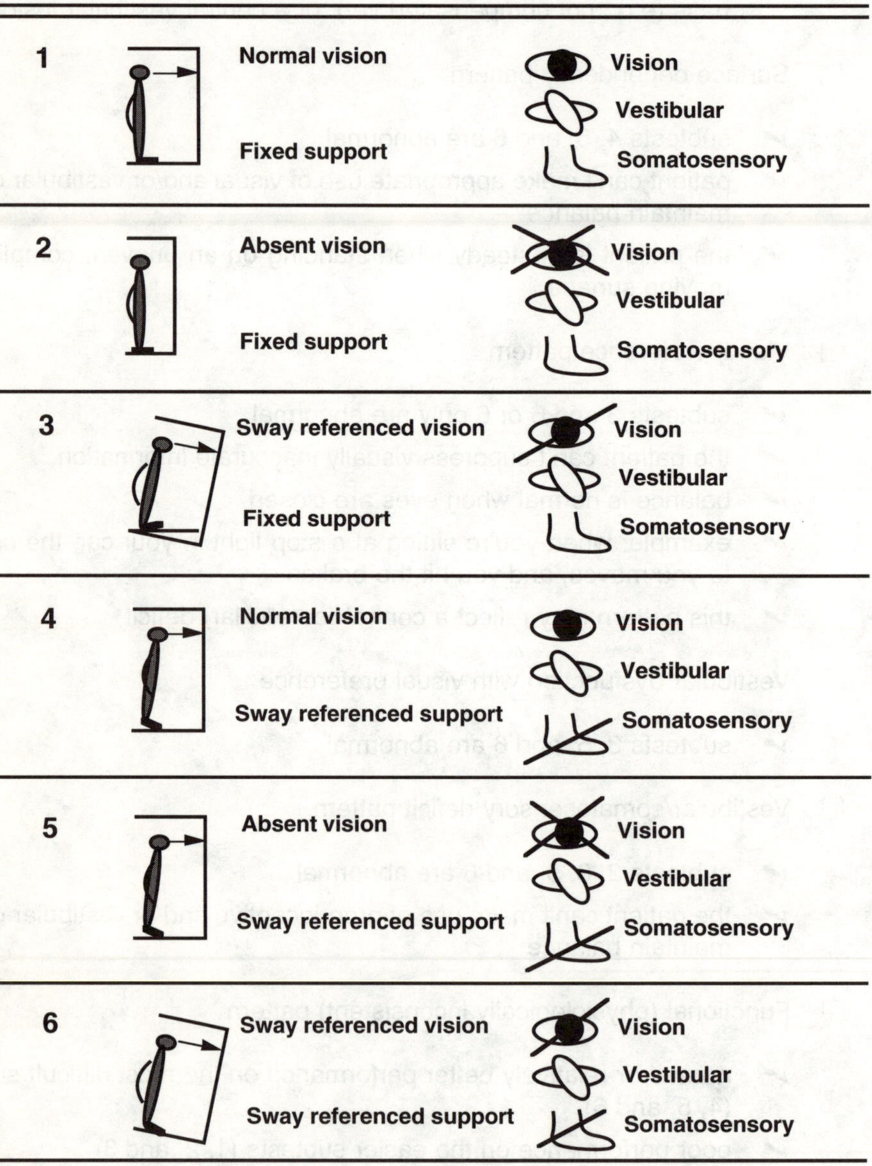

CHAPTER 15

Diseases and Syndromes

In This ADR Chapter

GENERAL INFORMATION

Seven Signs of Serious Ear Disease

Primary care providers are asked to evaluate and treat an ever-increasing number of both routine and complex medical problems. It is critical that the primary care provider be knowledgeable in a broad spectrum of routine medical problems, yet also recognize when the consultation of a specialist is indicated.

Seven signs of serious otologic (ear) disease that indicate the need for an evaluation by a specialist are:

1. Ear pain or fullness
2. Discharge or bleeding from the ear
3. Sudden or progressive hearing loss, even with recovery
4. Unequal hearing between ears or noise in the ear
5. Hearing loss after an injury, loud sound, or air travel
6. Slow or abnormal speech development in children
7. Balance disturbance or dizziness

1. **Ear pain or fullness**
   Ear pain (**otalgia**) may arise as a result of ear diseases or as a result of an illness elsewhere in the head and neck. **Otitis externa**, or swimmer's ear, is often a benign infection that responds well to topical therapy; but in cases of immunocompromise or diabetes, otitis externa may be the first sign of and eventually lead to skull base osteomyelitis. Acute **otitis media** is a frequent cause of otalgia and is usually effectively treated with antibiotics, but a middle ear infection can become complicated and lead to facial paralysis, intracranial abscess or meningitis. Referred otalgia, or pain referred to the ear from another source, may be due to **temporomandibular joint** (TMJ) dysfunction as well as **cancers** of the upper aerodigestive tract. **Tumors** in the pharynx and base of tongue have a particular tendency to cause referred otalgia through a neural network that innervates both the source of the cancer as well as the ear.
2. **Discharge or bleeding from the ear**
   Discharge or bleeding from the ear commonly results from infection or tumor. **Otitis externa** may lead to purulent discharge (otorrhea) or bleeding and is accompanied by severe otalgia. More diffuse disorders of the temporal bone include **chronic otitis media** and **cholesteatoma**. These are often associated with multiple episodes of ear drainage. Cholesteatoma is a slow growing lesion that erodes bone so that critical anatomy becomes vulnerable to erosion and infection over time. Complications of cholesteatoma include facial paralysis, labyrinthitis, meningitis, and brain abscess. Tumors of the external auditory canal, middle ear, and other regions of the temporal bone may present with bleeding from the ear. Bleeding from the ear may also be a result of trauma and can be a harbinger of more serious medical problems.

3. **Sudden or progressive hearing loss: even with recovery**
Sudden sensorineural hearing loss is often ascribed to a **viral infection** or an **ischemic event** but may be a symptom of a far more ominous pathology. Up to one-third of patients with **acoustic neuromas** experience a hearing loss at some point during their illness. These tumors most commonly present as a unilateral or asymmetric sensorineural hearing loss, often with tinnitus. Hearing loss with recovery or fluctuating sensorineural hearing loss is also frequently noted in patients with Ménière's disease along with whirling vertigo, aural fullness, and tinnitus. Progressive losses may also be caused by **immune disorders**, **syphilis** or **infections** at other sites in the body. Conductive hearing losses should be evaluated medically because of the risk of cholesteatoma and because most causes of conductive hearing loss can be readily treated.
4. **Unequal hearing between ears or noise in the ear**
Progressive asymmetric hearing loss or unilateral noise in the ear may be associated with acoustic **neuroma** or **other tumors**.
5. **Hearing loss after an injury, loud sound, or air travel**
Hearing loss after an injury may be conductive or sensorineural. Conductive hearing losses are due to a disruption of the free movement of the vibrating tympanic membrane and ossicular unit. Both blunt and penetrating trauma may lead to tympanic membrane perforation or ossicular discontinuity. Noise-induced sensorineural hearing loss may occur after a single extremely loud noise or after repeated exposures to loud sounds. Air travel is one cause of otologic barotrauma, scuba diving is another. Hearing loss again may be either conductive, as in the case of hemorrhage behind an intact tympanic membrane (hemotympanum), or sensorineural, as in the case of an inner ear membrane tear. The membranes that are most vulnerable to this type injury are the oval and round window membranes.
6. **Slow or abnormal speech development in children**
Abnormal speech development in children very frequently is a result of the child's inability to hear speech, recognize it, mimic it, and learn to use it appropriately. A common reason for hearing loss in young children may be otitis media with effusion that does not clear with treatment and leads to a significant conductive hearing loss. However, significant delays in speech acquisition are usually due to more serious, permanent sensorineural hearing losses. Abnormal speech development in children requires immediate action because speech and language are most efficiently acquired in early years of life.
7. **Balance disturbance or vertigo**
Balance disturbance or vertigo may originate from an otologic or a neurological source. A variety of specific otologic etiologies for vertigo are amenable to either medical or surgical treatment, as in Ménière's disease, or perilymphatic fistula. It is particularly important to exclude some specific potentially dangerous etiologies for vertigo including acoustic neuroma and other intracranial tumors, stroke, or demyelinating disease.

Conclusion

Primary care providers must be familiar with many types of diseases and decide which are to be treated in the primary care environment and which are to be referred to a specialist. The seven warning signs of serious ear disease were created to help in making that decision. Each warning sign should be a "red flag" and could indicate a potentially serious condition. When these warning signs appear, the patient should be referred to an otolaryngologist—head and neck surgeon to rule out serious disease of the ear, nose, or throat. The American Academy of Otolaryngology—Head and Neck Surgery is a resource that can be contacted and can supply a list of Academy members in a given region that may be of help.

Source: Reprinted with permission of the American Academy of Otolaryngology—Head and Neck Surgery, Alexandria, Virginia. American Academy of Otolaryngology-Head and Neck Surgery, Inc.

Common Pathogenic Organisms Responsible for Infectious Diseases

Code	Genus and Species	Gram Test	Associated Diseases
1	Streptococcus pneumoniae (pneumococcus)	positive	pneumonia
2	Streptococcus pyogenes	positive	respiratory disease, impetigo, scarlet fever, rheumatic fever
3	Streptococcus agalactiae	positive	meningitis and pneumonia in newborns
4	Streptococci Group D (enterococci)	positive	endocarditis, urinary tract infection
5	Streptococcus aureus	positive	epidermal skin diseases, dermatitis
6	Myobacterium tuberculosis	positive	tuberculosis
7	Haemophilus influenzae	negative	meningitis, otitis media, bronchitis, pneumonia, arthritis
8	Neisseria meningitidis (meningococcus)	negative	meningitis, upper respiratory infection
9	Neisseria gonorrhoeae (gonoccus)	negative	gonorrhea
10	Vibrio cholerae	negative	cholera
11	Escherichia coli	negative	diarrhea
12	Pseudomonas aeruginosa	negative	cystic fibrosis, serious infections, burn infections
13	Bacteroides fragilis	negative	various suppurative processes
14	Proteus	negative	numerous suppurative processes, cystitis
15	Krebsiella	negative	pneumonia, rhinoscleroma, rhinitis

Intracranial Tumors in Children versus Adults

Tumor Type	Children	Adults
Glioma	>75%	45–50%
Astrocytoma	>50%	>75%
Cerebellar	30%	—
Brain Stem	10%	—
Malignant	—	50–60%
Benign	—	25–30%
Oligodendroglioma	<2%	5%
Ependymoma	8%	5%
Medulloblastoma	25%	6%
Schwannoma	Rare	6%
Meningioma	Rare	15%
Hemangioblastoma	Rare	1–2%
Sarcoma	Rare	1–2%
Lymphoma	0%	<1%
Germ cell tumor	2–4%	1–2%
Dermoid, epidermoid	1–2%	<1%
Craniopharyngioma	5–10%	3%
Pituitary adenoma	Rare	5%

Note: About 15–20% of all intracranial tumors occur in childhood. Approximately 70% of intracranial tumors in children are located in infratentorial (e.g., brainstem) regions. In contrast, in adults approximately 70% are located supratentorially. See figures in Chapter 1 for details on central nervous system anatomy.

Source: Adapted from Okazaki H. *Fundamentals of neuropathology*. New York: Igaku-Shoin, 1983.

Vestibular Disorders

Commonly Used Medications

☐ Diuretics

- used when low-sodium diet restrictions fail
- aim is to drive the kidney to maintain a relatively constant urine output throughout the day
- hydrochlorothiazide, acetazolamide, etc.
- potassium levels must be monitored
- some diuretics (e.g., Lasix, ethacrynic acid) are ototoxic

Vestibular Suppressants

☐ Diazepam (Valium)

- psychotropic benzodiazepine
- very effective in most cases
- very addictive
- may temporarily decrease symptoms but may actually prolong underlying problem by interfering with compensatory mechanisms

☐ Meclizine (Antivert)

- must be taken continuously and at high doses
- dosing is titrated against side effects up to 150 mg/day
- side effects: drowsiness, dry mouth, double or blurred vision
- can be taken for years
- occasional weight gain

☐ Dimenhydrinate (Dramamine)

- drowsiness with continued use

☐ Promethazine (Phenergan)

- strong antiemetic properties

☐ Scopolamine (Transdermscop)

- diminished short-term memory and dry mouth

- ☐ Astemizole (Hismanal)
    - ✔ dryness of oral/nasal mucosa
    - ✔ less drowsiness

Vestibular Ablatants

- ☐ Aminoglycosides
    - ✔ mechanism of ototoxicity is increased permeability of hair cell membranes causing loss of magnesium
- ☐ Intramuscular Streptomycin
    - ✔ bilateral Ménière's disease with only hearing ear
    - ✔ first reported by Schuknecht in 1956. He administered 0.75–1.75 gm IM q12h which was continued until ice water caloric responses were abolished in 20 patients.
- ☐ Transtympanic Streptomycin or Gentamicin
    - ✔ placed through a cannula or repeated puncture
    - ✔ Streptomycin or Gentamicin given over a few days
    - ✔ very painful
    - ✔ vertigo controlled in >90%
    - ✔ high risk of hearing loss

Source: Courtesy of Jack A. Shohet, M.D.

Facial Palsy

Commonly Used Medications

- ☐ Corticosteroids (Prednisone)
    - ✔ anti-inflammatory effect
    - ✔ relieves pain and edema
    - ✔ serious side effects are uncommon
    - ✔ should not be used in diabetics, hypertensives, or those with peptic ulcer disease
    - ✔ common side effects: transient insomnia, mood swings, and GI upset

Source: Courtesy of Jack A. Shohet, M.D.

OTOLOGIC AND NEUROTOLOGIC DISEASES

Otitis Media

Common Micro-organisms and Commonly Used Medications

KEY TO ABBREVIATIONS:

A. = Aspergillus
E. = Escherichia
H. = Hemophilus
M. = Mycobacterium
N. = Neisseria
P. = Pseudomonadaceae
Pr. = Proteus
S. = Staphylococcus
St. = Streptococcus
T. = Treponema

MICRO-ORGANISMS

Otitis Media

☐ Acute Suppurative (arranged from most to least common)

- pneumococcus
- H. influenzae (flu)
- M. catarrhalis
- S. pyogenes
- S. aureus

☐ Acute Mastoiditis

- pneumococcus
- pyogenes
- S. aureus
- anaerobes
- M. tuberculosis

☐ Chronic with Effusion

- H. flu
- pneumococcus

- S. pyogenes
- M. catarrhalis

☐ Chronic Suppurative

- mixed aerobes and anaerobes

Otitis Externa

☐ Acute

- Pseudomonas aeruginosa
- Proteus
- Staph
- Strep

☐ Otomycosis

- Aspergillus niger
- Candida albicans

MEDICATIONS

Otitis Media

☐ Penicillins (Beta-lactams)

Advantages:

- inhibit synthesis of the cell wall
- Pen G DOC for pneumococcal and strep infections
- wide margin of safety
- excreted by kidney
- cross blood-brain barrier

Disadvantages:

- Pen G inactivated by gastric acid (pen V preferred oral)
- hypersensitivity reactions in approximately 5%
- inactivated by penicillinase, beta-lactamase
- penicillinase resistant penicillins developed for anti-staph (methicillin, dicloxacillin, nafcillin)

☐ Aminopenicillins *(Ampicillin, Amoxicillin)*

- identical spectrum of antimicrobial activity
- active against strep with increased activity against gram-negs. including H. flu., E. coli, Proteus
- inactivated by beta-lactamase
- gastric acid destroys ampicillin
- amoxicillin has highest middle ear fluid levels
- ampicillin associated with more rash-type reactions (7%)

☐ Augmented Penicillins

- Augmentin = amoxicillin + clavulanate
- Unasyn = ampicillin + sulbactam
- Timentin = ticarcillin + clavulanate
- broad spectrum which increases incidence of loose stools or diarrhea

☐ Antipseudomonas Penicillins *(Ticarcillin, Piperacillin)*

- effective against most strains as well as Proteus, E. coli, most H. flu
- Ticarcillin may prolong bleeding times with occasional anemia/neurtopenia
- valuable in malignant OE and other invasive pseudomonal infections
- often combined with another ABX for "double-coverage" (synergism)

☐ Cephalosporins (Beta-lactams)

- inhibit cell wall synthesis
- often safe alternative to PCN in penicillin-allergic patient
- categorized as first, second or third generation according to certain molecular configuration that affect their spectrum of activity

☐ Cephalosporins: *First generation*

- active against most gram-positive cocci
- Keflex, Ancef

☐ Cephalosporins: *Second generation*

- valuable against H. flu., strep, most anaerobes
- Ceclor, Ceftin
- nausea, diarrhea

- ☐ Cephalosporins: *Third generation*
  - gram negative bacilli, Pseudomonas
  - less activity against anaerobes and gram-positives
  - Fortaz, Claforan, Rocephin, Suprax, Vantin
- ☐ Erythromycin (a macrolide)
  - inhibits bacterial protein synthesis
  - H. flu. strains mostly resistant
  - GI distress in 10–15%
- ☐ Clarithromycin and Azithromycin (macrolides)
  - active against pneumococcus and H. flu.
  - expensive
- ☐ Clindamycin
  - inhibits protein synthesis
  - Gram-positives and anaerobes
  - side effects: gastroenteritis, diarrhea and rarely pseudomembranous colitis

Source: Courtesy of Jack A. Shohet, M.D.

Otitis Externa

Common Micro-organisms and Commonly Used Medications

- ☐ Ototopicals
  - ear canal must be debrided to facilitate penetration
  - acidic base because most pathogens prefer alkaline environment
  - white vinegar and alcohol are effective in many cases (Swim Ear, Aqua Ear, and Ear Magic)
  - most are a combination of several different drug types
- ☐ Antibiotics: *Neomycin*
  - contact dermatitis in 0.1%
  - active against S. aureus, Proteus

- Pseudomonas, anaerobes, and pneumococcus are resistant

- ☐ Polymyxin B
  - bactericidal against most gram-negatives
  - ototoxicity is theoretical

- ☐ Antifungals
  - acid is most important ingredient
  - very painful when they reach middle ear through a perforation
  - no currently available otic preparations
  - Amphotericin B (Funfizone), clotrimazole (Lotrimin), tolnafate (Tinactin) and nystatin (Mycostatin) topical preparations

- ☐ Anti-inflammatory agents
  - steroid-containing preparations useful in dermatosis such as psoriasis and seborrheic dermatitis
  - helpful for long-term therapy against itching and scaling
  - Orlex HC, VoSol HC, EarSol HC
  - added to antibiotic preparations to decrease mucosal and cutaneous edema bacterial infections
  - steroid-containing preparations useful in dermatoses such as psoriasis and seborrheic dermatitis

- ☐ Anesthetic Agents
  - Auralgan and Lidosporin contain benzocaine and lidocaine to reduce pain associated with OM
  - sometimes helpful in relief of the itching of external ear canal dermatitis

- ☐ Ceruminolytic Agents
  - carbamide peroxide in glycerol (Debrox) is the preferred agent for softening hard ear wax
  - may require treatment for several days
  - Cerumenex works within 15–30 minutes
  - severe allergic eczemoid reactions occasionally occur
  - should not be prescribed for at-home use

Source: Courtesy of Jack A. Shohet, M.D.

Otosclerosis

Commonly Used Medication

- ☐ Sodium Fluoride (Florical)
  - ✔ incorporated into skeletal bone rendering it more resistant to resorption
  - ✔ promotes bone formation
  - ✔ enzyme inhibitor of proteolytic enzymes sometimes found in perilymph
  - ✔ effectiveness is inconclusive
  - ✔ worthwhile for signs of progressive degradation of cochlear function

Source: Courtesy of Jack A. Shohet, M.D.

Clinical Concepts

Otosclerosis

- ☐ Excessive resorption of bone followed by abnormal formation of bone tissue
- ☐ New bony tissue is soft and hypervascular and may change into a dense sclerotic mass
- ☐ 96% of ears have fixation of the stapes at the oval window otolsclerosis will be found in other areas of the body in 49% of the patients (Schuknecht & Barber, 1985)
- ☐ Onset: 70% of patients first notice hearing losses between the ages of 11 and 30 years
- ☐ Family history: positive family history is reported in about 50% of cases
- ☐ Autosomal dominant transmission
- ☐ Usually occurs bilaterally; unilateral in about 10%
- ☐ No significant difference in occurance between the sexes
- ☐ Symptoms:
  - ✔ primarily conductive HL
  - ✔ degree of HL related to the degree of fixation of the stapes
  - ✔ vestibular disturbances can be associated with otosclerosis (e.g., hypoexcitability and elevated thresholds of angular acceleration and deceleration, directional preponderance, and positional nystagmus)

Courtesy of Donna Schwaber, M.CD.

Clinical Concepts

Paget's Disease

- ☐ Excessive bone destruction or resorption which is replaced by abnormal bony tissue
- ☐ Cause is unknown
- ☐ Usually affects middle-aged and elderly people
- ☐ Possible structural malformations of temporal bone:
  - thickening of petrous pyramid and narrowing of internal and external auditory canal
  - bony spurs in the epitympanic region of the middle ear space
  - pagetoid changes in the ossicles
  - ossification of the stapedial tendon
  - changes in the annular ligament
  - microfractures of the internal auditory canal, walls of the cochlea, semicircular canals, promontory and footplate (Schuknecht, 1993)
- ☐ Morphological changes
  - hair cell loss
  - atrophy of the tectorial membrane
  - atrophy of the stria vascularis
  - endolymphatic hydrops
  - vascular shunts
  - cochlear ossification (Schuknecht, 1993)
- ☐ Prevalence
  - increases with age
  - present in about 3% of persons >40 years and 5–10% of persons >89 years of age
  - higher prevalence in white than African-American persons
  - male-to-female ratio is about 4:3
- ☐ Hearing loss and vertigo
  - 70% of cases involve the skull
  - in about 50% of these there is hearing loss

- hearing loss is usually bilateral and mixed with a sloping configuration
- vertigo is present in 30% of patients

☐ Treatment

- calcitonin is used to lower both calcium and phosphate levels to relieve bone pain and stabilize hearing

Source: Courtesy of Donna Schwaber, M.CD.

Clinical Concepts

Perilymphatic Fistulae

☐ "Abnormal communications between the perilymphatic space and the middle ear" at either the oval or round windows or both (Schuknecht, 1993)

☐ Symptoms

- sudden hearing loss and/or
- sudden onset of mild to moderate vertigo in association with physical exertion, barotrauma, or head injury

☐ Testing that indicates side of involvement

- "eyes closed turning test"—patients tend to fall when turning toward the involved ear
- nystagmus with presentation of positive and negative pressure
- a positive Hennebert's sign
- positive positional tests when the involved ear is undermost

Source: Courtesy of Donna Schwaber, M.CD.

Clinical Concepts

Vascular Disorders

☐ Hemotympanum

- hemorrhage into the tympanomastoid compartment
- reddish-blue discoloration of the tympanic membrane is often visualized
- common with bleeding disorders: leukemia, thrombocytopenic purpura, hemophilia, and fracture of the temporal bone

☐ Hemolabyrinth

- hemorrhage into the inner ear
- caused by diseases that cause hemorrhages in the terminal stages
- trauma can cause hemolabyrinth without a fracture of the bony labyrinth
- bleeding from important nutrient vessels may cause ischemic necrosis of structures that are supplied by the vessels

Vascular Stasis or Occlusion

☐ Wallenberg's syndrome

- results from occlusion by embolism or thrombosis of either the posterior or vertebral inferior cerebellar artery
- symptoms, which may develop gradually or suddenly, include headache, pain in the side of the face, vertigo, vomiting, diplopia, dysphagia, dysphonia
- caloric testing may show directional preponderance to the side contralateral to the lesion
- hearing loss is not associated with Wallenberg's syndrome because the lesion is below the level of entry into the brain stem of the cochlear nerve

☐ Occlusion of anterior inferior cerebellar artery

- sudden onset of symptoms
- vertigo followed by facial paralysis, hearing loss, sensory disturbances and cerebellar asynergy
- vertigo and hearing loss are due to degenerative changes in the vestibular and auditory nuclei in the brain stem and ischemic necrosis of the membranous labyrinth
- occlusion is a result of hypertensive or arteriosclerotic vascular disease

☐ Vertebrobasilar ischemia

- decreased blood flow of the vertebral and basilar arteries
- most commonly caused by atherosclerosis
- may also be caused by mechanical compression of the vessels by cervical spondylosis with hyperextension or extreme rotation of the neck
- vertigo is the most common symptom and may be followed within a few days by visual sensory or somatic motor problems

Source: Courtesy of Donna Schwaber, M.CD.

Clinical Concepts

Otitis Media

- ☐ Acute otitis media
  - inflammation of the mucous membrane lining the middle ear space
  - sudden onset, limited duration, and usually a full recovery
  - highest incidence in the first 2 years of life
- ☐ Otitis media with effusion (OME)
  - "serous otitis"
  - results from Eustachian tube dysfunction
  - causes: infection, allergy
- ☐ Chronic serous otitis
  - results when an episode continues over several months
  - tympanic membrane becomes increasingly retracted, and the serous fluid becomes more viscous
- ☐ Prevalence
  - 80% of patients are >5 years old
  - chronic suppurative otitis media onset is 5–10 years of age
- ☐ Hearing loss
  - CHL can be acute or insidious
  - acute otitis media may involve earache, hearing loss, and rupture of the tympanic membrane
  - insidious onset presents with CHL, feeling of fullness in the ear, low-pitched tinnitus, crackling or popping sounds, fever and chills
  - 20–40 dB conductive hearing loss depending on the stage of the disease
  - chronic suppurative otitis media has a higher incidence of sensorineural hearing loss
- ☐ Complications
  - tympanic membrane perforation
  - tympanosclerosis
  - cholesteatoma

- mastoiditis
- labyrinthitis
- facial paralysis
- brain abscess
- meningitis

Source: Courtesy of Donna Schwaber, M.CD.

Clinical Concepts

Cholesteatoma

- ☐ Epidermoid cyst caused by accumulation of exfoliated keratin primarily found in the middle ear
- ☐ May also appear in pneumatized areas of the temporal bone
- ☐ Congenital cholesteatoma
  - probably due to epithelial remnants during the closure of the neural groove
  - most are first seen in children
  - can be seen behind a normal tympanic membrane
  - may be no history of middle ear disease
  - infection does not accompany unless the cholesteatoma erodes into the external auditory canal causing secondary infections
- ☐ Acquired cholesteatoma
  - occurs as a result of an epidermal invasion into a
  - perforation or retraction of Shrapnell's membrane
  - associated with recurrent acute or chronic otitis media
  - may also arise from entrapment of squamous epithelium as a result of injury or surgery
  - bone erosion may occur as the cholesteatoma increases in size; destruction of ossicles and invasion of the bony labyrinth or other areas adjacent to the temporal bone may also result
- ☐ Prevalence
  - may be either unilateral or bilateral
  - occurs in males more often than females

- ✓ prevalence is approximately 6:100,000

☐ Hearing loss

- ✓ dependent on the size and location of the cholesteatoma
- ✓ usually progressive conductive hearing loss
- ✓ may be complaints of pain, tinnitus, and foul-smelling discharge from the ear
- ✓ if cholesteatoma is in the attic area, there may be no hearing loss
- ✓ if cholesteatoma is in the internal auditory canal or
- ✓ cerebellopontine angle, there may be sensorineural hearing loss and facial palsy

Source: Courtesy of Donna Schwaber, M.CD.

Clinical Concepts

Labyrinthitis

☐ Serous (or toxic) labyrinthitis = "an irritation of the labyrinth caused by degradation of the tissue fluid environment in the inner ear" (Schuknecht, 1993)

☐ Pathogenesis usually from bacterial toxins

☐ May result from contamination of the perilymph with blood, tissue products, chemicals or air during surgery; may occur during acute or chronic otitis media or as a complication of meningitis

☐ Bacterial exotoxins enter the inner ear via the oval and round windows or via a bony labyrinthine fistula

☐ Symptoms

- ✓ various degrees of vertigo and hearing loss
- ✓ mild labyrinthitis usually with complete recovery
- ✓ serious labyrinthitis with partial to complete permanent loss
- ✓ of hearing and vestibular function

Source: Courtesy of Donna Schwaber, M.CD.

Clinical Concepts

Facial Nerve Disorders

- ☐ Bell's Palsy (idiopathic facial palsy)
- ☐ Believed to be a cranial neuropathy of viral etiology
- ☐ Some viruses include:
  - herpes simplex
  - varicella-zoster
  - Epstein-Barr virus
  - mumps
  - cytomegalovirus
  - influenza type B
- ☐ May be caused by an ischemia
- ☐ May be vasospasm resulting in venous stasis and nerve edema
- ☐ Swelling of facial nerve in the fallopian canal may cause compression and ischemia with temporary or permanent injury to the axons
- ☐ Complete recovery in 70-80% of patients with or without treatment
- ☐ 15% have some permanent weakness or dyskinesia
- ☐ < 5% have permanent severe or total paralysis
- ☐ Nystagmus and vertigo
- ☐ May occur as the facial nerve and superior division of the vestibular nerve have a close anatomic relationship in the internal auditory canal
- ☐ Nystagmus can be either spontaneous or positional
- ☐ Prevalence
  - occurs in about 2:100,000 persons
  - incidence changes with age
  - female to male ratio is about 1.2:1
  - familial tendency

Source: Courtesy of Donna Schwaber, M.CD.

Clinical Concepts

Neoplasms

Epidermoid carcinoma

- ☐ Prognosis
  - ✔ good for carcinomas of the auricle and external auditory canal
  - ✔ poor for carcinomas of the middle ear and mastoid
- ☐ Symptoms
  - ✔ otorrhea
  - ✔ hearing loss
  - ✔ pain
  - ✔ facial paralysis
  - ✔ mastoid swelling
  - ✔ vertigo

Adenomatous (glandular) neoplasms

- ☐ Occur in adults
- ☐ Symptoms: benign
  - ✔ painless mass
  - ✔ hearing loss
- ☐ Symptoms: malignant
  - ✔ hearing loss
  - ✔ otorrhea
  - ✔ pain
  - ✔ cranial nerve palsies

Glomus body tumor

- ☐ A mass of epithelioidlike cells with a rich vascular supply
- ☐ Located in the jugular, tympanic, carotid, and vagus nerve regions
- ☐ Can occur as an inherited, autosomal disease

- ☐ Increase of penetrance with age
- ☐ Symptoms usually begin in middle age
- ☐ More prevalent in white females
- ☐ Symptoms
  - conductive, sensorineural, or mixed hearing loss
  - pulsatile tinnitus (25%)
  - vertigo (25%)
- ☐ The tumor is highly vascular
- ☐ Reddish-blue pulsating mass behind the inferior portion of
- ☐ The tympanic membrane can often be seen
- ☐ Larger tumors may be seen in the floor of the external auditory canal

Cochleovestibular schwannoma (acoustic neuroma)

- ☐ A neoplastic growth arising from the vestibular nerve
- ☐ Prevalence
  - unilateral disease
  - incidence is about 2:100,000
  - accounts for 8–10% of all intracranial tumors and about
  - 78% of all tumors in the cerebellopontine angle
  - mean age at hospital admission is 45.1 years
- ☐ Order of symptoms
  - hearing loss
  - tinnitus
  - unsteadiness
  - occasional vertigo with nausea
  - with large tumors, there may be headaches located in the occipital or frontal lobes that are aggravated with stooping, straining, and sneezing
  - motor incoordination and nystagmus if the tumor presses on the cerebellar hemisphere
  - involvement of adjacent cranial nerves

Neurofibromatosis 1 (NF-1)

- ☐ a.k.a. von Recklinghausen's disease
- ☐ Autosomal dominant trait
- ☐ Incidence of 33:100,000
- ☐ Clinical manifestations:
  - onset in the first decade of life
  - multiple café au lait spots
  - intertriginous freckling
  - iris hamartoma
  - multiple neurofibromas
  - no more than 5% involve the cochleovestibular nerves
  - bilateral tumors are rare

Neurofibromatosis 2 (NF-2)

- ☐ Autosomal dominant with penetrance of over 95%
- ☐ Incidence of 1:100,000
- ☐ Clinical manifestations
  - signs of disease present during second or third decade
  - there may be café au lait spots
  - 75% develop other types of neoplasms of the CNS,
  - particularly meningiomas
  - bilateral vestibular schwannomas can be present

Source: Courtesy of Donna Schwaber, M.CD.

Clinical Concepts

Trauma

- ☐ Temporal bone fractures
  - ✔ longitudinal
  - ✔ transverse
  - ✔ mixed
- ☐ Longitudinal fracture
  - ✔ occurs when trauma is to the parietal and temporal regions
  - ✔ accounts for 80% of temporal bone fractures
  - ✔ fracture through the floor of the middle cranial fossa
  - ✔ parallel and adjacent to the anterior margin of the petrous pyramid
  - ✔ blood or cerebrospinal fluid may seep into the air space
  - ✔ of the middle ear and/or mastoid
- ☐ Symptoms
  - ✔ bleeding from the external auditory canal if the fracture line crosses the annulus tympanicus, causing a laceration of the tympanic membrane
  - ✔ facial weakness or paralysis, usually temporary
  - ✔ cerebrospinal otorrhea which subsides in a few days
  - ✔ dislocation of the incudomalleal and incudostapedial joints
  - ✔ conductive hearing loss if there is laceration of tympanic membrane, ossicular injuries, and hemotympanum
  - ✔ high-frequency sensorineural hearing loss which may improve during first 3 weeks
- ☐ Transverse fracture
  - ✔ usually caused by trauma to the occipital region
  - ✔ it passes across the temporal bone perpendicular to the long axis of the petrous pyramid
  - ✔ the fracture usually passes through the vestibule of the inner ear causing complete loss of cochlear and vestibular function
- ☐ Symptoms
  - ✔ severe vertigo with nausea and vomiting for several days (vertigo usually subsides within 2–3 weeks)
  - ✔ unsteadiness and a tendency to sway to the involved side when walking may persist for months
  - ✔ mild spontaneous nystagmus with the quick component to the opposite side of the lesion
  - ✔ may also be incomplete loss of auditory and vestibular function

Source: Courtesy of Donna Schwaber, M.CD.

Clinical Concepts

Ossicular Chain Discontinuity

- ☐ May result from congenital defects, skull trauma, or middle ear disease
- ☐ Trauma can be due to blows to the head, changes in barometric pressure, and penetrating objects
- ☐ Congenital discontinuity may be associated with branchial arch and facial anomalies (e.g., Pierre Robin and Treacher Collins syndromes and atresia/microtia)
- ☐ Common site of discontinuity is the incus and/or the incudostapedial joint
- ☐ Hearing loss: conductive hearing loss, usually unilateral, loss of 40–60 dB

Source: Courtesy of Donna Schwaber, M.CD.

Clinical Concepts

Autoimmune Disease

- ☐ Audiovestibular symptoms
  - sudden onset or gradually progressive
  - unilateral or bilateral
  - fluctuant hearing loss and spells of vertigo with nausea may mimic Ménière's disease
- ☐ More common in women and in patients with other autoimmune disease, for example:
  - rheumatoid arthritis
  - Cogan's syndrome
  - chronic ulcerative colitis
  - skin lesions
  - relapsing polychondritis

Source: Courtesy of Donna Schwaber, M.CD.

Clinical Concepts

Presbycusis

- ☐ Hearing loss due to degenerative changes associated with aging
- ☐ Four types of presbycusis:

1. Sensory prebycusis
   - ✓ cell loss at the basal end of the cochlea
   - ✓ initial loss of stereocilia followed by distortion and flattening of the organ of Corti and loss of supporting and sensory cells
2. Neural presbycusis
   - ✓ loss of cochlear neurons in the presence of a functional endorgan
   - ✓ progressive loss of word discrimination with stable pure-tone thresholds
3. Strial presbycusis
   - ✓ slowly progressive hearing loss
   - ✓ configuration of hearing loss is flat or slightly descending pure-tone thresholds with good word discrimination
   - ✓ patients respond well to amplification
   - ✓ hearing loss is due to patchy atrophy of the stria vascularis
4. Cochlear conductive presbycusis
   - ✓ gradually descending hearing loss with no greater than a 25 dB difference between any two adjacent frequencies and no other cochlear disease
   - ✓ hearing loss thought to be due to stiffening of the basilar membrane

Source: Courtesy of Donna Schwaber, M.CD.

Clinical Concepts

Sudden Idiopathic Sensorineural Hearing Loss

- ☐ Abrupt hearing loss without a known cause
- ☐ Clinical and pathologic evidence points to viral etiology
- ☐ Prevalence is 10.7:100,000
- ☐ Symptoms
  - ✓ hearing loss can occur instantaneously or over a period of days
  - ✓ hearing loss is usually unilateral and varies in degree
  - ✓ tinnitus is reported in 70 - 80% of patients
  - ✓ recovery of hearing also varies:

    25% = spontaneous recovery

    50% = partial return of hearing 25% –no recovery

    50% = experience vertigo, dizziness, or unsteadiness before, during, or following the hearing loss

Source: Courtesy of Donna Schwaber, M.CD.

Clinical Concepts

Ménières Disease

- ☐ An inner ear disorder associated with a dysfunction of the mechanism regulating the production and/or absorption of endolymph
- ☐ Three theories of cochlear dysfunction:
  - ✓ mechanical
  - ✓ metabolic
  - ✓ biochemical alterations
- ☐ Prevalence
  - ✓ .05–.15% of the population
  - ✓ third most common inner ear disorder after presbycusis and noise-induced hearing loss
  - ✓ onset at 40–60 years in 50% of subjects

- ☐ Symptoms include:
  - fluctuating sensorineural hearing loss
  - episodes of vertigo
  - tinnitus
  - sensation of pressure in the ear, vertigo, nausea, and vomiting become less severe with time, but hearing loss and tinnitus may worsen
- ☐ Characteristics of hearing loss
  - sensorineural hearing loss
  - loudness recruitment
  - decreased speech discrimination scores
  - acoustic distortion
  - loudness intolerance
  - fluctuant low-frequency hearing loss in early stages
  - flatter but slightly worse for very low and high frequencies in late stages

Variations of Ménière's disease:

- ☐ Lermoyez' syndrome:
  - hearing improves during and immediately following an attack of vertigo
- ☐ Vestibular Ménière's disease
  - vertigo is present without hearing loss
- ☐ Cochlear Ménière's disease
  - auditory symptoms are present without vertigo
- ☐ Otolithic catastrophe
  - person has abrupt falling attacks of fleeting duration

Source: Courtesy of Donna Schwaber, M.CD.

Clinical Concepts

Vestibular Disorders

Cupulolithiasis, also known as:

- ☐ Postural vertigo
- ☐ Positional vertigo
- ☐ Benign paroxysmal positional vertigo (BPPV)
- ☐ Caused by inorganic deposits of calcium or phosphorous
  - compounds on the cupula of the posterior semicircular canal; the organ is therefore sensitive to gravitational force and subject to stimulation with changes in the position of the head
- ☐ Etiologic factors
  - with no precipitating incident, the disorder is usually caused by degeneration and displacement of otoconia
  - most common vestibular disorder resulting from head injury
  - otitis media
  - ear surgery, particularly involving the stapes
  - vestibular neuritis
- ☐ Vertigo
  - sudden attacks of vertigo are precipitated by certain head positions
  - during testing, vertigo occurs when the injured ear is in the undermost position
  - usually 5–10 seconds in duration
  - the disorder usually subsides within a few weeks or months
  - sometimes there are remissions and recurrences over years

Source: Courtesy of Donna Schwaber, M.CD.

Syndromes Associated with Auditory Dysfunction

Syndrome	Category of Syndrome	Ear Malformation	Auditory Dysfunction
Abruzzo-Erickson (cleft palate, eye coloboma, short stature, hypospadias)	orofacial clefting	soft, prominent pinnae	MHL; SNHL
Acrodysostosis	skeletal dysplasia	otitis media (recurrent ear infections)	CHL
Acrocraniofacial dystosis	craniosynostosis	dysplastic ears	MHL
Acrofacial dysostosis (Reynold's syndrome)	head and neck	—	
Antley-Bixler	craniosynostosis	dysplastic ears, low-set protruding ears, EAC atresia	CHL
Apert (acrocephalosyndactyly)	head and neck	low-set ears, otitis media, congenital ossicular (stapes) fixation	CHL[a]
Auro-digital-anal	craniosynostosis	—	SNHL[a]
Baller-Gerold	craniosynostosis	dysplastic ears, low-set ears	CHL
Beckwith-Weidemann	overgrowth syndrome	ear lobe grooves, indented ear lesions on helix or concha	CHL
Branchio-oto-renal (BOR)	branchial arch	pre-auricular or helical pits, various forms of abnormal pinnae, narrow or atretic EAC, fused ossicles; inner ear malformations	CHL, SHL, MHL[a]
Campomelic	chondrodysplasia	otitis media	CHL
Camurati-Engelmann	connective tissue	—	MHL
Carpenter	craniosynostosis	low-set ears, preauricular pits	CHL, SHL, MHL
Cerebro-costo-mandibular	miscellaneous	—	SNHL?
Cervico-oculo-acoustic (Wildervanck)	branchial arch	preauricular tags; malformed pinnae; atretic EAC; ossicular abnormalities; inner ear and vestibular abnormalities;	CHL; SNHL; MHL[a]

(continued)

(continued)

Syndrome	Category of Syndrome	Ear Malformation	Auditory dysfunction
CHARGE (association)	miscellaneous association	E = ear anomalies; ears may be small, cup-shaped, lop-shaped	CHL, SHL, MHLL[a]
CHILD	limb defect	—	SNHL?
Cleft lip sequence	facial defects	middle ear dysfunction (otitis media)	CHL[a]
Cleft palate syndromes	orofacial clefting	large ears, otitis media, ossicular fixation	CHL[a]
Cleidocranial dystosis	osteochondrodysplasia	middle-ear dysfunction (incomplete mastoid air cell development)	CHL
Cornelia de Lange (Brachmann de Lange)	small stature	low-set ears	SNHL[a]
Crouzon	craniosynostosis	EAC atresia, otitis media (cleft palate)	CHL
Cockayne	senilelike appearance	—	SNHL
Craniodiaphyseal dysplasia	craniotubular disorder	—	MHL[a]
Craniometaphyseal dysplasia	osteochondroplasia	—	SNHL, CNS
del 18q	chromosomal abnormality	prominent antihelix and antitragus, narrow or atretic EAC	CHL
Diastrophic dysplasia	osteochondrodysplasia	EAC stenosis, ossicular fixation, otitis media (cleft palate)	CHL[a]
Dyskeratosis congenita	hemartoses	—	SNHL?
Ectrodactyly-ectodermal dysplasia-clefting (EEC)	facial-limb defects	small or malformed auricles, middle ear dysfunction (secondary to cleft palate), ossicular malformation	CHL; SNHL
Facio-audio-symphalangism	—		CHL[ab]
Facio-auriculo-radial dysplasia	—	dysplastic pinnae	CHL
Fanconi pancytopenia	limb defects	auricular anomaly	SNHL?
Fetal iodine deficiency effects	environmental agents	—	SNHL, CNS[a]
Fetal methyl mercury effects	environmental agents	—	SHL[a]

(continued)

Fetal trimethadione effects	environmental agent	poorly developed, cupped, or overlapping helix	CHL, SNHL?
FG	facial-limb defects	small, simple ears	SNHL, CNS
Fibrodysplasia ossificans progressiva	connective tissue disorder	—	SNHL?
Fountain	unusual facies	—	SNHL[a]
Fraser (cryptophthalmos)	head and neck	malformed pinnae, otitis media, stenotic EAC, ossicular defects	CHL
Frontometaphyseal dysplasia	osteochondroplasia	—	MHL, SNHL[ab]
Goldenhar	Facial-auriculo-vertebral spectrum (1st and 2nd branchial arch syndrome)	microtia, preauricular tags and/or pits, middle ear dysfunction	CHL, SHL, MHL[a]
Goltz-Gorlin (focal dermal hypoplasia)	skin disorder	—	MHL[a]
Hajdu-Cheney (acroosteolysis)	bone disorder	—	CHL; SNHL[a]
Hay-Wells syndrome of ectodermal dysplasia	facial-limb defects	cup-shaped ears; EAC atresia; middle ear dysfunction	CHL
Hunter (Mucopolysaccharidosis II)	storage disorder	—	SHL or MHL[ab]
Hurler-Scheie compound (Mucopolysaccharidosis I H/S)	storage disorders	otitis media	CHL; MHL
Hyperphosphatasemia	bone disorder	—	USHL
Hypertelorism-microtia—clefting (Bixler)		hypoplastic pinnae and EAC, atretic EAC, ossicular abnormalities	CHL
Johanson-Blizzard	small stature	—	SNHL[a]
Kartagener	miscellaneous sequences	middle ear dysfunction secondary to mastoiditis	CHL[a]
Keutel	miscellaneous	diffuse calcification of pinnae cartilage	MHL

(continued)

Syndrome	Category of Syndrome	Ear Malformation	Auditory Dysfunction
KID syndrome	skin disorder	K = keratosis; I = ichtyosis; D = deafness	SNHL[a]
Killian/Teschler-Nicole (tetrasomy 12p)	chromosomal abnormality	large ears with protruding lobules; stenosis of EAC	CHL, SNHL, MHL
Klippel-Feil sequence	miscellaneous	—	CHL, SHL[a]
Kniest dysplasia (metatropic dysplasia, type II)	skeletal disorder	otitis media	CHL; SHL[a]
LADD syndrome	L = lacrimo; A = auriculo; D = dento; D = digital	cup shaped pinnae	SNH[a]
Lenz-Majewski	bone disorder	—	SNHL[a]
LEOPARD syndrome (multiple lentigines syndrome)	L = lentigines; E = electrocardiographic abnormalities; O = ocular hypertelorism; P = pulmonic stenosis; A = abnormal genitalia; R = retardation of growth; D = deafness		SNHL[a]
Levy-Hollister	lacrimo-auriculo-dento-digital syndrome	small, cup-shaped ears; short helix	MHL, SNHL[a]
Mannosidosis (II)	storage disorder	—	SNL[a]
Marshall	facial defects	—	SHL[a]
Maxillofacial dysostosis, X-linked	craniofacial defects	prominant pinnae	MHL[a]
McCune-Albright	hemartoses (small spots or tumors)	narrowing of IAC	NHL
Melnick-Fraser	branchial arch anomalies	preauricular pits, malformed middle/inner ear	CHL, SHL, MHL[a]
Metaphyseal chondroplasia, Jansen type	osteochondrodysplasia	—	SNHL?
Miller (Postaxial acrofacial dysostosis)	facial-limb defects	hypoplastic cup-shaped ears (syndrome resembles Nager and Treacher Collins)	CHL

(continued)

Mohr	facial-limb defects	middle ear (ossicular) malformation	CHL[a]
Morateaux-Lamy (Mucopolysaccharidosis VI)	storage disorder	upper respiratory tract infections with otitis media	MHL, SHL[a]
Morquio (Mucopolysaccharidosis IV)	storage disorder	upper respiratory tract infections with otitis media	MHL, SHL[a]
Multiple lentigines	hamartoses (many tumors)	LEOPARD is acronym; D = deafness; prominent ears	SHL[a]
Multiple synostosis (Symphalangism)	skeletal dysplasia	fusion of middle ear ossicles (stapes fixation)	CHL[a]
Murcs association	miscellaneous	external ear defects	CHL, SHL
Nager	facial-limb defects	preauricular tags, aural atresia	CHL, MHL[a]
Neurofibromatosis II		—	NHL (bilateral)
Noonan	moderate small stature	low-set and/or abnormal auricles	SHL, NHL [a]
Oculodentodigital (Oculodentodigital dysplasia) type I (Lobstein disease)	facial-limbs defects	—	CHL
Oral-facial-digital		low-set ears	CHL
Otodental	head and neck	—	SHL[ab]
Oto-palato-digital, type I (Taybi syndrome)	facial-limb defects	cleft palate with middle ear dysfunction	CHL[a]
Osteopetrosis (Albers-Schonberg disease)	bone disorder	—	USHL
Osteopetrosis (benign autosomal dominant, Type I)	bone disorder	—	CHL

(continued)

Syndrome	Category of Syndrome	Ear Malformation	Auditory Dysfunction
Oto-palato-digital, types I and II	facial-limb defects	low-set ears, middle ear dysfunction (cleft palate)	CHL
Pallister-Killian (mosaic tetrasomy 12p)	chromosomal abnormality	fleshy pinnae	USHL
Postaxial acrofacial dysostosis (Miller syndrome; Wildervanck-Smith syndrome; Genee-Wiedemann syndrome)		cleft palate, cup shaped pinnae, malformed EAC and middle ear	CHL
Progeria (Hutchinson-Gilford)	senilelike appearance	middle ear dysfunction (ossicular fixation)	CHL, SHL, CNS
Rieger	miscellaneous	—	CHL
Robin sequence (Pierre Robin syndrome)	facial defects	middle ear dysfunction	CHL
Saethre-Chotzen	craniosynostosis	prominant ear crus, small ears, otitis media	CHL, SNHL
Sialidosis	storage disorder	—	USHL
Sanfillippo (Mucopolysaccharidosis III)	storage disorder	—	USHL
Scheie (Mucopolysaccharidosis I S)	storage disorder	—	SNHL?
Sclerotosis	osteochondroplasia	narrowing of internal auditory canal	NHL
Senter (Ichthyosiform Erythroderma)	ectodermal dysplasia	excessive EAC skin debris	SNH[a]
Shprintzen	facial-limb defects	minor auricular abnormalities; cleft palate (eustachian tube)	CHL[a]
Stickler	facial-limb defects	middle ear dysfunction (cleft palate)	CHL, SNHL, MHL[a]

(continued)

Townes (Townes-Brock)	facial-limb defects	large ears, poorly formed ears, or microtia; preauricular tags (resembles VATER syndrome and facio-auriculo-vertebral sequence)	SNHL
Treacher Collins	mandibulofacial dysostosis	malformed auricles; EAC defect; aural atresia/microtia	CHL, MHL[a]
Trisomy 13	chromosomal abnormality	abnormal helices; low set ears	SNHL
Trisomy 14	chromosomal abnormality	preauricular tags or pits; occasional EAC atresia	CHL
Trisomy 8	chromosomal abnormality	prominant cup-shaped ears with thick helices	CHL
Van Buchem disease	bone disorder	—	SNHL; MHL[b]
VATER association	miscellaneous	—	SNHL
Velocardiofacial (Shprintzen; Selackova)	head and neck	small auricles, thickened helices, otitis media (cleft palate)	CHL
Waardenburg (types I, II)	facial defects	—	SHL[a]
XO (Turner)	chromosomal abnormality	prominent and protruding auricles	SNHL[a]

Note: CHL = conductive hearing loss; SHL = sensory hearing loss; SNHL = sensorineural hearing loss; USHL = unspecified hearing loss; NHL = 8th cranial nerve involvement; MHL = mixed hearing loss; CNS = central nervous system involvement; EAC = external auditory canal

[a] Hearing loss is often a prominant feature of the syndrome.

[b] Progressive hearing loss.

CHAPTER 16

Diagnostic Medical Techniques and Surgical Procedures

In This ADR Chapter

GENERAL MEDICAL TESTS

Clinical Concept

Normal Pulse Rates

Age	Average Range (heartbeats/minute)
Neonate	120–160
2-year-old	80–140
5- to 12-year-olds	75–100
Adolescents and adults	60–100

Clinical Concept

Electroencephalography (EEG) Patterns

Pattern	Description
Alpha	Frequencies of 8–13 Hz, which may be lower in children. An alpha frequency is often present in posterior regions in the awake, alert individual with eyes closed. It disappears when the eyes are opened.
Beta	Symmetrical frequencies of 14–30 Hz with lower amplitude than alpha rhythm amplitude. Beta rhythms are normally found in the frontal areas.
Theta	Frequencies of 3–7 Hz. These slow waves are normal during sleep and are often associated with metabolic disorders and destructive cortical lesions.
Delta	Frequencies less than 3 Hz.
Sharp	Waves that are a brief high-voltage electrical discharge from a focal area of the brain. They are also referred to as "spike and dome" waves. An EEG feature of epilepsy.
Negative	EEG pattern representing a sudden burst of electrical activity from the brain surface which may be associated with epilepsy.
Asymmetric	EEG patterns representing large regions of the left and right hemispheres graphically displayed. The waves correspond to patterns of connections between electrodes montages. Asymmetric patterns reflect destructive lesions to one of the cerebral hemispheres.

Glasgow Coma Scale

Rating Severity of Brain and Head Injury

Response	Score
Eye opening	
None	1
To pain	2
To speech	3
Spontaneous	4
Verbal response	
None	1
Incomprehensible sounds	2
Inappropriate words	3
Confused conversation	4
Oriented conversation	5
Motor response	
None	1
Abnormal extension (decerebrate rigidity)	2
Abnormal flexion (decorticate rigidity)	3
Withdrawal	4
Localizes pain	5
Obeys commands	6
Total GCS:	**3–15**

Source: Adapted from Teasdale MJ, Jennett, B. Assessment of coma and impaired consciousness: A practical scale. *Lancet 11*: 81–84, 1974.

Rancho Los Amigos Cognitive Scale for Head Injury

Level	Indicators
I	No response to pain, touch, sound, or sight.
II	Generalized reflex response to pain.
III	Localized response. Blinks to strong light, turns toward/away from sound, responds to physical discomfort, inconsistent response to commands.
IV	Confused, inappropriate, and agitated. Alert, very active, aggressive or bizarre behaviors, performs motor activities but behavior is nonpurposeful, extremely short attention span.
V	Confused, inappropriate, and nonagitated. Gross attention to environment, highly distractible, requires continual redirection, difficulty learning new tasks, agitated by too much stimulation. May engage in social conversations but with inappropriate verbalizations.
VI	Confused, appropriate. Inconsistent orientation to time and place, retention span/recent memory impaired, begins to recall past, consistently follows simple directions, goal-directed behavior with assistance.
VII	Automatic, appropriate. Performs daily routine in highly familiar environment in a nonconfused but automatic manner. Skills noticeably deteriorate in unfamiliar environment. Lacks realistic planning for own future.
VIII	Purposeful, appropriate.

Source: From Hagen C, Malkmus D. (1979, November). *Intervention strategies for language disorders secondary to head injuries.* Paper presented at the American Speech-Language-Hearing Association Annual Convention, Atlanta, GA, November 1979, with permission as adapted by Golper, 1992.

RADIOLOGIC STUDIES

Summary of Current Radiologic Techniques

Studies of the Head and Brain

Conventional radiographs (X-rays)

- ☐ A view of the skull and contents within the skull
- ☐ X-ray beam is sent through the skull and received by an X-ray film
- ☐ Involves radiation of brain
- ☐ Tissues that absorb more X-rays appear brighter (e.g., bone and calcium-accumulating tissues)
- ☐ Clinical disadvantages
  - ✔ Presents only a two-dimensional representation of three-dimensional objects
  - ✔ Structures are differentiated only if they have large differences in absorbency of X-rays (e.g., gray matter and white matter are not detected, nor distinguished)
- ☐ Clinical advantages
  - ✔ Good for detecting bone (skull) fractures (inexpensively)
  - ✔ Relatively high spatial resolution (about 0.05 mm)
  - ✔ Useful for angiography (imaging of arteries and veins; description of cerebral vasculature)

Computerized tomography (CT)

- ☐ See figure illustrating principles of CT later in this chapter
- ☐ First described in 1973 (see Key References in this chapter)
- ☐ The original abbreviation CAT (computerized axial tomography) scan was dropped because the imaging wasn't always in the axial view (slices across the vertical axis of the head or body)
- ☐ A highly sophisticated, computer-intense process for measuring and analyzing multi-plane (multi-cut) X-rays
- ☐ Also based on differential absorption of X-rays

- ☐ X-ray absorption is measured over 180° along skull as X-ray detectors are also rotation on opposite side of skull
- ☐ Radiodensity of specific point within the skull is calculated by multiple measurements from different angles
- ☐ Spatial resolution of CT determined by distances between intersecting points among the various planes (see the figure)
- ☐ Within each section of the brain, thousands of absorption (radiation intensity) measures are used to compute a matrix of attenuation coefficients which appear as dark or light regions on the CT scan
- ☐ Early generation CT scans appeared "grainy" because resolution was poor due in part to relatively low computer power
- ☐ Clinical advantages
  - ✔ Resolution in soft tissue, like the brain, can be down to 1 mm or less
  - ✔ CT distinguishes between white and gray matter (more sensitive)
  - ✔ CT also distinguishes between brain, blood, and cerebrospinal fluid
  - ✔ When iodinated radiopaque material (highly absorbant) material is injected intravenously, the contrast between different types of brain tissues, such as blood vessels, abscesses, or tumors, is enhanced, and these structures are more easily and confidently identified
- ☐ Clinical disadvantages
  - ✔ expensive (in comparison to X-rays)
  - ✔ involves exposure to radioactivity
  - ✔ not optimal for imaging in brainstem region because of high concentration of bone with resulting artifacts
  - ✔ better for imaging bone than soft tissue

Magnetic resonance imaging (MRI)

- ☐ Also based on a computerized tomography type technique
- ☐ General magnetic resonance technology was first reported in the 1950s, but MRI was introduced as a clinical, computer-intensive radiologic technique in the early 1980s
- ☐ Different regions and tissues in the brain are distinguished by their individual chemical compositions, including the ventricular system
- ☐ Hydrogen atoms (with an odd atomic weight) are exposed to a strong magnetic field and are set into an aligned spinning motion along their axes
- ☐ The spin axes are upset (perturbed) by a brief radio wave impulse
- ☐ When the pulse is turned off, the nuclei begin to return to their spinning motion and release radio waves in the process

- ☐ Different brain tissues give off different radio wave frequencies due to their different chemical properties
- ☐ Also, various nuclei return to a lower-energy state (less spinning) at different rates. This is referred to as *relaxation*, and is defined by the corresponding time constant
- ☐ There are at least two types of relaxation (T_1 and T_2), which help to differentiate among brain tissues (e.g., gray versus white matter, normal tissue versus tissues)
- ☐ Clinical advantages
  - ✔ high spatial resolution
  - ✔ good images of soft tissue (e.g., brain and tumors)
- ☐ Clinical disadvantages
  - ✔ more expensive than CT
  - ✔ not as available as CT

Positron emission tomography (PET)

- ☐ Available first, mostly for research, about 1980
- ☐ Based on emission versus absorption of radiation
- ☐ Radio-isotope (manufactured by a cyclotron facility) is injected into major arteries leading to brain, or inhaled by patient
- ☐ Glucose (2-deoxyglucose) metabolism within neurons is measured and mapped throughout the brain, including the cerebrum, cortical sulci and gyri, subcortical regions (e.g., thalamus, caudate nucleus, etc.), the hippocampus (if memory is involved), the internal capsule, and the brainstem
- ☐ Clinical advantages
  - ✔ measures brain function versus structure
  - ✔ can objectively quantify and localize brain activation by sensory stimulation (e.g., hearing)
  - ✔ can be applied in the evaluation of cognition function
- ☐ Clinical disadvantages
  - ✔ involves the injection of a radioactive substance (can't be repeated often)
  - ✔ expensive
  - ✔ generally available only at large, research-oriented medical centers

Computerized Tomography (CT) Technique

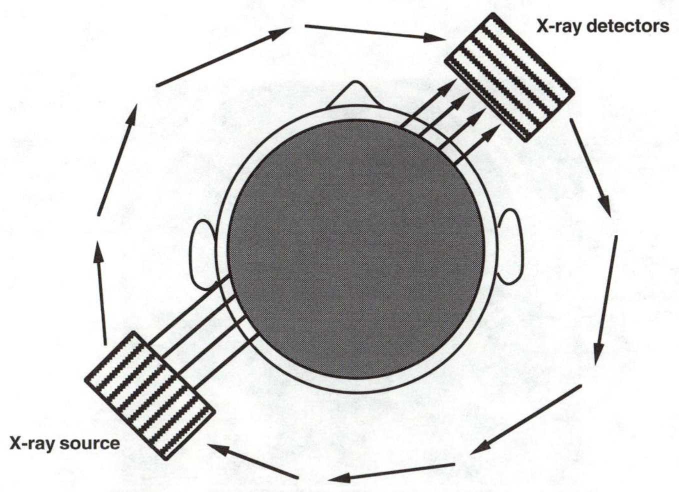

Sagittal MRI Image of Brain

Midline (top) and Off Midline (bottom)

Specific anatomic structures are labeled, including important auditory system structures such as the corpus callosum, midbrain (colliculi), pons, and medulla.

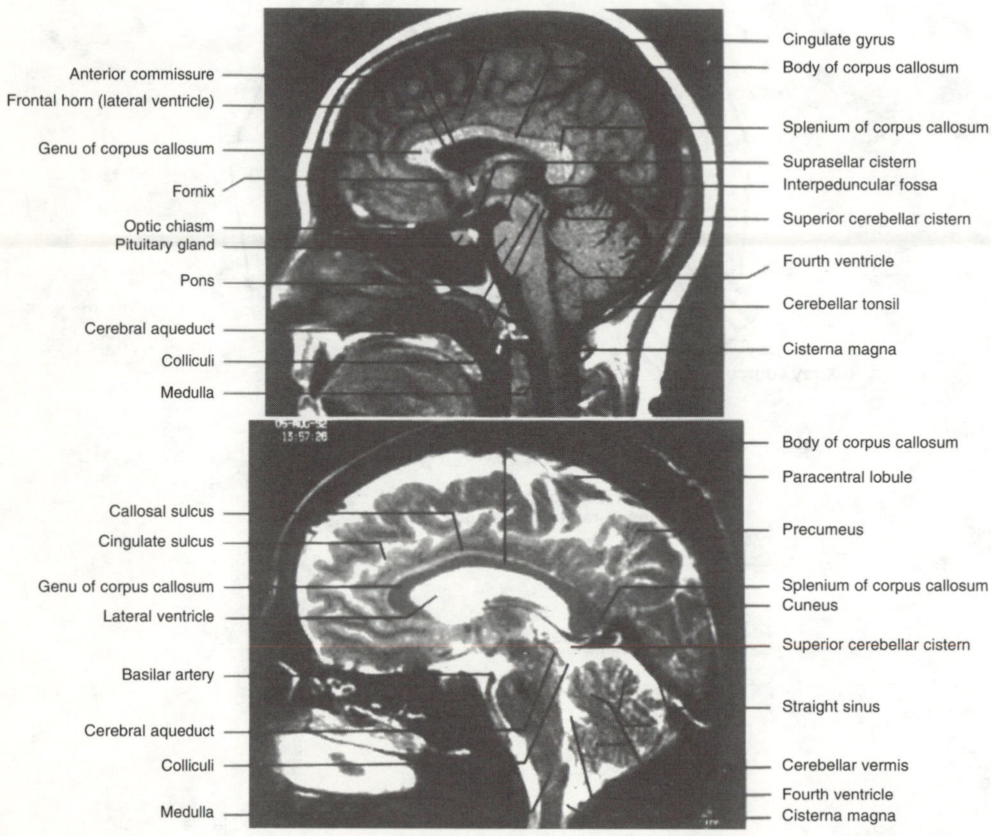

Sagittal MRI Image of Brain

Gyri and sulci, including auditory regions such as superior temporal gyrus and, specifically, Heschl's gyrus

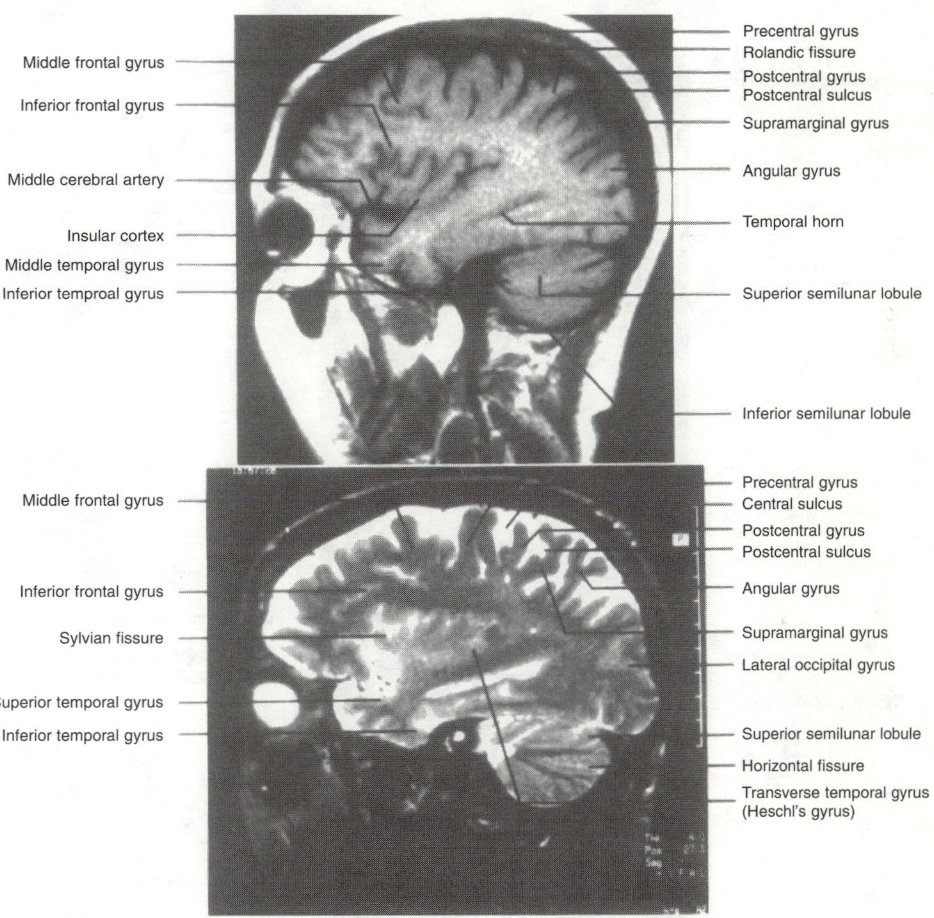

Coronal Image of Brain

Gyri, sulci, and structures and regions important to auditory function, such as the superior temporal gyrus, the basilar artery, the internal capsule, and the Sylvian fissure.

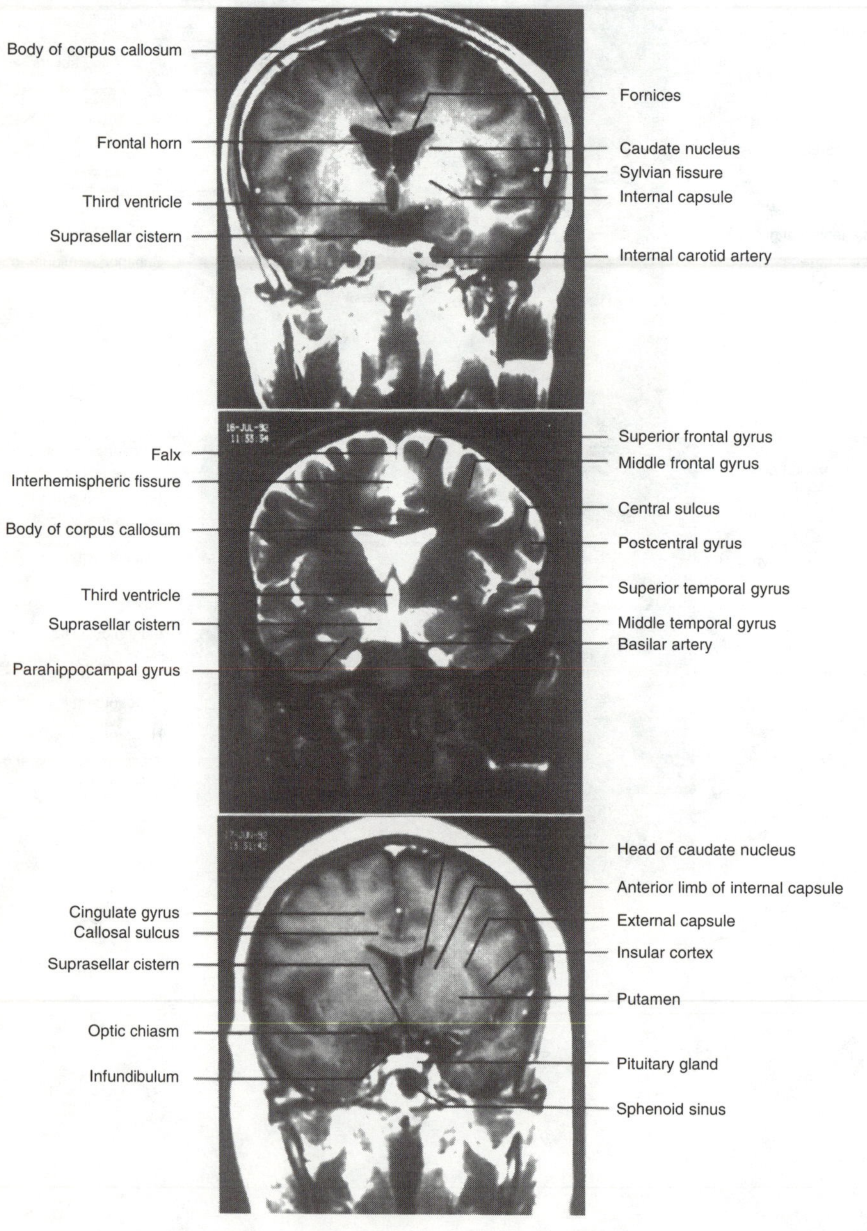

Coronal Image of Brain

Gyri, sulci, the ventricular system, and structures and regions important to auditory function, such as the superior temporal gyrus, the Sylvian fissure

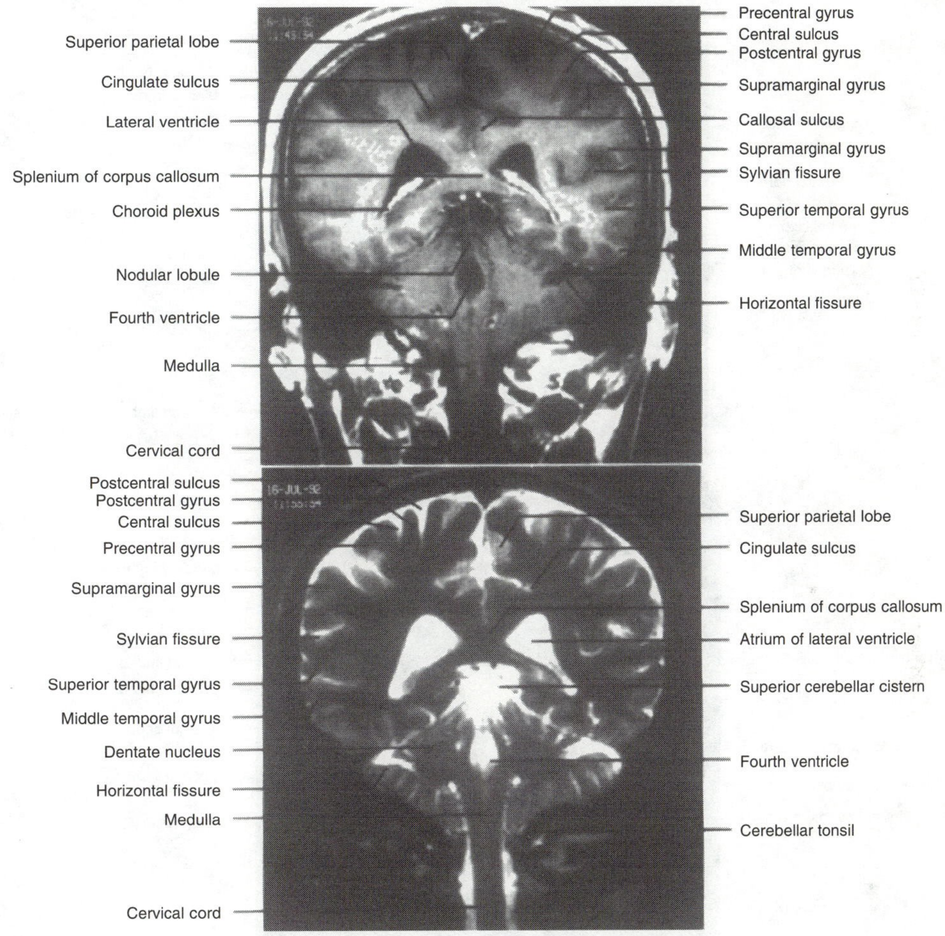

Coronal Image of Brain

Gyri, sulci, the ventricular system, and structures and regions important to auditory function, such as the superior temporal gyrus, the Sylvian fissure, the internal capsule, and the middle cerebral artery

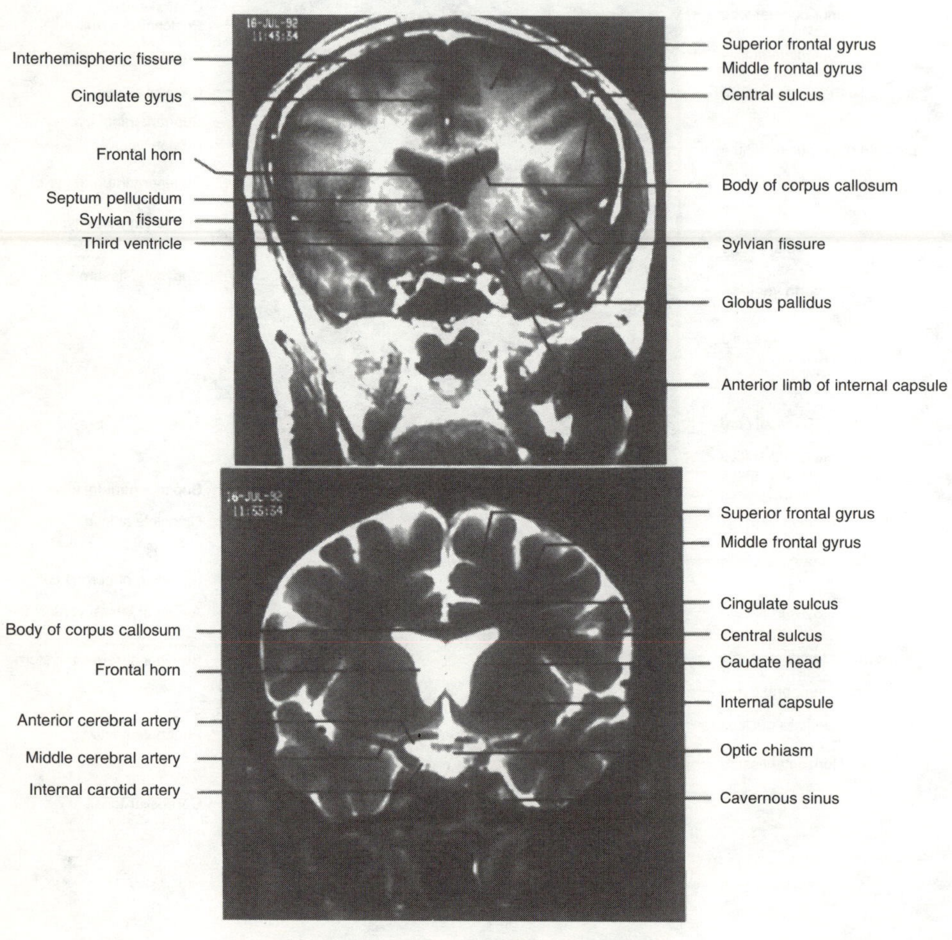

Axial View of Brain

Structures and regions important to auditory function, such as the thalamus, internal capsule, and the superior temporal gyrus

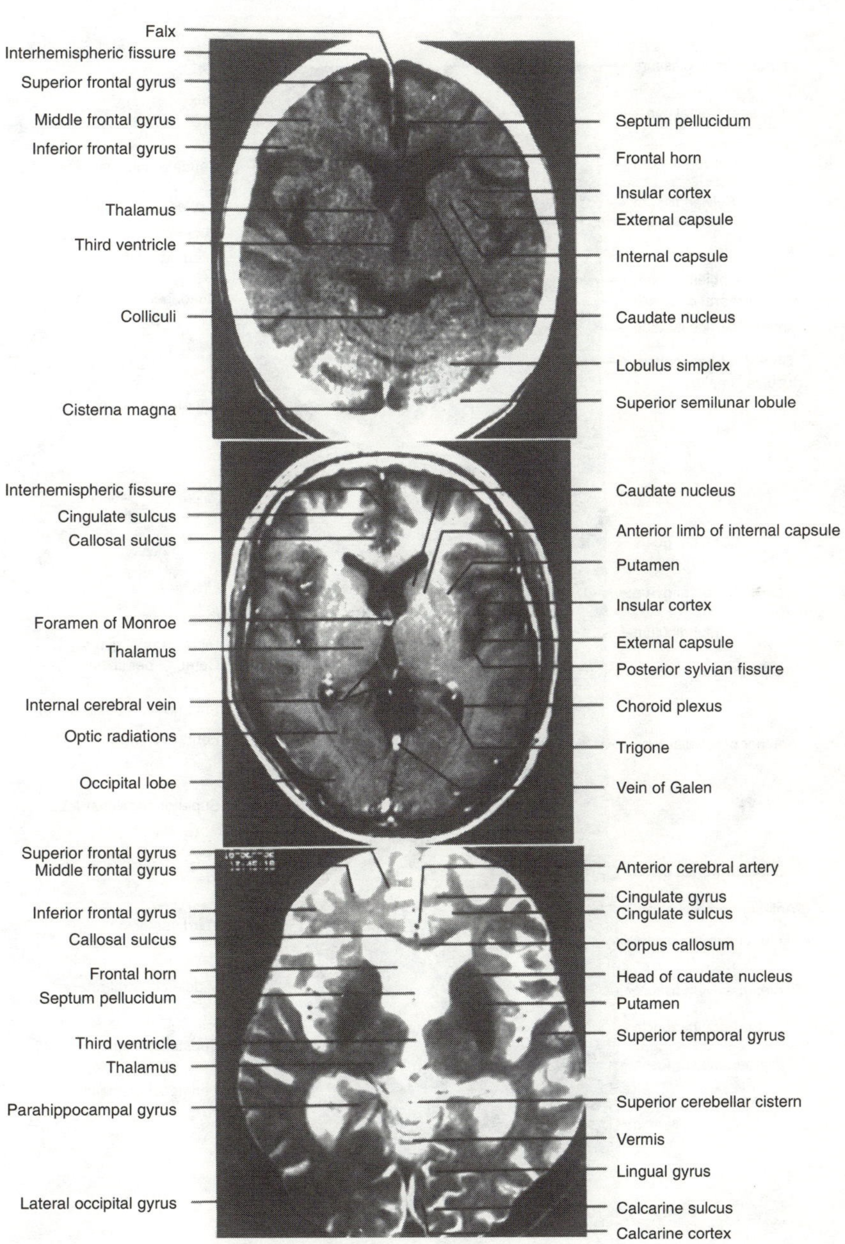

Axial View of Brain

Structures and regions important to auditory function, such as the Sylvian fissure, quadrageminal plate (region of inferior colliculus), middle cerebral artery, and the hippocampal gyrus

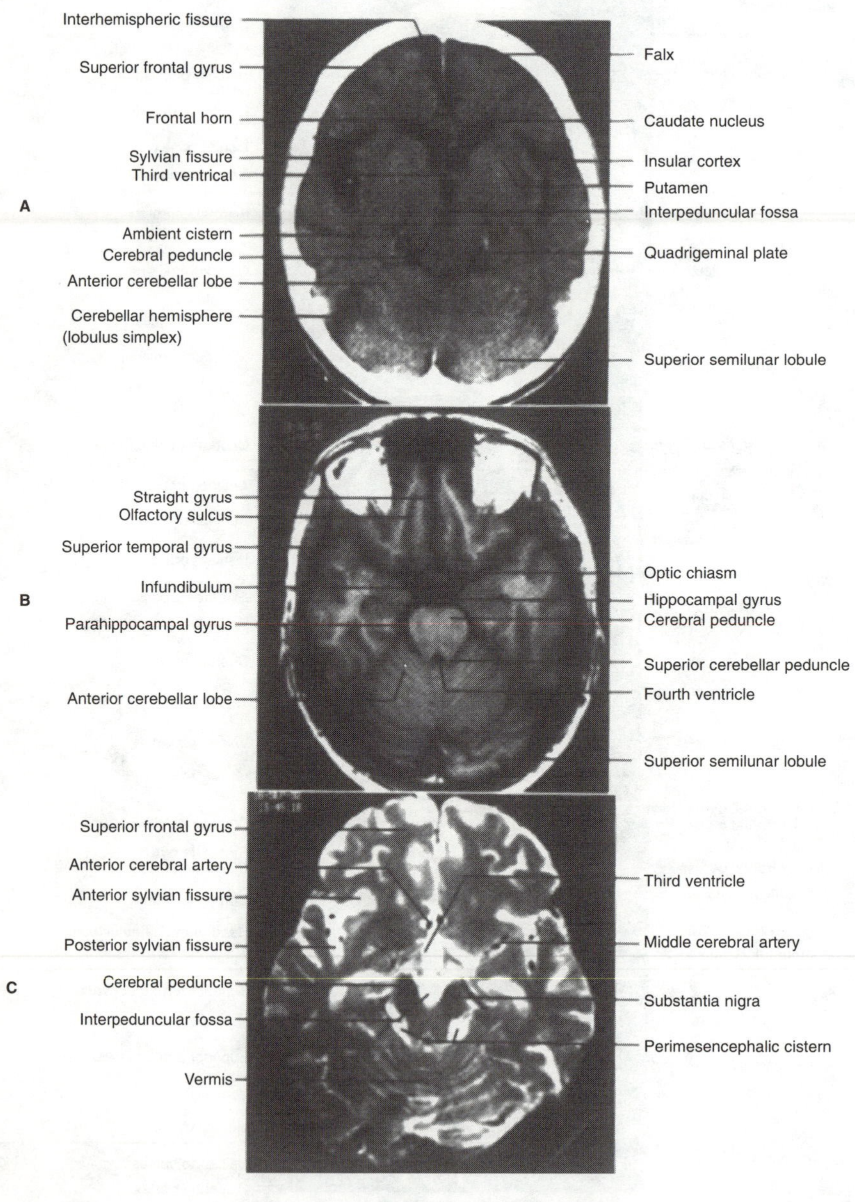

Axial View of Brain

Structures and regions important to auditory function, such as the Sylvian fissure, quadrageminal plate (region of inferior colliculus), middle cerebral artery, and the hippocampal gyrus.

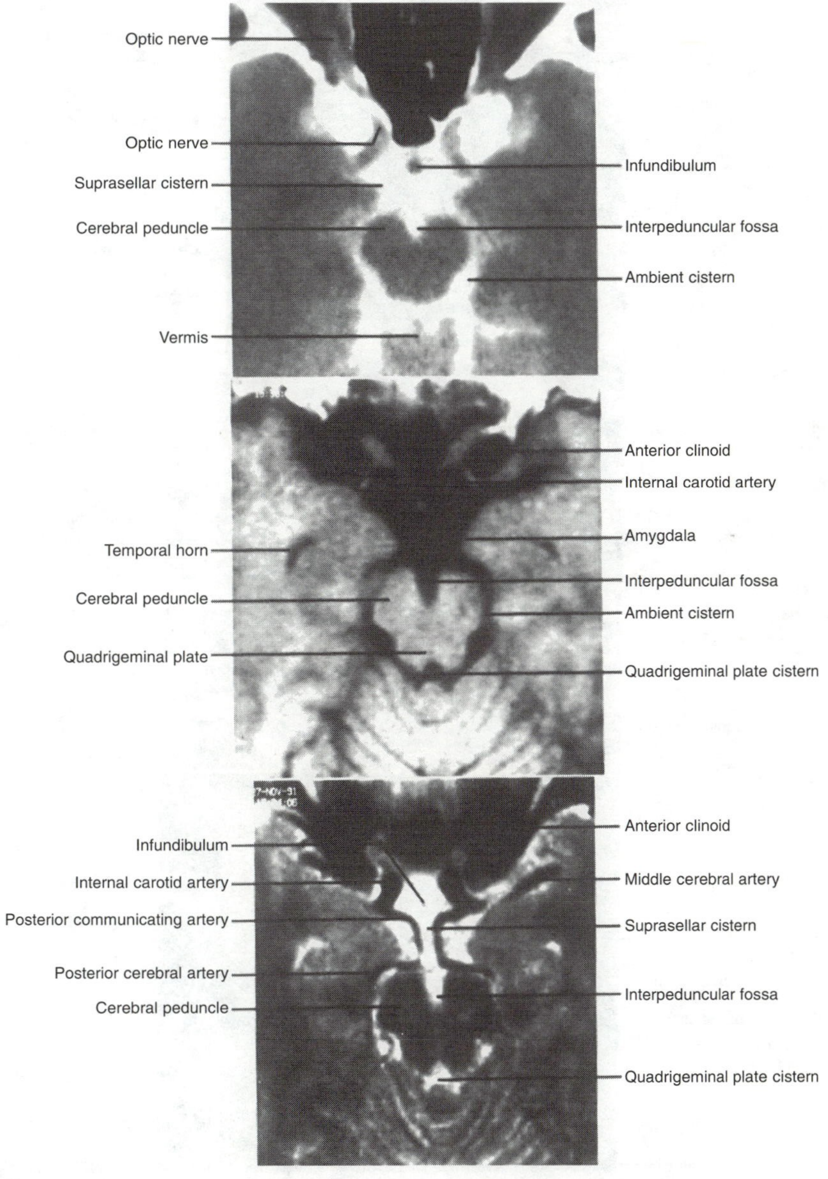

Enlarged View of Brain

Structures and regions important to auditory function, such as the Sylvian fissure, pons, posterior cerebral artery, the middle cerebral artery, and the temporal lobe

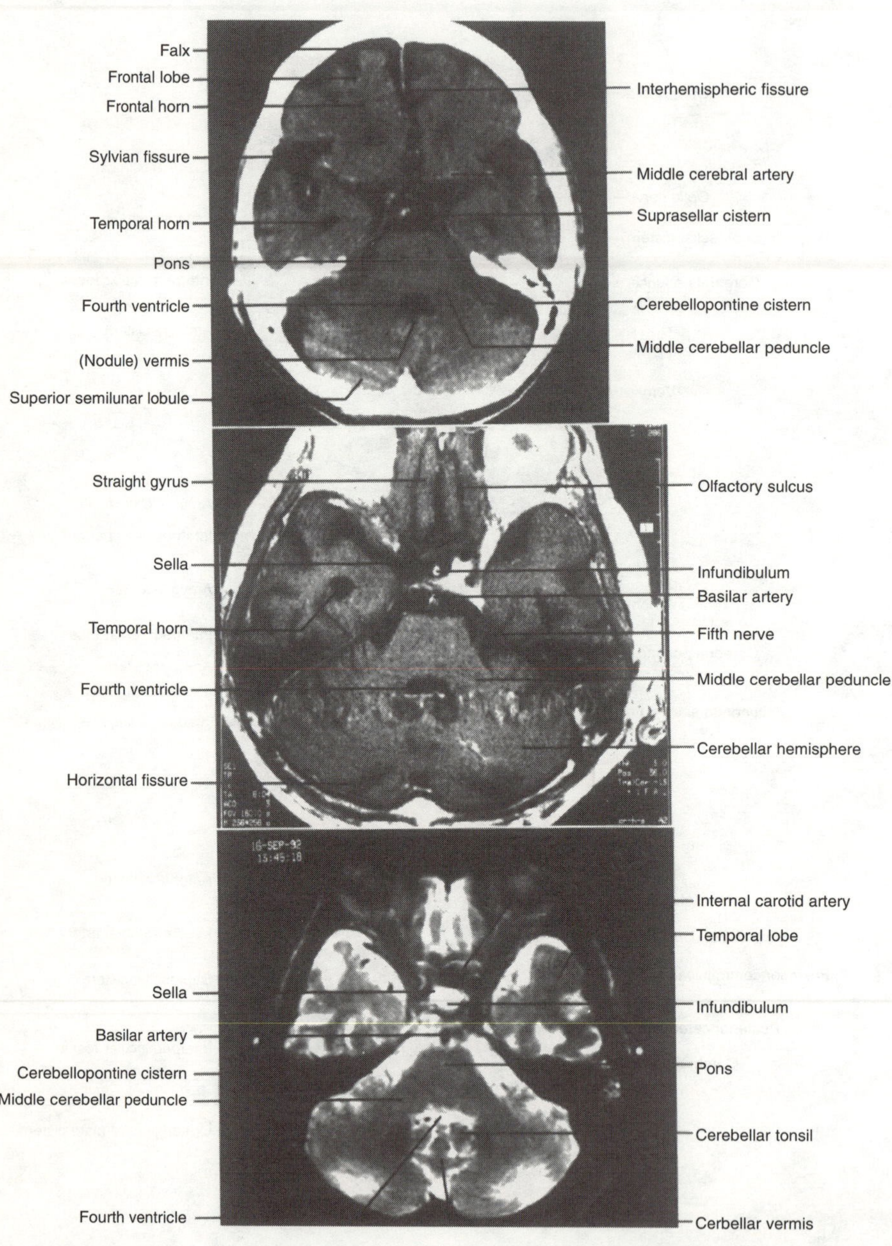

Axial View of Brain

Structures and regions important to auditory function, such as the corpus callosum, middle cerebral artery, and the superior temporal gyrus

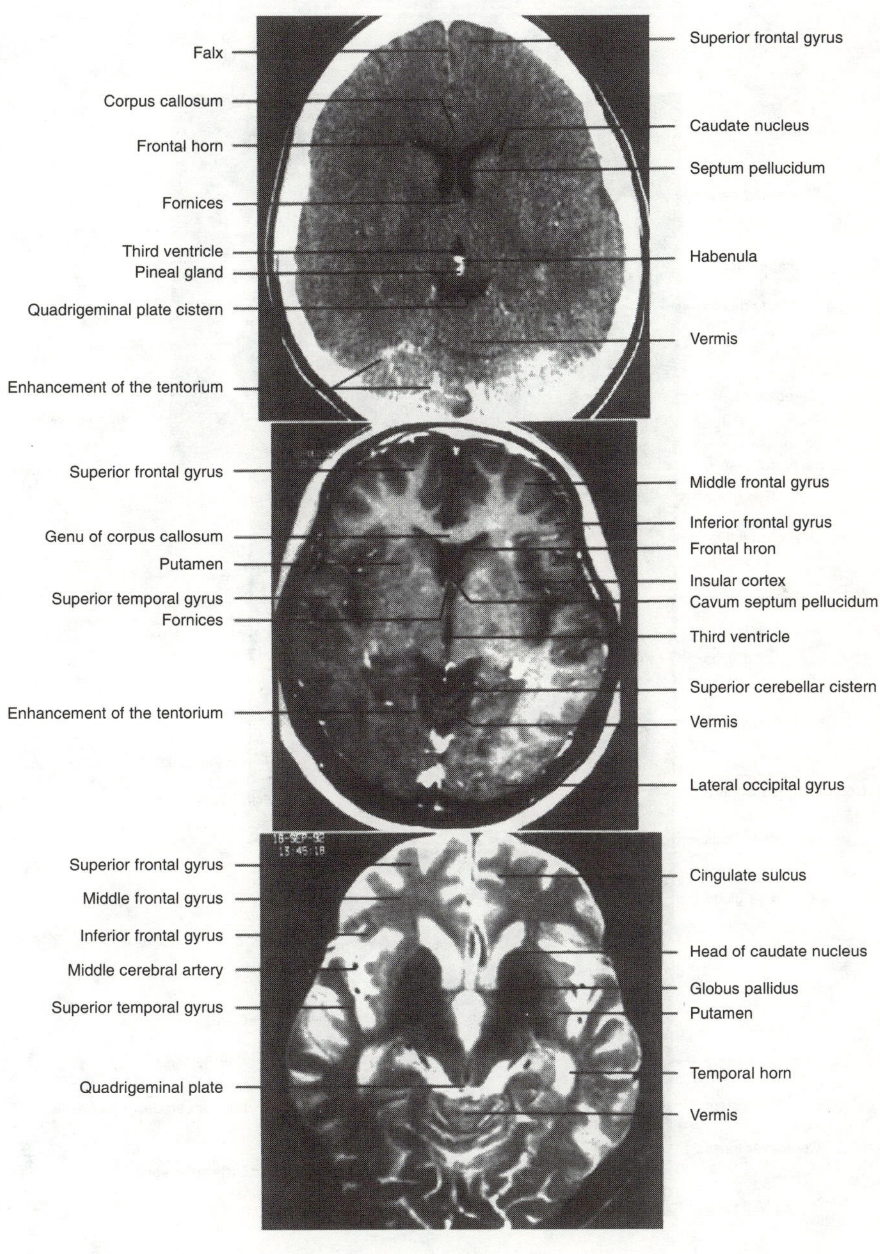

Caudal Axial View of Brain and Skull Base

Structures and regions important to auditory function, such as the mastoid cells, petrous bone, temporal lobe, and brain stem

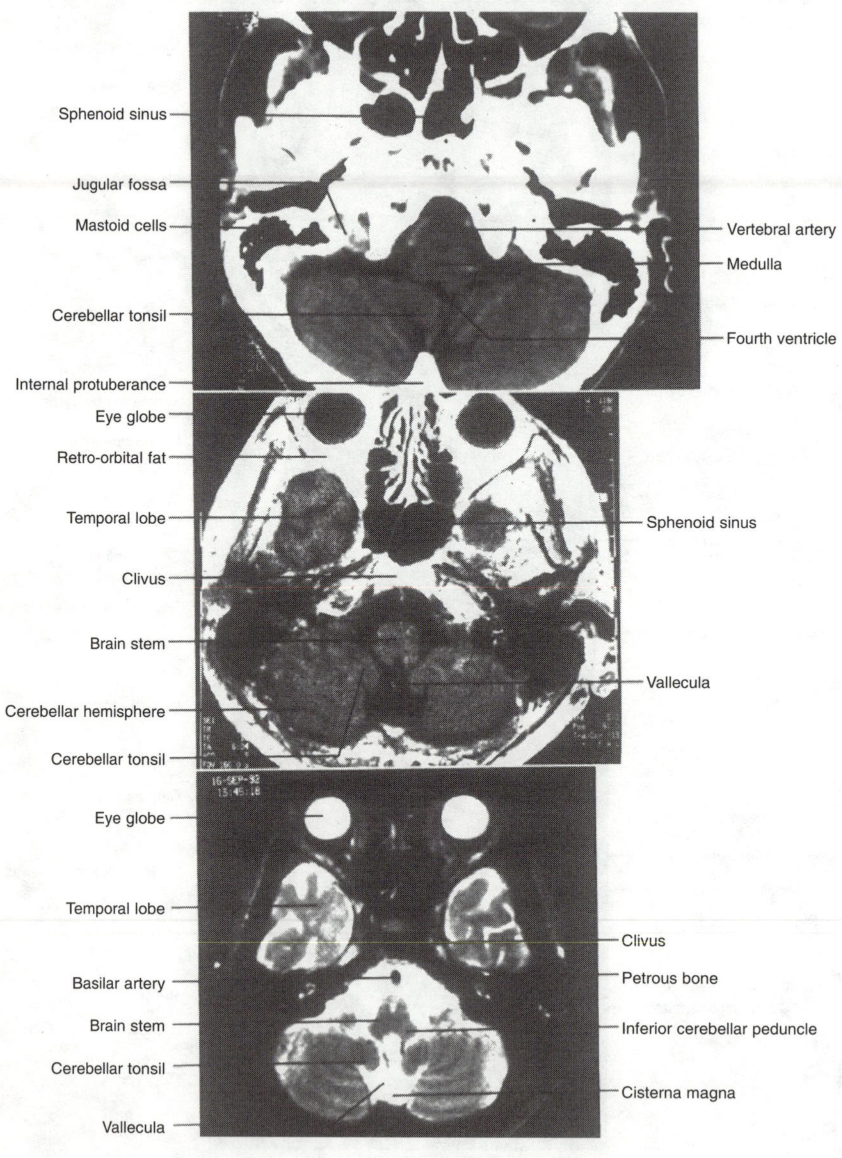

Did You Know?

Manufacturers of Radiologic Equipment

- ☐ Siemens, a major manufacturer of hearing aids, is also a major manufacturer of CT scanners and MRI devices
- ☐ One of the earliest companies involved in CT scanners was BMI (British Music Incorporated), the recording company at the time for the Fabuous Four (i.e., John, Paul, George and Ringo, aka The Beatles)

Key References

Radiography

Brownell GL, Budinger TF, Lauterbur PC, McGeer PL. Positron tomography and nuclear magnetic resonance imaging. *Science 215*: 619–626, 1982.

Hounsfield GN. Computerized transverse axial scanning (tomography): Part 1. Description of the system. *Brit Jour Radiol 46*: 1016–1022, 1973.

Moonen CTW, van Zijl PCM, Frank JA, Le Bihan D, Becker ED. Functional magnetic resonance imaging in medicine and physiology. *Science 250*: 53–61, 1990.

Posner MI, Petersen SE, Fox PT, Raichle ME. Localization of cognitive operations in the human brain. *Science 240*: 1627–1631, 1988.

LABORATORY TESTS AND VALUES

Clinical Concepts

Common Otologic Problems and Recommended Laboratory Tests

Childhood Middle Ear Effusion

Although routine blood studies contribute little to the diagnosis of otitis media, they are necessary for preoperative testing and may be useful in trying to establish subtle immune deficiencies as a cause of recurrent infection. In some cases, quantitative immunoglobin assay may reveal deficits in the amount of gamma subtypes. These tests, however, are not done routinely.

Ventilation Tube Drainage

A complete blood cell count with fasting blood glucose level is common.

Meningitis

Cerebrospinal fluid (CSF) studies. In most cases the CSF will indicate an intracranial suppurative process by the presence of leukocytes. A wide range of leukocyte and protein concentrations is recognized in meningitis, which makes absolute values of no particular help in distinguishing intracranial complications. A low CSF glucose concentration is usually seen in bacterial infections, but should the concentration remain low during the course of therapy, it is advisable to consider the potential of tuberculous meningitis. A history of tuberculosis contact or residence in an area with a high incidence of the disease should prompt this diagnosis. CSF testing can be helpful in distinguishing viral from bacterial meningitis.

Dizziness

Blood studies should be obtained routinely, especially in elderly patients. A complete blood cess count, fluorescent treponemal antibody test (FTA-ABS), thyroid function tests, and serum assays for electrolytes, glucose, and lipids may all reveal subtle causes of chronic dizziness. Rheumatoid factor and antinuclear antibody tests as well as triglyceride levels are also obtained. A hematocrit (Hct) level, to rule out the presence of anemia, is also common.

Allergic Labyrinthopathy

The following tests may be indicated:

- fluorescent treponemal antibody absorption test
- quantitative immunoglobins
- erythrocyte sedimentation rate (ESR)
- C-reactive protein level (CRP)

- total hemolyte complement assay
- cryoglobulins
- rheumatoid factor and antinuclear antibody tests may also be helpful in establishing the diagnosis of autoimmune ear disease.
- hypothyroidism and hyperthyroidism should also be ruled out

Once these disease processes are no longer in the differential diagnosis, allergy testing (IgE) should be considered.

Perilymphatic Fistula

Testing for syphilis and sedimentation rate (ESR) are warranted. If the patient's sedimentation rate is elevated, consider either an associated systemic disorder or an immune process affecting the ear.

Glomus Tumor

Catecholamine secretion—in the presence of hypotension one should suspect catecholamine secretion by the tumor and obtain 24-hour urinary studies for vanillymandelic acid and metanephrine, free catecholamine, and 5-hydroxyindoleacetic acid.

Sudden Sensorineural Hearing Loss

Blood tests are of limited value. Erythrocyte sedimentation rate (ESR) may be of prognostic value, but is not particularly helpful in establishing a definitive diagnosis. Syphilis is rarely unilateral, but fluorescent treponemal antibody absorption test should be performed.

Asymmetric Sensorineural Hearing Loss

If a patient is suspected of having syphilis, FTA-ABS and rapid plasma reagin (RPR) tests are in order. At other times an inner ear autoimmune problem may be suspected. In these cases an otologic immune profile is used which includes a complete blood count, urinalysis, antinuclear antibody test, rheumatoid factor, and immunoglobins A, M, and G. The lymphocyte transformation and leukocyte migration inhibition tests are difficult to obtain and costly but may be considered in diagnostic dilemmas. Genetic testing and evaluation may be necessary in patients with a familial history of hearing loss. Uncommonly, it is necessary to screen for systemic diseases. If there is a bilateral sensorineural loss and a strong family history of diabetes or symptoms of hypothyroidism, these diseases can be screened with laboratory tests.

Pulsatile Tinnitus

A complete blood count will rule out anemia in increased cardiac output. Vitamin A level and thyroid function tests should also be obtained to rule out disorders associated with benign intracranial hypertension syndrome (BIH).

Normal Ranges

Blood, Urine, and Cerebrospinal Fluid Analyses

BLOOD COUNTS AND CHEMISTRY

- albumin (Alb): 3.0–5.0 g/dL
- alkaline phosphatase (Alk. Pho.): 50–136 U/L
- amylase: 44–128 U/L
- bicarbonate (HCO_3): 24–30 mmol/L
- calcium: 8.5–10.5 mg/dL
- chloride (Cl): 100–106 mmol/L
- lipids (cholesterol) < 200 mg/dL
  HDL: 35–50 mg/dL
  LDL: < 159 mg/dL
  triglycerides: 35–200 mg/dL
- creatine phosphokinase (CPK): 3–350 U/L
- creatinine: 0.6–1.5 mg/dL
- iron (FE): 35–142 µg/dL
- glucose: 70–110 mg/dL (fasting)
- LDH: 300–650 U/L
- lipase: 40–210 U/L
- potassium (K): 3.4–5.3 mmol/L
- phosphate (PO_4): 2–4 mg/dL
- protein (total): 6.0–8.4 g/dL
- prealbumin (PAB): 17–42 mg/dL (well-nourished)
- magnesium (Mg): 1.4–2.4 mg/dL
- sodium (Na): 135–145 mmol/L
- transaminase (AST, SGOT): 0–50 U/L
- basal urea nitrogen (BUN): 5–25 mg/dL

BLOOD GASES

- oxygen saturation (arterial O_2 sat.): 96–100% (35–45 mm Hg)
- pH: 7.35–7.45
- partial pressure of arterial oxygen (PaO_2): 75–100 mm Hg
  [breathing room air; dependent upon age]
- HCO: −23 to −25 mmol/L

URINE ANALYSIS

✔ bacteria:	none; negative
✔ calcium (Ca):	100–250 mg/24 hrs
✔ chloride (Cl):	110–250 mmol/24 hrs
✔ creatinine:	15–25 mg/kg of body wt/24 hrs
✔ creatinine clearance:	140–180 liters/24 hrs
✔ glucose:	none; negative
✔ potassium (K):	40–80 mmol/24 hrs
✔ protein:	less than 150 mg/24 hrs
✔ sodium (Na):	130–200 mmol/24 hrs

HEMATOLOGIC VALUES

✔ differential cells	
segmenteds:	41–71%
eosinophils:	1–3%
basophils:	0–1%
lymphocytes:	24–44%
monocytes:	3–7%
stab neutrophils:	5–10%
✔ hemoglobin (HgB):	13–19 g/dL (males)
	12–16 g/dL (females)
✔ hematocrit (HCT):	45–52% (males)
	37–48% (females)
✔ erythrocytes (RBC):	4.2–5.9 million/mm^3
mean corpuscular hemoglobin (MCH):	27–32 pg
mean corpuscular volume (MCV):	80–94 μm^3
mean corpuscular hemoglobin concentration (MCHC):	33–37 g/dL
✔ erythrocyte sedimentation rate:	
male:	1–13 mm/h
females:	1–20 mm/h
✔ leukocytes (WBC):	4300–10,800/mm^3
✔ platelets:	150,000–35,000/mm^3

CEREBROSPINAL FLUID ANALYSIS

✔ bacteria:	none; negative
✔ cell count:	0–5 mononuclear cells (lymphs)
✔ glucose:	45–10 mg/dL

- pressure (initial): 70–180 mm of water
- protein: 1–5 mg/dL

Source: From Golper, LA. *Sourcebook for medical speech pathology*. San Diego, Calif: Singular Publishing Group, Inc., 1992, pp. 401–404, used with permission.

Clinical Concepts

General Laboratory Tests

ANTINUCLEAR ANTIBODIES (ANA) SERUM

Description of test:

The ANA test is a screening test for diagnosing systemic lupus erythematosus (SLE) and other collagen diseases.

Clinical implications of elevated level (>1:20):

- SLE
- progressive systemic sclerosis
- scleroderma
- rheumatoid arthritis
- leukemia, cirrhosis of the liver
- infectious mononucleosis
- myasthenia gravis
- malignancy

Drugs that may increase ANA level:

- antibiotics
- antihypertensives
- diuretics
- thiazides
- phenytoin
- oral contraceptives
- antiarrhythmias

Reference values:

- Adult: Negative

CATECHOLAMINES

Description of test:

Catecholamines are hormones (epinephrine and norepinephrine) secreted by the adrenal medulla. Catecholamine production increases after strenuous exercise; however, urinary levels are 3 to 100 times greater than normal in cases of pheochromocytoma. In some psychiatric clients, the urine catecholamine level increases only slightly. In children this test can be used to diagnose malignant neuroblastoma.

Clinical implications of elevated level:

- pheochromocytoma
- severe stress (shock)
- malignant neuroblastoma
- strenuous exercise
- manic-depressive disorder
- depressive neurosis

Reference Values:

- Adult:

  Total: <100 μg/24h
  Epinephrine: <20 μg/24h
  Norepinephrine: 10-90 μg/24h
- Child: Levels less than adult because of weight differences.

CEREBROSPINAL FLUID (CSF)

Description of test:

CSF/spinal fluid is obtained by a lumbar puncture (spinal tap) performed in the lumbar sac at S3-4 or at L4-5. First CSF pressure is measured, then fluid is aspirated and placed in sterile test tubes. Data from the analysis of the spinal fluid is important for diagnosing spinal cord and brain diseases.

Clinical implications of elevated level:

- intracranial pressure due to meningitis
- subarachnoid hemorrhage
- brain tumor
- brain abscess
- encephalitis
- viral infection

Reference values:

	Adult	Child	Premature Infant	Newborn
Pressure (mmH_2O)	75–175	50–100		
mm WBC	0–8	0–8	0–20	0–15
Protein (mg/dL)	15–45	4–45	<400	30–200
Chloride (mEq/L)	118–132	120–128		110–122
Glucose (mg/dL)	40–80	35–75		20–40

COMPLEMENT C3 AND C4 TEST (SERUM)

Description of test:

The complement system (a group of 11 proteins) is activated when the antibodies are combined with antigens. C3 is the most abundant component of the complement system and contributes about 70% of the total protein. Increased C3 levels occur in inflammatory disorders.

Clinical implications of decreased level:

- systemic lupus erythematosus
- lupus nephritis, protein malnutrition
- anemias
- multiple sclerosis
- cirrhosis of the liver

Clinical implications of elevated level:

- acute inflammatory disease
- acute rheumatic fever
- rheumatoid arthritis
- ulcerative colitis
- cancer

Reference levels:

- Adult:
  - C3: 83–177 mg/dL
  - C4: 15–45 mg/dL
- Elderly: Slightly higher than adult

C-REACTIVE PROTEIN (CRP) SERUM

Description of test:

CRP appears in the blood 6 to 10 hours after an acute inflammatory process or tissue destruction, or both, and it peaks within 48 to 72 hours. CRP is a non-specific test ordered for diagnostic reasons and in monitoring the effect of therapy. CRP elevates during bacterial infections but not viral infections. It is often used as an aid in differential diagnosis.

Clinical implications of elevated level:

- rheumatoid arthritis
- rheumatic fever
- inflammatory bowel disease
- bacterial infections
- acute myocardial infarction

Reference values:

- Adult: >1:2 titer, positive
- Child: not usually present

CREATININE PHOSPHOKINASE (CPK)

Description of test:

Creatinine phosphokinase (CPK) is an enzyme found in high concentration in the heart and skeletal muscles and in low concentrations in the brain tissue.

CPK has two types of isoenzymes: **M**, associated with muscle, and **B**, associated with the brain.

Electrophoresis separates the isoenzymes into three subdivisions, **MM** (in skeletal muscle), **MB** (in the heart), and **BB** (in brain tissue). When CPK is elevated, a CPK electrophoresis is done to determine which group of isoenzymes is elevated.

Clinical implications of elevated level:

- acute myocardial infarction
- skeletal muscle disease
- cerebrovascular accident

CPK-MM:

- muscular dystrophy
- delirium tremens
- crush injury/trauma
- hypothyroidism

CPK-MB:

- acute myocardial infarction
- cardiac ischemia
- severe angina pectoris

CPK-BB:

- CVA
- subarachnoid hemorrhage
- cancer of the brain
- acute brain injury
- pulmonary embolism and infarction

Reference values:

Adult Male:	30–180 IU/L
Adult Female:	25–150 IU/L
Newborn:	65–580 IU/L
Child, male:	0–70 IU/L
Child, female:	0–50 IU/L

CPK Isoenzymes:

CPK-MM:	94% to 100% (muscle)
CPK-MB:	0% to 6% (heart)
CPK-BB:	0% (brain)

CRYOGLOBULINS (SERUM)

Description of test:

Cryoglobulins are serum globulins (proteins) that precipitate from the plasma at 4° Celsius and return to dissolved status when warmed. They are present in IgG and IgM groups and are usually found in such pathologic conditions as leukemia, multiple myeloma, rheumatoid arthritis, systemic lupus erythematosus (SLE), and anemia.

Clinical implications of an elevated level:

- lymphocytic leukemia
- multiple myeloma
- Hodgkin's disease
- SLE
- rheumatoid arthritis

- acquired hemolytic anemias (autoimmune)
- cirrhosis

Reference Values:

- Adult: Negative to 6 mg/dL
- Child: Negative

ERYTHROCYTE SEDIMENTATION RATE (ESR)

Description of test:

The ESR test measures the rate at which red blood cells settle out of unclotted blood in millimeters per hour (mm/h). The ESR test is nonspecific.

The C-reactive protein (CRP) test is considered more useful than the ESR test because CRP increases more rapidly during an acute inflammatory process and returns to normal faster than ESR.

Clinical implications of a decreased level:

- polycythemia vera
- congestive heart failure
- sickle cell anemias
- infectious mononucleosis
- degenerative arthritis
- angina pectoris

Clinical implications of an elevated level:

- rheumatoid arthritis
- rheumatic fever
- cancer of the stomach
- colon
- breast
- liver and kidney
- Hodgkin's disease
- lymphosarcoma
- bacterial infections
- gout

Reference values:

- Adult, <50 years:

Male:	0–10 mm/h
Female:	0–20 mm/h

- Adult, >50 years:

Male:	0–20 mm/h
Female:	0–30 mm/h

- Child: 0–20 mm/h
- Newborn: 0–2 mm/h

FLUORESCENT TREPONEMAL ANTIBODY ABSORPTION SERUM (FTA-ABS)

Description of test:

The FTA-ABS uses the triponemal organism to produce and detect antibodies. The test is most sensitive, specific, and reliable for diagnosing syphilis. It is more sensitive than the Venereal Disease Research Laboratory (VDRL) or Rapid Plasma Reagin (RPR) test. Test results can remain positive after treatment or forever, and it does not indicate the stage and activity of the disease.

Clinical implications of reactive test outcome:

- primary and secondary syphilis
- lupus erythematosus
- pregnancy
- acute genital herpes

Reference values:

- Adult: Nonreactive (negative)
- Child: Nonreactive (negative)

GLUCOSE: FASTING BLOOD SUGAR (FBS)

Description of test:

A fasting blood sugar greater than 125 mg/dL might indicate diabetes or severe infection. When results are borderline or slightly elevated, a feasting (postprandial) blood sugar test may be ordered. A 2-hour feasting blood sugar is usually done to determine the patient's response to a high carbohydrate intake 2 hours after a meal. This test is a screening test for diabetes, normally ordered if the fasting blood sugar was high or abnormal.

Clinical implications of a decreased level:

- hypoglycemic reaction
- cancer

- adrenal gland hypofunction
- malnutrition
- alcoholism
- cirrhosis of the liver
- strenuous exercise

Clinical implications of an elevated level:

- diabetes mellitus
- diabetic acidosis
- adrenal gland hyperfunction (Cushing's syndrome)
- stress
- burns
- exercise
- infections
- acute pancreatitis
- acromegaly

Reference values:

- Adult: 70–110 mg/dL
- Elderly: 70–129 mg/dL
- Child: 60–100 mg/dL
- Newborn: 30–80 mg/dL

HAPTOGLOBIN (HP) SERUM

Description of test:

Haptoglobins are alpha globulins in the plasma. These globulin molecules combine with free hemoglobin during hemolysis (RBC destruction). A haptoglobin-hemoglobin complex occurs and the iron in the hemoglobin is able to be conserved. A decreased level of serum haptoglobin indicates hemolysis. After a hemolytic transfusion reaction, the serum haptoglobin level begins to fall within a few hours. It may take several days before the haptoglobin level returns to normal.

Clinical implications of a decreased level:

- hemolysis
- anemias
- liver disease

Clinical implications of an elevated level:

- inflammation
- acute infections
- malignancies
- Hodgkin's disease
- rheumatic fever

Reference values:

- Adult: 20–240 mg/dL
- Child: 0–10 mg/dL
- Infant: 0–30 mg/dL

HEMATOCRIT (HCT) BLOOD

Description of test:

The hematocrit is the volume of packed red blood cells in 100 ml (1 dL) of blood, expressed as a percentage. The purpose of the test is to measure the concentration of red blood cells in the blood.

Clinical implications of a decreased level:

- acute blood loss
- anemia
- leukemia
- Hodgkin's disease
- lymphosarcoma
- multiple myeloma
- chronic renal failure
- cirrhosis of the liver
- vitamin B and C deficiencies
- rheumatoid arthritis
- bone marrow failure

Clinical implications of an elevated level:

- dehydration
- severe diarrhea
- diabetic acidosis
- pulmonary emphysema
- transient cerebral ischemia
- burns

Reference values:

- Adult male: 40% to 54%
- Adult female: 36% to 46%
- Child 1–3 years: 29% to 40%
- Child 4–10 years: 31% to 43%
- Newborn: 44% to 65%

IMMUNOGLOBINS (IG) SERUM

Description of test:

Immunoglobins are classes of proteins referred to as antibodies. They are divided into five groups in gamma globulin (**IgG, IgA, IgM, IgD, IgE**) and can be separated by the process of immunoelectrophoresis. As individuals are exposed to antigens, immunoglobin (antibody) production occurs, and with further exposure to the same antigen, immunity results.

IgG:

IgG results from secondary exposure to the foreign antigen and is responsible for antiviral and antibacterial activity. This antibody passes through the placental barrier and provides early immunity for the newborn.

IgA:

IgA is found in secretions of the respiratory, GI, and genito-urinary tracts, tears, and saliva. It protects mucous membranes from viruses and some bacteria. IgA does not pass the placental barrier. Those having congenital IgA deficiency are prone to autoimmune disease.

IgM:

IgM antibodies are produced 48 to 72 hours after an antigen enters the body and are responsible for primary immunity. IgM does not pass the placental barrier. It is produced early in life, after 9 months.

IgD:

Unknown.

IgE:

Increases during allergic reactions.

Clinical implications of:

	Decreased Level	Elevated Level
IgG	Lymphocytic leukemia Agammaglobulinemia Amyloidosis	Infections (all types) Severe malnutrition Hyperimmunization Liver disease Rheumatic fever Sarcoidosis
IgA	Lymphocytic leukemia Agammaglobulinemia Malignancies	Autoimmune disorders Rheumatic fever Chronic infections Liver disease
IgM	Lymphocytic leukemia Agammaglobulinemia Amyloidosis	Lymphosarcoma Rubella virus in newborn Infectious mononucleosis
IgE		Allergic reactions Skin sensitivity

Reference values:

	Total Ig (mg/dL)	IgG (mg/dL)	IgA (mg/dL)	IgM (mg/dL)	IgE (mg/dL)
Adult	900-2200	650-1700	70-400	40-350	<40
6–16 yrs.	800-1700	700-1650	80-230	45-260	<62
4–6 yrs.	700-1700	550-1500	50-175	22-100	<25
1–3 yrs.	400-1500	300-1400	20-150	40-230	<10
6 mos.	225-1200	200-1100	10-90	10-80	
3 mos.	325-750	275-750	5-55	15-70	
Newborn	650-1450	700-1480	0-12	5-30	

LACTIC ACID (BLOOD)

Description of test:

Increased secretion of lactic acid following strenuous exercise, and acute or prolonged hypoxemia. A major cause of metabolic acidosis is excess circulating lactic acid.

Clinical implications of a decreased level:

- high lactic dehydrogenases (LDH) value

Clinical implications of an increased level:

- shock
- severe dehydration

- salicylate toxicity
- severe infections
- renal disease
- hepatic failure

Reference values:

- Adult: 0.5 to 2.0 mEq/L or 11.3 mg/dL
- Panic range: >5 mEq/L or >45 mg/dL

LIPOPROTEINS, LIPOPROTEIN, ELECTROPHORESIS, LIPIDS (SERUM)

Description of test:

The three main lipoproteins are cholesterol, triglycerides, and phospholipids. The two fractions of lipoproteins—alpha, high-density lipoproteins (HDL) and beta, low-density lipoproteins (LDL)—can be separated by electrophoresis. The beta groups are the largest contributors of atherosclerosis and coronary artery disease. HDL, called "friendly lipids," are composed of 50% protein and do aid in decreasing plaque deposits in blood vessels.

Clinical implications of an elevated level:

- hyperlipoproteinemia
- acute myocardial infarction (AMI)
- hypothyroidism
- diabetes mellitus
- nephrotic syndrome
- diet in high saturated fats

Drugs that may increase lipoprotein values:

- aspirin
- cortisone preparations
- oral contraceptives
- phenothiazines

Reference values:

- Adult:
  - Total: 400-800 mg/dL
  - Cholesterol: 150–240 mg/dL
  - Triglycerides: 10–190 mg/dL
  - Phospholipids: 150–380 mg/dL

LDL:	60–160 mg/dL
Risk for CHD:	
High:	>160 mg/dL
Moderate:	130–159 mg/dL
Low:	<130 mg/dL
HDL:	29–77 mg/dL
Risk for CHD:	
High:	<35 mg/dL
Moderate:	35–45 mg/dL
Low:	46–59 mg/dL
Very Low:	>60 mg/dL

RAPID PLASMA REAGIN (RPR) SERUM

Description of test:

The RPR test is a rapid-screening test for syphilis. A nontriponemal antibody test like VDRL, the RPR test detects reagin antibodies in the serum and is more sensitive but more specific than VDRL. Frequently it is used on donor's blood as a syphilis detection test. As with other nonspecific reagin tests, false positives can occur as the result of acute and chronic diseases. A positive RPR should be verified by VDRL and/or FTA-ABS tests.

Clinical implications of reactive (positive) test outcome:

Syphilis false positives

- tuberculosis
- pneumonia
- infectious mononucleosis
- chicken pox
- rheumatoid arthritis
- hepatitis
- pregnancy

Reference values:

- Adult: Nonreactive
- Child: Nonreactive

RHEUMATOID FACTOR (RF); RHEUMATOID ARTHRITIS (RA) FACTOR

Description of test:

The rheumatoid factor (RF), or rheumatoid arthritis (RA) factor, test is a screening test to detect antibodies (IgM, IgG, or IgA) found in the serum of patients with rheumatoid arthritis. The RF occurs in 53% to 94% of patients with rheumatoid arthritis. If the test is negative, it should be repeated.

Clinical implications of an elevated level:

- rheumatoid arthritis
- chronic infections
- lupus erythemastosis
- scleroderma
- infectious mononucleosis
- tuberculosis
- leukemia
- cirrhosis of the liver
- hepatitis
- syphilis
- renal disease

Reference values:

- Adult: <1:20 titer
  1:20-1:80 positive for rheumatoid and other conditions
  >1:80 positive for rheumatoid arthritis
- Elderly: Slightly increased
- Child: Not usually done

RUBELLA ANTIBODY DETECTION (SERUM)

Description of test:

Rubella (German measles) is a mild viral disease of short duration casing a fever and a transient rash. The rubella virus produces antibodies against future rubella infections, but the exact antibody titer is unknown. Hemagglutination inhibition measures rubella antibody titers and is considered to be a sensitive and reliable test. Women should be immune to rubella or should receive the rubella vaccine before marriage and definitely before pregnancy. When women contract rubella during the first trimester of pregnancy, serious congenital deformities of the fetus could result.

Clinical implications of a decreased level:

- <1:8 = susceptible to rubella

Clinical implications of an elevated level:

- >1:32 = immunity
- >1:64 = definite immunity

Reference values:

- Adult:
  Titer = <1:8
  Susceptibility to rubella = Titer 1:8 to 1:32
  Past rubella exposure and immunity = Titer 1:32 to 1:64
  Definite immunity = Titer >1:64

SALICYLATE (SERUM)

Description of test:

Salicylate levels are measured to check the therapeutic level, as in the treatment of rheumatic fever, and to check the levels caused by an accidental or deliberate overdose. Blood salicylate reaches its peak in 2 to 3 hours, and the blood level can be elevated for as long as 18 hours. Prolonged use of salicylates can cause bleeding tendencies because it inhibits platelet aggregation.

Clinical implications of an elevated level:

- >3 mg/dL = overdose or large, continuous doses of aspirin or drugs containing aspirin

Reference values:

- Adult:
  Normal = Negative
  Therapeutic = 5-30 mg/dL
  Mild toxic = >30 mg/dL
  Severe toxic = >50 mg/dL
  Lethal = >60 mg/dL
- Child: Toxic = >25 mg/dL
- Elderly: Mild toxic = >25 mg/dL

THYROID-STIMULATING HORMONE (TSH) SERUM

Description of test:

The anterior pituitary gland secretes thyroid-stimulating hormone (TSH) in response to thyroid-releasing hormone (TRH) from the hypothalamus. TSH stimulates the secretion of thyroxine (T_4) produced in the thyroid gland. TSH and T_4 levels are frequently measured to differentiate pituitary from thyroid dysfunctions. A decreased T_4 level and a normal or elevated TSH level can indicate a thyroid disorder. A decreased T_4 level with a decreased TSH level can indicate a pituitary disorder.

Clinical implications of a decreased level:

- secondary hypothyroidism (pituitary involvement)
- hyperthyroidism
- anterior pituitary hypofunction

Clinical implications of an elevated level:

- primary hypothyroidism (thyroid involvement)
- thyroiditis (Hashimoto's autoimmune disease)

Reference values:

- Adult: 2–5.4 mIU/ml
- Child: <25 mIU/ml by the third day of life

THYROXINE (T4) SERUM

Description of test:

Thyroxine (T_4) is the major hormone secreted by the thyroid gland and is at least 25 times more concentrated than T_3. The serum T_4 levels are commonly used to measure thyroid hormone concentration and to determine thyroid function. Other thyroid laboratory tests should be performed to verify and confirm thyroid gland disorders. In some institutions, the T_4 test is required for all newborns to detect a decreased thyroxine secretion, which could lead to irreversible mental retardation.

Clinical implications of an elevated level:

- hypothyroidism
- protein malnutrition
- anterior pituitary hypofunction
- renal failure

Clinical implications of an elevated level:

- hyperthyroidism
- acute thyroiditis
- viral hepatitis
- myasthenia gravis
- pregnancy

Reference values:

- Adult: 4.5–11.5 µg/dL
- Newborn: 11–23 µg/dL
- Newborn, 1–4 months: 7.5–16.5 µg/dL
- Newborn, 4–12 months: 5.5–14.5 µg/dL
- Child, 1–6 years: 5.5–13.5 µg/dL
- Child, 6–10 years: 5–12.5 µg/dL

TORCH SCREEN TEST

Description of test:

TORCH stands for toxoplasmosis, rubella, cytomegalovirus (CMV), and herpes simplex. It is a screening test to detect the presence of these organisms in the mother and newborn infant. The two common viruses that affect the infant most are CMV and rubella. During pregnancy, TORCH infections can cross the placenta and could result in mild to severe congenital malformation, abortion, or stillbirth. The most severe effects from these organisms occur during the first trimester. If the fetus is infected, the organism remains throughout the pregnancy.

The TORCH screening test is more frequently performed when congenital infection in the newborn is suspected. The IgG titers are compared with both the mother and newborn serum. If the IgG titer level is higher in the fetus than in the mother, congenital TORCH infection is likely.

Reference values:

- Maternal: IgG titer antibodies = Negative
  IgM titer antibodies = Negative
- Infants: Same as mother; infant should be tested under 2 months of age

TRIGLYCERIDES (SERUM)

Description of test:

Triglycerides are a blood lipid carried by the serum lipoproteins. Triglycerides are a major contributor to arterial diseases and are frequently compared with cholesterol with the use of lipoprotein electrophoresis. As the concentration of triglycerides increases, so will the very low-density lipoproteins increase, leading to hyperlipoproteinemia. Alcohol intake can cause a transient elevation of serum triglyceride levels.

Clinical implications of a decreased level:

- congenital beta-lipoproteinemia
- hyperthyroidism
- protein malnutrition
- exercise

Clinical implications of an elevated level:

- hyperlipoproteinemia
- acute myocardial infarction
- hypertension
- hypothyroidism

- cerebral thrombosis
- alcoholic cirrhosis
- uncontrolled diabetes mellitus
- Down's syndrome
- pregnancy
- high carbohydrate diet

Reference values:

- Adult

12–29 years:	10–140 mg/dL
30–39 years:	20–150 mg/dL
40–49 years:	30–160 mg/dL
>50 years:	40–190 mg/dL

- Child, 5–11 years: 10–135 mg/dL

TRIIODOTHYRONINE (T_3) SERUM

Description of test:

T_3 is one of the thyroid hormones, present in small amounts in blood and is shorter acting and more potent than thyroxine (T_4). Both T_3 and T_4 have similar actions in the body. Serum T_3 radioimmunoassay (RIA) measures both bound and free T_3. It is effective for diagnosing hyperthyroidism, in which T_3 is increased and T_4 is in the normal range. It is not as reliable for diagnosing hypothyroidism, for T_3 remains in normal range.

Clinical implications of a decreased level:

- severe illness and trauma
- malnutrition

Clinical implications of an elevated level:

- hyperthyroidism
- toxic adenoma
- Hashimoto's thyroiditis

Reference values:

- Adult: 80–200 mg/dL
- Child: 115–190 mg/dL
- Newborn: 90–170 mg/dL

URINALYSIS (ROUTINE)

Description of test:

Urinalysis is useful for diagnosing renal disease and urinary tract infection and for detecting metabolic disease not related to the kidneys. Many routine urinalyses are done in the physician's office.

Reference values:

	Adult	Newborn	Child
pH	4.5–8.0	5.0–7.0	4.5–8.0
Specific gravity	1.005–1.030	1.001–1.020	1.005–1.030
Protein	2–8 mg/dL		
Glucose	negative		negative
Ketones	negative		negative
WBC	3–4		0–4

UROBILINOGEN (URINE)

Description of test:

Urobilinogen test is one of the most sensitive tests for determining liver damage, hemolytic disease, and severe infections. In early hepatitis, mild liver cell damage, or mild toxic injury, the urine urobilinogen level will increase despite an unchanged serum bilirubin level. The urobilinogen test may be one of the tests performed during urinalysis.

Clinical Implications of a decreased level:

- biliary obstruction
- severe liver disease
- severe inflammatory disease

Clinical implications of an elevated level:

- cirrhosis of the liver
- infectious hepatitis
- anemia
- infectious mononucleosis

Reference values:

- Adult: 0.3-3.5 mg/dL
- Child: similar to adult

WHITE BLOOD CELLS (WBC)

Description of test:

WBCs (leukocytes) are divided into two groups, the polymorphonuclear leukocytes and the mononuclear leukocytes. Leukocytes are a part of the body's defense system; they respond immediately to foreign invaders by going to the site of involvement. An increase in WBCs is called leukocytosis, and a decrease in WBCs is called leukopenia.

Clinical implications of a decreased level:

- hematopoietic diseases (anemias)
- viral infections
- malaria
- agranulocytosis
- alcoholism

Clinical implications of elevated level:

- acute infection (pneumonia)
- meningitis
- appendicitis
- tuberculosis
- tissue necrosis
- leukemia
- collagen diseases
- parasitic diseases
- stress

Reference values:

Total WBC count

- Adult: 4500–10,000 μL
- Child: 6000–17,000 μL
- Newborn: 9000–30,000 μL

WHITE BLOOD CELL DIFFERENTIAL (BLOOD)

Description of test:

Differential WBC count, part of the complete blood count, is composed of five types of WBC—neutrophils, eosinophils, basophils, monocytes, and lymphocytes. The differential WBC count is expressed as cubic millimeters (uL) and percent of the total number of WBC. Neutrophils and lymphocytes make up 80% to 90% of the total WBC. Differential WBC count provides more specific information related to infections and disease process.

Neutrophils: Neutrophils are the most numerous circulating WBC, and they respond more rapidly to the inflammatory and tissue injury sites than other types of WBC. During an acute infection, the body's first line of defense is the neutrophils.

Eosinophils: Eosinophils increase during allergic and parasitic conditions. With an increase in steroids, either produced by the adrenal glands during stress or administered orally or by injection, eosinophils decrease in number.

Basophils: Basophils increase during the healing process. With an increase in steroids, the basophil count will decrease.

Monocytes: Monocytes are the second line of defense against bacterial infections and foreign substances. They are slower to react to infections and inflammatory diseases, but they are stronger than the neutrophils and can ingest larger particles of debris.

Lymphocytes: Increased lymphocytes occur in chronic and viral infections. Lymphocytes play a major role in the immune response system with B lymphocytes and T lymphocytes.

Reference Values:

	Percent	**μL**
Neutrophils	50–70	2500–7000
Eosinophils	1–3	100–300
Basophils	0.4–1.0	40–100
Monocytes	4–6	200–600
Lymphocytes	25–35	1700–3500

Courtesy of: Anne Strouse, M.A.,Vanderbilt University, Nashville, Tennessee

Laboratory Diagnosis in Otology

Preoperative Evaluation

- ☐ Complete blood count (CBC)
  - white blood cell count (WBC): 4–11,000
  - hemoglobin (HgB: 1–18
  - packed cell volume (PCV)
  - platelet count (Plt): 150–400,000
- ☐ Coagulation studies
  - prothrombin time (PT): 10–13
  - partial thromboplastin time (PTT): 25–40
  - type and screen/cross of blood
  - EKG (electrocardiogram)
  - CXR (chest X-ray)
  - urinalysis (U/A)
- ☐ SMA7 (SMA = sequential medical analysis or "blood chemistry lab tests")

Test	Range
Sodium (Na)	135–145
Potassium (K)	3–5.5
Chloride (Cl)	95–105
Bicarbonate (HCO)	23–30
Glucose (Glu)	70–110
Blood Urea Nitrogen (BUN)	5–25
Creatinine (Cr)	0.7–1.5

- ☐ SMA12

Test	Range
Creatinine (Cr)	0.7–1.5
Serum Glutamic Oxalacetic Transaminase (SGOT)	4–40
Lactate Dehydrogenase (LDH)	125–250
Alkaline Phosphatase	40–90
Total Bilirubin	0.2–1.2
Calcium (Ca)	8.5–10.5
Phosphorus	2.5–4.5
Total Protein	6–8

- Albumin 3.5– 5
- Uric Acid 2–7
- Total Cholesterol 160–40
- Triglycerides 55–280

Otitis Externa *("Swimmer's Ear")*

☐ History

- otalgia
- otorrhea
- itching
- hearing loss

☐ Physical examination

☐ Laboratory evaluation (if severe)

- Culture and sensitivity
- CBC

Malignant (Necrotizing) Otitis Externa

- otalgia for at least 1 month
- purulent otorrhea with granulation tissue
- immunocompromised stat
- diabetes melitis
- age
- cranial nerve involvement

Otitis Media with Effusion (OME)

☐ History

- otalgia
- otorrhea
- hearing loss
- constitutional symptoms

☐ Physical examination

☐ Audiometric evaluation

- baseline
- conductive hearing loss is most common

☐ Laboratory

- immune deficiency
- allergy

☐ Immunology

- IgA, IgG deficiencies (subclasses 2,3)
- complement deficiencies
- HIV
- defect in chemotaxis
- defect in phagocytosis (neutropenia)
- defect in bacterial killing (chronic granulomatous disease)

☐ Allergy

(NOTE: The role of allergy in the pathogenesis of OME is debated. There is no conclusive evidence linking the two conditions.)

Evidence for allergy

- concomitant allergic rhinitis and asthma
- positive skin tests or RAST testing
- elevated IgE levels in both middle ear and serum
- mast cells found in middle ear mucosa

Evidence against allergy

- OME most common in winter and early spring; major
- allergens (grasses, trees, molds) found in late spring and fall
- absence of eosinophils and few or none IgE-producing cells in middle ear mucosa in middle ear effusions
- most patients do no have marked improvement of their ear disease even though nasal and other symptoms may be markedly improved

Idiopathic Sudden Sensorineural Hearing Loss (ISSNHL)

☐ History

☐ Head and neck exam

☐ Full audiometric evaluation

☐ Radiologic studies if indicated

☐ Pertinent laboratory studies

- Differential Diagnosis of ISSHNL
  - trauma
  - vascular disorders
  - hypercoagulability
  - anterior inferior cerebellar artery
  - basilar artery thrombosis
  - tumors (acoustic neuroma)
  - viral labyrinthitis
  - perilymph fistula
  - metabolic
- Laboratory Evaluation of ISSHNL
  - CBC
  - Erythrocyte Sedimentation Rate (ESR)
  - Glucose, Hemoglobin A1c level
  - Lipid profile (cholesterol, triglyceride)
  - Fluorescent Treponemal Antibody Absorption Test (FTA-ABS)
  - Viral Titers (research purposes)

Luetic Labyrinthitis

- Ssyphilis (Treponema pallidum)
- Sensorineural hearing loss
  - congenital and acquired
  - often bilateral
- Vertigo
- Laboratory tests
  - FTA-ABS (fluorescent treponema—antibody absorbed)
  - MHA- TP (microhemagglutination assay—TP)
- False positives
  - connective tissue diseases
  - leprosy
  - infectious mononucleosis
  - pregnancy

Subjective Tinnitus

☐ Complete history

☐ Examination

☐ Audiometric evaluation

☐ Blood pressure in both arms

☐ Laboratory diagnosis

☐ Imaging studies

☐ Etiologic factors in subjective tinnitus: diseases

- otologic factors
- presbycusis
- noise-induced HL
- Ménière's disease
- otosclerosis
- acoustic neuroma (unilateral tinnitus)

☐ Etiologic factors in subjective tinnitus: metabolic function

- thyroid dysfunction
- hyperlipidemia
- vitamin deficiency

☐ Etiologic factors in subjective tinnitus: neurologic abnormalities

- skull fracture or closed head trauma
- whiplash injury
- multiple sclerosis
- meningitic effects

☐ Etiologic factors in subjective tinnitus: pharmacologic factors

- aspirin compounds
- nonsteroidal anti-inflammatory drugs
- aminoglycosides
- heavy metals

☐ Etiologic factors in subjective tinnitus: dental factors

- temporomandibular joint (TMJ) syndrome

☐ Etiologic factors in subjective tinnitus: psychologic factors

- depression
- anxiety

- ☐ Laboratory diagnosis of tinnitus
  - ✓ PCV
  - ✓ FTA-ABS (fluorescent treponema—antibody absorbed)
  - ✓ thyroid function tests
  - ✓ lipid profile

Dizziness

- ☐ History
- ☐ Etiologies requiring urgent management
- ☐ Location
  - ✓ central
  - ✓ peripheral
  - ✓ systemic changes
- ☐ Specific pathology

Peripheral Vestibular Disorders (Causes)

- ☐ sudden onset unilateral
  - ✓ labyrinthitis
  - ✓ labyrinthine or eighth nerve trauma
  - ✓ latrogenic injury (labyrinthectomy or eighth nerve section)
  - ✓ vascular labyrinthine lesion
  - ✓ perilymph fistula
  - ✓ cholesteatoma
- ☐ Sudden onset bilateral
  - ✓ ototoxicity
  - ✓ labyrinthitis from meningitis
  - ✓ bilateral trauma
- ☐ Gradual onset unilateral
  - ✓ eighth nerve neoplasm
  - ✓ degenerative and autoimmune disease
- ☐ Unilateral fluctuating
  - ✓ endolymphatic hydrops
  - ✓ benign paroxysmal positional vertigo

Central Vestibular Disorders (Causes)

- ☐ Degenerative
- ☐ Infectious
  - ✔ otogenic meningitis
  - ✔ epidural abscess
  - ✔ congenital syphilis
- ☐ Circulatory
  - ✔ vertebrobasilar insufficiency
  - ✔ Wallenberg's syndrome (lateral medullary infarction)
  - ✔ cerebellar hemorrhage
- ☐ Structural
  - ✔ Arnold-Chiari malformation
- ☐ Systemic
  - ✔ multiple sclerosis
- ☐ Carcinoma

Laboratory Evaluation for Dizzy Patients

- ☐ Routine screen
  - ✔ PCV
  - ✔ ESR
  - ✔ ANA (antinuclear antibody)
  - ✔ FTA-ABS (fluorescent treponema—antibody absorbed)
- ☐ 3-hour glucose tolerance test
- ☐ lipid profile
- ☐ EEG (electroencephalograpy)
- ☐ thyroid function tests

Other Diseases to Consider

- ☐ Influenza
- ☐ Parainfluenza
- ☐ Mumps
- ☐ Rubeola

- ☐ Rubella
- ☐ Herpes simplex 1 (HSV)
- ☐ Varicella-Zoster
- ☐ Adenovirus
- ☐ Respiratory Syncitial Virus (RSV)
- ☐ Mycoplasma pneumonia

Source: Courtesy of Grady L. Bryant, Jr. M.D.

OTOLOGIC SURGICAL PROCEDURES

Historical Reverberation

The Beginning of a New Era in Otologic Surgery

- ☐ Early surgical efforts at improvement of hearing in otosclerosis date back to the 19th century, mostly in Europe, by a variety of surgeons including the Germans Kessel (1878) and Passow (1897), Frenchmen Boucheron (1888) and Miot (1890), the Italian Faraci (1899), and the American Jack (1893). The primary technique then was mobilization of the fixed stapes footplate.
- ☐ The next big development was the beginning of an period of fenestra surgerical procedures in which the stapes footplate was avoided, and small openings were drilled in the horizontal canal to permit transmission of sound energy from the middle to inner ear. In the United States, Lempert, an otologist in New York City, really generated interest in this general approach in 1938 with a one-stage fenestration operation. Although stapes mobilization enjoyed another short-lived period of popularity thanks to Rosen (1955), an even better technique was just around the bend.
- ☐ The modern era in surgical treatment of otosclerosis was ushered in by the published description of the stapedectomy procedure by John Shea in 1958. He removed the stapes footplate, and then used a polyethylene strut prosthesis sealed to the oval window with a vein graft.
- ☐ Soon after, other otologists, among them Harold Schuknecht and Howard House, introduced the use of wire and fat, or wire and absorbable gelatin sponge (Gelfoam) prostheses techniques.
- ☐ The technique has undergone refinement over the years have occured in three general ways:
  - ✔ prosthesis design, especially the piston prosthesis in 1961
  - ✔ strategies for seal of the oval window
  - ✔ a small fenestra technique (mostly in Europe)

References: House HP, Greenfield EC. Five year study of wire-loop absorbable gelatin sponge technique. *Arch Otolaryngol 89:* 420–421, 1969; Lempert J. Improvement in hearing in cases of otosclerosis: A new, one stage surgical technique. *Arch Otolaryngol Head Neck 28*: 42, 1938; Rosen S. Restoration of hearing in otosclerosis by mobilization of the fixed stapedial footplate, an analysis of results. *Laryngoscope 65*: 224–269, 1955; Schuknecht H. Stapedectomy and graft prosthesis operation. *Acta Otolaryngol 51*: 241–243, 1960; Shea JJ. Fenestration of the oval window. *Ann Otol Rhinol Laryngol 67*: 932–951, 1958.

Instruments and Equipment Used in Otologic Surgery

General Operating Equipment

1. 3M 1000 plastic adhesive drapes
2. 3M 1020 aperture drapes
3. 3M Steri-Drape, Ioban drape, or cranial-incise drape
4. Pharmaseal preoperative skin preparation tray No. 4480
5. Dow-Corning flexible surgical tubing
6. Suction canisters
7. Elecrocautery unit

Stapes Surgery

1. Assorted Farrior speculums
2. Finger-control Luer-Lok syringe
3. 1.5 inch 25-gauge needle
4. Small Weitlaner retractor
5. Sheehy fascia press
6. House cutting block
7. Scalpel, No. 15 Bard-Parker blade
8. Adson issue forceps
9. Iris scissors
10. House-Baron suction tubes No. 3 Fr through No. 7 Fr
11. House suction tube adapter
12. Rosen suction tubes 18- through 24-gauge
13. Sickle knife (No. 1 knife)
14. Lancet knife (No. 2)
15. Robinson knife
16. Sheehy-House weapon (large and small)
17. Rosen needle
18. House elevator
19. Gimmick annulus elevator
20. House stapes curette
21. Incudostapedial joint knife
22. Bellucci scissors
23. Straight Barbara pick
24. Measuring struts, 4.0 mm through 5.0 mm
25. Measuring disk, 0.6 mm
26. Hough hoe
27. Obtuse 30 degree, 0.25 mm hook
28. Pick, 0.3 mm, 90 degree
29. Strut guide
30. Footplate chisel
31. Skeeter drill; 1.0 mm, 0.7 mm, 0.6 mm burrs

32. House strut forceps (nonserrated)
33. McGee wire closing forceps (crimper)
34. Kos-House ointment
35. Cotton balls, Band-Aids, mastoid dressing

Chronic Ear Surgery

1. Assorted Farrior speculums
2. Finger-control syringe
3. 1½ inch 25-gauge needle
4. Small Weitlaner retractor
5. Large self-retaining retractor
6. Scalpel, #15 Bard-Parker blade
7. No. 64 or 67 Beaver blade
8. House cutting block
9. Shehy fascia press
10. House-Baron suction tubes No. 3 Fr. through No. 7 Fr.
11. Adson forceps
12. Iris scissors
12. Iris scissors
13. Small Metzenbaum scissors
14. Sickle knife
15. Lancet knife
16. Robinson knife
17. Sheehy-House weapon (small and large)
18. Rosen needle
19. Gimmick
20. Crabtree dissector (large and small)
21. Lempert elevator
22. House narrow elevator
23. Pick, right angle, 0.6 mm
24. Pick, right angle, 1.5 mm
25. Pick, right angle, 3 mm
26. Bellucci scissors
27. Hartmann forceps
28. House alligator forceps
29. House cup forceps
30. House-Dieter malleus nipper
31. Zini mirrors
32. Sheehy ossicle holder
33. Speculum, endaural (or nasal)
34. Drill with assortment of cutting and diamond burrs
35. House suction-irrigators
36. Needle holder, Webster
37. Suture scissors
38. Suture, 2.0 chromic and 4.0 Dexon (or Vicryl)
39. Gelfoam
40. Adaptic gauze
41. Silastic sheeting

42. Steri-Strips
43. Mastoid dressing
44. Bone wax
45. Surgicel
46. Sheehy bone pate collector

Endolymphatic Sac Surgery

1. Finger-control syringe
2. 1.5 inch 25-gauge needle
3. Scalpel, No. 15 Bard-Parker blade
4. Large self-retaining retractor
5. Lempert elevator
6. House narrow elevator
7. Drill and burrs
8. House suction-irrigators
9. Brackmann suction-irrigators
10. Stapes curette
11. Gimmick
12. Insulated gimmick
13. Bone wax
14. Surgicel
15. Malis bipolar cautery
16. Bacitracin irrigation solution
17. Beaver ophthalmic blade
18. Pick, right angle, 1.5 mm
19. Hook, right angle, blunt
20. Rosen needle
21. House alligator forceps
22. Shunt tube or material
23. Suture, 2.0 chromic and 4.0 Dexon (or Vicryl)
24. Steri-Strips
25. Mastoid dressing

Neurotologic Surgery

1. Finger-control syringe
2. 1.5 inch 25-gauge needle
3. Scalpel
4. Large self-retaining retractor
5. Lempert elevator
6. House narrow elevator
7. Drill and burrs
8. House suction-irrigators
9. Brackmann suction-irrigators
10. Stapes curette
11. Gimmick
12. Insulated gimick
13. Bone wax

14. Surgicel
15. Malis bipolar cautery
16. Bacitracin irrigation solution
17. SK-100 Surgi-Kit
18. Suture scissors
19. House-Urban dissector
20. Pick, right angle, 1 mm
21. Pick, right angle, 1.5 mm
22. Hook, right angle, blunt, 1.5 mm
23. Bellucci scissors
24. House cup forceps
25. Blakesle nasal forceps
26. House alligator forceps
27. Myringoplasty knife
28. Jacobson scissors
29. Malis scissors
30. Allis forceps
31. Bayonet forceps
32. Adson tissue forceps
33. Microclip applicator
34. Assorted hemostats
35. Metzenbaum scissors
36. Senn retractor
37. U.S. Army retractor
38. Pediatric rib retractor
39. Fisch microraspatory
40. Woodson elevator
41. Fisch microraspatory
42. Sagittal saw
43. Needle holder, Castroviejo
44. Needle holder, Crile-Wood
45. Needle holder, Webster
46. Avitene
47. Drains, Penrose and Jackson-Pratt
48. Vessel loops
49. Suture, 5.0 and 6.0 vascular Prolene
50. Suture, 0 and 2.0 Chromic
51. Suture, 0 and 2.0 silk
52. Suture, 9.0 nylon and Prolene
53. Suture, 4.0 Dexon and Vicryl
54. Assorted neurosurgical Cottonoids
55. Steri-Strips
56. Mastoid dressing

Indications and Contraindications for Stapes Surgery

Indications

- ☐ Purpose of surgery is to improve patient's hearing
- ☐ Reasonably good health for surgery requiring general anesthesia, although age is not a factor (young or old)
- ☐ The ear with poorer hearing is selected for surgery
- ☐ Surgery may be indicated for unilateral or bilateral hearing loss of any degree. Bilaterally normal hearing is the normal human condition.
- ☐ Minimum air-bone gap of 15 dB HL
- ☐ Speech discrimination is considered, but is not a major factor

Contraindications

- ☐ Poor physical health
- ☐ Presence of an active vestibular disorder (e.g., Ménière's disease)
- ☐ A pre-existing tympanic membrane perforation
- ☐ Active external or middle ear infection
- ☐ Small (less than 15 dB) air-bone gap in pure tone thresholds

Source: Adapted from House HP, Kwartler JA. Total stapedectomy. In Brackmann DE, Shelton C, Arriaga MA. (eds). *Otologic Surgery*. Philadelphia: WB Saunders, 1994.

Neuro-otologic Surgical Approaches

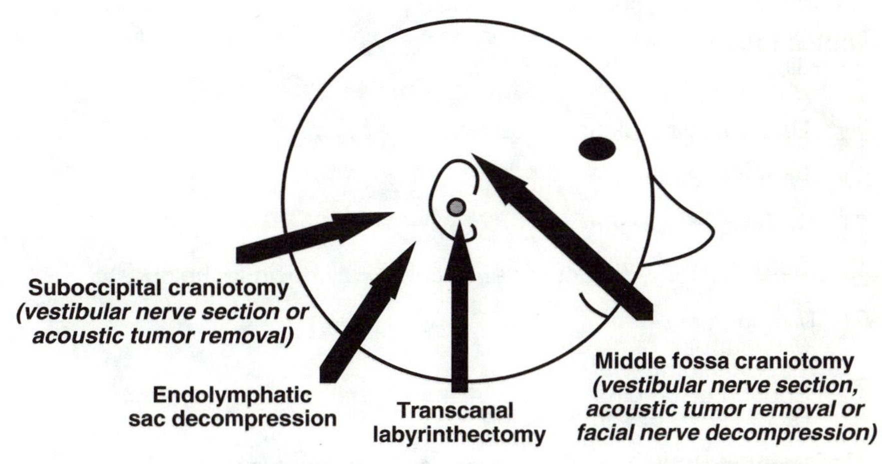
Suboccipital craniotomy
(vestibular nerve section or
acoustic tumor removal)
Endolymphatic
sac decompression
Transcanal
labyrinthectomy
Middle fossa craniotomy
(vestibular nerve section,
acoustic tumor removal or
facial nerve decompression)

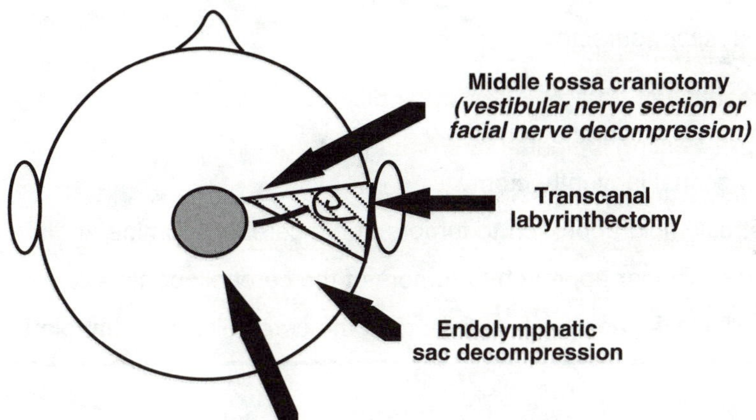
Middle fossa craniotomy
(vestibular nerve section or
facial nerve decompression)
Transcanal
labyrinthectomy
Endolymphatic
sac decompression
Suboccipital craniotomy or retrosigmoid
(vestibular nerve section or acoustic tumor removal)

Otologic Surgical Procedures

Audiologists may perform pre- and postoperative hearing, vestibular, or facial nerve assessments for patients undergoing these procedures. Audiologists may also perform intraoperative monitoring of auditory system and/or facial nerve function for selected procedures.

- ☐ Abnormally patulous eustachian tube
- ☐ Tympanoplasty
- ☐ Chronic ear surgery
- ☐ Mastoidectomy (intact canal or canal wall down techniques)
- ☐ Myringotomy
- ☐ Stapedectomy
- ☐ Facial nerve decompression
- ☐ Endolymphatic sac decompression and shunt insertion
- ☐ Vestibular neurectomy
- ☐ Cochleosacculotomy
- ☐ Chemical labyrinthectomy
- ☐ Transcanal labyrinthectomy
- ☐ Retrosigmoid approach to tumors of the cerebellopontine angle (CPA)
- ☐ Transcochlear approach to tumors of the cerebellopontine angle (CPA)
- ☐ Middle fossa approach to tumors of the cerebellopontine angle (CPA)

Key References

Otology

Britton BH. *Common problems in otology*. Chicago: Mosby Year Book,1991.

Kee, JL. *Handbook of laboratory and diagnostic tests with nursing implications*. Norwalk: Appleton & Lange, 1994.

Lee, KJ. *Essential otolaryngology: Head and neck surgery* (5th ed.). New York: Medical Examination Publishing Company, 1991.

Paparella MM, Shumrick DA, Gluckman JL, & Meyerhoff WL. *Otolaryngology. I. Basic sciences and related principles* (3rd ed.). Philadelphia: W. B. Saunders Company, 1991.

Paparella MM, Shumrick DA, Gluckman JL., & Meyerhoff WL. *Otolaryngology. II. Otology and neuro-otology* (3rd ed.). Philadelphia: W. B. Saunders Company, 1991.

CHAPTER 17

Drugs and Clinical Pharmacology

In This ADR Chapter

GENERAL CLINICAL PHARMACOLOGY

Medications and Side Effects

Related to Hearing, Auditory Function, Vestibular Function and Central Nervous System Function

Compiled by DiSorga RM, Weir, K. *Audiology Today 5*:32–35, 1993.

Side Effects

1. Auditory acuity, decrease
2. Auditory canals, small or absent, fetal
3. Auditory disturbances
4. Bell's palsy
5. Carcinoma, ear
6. Cerebral arterial insufficiency, symptoms
7. Cerebrovascular disorders
8. Circulatory collapse
9. Circulatory collapse, peripheral
10. Circulatory depression
11. Circulatory failure
12. Cochlear lesion
13. Confusion
14. CNS depression
15. CNS depression, neonatal
16. CNS reactions
17. CNS stimulation
18. CNS stimulation, paradoxical
19. CNS toxicity
20. Deafness
21. Disorientation
22. Dizziness
23. Ear discomfort
24. Ear drainage
25. Ear, external abnormalities, fetal
26. Ears, blocked
27. Echoacousia
28. Edema, cerebral
29. Edema, facial
30. Encephalitis
31. Encephalopathy
32. Encephalopathy, hepatitis
33. Encephalopathy, hypertensive
34. Encephalopathy, post-viral
35. Encephalopathy, toxic
36. Face, rhythmical involuntary movements
37. Facial cramps
38. Facial features, coarsening
39. Facial swelling
40. Flushing, ears
41. Hallucinations, auditory
42. Hearing decrease
43. Hearing disturbances
44. Hearing, impaired
45. Hearing, loss of
46. Hearing loss, reversible
47. Hyperacusis
48. Infection, ears
49. Labyrinthitis
50. Labyrinthitis hysteria, acute
51. Memory impairment
52. Memory loss, short term
53. Ménière's disease
54. Mental acuity, loss of
55. Mental clouding
56. Mental perception, altered
57. Mental performance, impaired
58. Mental slowness
59. Mental status, altered
60. Moro reflex, depressed
61. Nerve deafness
62. Neurotoxicity
63. Numbness, facial
64. Nystagmus
65. Otitis externa
66. Otitis media

67. Ototoxicity
68. Pain, ear
69. Psychiatric disturbances
70. Rhinitis
71. Rhinorrhea
72. Sensory disturbances
73. Sinusitis
74. Speech, incoherent
75. Speech, slurred
76. Speech difficulties
77. Speech disturbances
78. Tingling ears
79. Tinnitus
80. Vasoconstriction
81. Vascular collapse
82. Vasodilation
83. Vertigo

Drugs	Side Effects
Accutane Capsules	2, 22, 25, 79
Actibine	21
Actifed w/Codeine Cough Syrup	14, 22, 49, 79, 83
Actigall Capsules	70
Actimmune	21
Adipex-P Tablets & Caplets	17, 22
AeroBid Inhaler Syrup	22, 23, 48, 69, 71, 73, 83
AK-Pentolate	21, 74
AK-Taine	14, 17
Akineton	21
Aldactazide	22, 79
Aldoclor Tablets	4, 7, 22, 57, 69, 79
Aldomet Ester HCl Injection	4, 7, 22, 57, 69
Aldomet Oral	4, 7, 22, 57, 69
Aldoril Tablets	4, 7, 22, 57, 69, 79
Alfenta Injection	22
Alferon-N Injection	22, 57, 79
Altace Caplets	22, 45, 79, 83
Alurate Elixir	14, 22, 69
Amicar Syrup, Tablets, & Injection	22, 79
Amikin Injection	20, 45, 67
Aminophylin Tablets	11
Amocil	22
Anadrol-50 Tablets	17
Anafranil Caplets	20, 22, 31, 47, 51, 57, 64, 66, 68, 69, 70, 72, 73, 77, 83
Ana-Kit Anaphylaxis Emergency Treatment Kit	14, 22
Anaprox/Anaprox DST	22, 42, 70, 79, 83
Ancobon Capsules	45, 83
Anestacon Solution	16, 22, 79
Anexsia 5/500 Tablets	22, 55, 57
Anexsia 7.5/650 Tabs	22, 55, 57
Ansaid Tablets	14, 17, 22, 23, 46, 70, 79, 82
Antivenon	29
Antivenin (Crotalidae) Polyvalent	29
Apresazide Capsules	21, 22, 83
Apresoline-Esidrix Tablets	21, 22, 69, 83
Apresoline HCl Parenteral	21, 22
Apresoline HCl Tablets	21, 22
Aralen HCl Injection	3, 20, 42, 45, 69, 79
Aralen Phosphate with Primaquine Tablets	3, 20, 42, 45, 69, 79
Aralen Phosphate Tablets	3, 20, 42, 45, 69, 79
Arthritis Strength Bufferin Analgesic Capsules	44
Arthritis Strength BC Powder	44, 79
Aristocort Suspension	44, 83
Aristospan Suspension	83
Asbron G	11
Ascriptin A/D Capsules	45, 79
Asendin Tablets	13, 21, 22, 57, 79
Atabrine HCl Tablets	21, 69, 83
Atgam Sterile Solution	13, 21, 22, 30, 34
Ativan Injection	13, 14, 21, 22, 42, 57
Atrohist Sprinkle Capsules	14, 21
Attenuvax	16, 30
Augmentin Tablets, Powder, or Oral Suspension, Chewable Tablets	13, 21
Axid Pulvules	13
Azactam for Injection	13, 21, 79, 83
Azdone Tablets	13, 21, 55, 57, 71
Azmacort Inhaler	29
Azo Gantanol Tablets	79, 83
Azo Gantrisin Tablets	21, 22, 45, 79, 83
Azulfidine Tablets, EN-Tabs, Oral Suspension	45, 79, 83

Bactrim DS Tablets	79, 83
Bactrim I.V. Infusion	79, 83
Bactrim	79, 83
BAL in Oil Ampules	71
Bayer-Children's Chewable Aspirin	45, 79
Bayer-Aspirin Tablets & Caplets	45, 79
Bayer-Aspirin Max. Tablets & Caplets	45, 79
Bayer Plus Aspirin Tablets	45, 79
Therapy Bayer Aspirin Caplets	45, 79
8 Hr. Bayer Time-Release Aspirin, BC Powder	21, 45, 79
Beconase AQ Nasal Spray	71
Beconase Inhalation Aerosol & Refill	71
Benadryl Capsules	13, 21, 50, 79, 83
Benadryl Injection	13, 21, 50, 79, 83
Bentyl	13, 21, 57, 77
Betoptic Sterile Ophthalmic Solution	21, 28, 83
Betoptic S Sterile Ophthalmic Suspension	21, 28, 83
Biavax ii	16, 21, 30, 61
Blenoxane	13
Blocarden Tablets	21, 52, 79, 83
Brethaire Inhaler	17, 83
Bretylol Injection	13, 21, 83
Brevibloc Injection	13, 21, 73, 77
Breviblok	21
Brevicon	7, 21
Brevital Sodium Vials	10, 70, 81
Bumex	21, 23, 31, 44, 45, 67, 83
BuSpar	13, 16, 21, 29, 75, 79
Butalzolidin Capsules & Tablets	13, 45, 79
Butisol Sodium Elixir & Tablets	13, 14, 21
Calan SR Caplets	13, 21
Calan Tablets	13, 21
Calcijex Calcitriol Injection	70
Calciparine Injection	70, 71
Calderol Capsules	71
Cama Arthritis Pain Reliever	21, 45, 79
Cantil Tablets	13, 21
Capastat Sulfate Vials (approximately 11%)	1, 45, 79, 83
Capoten	13, 70
Capozide	13, 70, 83
Carafate Tablets	70, 83
Carbocaine	14, 17, 39, 72, 79
Carbocaine Hydrochloride Injection	14, 17, 39, 72
Cardene Capsules	13, 70, 73, 79, 83
Cardioquin Tablets	1, 13, 45, 79, 81, 83
Cardizem SR Capsules (60 mg, 90 mg, 120 mg)	79
Cardura Tablets	13, 29, 57, 66, 70, 73, 79, 83
Cartrol Tablets	52, 70, 73, 79, 82
Catapres-TTS	41
Ceclor Pulvules and Suspension	13
CeeNU	21
Celestone Soluspan Suspension	83
Celontin	13, 58
Centrax	13, 57
Ceptaz for Injection	31
CHEMET	26, 66, 71
Children's Advil Suspension	13, 45, 70, 79
Chloromycetin Kapseals	13
Chloromycetin Palmitate Oral Suspension	13
Chloromycetin Sodium Succinate	13
Choledyl Pediatric Elixir	11, 17
Choledyl Tablets	11, 17
Choledyl SA Tablets	11, 17
Cholybar	79, 83
Cibacalcin Double-chambered Syringes	40
Cibalith–S	9, 13, 57, 64, 75, 79, 83
Cipro I.V.	13, 17, 29, 45, 64, 79
Cipro Tablets	13, 17, 29, 45, 64, 79
Clinoril Tablets	42, 69, 79, 83
Clozaril Tablets	13, 52, 57, 59, 64, 71, 73, 74, 76, 83
Cocaine Hydrochloride Topical Solution	17, 80
Cogentin	13, 51, 69
Colestid Granules	83
Coly-Mycin	83
Coly-Mycin M Parenteral	83
Colyte	71

(continued)

Medications and Side Effects *(continued)*

Medication	Side Effects
Combipres Tablets	33, 41, 83
Compazine	16, 28, 36, 55, 57
Constant-T Tablets	11
Corgard Tablets	39, 52, 75, 79
Cortenema	83
Cortifoam	39
Cortisporin Cream	67
Cortisporin Ointment	67
Cortisporin Otic Suspension Sterile	67
Cortone Acetate Sterile Suspension	69, 83
Cortone Acetate Tablets	69, 83
Cuprimine Capsules	69, 79
Cyclogyl	21, 74, 82
Cyclomydril	21, 74, 82
Cycrin	7
Cylert Tablets	64
Cytosar-U Sterile Powder	19, 62
Cytotec	20, 23, 79
Cytovene Sterile Powder	13
Dalalone D.P. Injectable	64, 83
Dalgan Injection	13, 26, 75, 79, 83
Dalmane Capsules	13, 21, 75
Damason-P	55, 57, 71
Danocrine Capsules	16
Dantrium Capsules	13, 77
Dapsone USP	79, 83
Daranide Tablets	13, 21, 79
Darbid Tablets	13
DDAVP	70, 82
Decadron Elixir	64, 69, 83
Decadron-LA Sterile Solution	64, 69, 83
Decadron Phosphate Injection	64, 69, 83
Decadron Phosphate Respihaler	64, 69, 83
Decadron Phosphate Turbinaire	64, 69, 83
Decadron Phosphate w/Xylocaine Injection, Sterile	64, 69, 83
Decadron Tablets	64, 69, 83
Deconamine	13, 14, 17, 79, 83
Deconsal	14
Deltasone Tablets	83
Demerol Tablets	10, 21, 57
Demser Capsules	13, 21, 76
Demulen	3, 7, 70
Depakene Capsules & Syrup	64
Depakote Sprinkle Capsules	14
Depen Titratable Tablets	25, 79
Depo-Medrol Sterile Aqueous Suspension	69, 70, 72, 83
Deprol Tablets	16, 75, 83
Desferal Vials	1, 44, 45, 79
Desyrel & Desyrel Dividose	13, 16, 21, 51, 57, 75, 79, 82, 83
Diamox Parenteral	13, 43, 44, 79
Diamox Sequels	13, 43, 44, 79
Diamox Tablets	13, 43, 44, 79
Diapid Nasal Spray	71
Dilantin Infatabs	13, 14, 38, 64, 75
Dilantin Kapseals	13, 14, 38, 64, 75
Dilantin Parenteral	13, 14, 38, 64, 75
Dilantin-30	13, 14, 38, 64, 75
Pediatric/Dilantin-125	13, 14, 38, 64, 75
Dilantin	13, 14, 38, 64, 75, 83
Dilantin w/Phenobarbital Kapseals	13, 14, 38, 64, 75, 83
Dilatrate-SR	82
Dilaudid	10, 11, 13, 57, 64
Dilaudid-HP Injection	10, 11, 13, 21, 64
Dilaudid Cough Syrup	10, 11, 13, 57, 64
Dilor	11, 17
Dilor-G Tablets & Liquid	11, 17
Dipentum Capsules	83
Diphtheria and Tetanus Toxoids and Pertussis Vaccine Adsorbed USP	
Adult	31
Pediatric Use	12
Diprivan Injection	13, 68, 79
Disalcid	44, 79, 83
Ditropan	13, 82
Diucardin Tablets	83
Diulo	83
Diupres Tablets	16, 20, 60, 83
Diuril Oral Suspension	83
Diuril Sodium Intravenous	83
Diuril Tablets	83
Dolobid Tablets	13, 21, 79, 83
Dolophine Hydrochloride Ampoules and Vials	10, 21
Dolophine Hydrochloride Tablets	10, 21

Side Effects listed on pages 789–790

Drug	Side Effects
Dopram Injectable	21
Doral Tablets	
Dorcol Children's Cough Syrup	16
Dorcol Children's Decongestant Liquid	16
Dorcol Children's Liquid Cold Formula	16
Doxorubicin Hydrochloride for Injection, USP	26
Dristan Long Lasting Nasal Spray	71
Dristan Long Lasting Nasal Spray, Dose Pump	71
Duragesic Transdermal System	13, 77, 83
Duranest Injections	13, 79
Dyazide Capsules	83
Dyclone 0.5% and 1% Topical Solutions, USP	13, 79
Easprin	13, 46, 79, 83
Ecotrin	44, 79
Edecrin	13, 20, 79, 83
E.E.S.	13, 46, 83
Elavil	13, 21, 29, 57, 79
Eldeprl	13, 21, 51, 59, 77, 79, 83
Elspar	13
Emcy Capsules	79
Eminase	83
Empirin with Codeine Phosphate	13, 45, 71, 79
E-Mycin Tablets	46
Endep Tablets	13, 21, 29, 57, 79
Enduron Tablets	83
Enduronyl	20, 83
Engerix-B Unit-Dose Vials	4, 83
Enovid	3, 7, 70
Epogen for Injection	33
Equagesic Tablets	57, 75, 79, 83
Ergamisol Tablets	13, 31, 52, 64
EryPed	13, 46, 83
Ery-Tab Tablets	13, 46, 83
Erythrocin Stearate Filmtab	13, 46, 83
Erythromycin Base Filmtab	13, 46, 83
Erythromycin Delated-Release Capsules, USP	13, 46, 83
Esgic-Plus Tablets	13
Esgic Tablets & Capsules	13
Esidrix Tablets	83
Esimil Tablets	83
Eskalith	9, 13, 51, 57, 64, 75, 79, 83
Ethmozine Tablets (less than 2%)	7, 13, 52, 64, 73, 76, 79, 82, 83
Etrafon	11, 13, 21, 28, 29, 36, 57, 75, 79
Eulexin Capsules	13, 32
4-Way Fast Acting Nasal Spray-Original	71
4-Way Long Lasting Nasal Spray	71
Fansidar Tablets	79, 83
Fedahist Gyrocaps	14
Fedahist Timecaps	4
Feldene Capsules	13, 45, 79, 83
Fioricet Tablets	13
Flagyl I.V.	13, 83
Flexeril Tablets	4, 21, 29, 79, 82, 83
Florinal with Codeine Capsules	21, 68, 75, 79, 83
Floxin Tablets	13, 45, 64, 71, 82, 83
Fluorouracil Injection	13, 21, 64
FUDR (Sterile)	13, 21, 64
Fulvicin P/G Tablets	13, 57
Fulvicin P/G 165 & 330 Tablets	13, 57
Fulvicin-U/F Tablets	13, 57
Fungizone Intravenous	45, 79, 83
Ganite Injection	1, 13, 79
Gantanol	79, 83
Gantrisin Ophthalmic Ointment/Solution	79, 83
Gantrisin	79, 83
Garamycin Injectable	13, 31, 45, 62, 67, 79, 83
Gelfoam Sterile Sponge	45
GoLYTELY	71
Grifulvin V Tablets/Suspension	13, 57
Grisactin	13, 57
Grisactin Ultra Tablets	13, 57
Gris-PEG Tablets, 125 mg and 250 mg	13
Halcion Tablets	13, 18, 21, 51, 55, 75, 79
Haldol Decanoate	13, 83
Haldol Injection, Tablets and Concentrate	13, 83

(continued)

Medications and Side Effects *(continued)*

Medication	Side Effects
Harmonyl Tablets	16, 20
Heparin Lock Flush Solution	70
Heparin Sodium Vials	70
Heparin Sodium Injection, USP, Sterile Solution	70
Hexalen Capsules	16, 62, 83
Hibiclens Antimicrobial Skin Cleanser	20
Hibistat	20
Humulin 70/30, 100 units	13
Humulin BR, 100 units	13
Humulin L, 100 units	13
Humulin U, 100 units	13
Hycodan Syrup, Tablets	55, 57
Hycomine Compound Tablets	55, 57
Hycomine Syrup	55, 57
Hycotuss Expectorant Syrup	55, 57
Hydeltrasol Injection, Sterile	69, 83
Hydeltra-T.B.A. Sterile Suspension	69, 83
Hydrea Capsules	21
Hydrocet Capsules	16, 55, 57
Hydrocortone Acetate Sterile Suspension	69, 83
Hydrocortone Phosphate Injection Sterile	69, 83
Hydrocortone Tablets	69, 83
HydroDIURIL Tables	83
Hydromox Tablets	15, 83
Hydromox R Tablets	15, 83
Hydropres Tablets	16, 20, 60, 83
Hylorel Tablets	13, 69
Hyperstat I.V. Injection	13, 45, 79, 82
Hytrin Tablets	29, 70, 73, 79, 82
Idamycin for Infection	59
IFEX	13, 21
Ilasone	45, 79
Ilotycin Gluceptate, IV Vials	45
Inderal	52
Inderal LA Long Acting Capsules	52
Inderide Tablets	52, 83
Inderide LA Long Acting Capsules	52, 83
Indocin	13, 20, 43, 69, 79, 83
Indocin Capsules	13, 20, 43
Indocin I.V.	13, 20, 43, 62
INH Tablets	35, 51
Intal Capsules	83
Intal Inhaler	83
Intron A	13, 16, 29, 43, 57, 68, 70, 71, 73, 77, 79, 83
Inversine Tablets	57
ISMOTIC	13, 21, 83
Isoptin Injectable	13, 64, 83
Isoptin Oral Tablets	13, 64
Isopin SR Sustained Release Tablets	13, 64
Jenest-28 Tablets	7, 22
Keflex Pulvules/Oral Suspension	13, 22
Keftab Tablets	13, 22
Kefurox Vials, Faspak and ADD-Vantage	44
Kemadrin	22
Kenalog-10 Injection	69, 83
Kenalog-40 Injection	69, 83
Kerlone Tablets (less than 2%)	7, 13, 20, 22, 23, 29, 52, 70, 73, 77, 79
Ketalar	64
Klonopin Tablets	13, 14, 29, 51, 64, 71, 75, 83
Klorvess Effervescent Granules	13
Klorvess Effervescent Tablets	13
Klorvess 10% Liquid	13
K-Lyte	13
K-Phos M.F. Tablets	13, 22
K-Phos Neutral Tablets	13, 22
K-Phos Original Formula 'Sodium Free' Tablets	13, 22
K-Phos No.2 Tablets	13, 22
Kwell Cream	17, 22
Kwell Lotion	17, 22
Kwell Shampoo	17, 22
Lanoxicaps	16, 22
Lanoxin Elixir Pediatric	16, 22
Lanoxin Injection	16, 22
Lanoxin Injection Pediatric	16, 22
Lanoxin Tablets	16, 22
Lariam Tablets	13, 16, 22, 31, 79, 83
Larodopa Tablets	13, 22
Lasix	4, 22, 45, 79, 83

Side Effects listed on pages 789–790

Lasix Oral Solution	4, 45	Marinol (Dronabinol) Capsules	22, 57
Legatrin	20, 79	Marplan Tablets	13, 22, 51, 83
Leukeran Tablets	13	Matulane Capsules	13, 22, 45, 64, 75
Leukine for IV Infusion	16	Maxair Inhaler	13, 22
Levatol	22, 52	Maxzide	22, 83
Levlen/Tri-Levlen	7, 22	Mebaral Tablets	13, 14, 22, 64, 57, 69, 75
Levsin/Levsinex	13, 22, 77	Meclomen Capsules	22, 79
Levo-Dromoran	22	Medrol	22, 83
Lebrax Capsules	13	Mellaril	36, 59
Lebritabs Tablets	13, 18, 57	Menrium Tablets	13, 22
Librium Capsules	13, 18	Mepergan Injection	10, 21, 22
Librium Injectable	13, 18	Mesantonin Tablets	22, 64
Limbitrol	13, 22, 29, 57	Methadone Hydrochloride Diskets	10, 21, 22, 71
Lincocin	79, 83	Methadone Hydrochloride Oral Solution/Tablets	10, 13, 21, 22, 71
Lioresal Tablets	13, 22, 64, 75, 79	Methergine	79
Lithane Tablets	9, 13, 22, 64, 75, 79, 83	Methotrexate Tablets, Parenteral, LP	13, 22, 31, 79
Lithium Carbonate Capsules & Tablets	9, 13, 22, 64, 75, 79, 83	Metubine Iodide Vials	11
Loestrin	7, 22	Mevacor Tablets	22, 69
Lomotil	13, 22	Mexitil Capsules1	3, 22, 52, 76, 79
Lopid Capsules and Tablets	13, 22, 83	Micronor Tablets	7, 22
Lopressor Ampuls	22, 51, 52, 68, 79, 83	Midamor Tablets	13, 22, 31, 79, 83
Lopressor HCT Tablets	22, 51, 52, 68, 79, 83	Miltown Tablets	13, 22, 75, 83
Lopressor Tablets	13, 22, 51, 52, 68, 79, 83	Minipress Capsules	22, 79, 83
Lorelco Tablets	22, 79	Minizide Capsules	22, 79, 83
Lortab ASA Tablets	13, 22, 55, 57, 71	Minocin Intravenous	22, 83
Lortab	22, 55, 57, 71	Minocin Oral Suspension	22, 83
Lotensin Tablets	22, 73	Minocin Pellet-Filled Capsules	22, 83
Loxitane	13, 22, 29, 57, 75	Mintezol	22, 69, 79
Lozol Tablets	22, 71, 83	M-M-R	20, 22, 30, 31, 61, 66
Ludiomil Tablets	13, 21, 22, 51, 79	M-R-VAX	22, 30, 31
Lufyllin & Lufyllin-400 Tablets	11, 17	Mobran Tablets & Concentrate	59
Lufyllin-GG Elixir & Tablets	11, 17	Modicon	7, 22
Lupron Depot 7.5 mg	5, 22, 39, 43, 51	Moduretic Tablets	13, 22, 31, 79, 83
Lupron Injection (less than 5%)	5, 22, 39, 43, 51	Mono-Gesic Tablets	13, 45, 79, 83
Lysodren	14, 22, 83	Monopril Tablets	13, 22, 51, 70, 73, 79
Macrodantin Capsules	22, 64, 83	Motofen Tablets	13, 22
Marax Tablets & DF Syrup	16, 83	Motrin Tablets	13, 14, 22, 45, 70, 79
Marcaine Hydrochloride 0.5% with Epinephrine	19, 22, 39, 74, 79, 82	MS Contin Tablets	10, 21, 22, 64
Marcaine Hydrochloride with Epinephrine	19, 22, 39, 74, 79, 82	MSIR	10, 21, 22, 64
Marcaine Spinal	19, 22, 39, 74, 79, 82	Mumpsvax	30, 61, 70
		Mustargen	44, 79, 83
		Mutamycin	13
		Myambutol Tablets	13, 21, 22
		Mykrox 2 mg Tablets	22, 54, 79

(continued)

Medications and Side Effects *(continued)*

Medication	Side Effects	Medication	Side Effects
Myochrysine Injection	13, 22	Novafed A Capsules	14, 22
Mysoline (Occasional) Pediatric Drops/Syrup	14, 22	Novafed Capsules	14, 22
Nalfon Pulvules & Tablets	13, 21, 22, 42, 79	Novahistine DH	14, 22
Naphcon-A Ophthalmic Solution	14, 22	Novahistine DMC	14, 22
Naprosyn	4, 14, 22, 42, 79, 83	Novahistine Elixir	14, 22
Naprosyn Suspension	4, 14, 22, 42, 57	Novantrone for Injection Concentrate	16
Nardil	22, 64	Novocain Hydrochloride for Spinal Anesthesia	22, 82
Naturetin Tablets	22, 83	Nubain Injection	13, 22, 76, 83
Navane Capsules and Concentrate	28, 59	NuLYTELY	71
Navane Intramuscular	28, 59	Oculinum for Injection	21
Nebcin Vials, Hyporets & ADD-Vantage	13, 21, 22, 45, 62, 67, 79, 83	Ogen	22
NebuPent for Inhalation Solution	13, 22, 52, 70, 82, 83	OMIU	64
NegGram	22, 83	Omnipaque	13, 16, 21, 22, 27, 37, 43, 46, 57, 70, 77, 79, 82, 83
Nembutal Sodium Capsules	13, 14, 22, 83	Oncovin Solution Vials & Hyporets	62
Nembutal Sodium Solution	13, 14, 22, 83	Optimine Tablets	13, 22, 49, 79, 83
Nembutal Sodium Suppositories	13, 14, 22, 83	OpiPranolol Sterile Ophthalmic Solution	22, 71
NeoDecadron Topical Cream	22, 67	Oramorph SR (Morphine Sulfate Sustained Release Tabs)	10, 13, 21, 22, 64
Neosporin Cream	67	Orap Tablets	16, 22, 36, 57, 59
Neosporin G.U. Irrigant Sterile	67	Oretic Tablets	22, 83
Neosporin Ointment	67	Oreticyl	22, 83
Neptazane Tablets	13, 83	Ornade Spansule Capsules	13, 22, 49, 79, 83
Nescaine/Nescaine MPF	22, 79	Ornex	22
Netromycin Injection 100 mg/ml	21, 22, 31, 45, 53, 62, 64, 67, 79, 83	Orthoclone OKT3 Sterile Solution	13, 21, 31, 59
Nicorette	13, 22, 79	Ortho Novum	7, 22
Nipride I.V. Infusion	13, 22, 62, 79	Orudis Capsules	13, 16, 22, 29, 44, 70, 79, 82, 83
Nitro-Bid Ointment	22, 82	OSM GLYN	13, 21
Nitrostat Tablets	22, 82	Ovcon	7, 22
Nizoral Tablets	22, 82	P-A-C Analgesic Tablets	79
Norethin	3, 22, 70	Pamelor	13, 21, 22, 29, 79
Norgesic	13, 22	Papaverine HCl Vials/Ampoules	83
Norinyl	7, 22	Paradione Capsules	83
Norisodrine Aerotrol	17, 83	Paraplatin for Injection	16, 62, 67
Normodyne Injection	22, 52, 83	Parlodel	13, 19, 22, 78, 83
Normodyne Tablets	22, 52, 83	Parnade Tablets	22, 79
Normozide Tablets	22, 52, 70, 83	Pavabid Capsules	83
Noroxin Tablets	13, 16, 17, 22, 29, 46, 69	Pavabid HP Capsulets	83
Norpramin Tablets	13, 21, 22, 29, 57, 79	PBZ Tablets & Elixir	13, 22, 79, 83
Norzine	13, 22, 79	PBZ-SR Tablets	13, 22, 57, 79, 83

Side Effects listed on pages 789–790

Drug	Codes
PCE Dispertab Tablets	13, 22, 46, 83
Pediapred Oral Liquid	22, 83
PediaProfen Suspension	13, 14, 22, 45, 70, 79
Pedeazole	46, 79, 83
PediOptic Suspension Sterile	67
Pedvax HIB	48, 66
Peganone Tablets	22, 64
Penam 300 Injection	13, 22
Pepcid	13, 22, 29, 79, 83
Pepto-Bismol Liquid & Tablets	79
Percodan	22
Periactin	13, 22, 49, 79, 83
Permax Tablets	4, 13, 20, 22, 28, 29, 66, 68, 70, 73, 77, 79, 82, 83
Pfizerpen- AS Aqueous Suspension	13, 83
Phenergan w/Codeine	10, 13, 14, 21, 22, 57, 79
Phenergan VC w/Codeine	10, 13, 14, 21, 22, 57
Phenergan with Dextromethorphan	10, 13, 14, 21, 22, 57, 79
Phenergan Suppositories	10, 13, 14, 21, 22, 57
Phenergan Syrup	10, 13, 14, 21, 22, 57
Phenergan VC	10, 13, 14, 21, 22, 57, 79
Phenergan VC w/Codeine	10, 13, 14, 21, 22, 44, 57
Phenobarbital Elixir and Tablets	9, 13, 14, 22, 83
Phenurone Tablets	22, 83
PhosLo Tablets	13
Phrenilin	13
Pipracil	22
Pitressin Synthetic, Ampoules	83
Placidyl Capsules	22, 63
Plaquenil Sulfate Tablets	20, 22, 61, 64, 79, 83
Platinol	20, 29, 45, 62, 67, 79
Platinol-AQ Injection	20, 29, 45, 62, 67, 79
Plendil Extended-Release Tablets PMB 200 and PMB 400	22, 29, 57, 70, 71, 73, 75, 79
Polaramine	13, 22, 49, 79, 83
Polycitra Syrup	13
Polycitra-K	13
Polycitra-LC — Sugar Free	13
Polymyxin B Sulfatel, Aerosporin Brand Sterile Powder	22, 62
Pondimin Tablets	13, 22
Ponstel	22, 23, 29
Pontocaine Hydrochloride for Spinal Anesthesia	16, 17, 22, 79
Prilu	22
Prilosec Delayed-Release Capsules	13, 22, 79, 83
Primaxin I.M.	13, 22, 29, 31, 46, 79, 83
Primaxin I.V.	13, 22, 29, 31, 46, 79, 83
Prinivil Tablets	13, 22, 83
Prinzide Tablets	13, 22, 39, 68, 70, 73, 79, 83
Pro-Banthine Tablets	13, 22
Procan SR Tablets	13, 22
Procardia XL Tablets	22, 29, 73, 79, 83
Procrit for Injection	22, 3
Prolixin Decanoate	28, 36
Prolixin Elixir	28, 36
Prolixin Enanthate	28, 36
Prolixin Injection	28, 36
Prolixin Oral Concentrate	28, 36
Prolixin Tablets	28, 36
Pronestyl Capsules/Tablets	22
Pronestyl Injections	22
Propagest	22
ProSom Tablets	13, 15, 22, 42, 64, 68, 70, 73, 79
Protamine Sulfate Ampoules & Vials	8
Protopam	22
Protostat Tablets	13, 22, 83
Proventil Inhalation Aerosol	17, 22, 79, 83
Proventil Repetabs Tablets	17, 22, 79, 83
Proventil Syrup	17, 22, 83
Proventil Tablets	17, 22, 83
Prozac Pulvules	14, 17, 20, 22, 29, 57, 64, 68, 70, 73, 79, 83
Quadrinal Tablets	11, 13, 22
Quarzan Capsules	13, 22
Questran Light	22, 79, 83
Questran Powder	22, 79, 83
Qulbron Capsules	11, 22

(continued)

Medications and Side Effects *(continued)*

Quibron-T	11, 22	Ru-Tuss II Capsules	14, 49, 79
Quibron-T/SR	11	Ryna	57
Quinaglute Dura-Tabs Tablets	1, 13, 44, 79, 82, 83	Rythmol Tablets	13, 52, 79, 83
Quinamm Tablets	13, 20, 29, 79, 83	Salflex	22, 44, 45, 46, 79, 83
Quinidex Extentabs	1, 13, 22, 45, 79, 82, 83	Saluron	22, 83
Q-vel Muscle Relaxant Pain Reliever	20, 79	Salutensin/Salutensin-Demi	20, 22, 83
Raudixin Tablets	20, 22	Sandimmune	13, 45, 73, 79, 83
Rauzide Tablets	16, 20, 22, 57, 83	Sandostatin Injection (less than 1%)	4, 16, 22, 51, 60, 71, 83
Recombivax HB	4, 68, 70, 79	Seconal Sodium Pulvules	13, 14, 22, 83
Reglan	13, 22, 36	Sectral Capsules	22, 52, 70
Renese	20, 22, 83	Sedapap Tablets 50 mg/650 mg	13, 22
Renese-R Tablets	13, 20, 22, 83	Seldane Tablets	13, 14, 21, 22
Respbid Tablets	11	Seldane-D Extended-Release Tablets	13, 14, 21, 22
Restoril Capsules	13, 18, 22, 57	Sensorcaine	22, 74, 79
Retrovir Capsules	13, 22, 45, 65, 70, 73, 82, 83	Sensorcaine-MPF Spinal	22, 74, 79
Retrovir I.V. Infusion	13, 22, 45, 65, 70, 73, 82, 83	Septra	22, 79, 83
Retrovir Syrup	22, 45, 5, 70, 73, 82, 83	Septra I.V. Infusion	22, 79, 83
Rheumatrex Methotrexate Dose Pack	13, 22, 31, 79	Septra I.V. Infusion ADD-Vantage Vials	22, 79, 83
Rithmol Tablets	77	Ser-Ap-Es Tablets	20, 21, 22, 83
Rifadin	13, 22, 29, 57	Serax Capsules	21, 75, 51, 83
Rifamate Capsules	13, 22, 35, 51, 57	Serax Tablets	21, 75, 51, 83
Rimactane Capsules	13, 22, 57	Serentil	13, 75
Robaxin Injectable	22, 64, 83	Seromycin Pulules	13, 21, 51, 83
Robinul Forte Tablets	13, 22	Serpasil Tablets	20, 21, 22, 83
Robinul Injectable	13, 22	Serpasil Apresoline Tablets	20, 22, 83
Robinul Tablets	13, 22	Serpasil Esidrix Tablets	20, 22, 83
Rocaltrol Capsules	71	Silvadine Cream 1%	16
Roferon-A Injection	13, 16, 22, 31, 51, 59 68, 70, 73, 77, 83	Sinemet Tablets	13, 21, 22, 54, 59
Rogaine Topical Solution	22, 29, 48, 70, 73, 83	Sinemet CR Tablets	13, 21, 22, 51, 54, 59
Rondec	17, 22	Sinequan	13, 21, 79
Rondec-DM	17, 22	Slo-bid Gyrocaps	11, 22
Rondec-TR Tablets	17, 22	Solganal Suspension	30
Roxanol	13, 21, 22	Solu-Cortef Sterile Powder	83
Roxicodone Tablets, Oral Solution & Intensol	13, 22	Solu-Medrol Sterile Powder	83
Rufen Tablets	13, 22, 45, 70, 79	Soma Compound with Codeine Tablets	13, 21, 22, 70, 79, 83
Ru-Tuss II Capsules	13, 14, 22, 49, 79, 83	Soma Compound	13, 21, 22, 70, 79, 83
Ru-Tuss DE Tablets	14, 49, 79	Soma Tablets	13, 21, 22, 70, 83
Ru-Tuss w/Hydrocone	14, 22, 49, 79	Sorbitrate	82
		SSD RP Cream	16
		Stadol	13, 83

Side Effects listed on pages 789–790

Stelazine	16, 28, 36, 39, 59
Surital Ampoules, Steri-Vials	11, 22
Surmonil Capsules	13, 21, 22, 29, 57, 79
Symmetrel Capsules & Syrup	13, 22, 57
Synalgos-DC Capsules	57
Syntocinon Nasal Spray	22, 71
T-PHYL (Uniphyl) 200 mg Tablets	11, 22
Tacaryl	22, 79
Tagamet	13, 21
Talacen	13, 21, 29, 79
Talwin Compound	10, 13, 21, 22, 29, 64, 79
Talwin Injection	10, 13, 21, 22, 29, 64, 79
Talwin Nx	10, 13, 21, 22, 29, 64, 79
Tambocor Tablets	13, 22, 39, 64, 77, 79, 83
Tapazole Tablets	22, 31, 83
Taractan	28, 36
Tavist Syrup	13, 22, 49, 79, 83
Tavist Tablets	13, 22, 49, 79, 83
Tavist-D Tablets	13, 22, 49, 79, 83
Tegison Capsules	22, 23, 24, 45, 48, 65, 71
Tegral-D	17, 22
Tegretol Chewable Tablets	6, 13, 22, 47, 64, 77, 79
Tegretol Suspension	6, 13, 22, 47, 64, 77, 79
Tegretol Tablets	6, 13, 22, 47, 64, 77, 79
Temaril Tablets, Syrup, Spansule Sustained Release Capsules	22, 79
Tenex Tablets	13, 22, 70, 79, 83
Tenoretic Tablets	22, 52, 83
Tenormin Tablets and I.V. Injection	22, 52, 83
Thalitone Tablets	22, 83
Theo-24	11
Theo-Dur Sprinkle	11
Theo-Dur Extended-Release Tablets	11
Theolair	11
Theolair-SR Tablets	11
Theo-Organidin Elixir	17
TheoX Extended-Release Tablets	17
Thera-Gesic	79
Thiosulfil Forte Tablets	79, 83
Thorazine	22, 28, 36
Tigan	21, 22
Timolide Tablets	13, 22, 51, 57, 68, 79, 82, 83
Timoptic in Ocudose	13, 21, 22, 52, 57, 79, 82, 83
Timoptic Sterile Ophthalmic Solution	13, 21, 22, 52, 57, 79, 82, 83
Tofranil Ampuls	13, 21, 22, 29, 79
Tofranil Tablets	13, 21, 22, 29, 79
Tofranil-PM Capsules	13, 21, 22, 29, 79
Tolectin (200, 400, 600 mg)	22, 79
Toinase Tablets	22, 83
Tonocard Tablets	13, 21, 22, 45, 51, 58, 64, 75, 77, 79, 83
Toradol IM Injection	22, 82, 83
Torecan	13, 22, 29, 79
Tracrium Injection	82
Trancopal Caplets	13, 22
Trandate Tablets	21, 22, 51, 52, 70, 83
Trandate HCT Tablets	22, 52, 70, 83
Tansderm Scop Transdermal Therapeutic System	13, 22, 51
Tranxene	13, 22, 75
Trecator-SC Tablets	22, 83
Trental	13, 22, 68
Trexan Tablets	13, 21, 33, 36, 71, 73, 79
Triaminic Cold Tablets	13, 14, 16, 17, 22, 49, 83
Triaminic-DM Syrup	14, 16, 17, 22, 49, 83
Triaminic Expectorant DH	13, 14, 16, 17, 22, 49, 79
Triaminic Oral Infant Drops	13, 14, 16, 17, 22, 49, 79, 83
Triaminic Repetabs Tablets	14, 16, 17, 22, 49
Triaminic Syrup	14, 16, 17, 22, 49
Triaminicol Multi-Symptom Relief	16, 22
Triavil Tablets	13, 21, 22, 28, 29, 59, 79
Tridione	83

(continued)

Medications and Side Effects *(continued)*

Medication	Side Effects	Medication	Side Effects
Tri-Immunol Diphtheria & Tetanus Toxoids & Pertussis Vaccine, Adsorbed	31	Vistaril Intramuscular Solution	57
Trilifon	11, 22, 28, 75	Vivactil Tablets	13, 22, 21, 79
Trilisate	13, 22, 44, 45, 79	Voltaren Tablets	21, 22, 46, 51, 79
Trinalin	13, 14, 22, 49, 79, 83	Vontrol Tablets	13, 22, 21, 41
Trinalin Repetabs Tablets	13, 14, 22, 49, 83	Wellbutrin Tablets	3, 13, 22, 51, 79, 83
Tri-Norinyl 28-day Tablets	7, 22	Wygesic Tablets	22, 57
Tussionex Extended-Release Suspension	22, 55, 57	Xanax Tablets	13, 14, 22, 51, 57, 75, 79
Tylox Capsules	22, 57	Xylocaine Injections	13, 14, 18, 22, 79
Unasyn	39	Xylocaine Injections for Ventricular Arrhythmias	13, 14, 18, 22, 79
Uniphyl 400 mg Tablets	11	Xylocaine 2% Jelly	13, 14, 18, 22, 79
Uricholine	22	Xylocaine 5% Ointment	13, 14, 18, 22, 79
Urised	22	Xylocaine 10% Oral Spray	13, 14, 18, 22, 79
Urispas Tablets	13, 83	4% Xylocaine-MPF Sterile Solution	13, 14, 18, 22, 79
Uroqid-Acid	13, 22	Xylocaine 2% Viscous Solution	13, 14, 18, 22
Ursinus Inlay-Tabs	22, 79	Yodoxin	83
Valium Injectable	13, 64, 75, 83	Yohimex Tablets	22, 71
Valium Tablets	13, 64, 75, 83	Zantac	13, 22, 83
Valpin-50 Tablets	13, 22	Zantac Injection/ Zantac Injected Premixed	13, 22, 83
Valrelease Capsules	13, 75, 83	Zarontin Capsules	22, 57, 83
Vancenase AQ Nasal Spray	71	Zarontin Syrup	22, 57, 83
Vancenase Nasal Inhaler	71	Zaroxolyn Tablets	22, 83
Vancocin HCl, Oral Solution & Pulvules	22, 45, 67, 79, 83	Zestoretic	13, 22, 39, 68, 70, 73, 79, 83
Vancocin HCl, Vials & ADD-Vantage	22, 45, 67, 79, 83	Zestril Tablets	13, 22, 39, 73, 83
Vascor Tablets	22, 70, 79, 82, 83	Zestoretic Capsules	22, 68, 73
Vaseretic Tablets	13, 22, 71, 79, 83	Zidone Capsules	22
Vasotec I.V.	13, 22, 71, 79, 83	Zinacef	45
Vasotec Tablets	13, 22, 71, 79	Zorprin Tablets	70, 79
Velban Vials	22, 62	Zovirax	13, 22, 31
Ventolin	17, 22, 83	Zovirax Capsules	13, 31
Verelan Capsules	13, 22	Zovirax Sterile Powder	13, 22, 31
Versed Injection	13, 15, 22, 23, 26, 64, 75	Zydone Capsules	22, 55, 57
Vicodin Tablets	22, 55, 57	Zyloprim Tablets	13, 22, 29, 70, 79, 82, 83
Vicodin ES Tablets	22, 55		
Vira-A for Injection	13, 22, 31		
Visken Tablets	22, 52		

Side Effects listed on pages 789–790

Clinical Concepts

Pharmacological Therapy and Analgesia in Otolaryngology

I. ANTIBIOTIC (ANTIMICROBIAL) THERAPY

Antibiotics are used to treat infectious diseases caused by pathogenic microorganisms. The existence of an infection indicates that the defenses of the immune system have been breached. To survive, the pathogenic organism must evade phagocytosis by neutrophils. This is accomplished in a number of ways by different organisms. Antibiotic drugs generally function by impairing the synthesis and/or maintenance of the pathogenic organism's cell structure (usually the cell wall). One of the most difficult aspects of antibiotic therapy is that a given microorganism may be susceptible to one antibiotic, but not another; and certain drugs are more effective against one pathogen than another. Thus, knowledge of the pathogenic organism underlying the disease process is critically important in selecting the most efficacious antibiotic.

A listing of common pathogenic organisms can be found in the table on page 812. Diseases frequently associated with each pathogen are listed for each organism. In addition, each organism is designated as either gram-negative or gram-positive based on Gram's method. Gram-negative organisms lose their crystal violet stain in the presence of alcohol, whereas gram-positive organisms retain the stain. Pathogenic organisms are often classified by this distinction. Accordingly, antibiotics are classified as being effective against particular gram-negative or gram-positive organisms.

The listing of antibiotics in the table beginning on page 813 is arranged by class. The pathogenic organisms (from the table on page 812) against which the drug is effective or ineffective are listed along with diseases which may result from infection by that organism.

A. Sulfonamides

The sulfonamides were the first chemotherapeutic agents used to treat bacterial infections in humans. This class of antibiotics is active against gram-positive and gram-negative organisms, although many strains have become resistant to sulfonamide therapy. The bacteriostatic action of these drugs is accomplished by preventing bacteria from incorporating para-aminobenzoic acid (PABA) into the folic acid molecule. Thus, bacteria that do not require folic acid are not affected by the antagonistic action of the drug. Sulfonamides are often used in combination with other antibiotics to increase the effectiveness of the therapy.

Common otolaryngologic indications are:

- acute otitis media and prophylaxis
- bronchitis
- acute sinusitis

B. Beta-Lactams

This large group of antibiotics includes the penicillins, cephalosporins, carbapenems, and the monobactams. These agents generally are effective against a broad range of gram-positive and gram-negative organisms with a few exceptions. The beta-lactams are considered bactericidal. This action is achieved by inhibiting bacteria cell wall synthesis and maintenance.

1. Penicillins

Since penicillin was first introduced in the 1950s, several generations of penicillins have been developed with extended spectra of actions. Like most antibiotics, some agents are more effective than others against a particular microbe.

Common otolaryngologic indications are:

- acute otitis media
- furuncle of ear canal
- pharyngitis
- acute and chronic mastoiditis
- bacterial laryngitis

2. Cephalosporins

These antibiotics are often used as alternatives to penicillin when an allergic reaction is anticipated. The cephalosporins are effective against a broad range of gram-positive and gram-negative organisms. Like the penicillins, the cephalosporins are considered bactericidal because they inhibit bacterial cell wall synthesis.

Common otolaryngologic indications are:

- acute and chronic sinusitis
- tonsilloadenoiditis
- pharyngitis
- acute otitis media
- acute mastoiditis
- meningitis
- malignant otitis externa

3. Carbapenems

This class of antibiotics is relatively new. Imipenem, a frequently used member of this class in otolaryngology, has the broadest spectrum of the beta-lactam antibiotics. It is effective against gram-positive and gram-negative aerobic and anaerobic bacteria. It is bactericidal even against bacteria which are resistant to the aminoglycosides and cephalosporins.

Common otolaryngologic indications are:

- acute and chronic mastoiditis
- pneumonia
- surgical infections
- skin infections
- osteomyelitis
- hospital (nosocomial) infections

4. Monobactams

Aztreonam is the first drug in this new class of beta-lactam antibiotics. Unlike most beta-lactams, aztreonam is ineffective against most gram-positive organisms. It is primarily active against aerobic gram-negative bacteria common in nosocomial infections. Like most beta-lactams, the monobactams interfere with bacterial cell wall synthesis. It is an effective alternative to the aminoglycosides with fewer side effects.

Common otolaryngologic indications are:

- acute and chronic mastoiditis
- malignant otitis externa
- acute sinusitis
- orbital cellulitis
- epiglottitis

C. Glycopeptides

Vancomycin is a glycopeptide antibiotic effective against gram-positive bacteria at minimal concentrations. At lower concentrations it is bacteriostatic, but becomes bactericidal at higher concentrations. Most gram-negative bacteria, mycobacteria, and fungi are resistant to this agent. It has very few side effects and is considered one of the safest antibiotics available. Ototoxicity and nephrotoxicity are among the side effects that require monitoring of serum levels during therapy.

Common otolaryngologic indications are:

- acute mastoiditis
- acute sinusitis
- orbital cellulitis
- parotitis
- serious CNS infections

D. Aminoglycosides

The aminoglycosides are bactericidal and bacteriostatic. They penetrate the bacterial cell wall and cytoplasmic membrane to inhibit protein synthesis on ribosomes, resulting in cell death. Unfortunately, the aminoglycosides are well known for being highly ototoxic and nephrotoxic. Gentamicin and tobramycin are the most nephrotoxic. Amikacin and gentamicin are the most cochleotoxic. Netilmicin is the least toxic to the kidneys, cochlea, and vestibular system. Despite the undesirable side effects, these agents are very important in the treatment of serious infections involving highly resistant bacteria. The aminoglycosides are often used in combination with other antibiotics (e.g., penicillin G, ampicillin, vancomycin, tetracycline) to increase the effectiveness of the therapy.

Common otolaryngologic indications are:

- tuberculosis
- the plague
- hepatic coma and prophylaxis
- meningitis
- acute and chronic mastoiditis
- necrotizing abcesses
- malignant otitis externa
- chronic suppurative otitis media
- acute diffuse otitis externa

E. Nitroimidazoles

This class of antibiotics is bactericidal. An important member of this class in otolaryngological applications is metronidazole. This agent is effective against gram-negative bacteria and many parasites which resist traditional antibiotic therapy.

Common otolaryngologic indications are:

- acute and chronic mastoiditis
- deep neck abcess
- chronic sinusitis
- infected cholesteatoma
- malignant otitis externa
- tonsillitis
- intracranial infections
- brain abcess

F. Rifampin

Rifampin is bactericidal against numerous gram-positive and gram-negative microbes. It is extremely important in the treatment of pulmonary tuberculosis and as a prophylactic agent in the prevention of meningitis in children and infants. It is also used in combination with aminoglycosides and cephalosporins to treat severe staphylococcal infections.

Common otolaryngologic indications are:

- tuberculosis
- malignant otitis externa
- nasopharyngeal and nasal infections

G. Macrolides

The most important member of the macrolide class of antibiotics in otolaryngology is erythromycin. Although it is similar in structure to some aminoglycosides, it does not belong to that class. It is considered bacteriostatic, inhibiting protein synthesis in the bacterial cell. Erythromycin is effective against most gram-positive bacteria and microbes causing diphtheria, tetanus, and pertussis. Most gram-negative bacteria are resistant. Erythromycin is often used to treat infections when beta-lactam antibiotics cannot be used because of allergy or resistance. Ototoxicity is a potential side effect.

Common otolaryngologic indications are:

- acute otitis media
- sinusitis
- pharyngitis
- bronchitis
- bacterial laryngitis
- tracheobronchitis
- surgical prophylaxis

H. Lincosamides

These antiobiotics are similar to the macrolides in structure and function. They are active against most gram-positive bacteria and most anaerobes. Gram-negative bacteria are generally resistant. Like the macrolides, the lincosamides are bacteriostatic, effective by inhibition of peptide chain synthesis in the bacteria cell.

Common otolaryngologic indications are:

- malignant otitis externa
- chronic sinusitis
- tonsilloadenoiditis
- chronic suppurative otitis media
- deep neck abcess
- parotitis

I. Tetracyclines

The tetracyclines are active against many gram-positive and gram-negative bacteria with notable exceptions. These agents are bacteriostatic; however, many strains are now resistant to treatment with these drugs. Numerous side effects have been reported including nephrotoxicity, hepatotoxicity, vestibular toxicity, and discoloration of teeth in children.

Common otolaryngologic indications are:

- acute and chronic sinusitis
- bacterial tracheobronchitis
- rhinoscleroma

J. Chloramphenicol

Chloramphenicol is a bacteriostatic antibiotic similar in activity to tetracycline. It is active against many gram-positive and gram-negative organisms. It is one of the most effective antibiotics in penetrating the blood-brain barrier and is well-distributed throughout the body. Its action appears to be primarily bacteriostatic. It can be ototoxic when given in high doses; therefore, serum blood monitoring is recommended.

Common otolaryngologic indications are:

- acute mastoiditis
- epiglottitis
- suppurative labyrinthitis
- topical otic and ophthalmic uses

K. Polymyxins

These agents are actually cationic detergents, exhibiting a bactericidal effect by disrupting the cell wall membrane complex. Systemic administration is rarely employed except in life-threatening infections caused by Pseudomonas aeruginosa. More often the polymyxins are used topically in the form of drops (e.g., otic drops).

Common otolaryngologic indications are:

- chronic suppurative otitis media
- acute diffuse otitis externa
- serious life-threatening infections

L. Quinolones

These antibiotics are extremely effective against most gram-postive and gram-negative bacteria, but are resisted by most anaerobes. Their action is bactericidal, inhibiting cell wall synthesis and maintenance. Ciprofloxacin is commonly used in otolaryngologic applications.

Common otolaryngologic indications are:

- malignant otitis externa
- chronic sinusitis

M. Antifungal Agents

A number of systemic infections are caused by fungi (e.g., aspergillus, mucor, candida), particularly in the lungs and mucosal membranes. These infections are typically difficult to eradicate.

Common otolaryngologic indications are:

- otomycosis (fungal infections of the external auditory canal and meatus)
- chronic sinusitis

Antiviral Agents

Viral infections are problematic in medicine. No "cures" are available. Antibiotic therapy is usually employed to prevent secondary bacterial infection. There are, however, agents that have some antiviral effects, particularly against herpes and influenza A.

Common otolaryngologic indications are:

- viral tracheobronchitis
- various herpes infections

II. ANTIHISTAMINES

Approximately 17% of the U.S. population suffer from allergic disease. An allergen is an antigen which causes an allergic reaction. An allergic reaction is an immune response with an undesirable effect on the patient. There are several types of allergic reactions which differ based on the precise immune response process involved. Although a few immunologic agents have been developed, most pharmacotherapy is limited to treatment of the symptoms. Antihistamines counteract the effect of histamines which are released by cells during an allergic reaction by occupying the histamine receptor site on effector cells. Histamine (H1) receptors mediate bronchial and gastrointestinal smooth muscle contraction, vasodilation, and stimulation of sensory nerve endings. Histamines are a powerful dilator of the capillaries and responsible for the discomfort experienced with most allergic reactions.

Sedation is the most common side effect associated with antihistamine use. Newly developed agents (e.g., astemizole, cetirizine, loratadine) are nonsedating, but expensive. Patients vary in their response to the therapeutic and adverse effects of the different classes of H1 antihistamines. Over-the-counter preparations are a good first choice. Changing to a different class of antihistamine may be necessary to avoid adverse side effects which limit usefulness. (See the table on page 822.)

Common otolaryngologic indications are:

- allergic reaction
- motion sickness
- post-operative nausea

III. DECONGESTANTS (VASOCONSTRICTORS)

Decongestants cause vasoconstriction in the mucosa, decreasing hyperemia, congestions, edema, and nasal congestion. Systemic decongestants are often combined with antihistamines to reduce symptoms and counteract the sedation often caused by antihistamines. The table on page 822 lists decongestants often used in otolaryngology.

Common otolaryngologic indications are:

- allergic reactions
- acute non-suppurative otitis media

IV. ANTICHOLINERGIC AGENTS

The anticholinergics are the most effective drugs for the prevention and treatment of motion sickness. Scopolamine is the most effective drug for motion sickness with fewer side effects than others in its class. All of these agents should be given prophylactically because they are much less effective after nausea or vomiting has developed. Classic side effects are: tachycardia, drowsiness, headache, gastrointestinal upset, nightmares, blurred vision, acute glaucoma, urinary retention, and xerostomia (dry mouth). Commonly used anticholinergics are listed on page 825.

Common indications are:

- motion sickness
- cardiac bradydysrhythmias

V. STEROIDS

Steroids are chemically similar to cholesterol and have a wide variety of therapeutic uses. In otolaryngology they are used primarily to reduce allergic hypersensitivity, reduce inflamation, and promote healing of the skin (e.g., rashes, scars, infections). There are many agents in use, each with a unique property. Commonly used steroids are listed on page 825 along with their indications.

Common otolaryngologic indications are:

- eczema
- sudden idiopathic hearing loss
- intranasal (allergic reactions)

VI. VASODILATORS

Vasodilators are used in the treatment of Ménière's disease to maintain normal endolymphatic pressure. The most frequently used vasodilators are listed on page 826.

VII. DIURETICS

Diuretics promote the secretion of urine. In otolaryngology, diuretics are sometimes used to maintain electrolyte water balance, as in the treatment of Ménière's disease. The loop diuretics are well-known for their ototoxic and vestibulotoxic properties, most of which are reversible. The most widely used loop diuretics are listed on page 826 along with their toxic properties.

VIII. ANTI-INFLAMMATORY

The most widely-used anti-inflammatory is aspirin. Its use in otolaryngology is varied, but it is listed here because of potential ototoxicity. In high doses, tinnitus and sensory neural hearing loss often appear. The effect is apparently reversible on cessation of aspirin use.

IX. ANTI-MALARIAL

The treatment of malaria is associated with the use of ototoxic agents. Quinine and chloroquine produce reversible and permanent tinnitus and sensory-neural hearing loss. These effects appear to be dose-dependent. Congenital hearing loss and cochlear hypoplasia have also been reported to be associated witht the use of quinine (see page 827).

X. CHEMOTHERAPEUTIC AGENTS

Chemotherapy is used primarily when surgery and/or irradiation is not possible or has failed. Chemotherapy is commonly administered by the oncologist, but the otolaryngologist and audiologist should be aware of the agents being used and their effect on the structures of the head and neck. The table beginning on page 828 lists the chemotherapeutic agents by class along with typical indications. Among these agents, Cisplatin, Methotrexate, and Bleomycin are thought to be the best single agents for the treatment of head and neck cancer. They are also ototoxic.

XI. NEUROLOGIC MEDICATIONS

A number of neurologic medications are used in otolaryngology. Indications are broad, but include: seizure prevention, muscle relaxation, vasoconstriction, and analgesia. The use of neurologic medications is often an important adjunct to other procedures (e.g., surgery). See Agents Used with Other Treatments (page 832).

XII. ANTIEMETIC AGENTS

Severe nausea and vomiting associated with anesthetic drugs may significantly threaten the result of surgical head and neck procedures. In the chemotherapeutic treatment of head and neck cancer, associated nausea and vomiting may defer completion of planned therapy. Modulation of this process is, therefore, extremely important. Several commonly used antiemetics are listed on page 832.

XIII. ANESTHETICS, ANALGESICS, AND AGENTS USED IN SURGERY

A. Short-acting Agents

The short-acting agents listed on page 834 are frequently used in outpatient or same-day surgery when a local or general anesthetic regimen is not appropriate for the procedure required. Most of these agents are analgesic or function as a neuromuscular blocker to permit completion of the procedure.

B. Local Anesthetics

Local anesthesia is the blockage of sensation in a circumscribed area. These anesthetics impede nerve conduction by interfering with ionic exchange and inhibiting action potentials. Most clinically-useful local anesthetics have the following properties:

- reversible nerve block
- onset and duration of blockage is predictable

- the drug is not irritating to the tissue
- the drug is permeable and diffusable
- the drug is highly therapeutic
- the drug is water soluble and chemically stable

A number of local anesthetics are listed on pages 834–835 along with common indications for their use.

C. Premedication

Preparation for surgical and anesthetic procedures often requires the use of medication. The patient must be in a state conducive to the procedure to maximize effectiveness and efficiency. Thus, the premedication regimen is selected individually to meet the needs of the patient and the subsequent procedure. Premedication is selected with the following goals in mind:

- relief of anxiety
- relief of pain
- provision of amnesia
- reduction of salivary and gastric secretions
- avoidance of noxious cardiovascular reflexes

Tranquilizers, barbiturates, narcotics, and anticholinergics are among the medications frequently employed to prepare the patient for anesthesia and surgery. These are listed on pages 836–837 along with common indications.

D. Supplemental Intravenous Sedation

Intravenous sedation is used to premedicate and supplement general anesthesia. Some of these agents are also used to induce anesthesia. Appropriate sedation is selected with the following goals in mind:

- calm, drowsy patient who is easily aroused by spoken commands
- antiemesis
- some degree of amnesia
- avoidance of cardiovascular and respiratory depression

Many of the same agents used to premedicate are also used to sedate the patient before induction of general anesthesia. These agents are listed on pages 839–840.

E. General Anesthesia

General anesthesia is defined as a chemically induced reversible loss of consciousness. Most of these agents block multisynaptic pathways, such as the reticular activating system in the brain. General anesthetics act on almost every cell affecting all organs and systems in the body. The most commonly used general anesthetics (inhalation and intravenous) and neuromuscular blockers are listed on pages 841–842.

F. Postoperative Analgesia

Postoperative pain management is accomplished through the use of a number of agents that have analgesic and/or anti-inflammatory properties. Many of these medications are administered under patient control. See page 843 for a list of these drugs and their indications.

Common otolaryngologic indications:

- chronic sinusitis

Source: Courtesy of Troy A. Hackett, Ph.D.

Common Microbes (Pathogenic Organisms) Responsible for Infectious Diseases

Code	Genus and Species	Gram Test	Associated Diseases
1	Streptococcus pneumoniae (pneumococcus)	positive	pneumonia
2	Streptococcus pyogenes	positive	respiratory disease, impetigo, scarlet fever, rheumatic feve"
3	Streptococcus agalactiae	positive	meningitis and pneumonia in newborns
4	Streptococci Group D (enterococci)	positive	endocarditis, urinary tract infection
5	Staphylococcus aureus	positive	epidermal skin diseases, dermatitis
6	Myobacterium tuberculosis	positive	tuberculosis
7	Haemophilus influenzae	negative	meningitis, otitis media, bronchitis, pneumonia, arthritis
8	Neisseria meningitidis (meningococcus)	negative	meningitis, upper respiratory infection
9	Neisseria gonorrhoeae (gonoccus)	negative	gonorrhea
10	Vibrio cholerae	negative	cholera
11	Escherichia coli	negative	diarrhea
12	Pseudomonas aeruginosa	negative	cystic fibrosis, serious infections, burn infections
13	Bacteroides fragilis	negative	various suppurative processes
14	Proteus	negative	numerous suppurative processes, cystitis
15	Krebsiella	negative	pneumonia, rhinoscleroma, rhinitis

Source: Courtesy of Troy A. Hackett, Ph.D.

Antibiotic (Antimicrobial) Therapy

Antibiotic Agent (See Table of Microbes on page 812)				
Generic Name *(trade name)*	**Effective Against**	**Ineffective Against**	**Indications (Infections)**	**Otologic/CNS Side Effects**
A. SULFONAMIDES				
sulfisoxazole *(gantrisin)*	G+, G-, 7, 11, 14, 15	1, 2, 3, 4	meningitis acute otitis media	tinnitus, vertigo
sulfamethoxazole *(gantanol)*	G+, G-, 7, 11, 14, 15	1, 2, 3, 4	otitis media prophylaxis	tinnitus, vertigo
sulfacetamide *(blephamide)*	G+, G-, 5, 7, 11, 15	8, 9, fungi	ophthalmic conjunctivitis	
mafenide acetate *(sulfamylon cream)*	G+, G-, 12	fungi	burns (prophylaxis)	
silver sulfadiazine *(SSD cream)*	G+, G-, 11, 12, 14, 15	clostridium	infected burns	CNS reactions
trimethoprim-sulfamethoxazole *(bactrim-DS, septra-DS)*	G+, G-, 1, 7, 11, 14, 15	12, 13	bronchitis, acute otitis media acute sinusitis, urinary tract	tinnitus, vertigo
B. BETA-LACTAMS				
1. Penicillins				
Generation 1				
penicillin G *(pfizerpen, bicillin)*	G+, 9, 11, 15	G-, 5	furuncle of ear canal pharyngitis, tonsilloadenoiditis	confusion, vertigo
penicillin V *(pen vee K)*	G+, 9, 11, 15	G-, 5	furuncle of ear canal pharyngitis, tonsilloadenoiditis	

(continued)

Antibiotic Agent (See Table of Microbes on page 812)				
Generic Name ***(trade name)***	**Effective Against**	**Ineffective Against**	**Indications (Infections)**	**Otologic/CNS Side Effects**
nafcillin *(unipen, nafcil)*	G+, 1, 2	5	acute/chronic mastoiditis from acute/chronic otitis media subglottic bacterial croup	
dicloxacillin *(dynapen, pathocil)*	G+, 1, 2	5	chronic sinusitis, tonsillitis	
Generation 2				
ampicillin *(omnipen, unasyn)*	G+, G-, 1, 2, 7, 11, 14, 15	5	acute otitis media, acute sinusitis, prophylaxis	facial swelling
amoxicillin *(amoxil)*	G+, G-, 1, 2, 7, 11, 14	5, clostridia	acute otitis media, acute sinusitis	dizziness
amoxicillin with clavulanic *(augmentin)*	G+, G-, 5, 7, 11, 15	clostridia	acute otitis media acute sinusitis bacterial laryngitis	dizziness, confusion, CNS depression
bacampicillin *(spectrobid)*	G+, G-, 7, 11, 14	12	chronic bronchitis, upper/lower respiratory infection	
Generation 3				
ticarcillin *(timentin, ticar)*	most G+, G-, 12	5	acute or chronic mastoiditis acute or chronic respiratory malignant otitis externa	
carbenicillin *(pyopen, geopen)*	G+, G-, 12	some 12, 15	urinary tract	

Antibiotic Agent (See Table of Microbes on page 812)				
Generic Name *(trade name)*	**Effective Against**	**Ineffective Against**	**Indications (Infections)**	**Otologic/CNS Side Effects**
Generation 4				
mezlocillin *(mezlin)*	G+, G-, 7, 11, 12, 13, 14, 15	5	lower respiratory, serious infections	
azlocillin	G+, G-, 7, 12	5	malignant otitis externa	
piperacillin *(pipracil)*	G+, G-, 7, 12, 13, 14, 15	5	lower respiratory, cystic fibrosis, bone, prophylaxis	
2. CEPHALOSPORINS				
Generation 1				
cephalexin *(keflex)*	G+, 1, 5, 7, 11, 14, 15	12, 13	otitis media, chronic sinusitis tonsilloadenoiditis, pharyngitis	confusion, dizziness
cefadroxil (*duricef, ultracef)*	G+, 1, 5, 11, 14, 15	12, 13	chronic sinusitis, tonsillo adenoiditis pharyngitis	
cefazolin *(ancef, kefzol)*	G+, 1, 5, 11, 14, 15	12, 13	subglottic bacterial croup pharyngeal, surgical prophylaxis	
Generation 2				
cefoxitin *(mefoxin)*	G+, G-, 7, 9, 11, 13, 14, 15	12, 13	acute sinusitis, croup epiglottitis, suppurative parotitis	
cefaclor *(ceclor)*	G+, G-, 7, 9, 15	12, 13	acute otitis media, acute sinusitis, croup, epiglottitis, bacterial laryngitis	confusion
cefamandole *(mandol)*	G+, G-, 5, 7, 9, 11, 14, 15	12, 13	acute sinusitis, croup, epiglottitis lower respiratory	
cefonicid *(monocid)*	G+, G-, 5, 7, 11, 14, 15	12, 13	acute sinusitis, croup, epiglottitis lower respiratory	
cefuroxime *(ceftin, zinacef)*	G+, G-, 5, 7, 13, 14, 15	12, 13	acute otitis media, acute sinusitis croup, epiglottitis bacterial laryngitis pharyngitis, tonsillitis	

(continued)

Antibiotic Agent (See Table of Microbes on page 812)				
Generic Name *(trade name)*	**Effective Against**	**Ineffective Against**	**Indications (Infections)**	**Otologic/CNS Side Effects**
Generation 3				
cefotaxime *(claforan)*	G+, G-, 5, 7, 11, 12 12, 13, 14, 15	some 12 and 13	lower respiratory, meningitis, ventriculitis	
cefixime *(suprax)*	G+, G-, 7, 9, 14, 15	12, 13	acute otitis media	
cefoperazone	G+, G-, 5, 7, 9, 12, 13, 14, 15		respiratory tract, septicemia (cefobid)	
ceftriaxone *(rocephin)*	G+, G-, 5, 7, 9, 12 13, 14, 15		acute mastoiditis, meningitis, sinusitis, orbital cellulitis (good CSF penetration)	
Generation 4				
ceftazidime *(ceptaz, fortaz, pentacef, tazicef)*	G+, G-, 5, 7 , 12, 14, 15	13	malignant otitis externa	dizziness
3. CARBAPENEMS				
imipenem *(primaxin)*	most G+ and G-		acute or chronic mastoiditis, pneumonia, osteomyelitis , surgical, nocosomial infections, skin, urinary tract	confusion, dizziness, facial edema, vasodilation, reversible hearing loss tinnitus
4. MONOBACTAMS				
aztreonam *(azactam)*	G-, 7, 11, 12, 14, 15	G+	acute/chronic mastoiditis, malignant otitis externa, epiglottitis, acute sinusitis, orbital cellulitis	confusion, disorientation, tinnitus

Antibiotic Agent (See Table of Microbes on page 812)				
Generic Name ***(trade name)***	**Effective Against**	**Ineffective Against**	**Indications (Infections)**	**Otologic/CNS Side Effects**
C. GLYCOPEPTIDES				
vancomycin (vancocin)	most G+	most G-	acute mastoiditis, acute sinusitis, orbital cellulitis, parotitis	dizziness, hearing loss, ototoxicity, tinnitus, vertigo
D. AMINOGLYCOSIDES				
streptomycin	G-, 12, 14, 15	G+ and anaerobes	tuberculosis, tularemia, plague, brucellosis	hearing loss, vertigo, ototoxicity, tinnitus
kanamycin	G-, 12, 14, 15	G+ and anaerobes	tuberculosis, hepatic coma, prophylaxis	
amikacin (amikin)	G-, 12, 14, 15	G+ and anaerobes	meningitis, respiratory, burns	deafness, hearing loss, ototoxicity
gentamicin (garamycin)	G-, 5, 12, 14, 15	G+ and anaerobes	meningitis, acute/chronic mastoiditis, necrotizing abcess, malignant otitis externa, chronic suppurative otitis media	confusion hearing loss ototoxicity, neurotoxicity encephalopathy, tinnitus, vertigo

(continued)

Antibiotic Agent (See Table of Microbes on page 812)				
Generic Name ***(trade name)***	**Effective Against**	**Ineffective Against**	**Indications (Infections)**	**Otologic/CNS Side Effects**
tobramycin *(nebcin)*	G-, 11, 12, 14, 15	G+ and anaerobes	meningitis, lower respiratory, urinary	confusion, disorientation, dizziness, hearing loss, facial numbness, neurotoxicity, ototoxicity, tinnitus, vertigo
netilmicin *(netromycin)*	G-, 12	G+ and anaerobes	gentamicin-resistant strains	cochlear lesion, disorientation, dizziness, encephalopathy, hearing loss, Ménière's disease, nystagmus, ototoxicity, tinnitus, vertigo
neomycin *(colymycin s otic, neosporin)*	most G-, 11, 12, 15	G+ and anaerobes	chronic suppurative otitis media, acute diffuse otitis externa, hepatic coma, prophylaxis	ototoxicity, vertigo

Antibiotic Agent (See Table of Microbes on page 812)				
Generic Name ***(trade name)***	**Effective Against**	**Ineffective Against**	**Indications (Infections)**	**Otologic/CNS Side Effects**
E. NITROIMIDAZOLES				
metronidazole *(flagyl)*	anaerobes, 13	1, 2, 5	acute/chronic mastoiditis, neck abcess, chronic sinusitis infected cholesteatoma, malignant otitis externa, tonsillitis, intracranial infections, brain abcess	confusion, vertigo
F. RIFAMPIN				
(rifampin)	1, 2, 5, 7, 8, 9		malignant otitis externa, tuberculosis, prophylaxis infections	confusion, dizziness, facial edema, impaired mental performance
G. MACROLIDES				
erythromycin *(erythrocin,EES-400, robimycin, E-mycin)*	G+, 7, diphtheria, tetanus, pertussis	most G	surgical prophylaxis, acute otitis media, sinusitis pharyngitis, tracheobronchitis, bronchitis, bacterial laryngitis,	confusion, reversible hearing loss, vertigo
H. LINCOSAMIDES				
lincomycin *(lincocin)*	G+, 13	G-, 7, 8, 9	serious infections	tinnitus, vertigo
clindamycin *(cleocin)*	G+, 1, 2, 5, 13	clostridia	malignant otitis externa, chronic sinusitis, tonsilloadenoiditis, chronic suppurative otitis media, deep neck abcess, parotitis	

(continued)

Antibiotic Agent (See Table of Microbes on page 812)				
Generic Name *(trade name)*	**Effective Against**	**Ineffective Against**	**Indications (Infections)**	**Otologic/CNS Side Effects**
I. TETRACYCLINES				
tetracycline *(achromycin, robitet, terramycin, tetrex)*	G+, G-	1, 2, 11, 12, 13, 15	bacterial tracheobronchitis, rhinoscleroma	
doxycycline *(vibramycin, vibra-tabs)*	G+, G-, 7, 9	1, 2, 11, 12, 13, 15	acute/chronic sinusitis	
J. CHLORAMPHENICOL				
chloramphenicol *(chloromycetin)*	G+, G-, 7, 8, 12		acute mastoiditis, epiglottitis, topical otic and ophthalmic	confusion
K. POLYMYXINS				
(cortisporin otic)	5, 7, 8, 9, 11, 12, 15	1	chronic suppurative otitis media, acute diffuse otitis externa, life-threatening infections	ototoxicity
L. QUINOLONES				
ciprofloxacin *(cipro)*	most G+ and G-	anaerobes	malignant otitis externa, chronic sinusitis	confusion, facial edema, CNS stimulation, hearing loss, nystagmus, tinnitus
M. ANTIFUNGAL				
amphotericin B *(fungizone)*	aspergillosis mucormycosis	P. boydii fusarium	life-threatening fungal infections (e.g., pulmonary)	hearing loss, tinnitus, vertigo
nystatin *(mycostatin)*	candidia	bacteria	otomycosis	

Antibiotic Agent (See Table of Microbes on page 812)				
Generic Name ***(trade name)***	**Effective Against**	**Ineffective Against**	**Indications (Infections)**	**Otologic/CNS Side Effects**
clotrimazole *(lotrimin)*	candidia trichophyton	C. guilliermondi	otomycosis, dermal	
ketoconazole *(nizoral)*	candidiasis H. Capsulatum		chronic sinusitis	dizziness, vertigo
N. ANTIVIRAL				
acyclovir *(zovirax)*	herpes 1 and 2 cytomegalovirus		herpes zoster, varicella	confusion, dizziness, encephalopathy
amantadine *(symmetrel)*	influenza A		viral tracheobronchitis, Parkinson's disease	confusion, dizziness, impaired mental performance

Source: Courtesy of Troy A. Hackett, Ph.D.

Nonantimicrobial Therapeutic Agents

Therapeutic Agent	Comments	Side Effects
I. Antihistamines		
ALKYLAMINES		
brompheniramine *(dimetane, bromfed)*	short-acting, prounced anticholinergic, stimulation	
chlorpheniramine *(chlor-trimeton, tylenol cold)*	short-acting, prounced anticholinergic, mild sedation	
ETHANOLAMINES		
diphenhydramine *(benadryl)*	motion sickness, pronounced sedation	confusion, disorientation, acute labyrinthitis hysteria, tinnitus, vertigo
dimenhydrinate *(dramamine)*	motion sickness, pronounced sedation	
clemastine *(tavist)*	pronounced sedation	confusion, dizziness, labyrinthitis, tinnitus, vertigo
ETHYLENEDIAMINES		
pyrilamine *(ru-tuss, triaminic)*	mild sedation	confusion, CNS depression, CNS reactions, CNS stimulation, dizziness, labyrinthitis, tinnitus, vertigo
pyribenzamine		
tripelennamine *(PBZ)*	pronounced sedation	confusion, dizziness, impaired mental performance, tinnitus, vertigo
PHENOTHIAZINES		
prochlorperazine *(compazine)*	post-operative nausea	CNS reactions, cerebral edema, rhythmical involuntary facial movements, mental clouding, impaired mental performance

Therapeutic Agent	Comments	Side Effects
prochlorperazine *(compazine)*	post-operative nausea	CNS reactions, cerebral edema, rhythmical involuntary facial movements, mental clouding, impaired mental performance
promethazine *(phenergan)*	controls motion sickness, post-op nausea sedation	circulatory depression, confusion, CNS depression, disorientation, dizziness, impaired mental performance, tinnitus
PIPERAZINES		
meclizine *(antivert, bonine)*	controls vertigo, motion sickness and symptoms	
PIPERIDINES		
azatadine *(optimine, trinalin)*	eustachian tube congestion; long acting	confusion, CNS depression, dizziness, labyrinthitis, tinnitus, vertigo
BUTYROPHENONES *(seldane)*	terfenadine, nonsedating, long-acting	confusion, CNS depression, disorientation, dizziness
TRICYCLICS		
astemizole *(hismanal)*	nonsedating, long-acting	
cetirizine *(zytec)*	nonsedating, long-acting	
loratadine *(claritin)*	nonsedating, long-acting	
ketotifen *(zaditen)*	long-acting	
OTHER		
cyproheptadine *(periactin)*		confusion, dizziness, labyrinthitis, tinnitus, vertigo

(continued)

Therapeutic Agent	Comments	Side Effects
II. Decongestants (vasoconstrictors)		
epinephrine (*epi-pen, sus-phrine*)	decreases uptake of local anesthetic prolonging effect	
ephedrine (*quadrinal, broncholate, mudrane*)	systemic/topical decongestant	circulatory failure, confusion, dizziness
pseudoephedrine (*sudafed*)	systemic decongestant	
phenylpropanolamine (*entex*)	systemic decongestant	
cocaine	topical application	CNS stimulation, vasoconstriction
oxymetazoline (*afrin*)	topical application, decongestant	
phenylephrine (*neo-synephrine*)	topical application	
propylhexedrine (*benzedrex*)	topical application	
naphazoline (*privine*)	topical application	
tetrahydrozoline (*tyzine*)	topical application	
xylometazoline (*otrivin*)	topical application	
Combined Antihistamine-Decongestant		
azatidine-pseudoephedrine (*trinalin*)	eustachian tube congestion	confusion, CNS depression, dizziness, labyrinthitis, tinnitus, vertigo

Therapeutic Agent	Comments	Side Effects
clemastine-phenypropanolamine *(tavist-D)*	allergic rhinitis	confusion, dizziness, labyrinthitis, tinnitus, circulatory collapse
dexbrompheniramine-isoephedrine *(drixoral)*		
brompheniramine-phenylephrine *(dimetapp)*		
III. Anticholinergic		
atropine *(lomotil, donnatal)*	motion sickness, cardiac bradydysrhythmias	confusion, dizziness
scopolamine *(hyoscine)*	the most effective drug for motion sickness	
glycopyrrolate *(robinul)*	prophylactic motion sickness	confusion, dizziness
IV. Steroids		
hydrocortisone *(solucortef, cortef)*	systemic, herpes simplex, eczema (topical)	vertigo
prednisone *(deltasone)*	sudden idiopathic hearing loss; systemic	vertigo
prednisolone *(delta-cortef)*	systemic	vertigo
triamcinolone *(kenalog, remiderm, nasacort)*	systemic, eczema, topical intranasal	psychiatric disturbances, vertigo
dexamethasone *(decadron, turbinaire)*	intranasal, systemic	nystagmus, psychiatric disturbances, vertigo
methylprednisolone *(medrol, solumedrol)*	systemic	vertigo

(continued)

Therapeutic Agent	Comments	Side Effects
beclomethasone *(vancenase, beconase)*	intranasal	rhinorrhea
betamethasone *(celestone)*	systemic	vertigo
flunisolide *(nasalide)*	intranasal	
budesonide *(rhinocort)*	intranasal	
fluocortin *(rhinolar)*	intranasal	
fluticasone *(flixonase)*	intranasal	
V. Vasodilators		
betahistine hydrochloride	Ménière's disease	
nicotinic acid *(niacor, slo-niacin)*	Ménière's disease	
lipoflavanoid capsules	Ménière's disease	
VII. Diuretics		
ethacrynic acid	loop diuretic, ototoxic, vestibulotoxic	
furosemide *(lasix)*	loop diuretic, ototoxic and vestibulotoxic (reversible?) Ménière's disease (electrolyte water balance)	dizziness, impaired hearing, tinnitus, vertigo
bumetanide *(bumex)*	loop diuretic, mild ototoxicity	disorientation, ear discomfort, encephalopathy, hearing loss, ototoxicity, vertigo
VIII. Anti-Inflammatory		
acetylsalicylic acid *(aspirin)*	reversible tinnitus	high-frequency sensorineural hearing loss in high doses

Therapeutic Agent	Comments	Side Effects
IX. Anti-Malarial		
quinine *(quinamm)*	reversible and permanent tinnitus and hearing loss in high doses; congenital hearing loss; cochlear hypoplasia	confusion, facial edema, tinnitus, vertigo
chloroquine *(aralen)*	reversible and permanent tinnitus and hearing loss in high doses; congenital hearing loss; cochlear hypoplasia	auditory disturbances, impaired hearing, psychiatric disturbances, tinnitus

Chemotherapeutic Agents

Therapeutic Agent	Comments	Side Effects
ALKYLATING AGENTS		
cisplatin *(platinol)*	head and neck, ovary, testicle, lung	hearing loss, facial edema, neurotoxicity, ototoxicity, tinnitus
carboplatin *(paraplatin)*	ovary , testicle, lung	CNS reactions, neurotoxicity, ototoxicity
mechlorethamine *(nitrogen mustard, Mustargen)*	lymphoma, lung cancer	hearing impairment, tinnitus, vertigo
chlorambucil *(leukeran)*	lymphoma, leukemia	confusion
cyclophosphamide *(cytoxan, endoxan neosar)*	lymphoma, breast, myeloma, lung	
ifosfamide *(ifex)*	lymphoma, lung sarcoma	confusion, disorientation
melphalan *(alkeran, L-PAM)*	myeloma, ovary	
triethylene thiophosphoramide *(thiopeta)*	ovary, bladder	
busulfan *(myleran)*	leukemia	
dacarbazine *(DTIC-dome)*	melanoma, sarcoma	
estramustine *(estracyt)*	prostate	
dibromodulcitol *(mitolactol)*	breast, leukemia	

Therapeutic Agent	Comments	Side Effects
NITROSOUREAS		
camustine *(BiCNU, BCNU)*	brain, lymphoma, myelo	
lomustine *(CeeNU, CCNU)*	brain, lymphoma, lung	disorientation
semustine *(methyl-CCNU)*	gastrointestinal (experimental)	
streptozocin *(zanosar, streptozotocin)*	carcinoid, pancreas	
ANTIMETABOLITES		
5-azacitidine	leukemia (experimental)	
cytarabine *(Cytosar-U, Ara-C)*	leukemia, lymphoma	CNS toxicity, neurotoxicity
5-fluorouracil *(adrucil)*	gastrointestinal, breast	ototoxicity, CNS toxicity, ataxia
floxuridine *(FUDR)*	colon	confusion, disorientation, nystagmus, CNS toxicity
hexamethylmelamine	ovary,neurological toxicity	
fludarabine *(fludara)*	leukemia,neurological toxicity	
6-mercaptopurine *(purinethol)*	acute & chronic leukemia	
6-thioguanine	leukemia, (tabloid)	
methotrexate** *(folex, MTX)*	head & neck, breast, leukemia osteosarcoma, trimetrexate, head & neck, lung, breast (experimental)	ototoxicity

(continued)

Therapeutic Agent	Comments	Side Effects
triazinate *(Baker's antifol)*	breast, colon (experimental)	
2-deoxycoformycin *(pentostatin)*	hairy cell leukemia, chronic lymphocytic leukemia (experimental)	
hydroxyurea *(hydrea)*	leukemia	disorientation
MITOTIC INHIBITORS		
vinblastine *(velban)*	lymphoma, testicular, breast	
vincristine *(oncovin)*	lung, sarcoma, lymphoma, leukemia	neurotoxicity
vindesine *(eldisine)*	lung, lymphoma, breast (experimental)	
teniposide *(VM-26)*	lymphoma, leukemia (experimental)	
etoposide *(vepesid, VP 16-213)*	lung, lymphoma, leukemia	
ANTITUMOR ANTIBIOTICS		
dactinomycin *(cosmegen, actinomycin D)*	Wilms' tumor, sarcoma	
mitomycin *(mutamycin)*	gastrointestinal, breast, bladder	confusion
plicamycin *(mithracin, mithramycin)*	testicular, hypercalcemia	
daunorubicin *(cerubidine, daunomycin)*	leukemia	

Therapeutic Agent	Comments	Side Effects
doxorubicin *(adriamycin)*	lymphoma, gastrointestinal, sarcom	
breast	leukemia	
bleomycin** *(blenoxane)*	head & neck, lymphoma, testicular	confusion, ototoxicity
ANTINEOPLASTIC		
mitotane *(lysodren)*	adrenal cortical	CNS depression, dizziness, vertigo
levamisole *(ergamisol)*	colon	
procarbazine *(matulane)*	lymphoma	confusion, dizziness, hearing loss, nystagmus, slurred speech
L-asparaginase *(elspar)*	leukemia	confusion
mitoxantrone *(novantrone)*	acute leukemia, breast	CNS reactions

** Best single agents for head and neck cancer
Source: Courtesy of Troy A. Hackett, Ph.D.

Agents Used With Other Treatments

Therapeutic Agent	Comments and Indications	Side Effects
Neurologic		
diphenylhydantoin *(dilantin)*	antiseizure	confusion, CNS depression, coarsening facial features, nystagmus, slurred speech
carisoprodol *(soma)*	muscle relaxant	confusion, disorientation, dizziness, rhinitis, tinnitus, vertigo
ergotamine *(sansert)*	cerebral vasoconstrictor for migraine	
carbamazepine *(tegretol)*	trigeminal neuralgia	symptoms of cerebral artery insufficiency, confusion, dizziness, hyperacusis, nystagmus, speech disturbances, tinnitus
Antiemetic		
metaclopramide *(reglan)*	dopamine and 5-HT3 antagonist	confusion, dizziness, rhythmical involuntary movements of face
prochlorperazine *(compazine)*	dopamine antagonist	CNS reactions, cerebral edema, rhythmical involuntary movements of face, mental clouding, impaired mental performance
promethazine *(phenergan)*	dopamine antagonist	circulatory depression, confusion, CNS depression, disoriention, dizziness
diphenhydramine *(benadryl)*	H1 antihistamine	confusion, disorientation, tinnitus, vertigo
scopolamine *(atrohist, donnatol)*	muscarinic anticholinergic	CNS depression, disorientation

Therapeutic Agent	Comments and Indications	Side Effects
Antiseptic		
chlorohexidine *(betasept, hibiclens)*	pre-op skin preparation; ototoxic	deafness, ototoxicity
povidone-iodine	pre-op skin preparation; ototoxic	ototoxicity
ethyl alcohol	pre-op skin preparation; ototoxic	ototoxicity
Miscellaneous		
cromolyn sodium *(intal, gastrocrom)*	symptoms of allergic rhinitis, mast cell stabilize	vertigo
iodinated glycerol *(organidin)*	mucolytic expectorant	
hyaluronidase *(widase)*	enhances anesthetic absorption	
nicotine polyacrilex gum *(nicorette)*	cigarette withdrawal	confusion, dizziness, tinnitus

Source: Courtesy of Troy A. Hackett, Ph.D.

Short-acting and Local Anesthetics and Analgesics

Therapeutic Agent	Comments	Side Effects
SHORT-ACTING AGENTS		
midazolam *(versed)*	benzodiazepine	confusion, CNS depression, dizziness, ear discomfort, blocked ears, nystagmus, slurred speech
trazolam	benzodiazepine	confusion, paradoxic CNS stimulation, disorientation, memory impairment, mental clouding, slurred speech, tinnitus
fentanyl *(sublimaze, duragesic)*	analgesia; induction of anesthesia	confusion, speech disturbances, vertigo
vecuronium *(norcuron)*		
atracurium *(tracrium)*	neuromuscular blocker	
pancuronium *(pavulon)*	neuromuscular blocker	
botulinum-A toxin *(oculinum)*	cholinergic neuromuscular blocker hemifacial spasm	disorientation
LOCAL ANESTHETICS		
Esters		
cocaine	topical local	CNS stimulation, vasoconstriction
procaine hydrochloride *(novocaine)*	short-acting local	dizziness, vasodilation
tetracaine hydrochloride *(pontocaine)*	long-acting local	CNS reactions, CNS stimulation, dizziness, tinnitus

Therapeutic Agent	Comments	Side Effects
chloroprocaine *(nesacaine)*	short-acting local	dizziness, tinnitus
hexylcaine *(cyclaine)*		
benzocaine *(americaine, hurricaine)*	short-acting topical local	
piperocaine *(metycaine)*		
Amides		
lidocaine hydrochloride *(xylocaine)*	intermiediate-acting regional	confusion, CNS depression, paradoxic CNS stimulation, dizziness
mepivacaine hydrochloride *(carbocaine)*	intermediate-acting regional	CNS depression, CNS stimulation, facial swelling, sensory disturbances
prilocaine hydrochloride *(citanest)*		
bupivacaine *(marcaine)*	long-acting regional	CNS toxicity, dizziness, facial swelling, incoherent speech, tinnitus, vasodilation
dibucaine hydrochloride *(nupercaine)*		
etidocaine *(duranest)*	long-acting regional	confusion, tinnitus
Piperidines		
dyclonine hydrochloride *(dyclone)*		confusion, tinnitus

Source: Courtesy of Troy A. Hackett, Ph.D.

Premedications (Pre-operative and Pre-anesthesia)

Therapeutic Agent	Comments	Side Effects
Tranquilizers		
chlorpromazine *(thorazine)*	phenothiazine: sedative, antiemetic,* antihistaminic	dizziness, cerebral edema, facial movements
prochlorperazine *(compazine)*	phenothiazine: sedative, antiemetic, antihistaminic	CNS reactions, cerebral edema, mental clouding, rhythmical involuntary movements, impaired mental performance
promethazine theoclate *(avomine)*	phenothiazine: sedative, antiemetic, antihistaminic Ménière's disease	
promethazine hydrochloride *(phenergan)*	phenothiazine: sedative, antiemetic, antihistaminic Ménière's disease	circulatory depression, confusion, tinnitus, CNS depression, disorientation, dizziness, impaired mental performance
diazepam *(valium)*	benzodiazepine: reduces anxiety, seizures Ménière's disease	confusion, nystagmus, slurred speech, vertigo
chlordiazepoxide *(librium)*	benzodiazepine: reduces anxiety, seizures	confusion, paradoxical CNS stimulation
lorazepam *(ativan)*	benzodiazepine: reduces anxiety, seizures	confusion, CNS depression, diorientation, dizziness, decreased hearing, impaired mental performance
midazolam *(versed)*	benzodiazepine: reduces anxiety, seizures	confusion, neonatal CNS depression, dizziness, ear discomfort, blocked ears, nystagmus, slurred speech
hydroxyzine *(atarax, marax)*	antihistamine: enhances narcotic effects	CNS reactions, vertigo

Therapeutic Agent	Comments	Side Effects
droperidol *(inapsine, innovar)*	antiemetic and sedative properties	
haloperidol *(haldol)*	antiemetic and sedative properties	confusion, vertigo
Barbiturates		
pentobarbital *(nembutal)*	cortical depressant	confusion, CNS depression, dizziness, vertigo
secobarbital *(seconal)*		confusion, CNS depression, dizziness, vertigo
Narcotics		
morphine sulfate *(MSIR, roxanol, oramorph, MS contin)*	pre-operative or ICU analgesia	circulatory depression, confusion, disorientation, dizziness, nystagmus
meperedine *(demerol)*	pre-operative analgesia	circulatory depression, disorientation, impaired mental performance
fentanyl *(sublimaze, duragesic)*	pre-operative analgesia, induction	confusion, speech disturbances, vertigo
Anticholinergics	used to dry secretions of upper airway	
atropine *(arco-lase, atrohist, donnatal, lomotil, motofen, ru–tuss, urised)*	antimuscarinic	confusion, CNS depression, disorientation, dizziness, labyrinthitis, tinnitus
scopolamine *(atrohist, donnatal, rut–uss)*	antimuscarinic	confusion, CNS depression, vertigo, disorientation, dizziness, labyrinthitis, tinnitus
glycopyrrolate *(robinul)*	antimuscarinic	confusion, dizziness

(continued)

Therapeutic Agent	Comments	Side Effects
Hemodynamic Support		
dobutamine hydrochloride *(dobutrex)*	tachycardia, dysrhythmias	
dopamine hydrochloride *(intropin)*	dysrhythmias	
ephedrine sulfate *(marax, pazo)*	dysrhythmias	CNS reactions, vertigo
epinephrine *(epipen, sus-phrine)*	dysrhythmias	
amrinone lactate *(inocor)*		
norepinephrine bitartrate *(levophed bitartrate)*	renal protection	
phenylephrine hydrochloride *(atrohist, deconsal, phenergan, ru-tuss)*		circulatory depression, confusion, CNS depression, disorientation, dizziness, labyrinthitis, impaired mental performance, tinnitus, vertigo
Antacids	increase gastric pH above 2.5	
cimetidine *(tagamet)*		confusion, disorientation
rantidine *(zantac)*		confusion, dizziness, vertigo
Other		
chloral hydrate *(aquachloral)*	hypnotic; conscious sedative; when barbiturates are contraindicated	
metoclopramide *(reglan)*	dopamine antagonist: used to hasten gastric emptying	confusion, dizziness, rhythmical involuntary facial movements

* antiemetic = a drug that will reduce or prevent vomiting

Supplemental Intravenous Sedation

Therapeutic Agent	Side Effects
Benzodiazepines	
diazepam *(valium)*	confusion, nystagmus, slurred speech, vertigo
midazolam *(versed)*	confusion, neonatal CNS depression, dizziness, ear discomfort, blocked ears, nystagmus, slurred speech
lorazepam *(ativan)*	
Narcotics	
fentanyl *(sublimaze, duragesic)*	confusion, speech disturbances, vertigo
sufentanil *(sufenta)*	
alfentanil *(alfenta)*	dizziness
innovar (droperidol + fentanyl)	confusion, speech disturbances, vertigo
Barbiturates	
sodium thiopental *(pentothal)*	
pentobarbital *(nembutal)*	confusion, CNS depression, dizziness, vertigo
secobarbital *(seconal)*	confusion, CNS depression, dizziness, vertigo
methohexital *(brevital)*	circulatory depression, rhinitis, vascular collapse

(continued)

Therapeutic Agent	Side Effects
Butyrophenones	
droperidol *(inapsine)*	
Induction Agents	
propofol *(diprivan)*	confusion, ear pain, tinnitus
ketamine	
etomidate	
fentanyl citrate *(innovar, sublimaze)*	
sufentanyl citrate *(sufenta)*	

Source: Courtesy of Troy A. Hackett, Ph.D.

General Anesthetics and Post-operative Analgesics

Therapeutic Agent	Comments	Side Effects
Inhalation Anesthetics		
nitrous oxide		
diethyl ether		
cyclopropane		
halothane *(fluothane)*		
enflurane *(ethrane)*		
isoflurane *(forane)*		
desflurane *(suprane)*		
Intravenous Anesthetics		
thiopental		
ketamine		
etomidate		
propofol *(diprivan)*		confusion, ear pain, tinnitus
butorphanol *(stadol)*		confusion, vasodilation
nalbuphine *(nubain)*		confusion, dizziness, speech difficulties, vertigo
diazepam *(valium)*		confusion, nystagmus, slurred speech, vertigo

(continued)

Therapeutic Agent	Comments	Side Effects
midazolam *(versed)*		confusion, neonatal CNS depression, dizziness, ear discomfort, blocked ears, nystagmus, slurred speech
Neuromuscular Blockers		
succinylcholine chlorid *(anectine)*	muscle relaxation; short-acting; usually for intubation	
d-tubocurarine		
pancuronium *(pavulon)*	muscle relaxation; intermediate acting	
pipercuronium *(adruan)*	muscle relaxation; long-acting	
vecuronium *(norcuron)*	muscle relaxation; intermediate acting	
atracurium *(tracium)*	muscle relaxation; intermediate acting	vasodilation
curare	muscle relaxation; intermediate acting	
Antihypertensives		
hydralazine *(apresazide, apresoline, ser-ap-es)*	vertigo	disorientation, dizziness, psychiatric disturbances,
nifedipine *(adalat, procardia)*		dizziness, facial edema, sinusitis, tinnitus, vertigo
nitroglycerine *(nitrostat, nitro-bid)*		dizziness, vasodilation, vertigo
nitroprusside		
esmolol hydrochloride *(brevibloc)*		confusion, disorientation, sinusitis, speech disturbances
labetalol hydrochloride *(normodyne, trandate)*		dizziness, short term memory loss, rhinitis, vertigo

Therapeutic Agent	Comments	Side Effects
Postoperative Analgesia		
butorphanol tartrate *(stadol)*	analgesia	confusion, vertigo
ketorolac *(toradol)*	anti-inflammatory; no CNS depression	dizziness, vasodilation, vertigo
nalbuphine hydrochloride *(nubain)*	analgesia, sedation	confusion, dizziness, speech difficulties, vertigo
fentanyl *(sublimaze)*	analgesia; induction of anesthesia	confusion, speech disturbances, vertigo
meperidine hydrochloride *(demerol)*	analgesia	circulatory depression, disorientation, impaired mental performance
morphine sulfate *(MSIR, roxanol, oramorph, MS contin)*	analgesia	circulatory depression, confusion, disorientation, dizziness, nystagmus
sufentanil citrate *(sufenta)*	analgesia, induction of anesthesia	
alfentanil hydrochloride *(alfenta)*	analgesia; supplement general anesthesia	dizziness
naloxone hydrochloride *(narcan)*	sedation, narcotic depression reversal	

Source: Courtesy of Troy A. Hackett, Ph.D.

Key References

Clinical Pharmacology in Otolaryngology

Bjoraker, DG, Modell JH. Planning and managing anesthesia. In: Polk HC, Gardner B, Stone HH (eds): *Basic Surgery.* St. Louis. Quality Medical Publishing, pp. 28–60, 1993.

Cipolle, RJ, Canafax DM. Principles of pharmacotherapy. In: Paparella, MM, Shumrick, DA, Gluckman, JL, Meyerhoff, WL (eds). *Otolaryngology.* Vol *1*, 3rd ed. Philadelphia : Saunders, pp. 599–604, 1991.

DeLacure MD, Lee KJ. Pharmacology and therapeutics. In: Lee KJ (ed): *Essential Otolaryngology.* 5th ed. New York: Elsevier Science Publishing, pp. 955–970, 1991.

Fischer DS. Cancer chemotherapy. In: Lee KJ (ed). *Essential Otolaryngology.* 5th ed. New York: Elsevier Science Publishing, pp. 255–372, 1991.

Houck JR. Immunology and Allergy. In: Lee KJ (ed): *Essential Otolaryngology.* 5th ed. New York: Elsevier Science Publishing, pp. 273–296, 1991.

Fairbanks DNF. Microbiology, infections, and antibiotic therapy. In: *Head and Neck Surgery—Otolaryngology.* Bailey BJ (ed): Philadelphia: JB Lippincott, pp. 52–62, 1993

Katz JD, Lee KJ. Anesthesia for head and neck surgery. In: Lee KJ (ed): *Essential Otolaryngology.* 5th ed. New York: Elsevier Science Publishing, pp. 875–900, 1991.

Mabry RL. (1993) Principles of pharmacology and medical therapy. In: Bailey BJ (ed): *Head and Neck Surgery—Otolaryngology.* Philadelphia: JB Lippincott, pp. 44–51, 1993.

Matz GJ, Ryback LP. (1993) Ototoxic drugs. In: *Head and Neck Surgery—Otolaryngology*, Bailey, BJ (ed): Philadelphia: JB Lippincott, pp. 1793–1801, 1993.

Physicians Desk Reference. Montvale, NJ: Medical Economics Data Production Company, 1994.

von Roemling RW, Hrushesky WJM. Principles of chemotherapy and immunotherapy for head and neck cancer. In: *Otolaryngology.* vol. *2*, 3rd edition, Paparella MM, Shumrick DA, Gluckman JL, Meyerhoff WL. (eds): Philadelphia: WB Saunders, pp. 1653–1669, 1991.

Rybak, LP. Antibiotics. In *Otolaryngology,* vol. *2*, 3rd edition, Paparella, M.M., Shumrick, D.A., Gluckman, J.L., Meyerhoff, W.L. (eds): Philadelphia: WB Saunders, pp. 605–615, 1991.

Stringer SP, Meyerhoff, WL, Wright CG. (1991) Ototoxicity. In: Paparella, MM, Shumrick, DA, Gluckman, JL, Meyerhoff, WL. (eds): *Otolaryngology.* vol *2*, 3rd ed. Philadelphia: WB Saunders, pp. 1653–1667, 1991.

Yanagisawa E. (1991) Infections of the ear. In: Lee, K.J. (ed): *Essential Otolaryngology.* 5th ed. New York: Elsevier Science Publishing, pp. 581–616, 1991.

Yanagisawa E, Lee KJ. (1991) Noninfectious diseases of the ear. In: Lee KJ. (ed): *Essential Otolaryngology.* 5th ed. New York: Elsevier Science Publishing, pp. 617–646, 1991.

OTOTOXICITY

Classic Quotes

Ototoxicity

"One who pours drugs of which he knows little into a body of which he knows less."

Voltaire's definition of a physician

"The remedy is worse than the disease."

Francis Bacon [1597–1625]
Essays

"I find the medicine worse than the malady."

Beaumont and Fletcher [1647]
Love's Cure

Clinical Concept

1994 Joint Committee on Infant Hearing Statement on Ototoxicity

"Indicators associated with sensorineural hearing loss:

Ototoxic medications including, but not limited to, the aminoglyscosides, used in multiple courses or in combination with loop diuretics."

Common Ototoxic Drugs

Drug	General Therapeutic Application(s)
Aminoglycoside antibiotics	treatment of infections
amikacin	
gentamicin	
kanamycin	
livodomycin	
neomycin	
netilmicin	
sisomycin	
streptomycin	
tobramycin	
Antineoplastic drugs	treatment of cancer and tumors
cisplatin	
carboplatin	
nitrogen mustard	
Diuretics and loop diuretics	treatment of congestive heart failure, pulmonary edema
furosemide (lasix)	
ethacrynic acid	
bumetanide	
Salicylates	treatment of arthritis, rheumatic fever, and connective tissue disorders
aspirin	
Quinine	uncommon, treatment of malaria
Deferoxamine	iron-overloaded patients who require multiple blood transfusions due to severe anemia (e.g. thalassemia)
Environmental chemicals	
arsenic	
mercury	
tin	
lead	
manganese	

Technical Tip

Mechanisms of Ototoxicity

Aminoglycosides

- ☐ Cochlear damage is by a toxic metabolite (with contribution from the liver).
- ☐ Drugs cause calcium antagonism and blockage of ion channels.
- ☐ Maternal inheritance may play a role.
- ☐ Toxic effects may be delayed or prolonged.
- ☐ Some drugs (e.g., Glutathione) may block toxin formation or increase detoxification and prevent aminoglycoside ototoxicity.

Cisplatin

- ☐ Morphologic, biochemical, and electrophysiologic basis of toxicity is not known.
- ☐ Considerable differences in individual susceptability.
- ☐ More severe in pediatric populations.
- ☐ May be enhanced by prior cranial irradiation.
- ☐ Effects documented for stria vascularis and organ of Corti.
- ☐ Outer hair cell degeneration, plus changes in supporting cells and Reissner's membrane.

Loop diuretics

- ☐ Act on epithelial cells in the loop of Henle of the kidney.
- ☐ Among eight different types, furosemide (or lasix) is the most common.
- ☐ Direct effects on the stria vascularis.
- ☐ Changes in outer hair cells.
  - ✓ Impairment of oxidative metabolism
  - ✓ Splaying of stereocilia
  - ✓ Breakage of tip links and cross-links between stereocilia
- ☐ Effects on auditory function include:
  - ✓ Reduced sharpness in tuning curves
  - ✓ Reduced cochlear potentials
  - ✓ Depressed ECochG and ABR

Technical Tip

Principles of Ototoxicity

- ☐ Ototoxicity is related to:
  - Dosage
  - Duration of continuous administration
- ☐ Ototoxic effects of more than one drug may be synergistic:
  - Risk is compounded by concomitant administration of multiple ototoxic agent.
  - For example, aminoglycosides increase hair cell membrane permeability which enhances penetration of loop diuretics in higher concentrations resulting in more ototoxicity.
- ☐ Ototoxic effects are greatly enhanced in patients with impaired renal function.

Terminology

Ototoxicity

Pharmacokinetics = changes in drug concentration (dC) with the body over time; that is, the rate of removal of drug from circulation.

Pharmacokinetics are described or expressed by forumlae, such as $C = (-k_o)(t)$, where k_o is the elimination rate constant and t is the unit of time (minutes or hours).

Half-life = the time for a drug concentration to decrease by one-half, that is, a first-order kinetic process where the same proportion or fraction of the drug is removed during equal time periods.

Did You Know?

Vancomycin and why it may not be quite so ototoxic as we think

- ☐ Background information about vancomycin
  - first introduced in the late 1950s
  - glycopeptide, not an aminoglycoside
  - treatment for resistant Staphylococcus aureus infections
  - first report of ototoxicity was in 1958
- ☐ Good general reference
  - Brummett RE. Ototoxicity of vancomycin and analogues. *Otolaryngologic Clinics of North America 26:* 1993.
- ☐ Reasons to doubt the reputation of ototoxicity:
  - often confused aminoglycosides
  - patients in most of the many reports of ototoxicity also concurrently or previously received other ototoxic drugs
  - some patients also were in renal failure or end-stage renal disease
- ☐ Vancomycin may augment the ototoxicity of aminoglycoside antibiotics.

Clinical Concept

Rationale for Audiologic Monitoring of Ototoxicity

- ☐ Document early evidence of hearing loss, and perhaps:
  - limit the dose of the drug
  - change therapy to an alternate drug
  - prevent or reduce severity of ototoxicity
- ☐ When planned therapy is mandatory, early detection of hearing loss provides:
  - parent/patient counseling
  - prompt audiologic management
  - initial implementation of amplification and assistive listening device

Protocol

Audiologic Test Battery for Monitoring Ototoxicity

- ☐ Immittance measurement
  - to rule out middle ear dysfunction (may be related to irradiation)
  - objective confirmation of auditory status
- ☐ Pure tone audiometry
  - air conduction thresholds, including above 8000 Hz, if possible
  - bone conduction thresholds, as indicated by immittance measures
- ☐ Speech audiometry
  - speech thresholds, especially in children
  - word recognitions scores (may be unusually poor)
- ☐ Otoacoustic emissions
  - the most sensitive and earliest detector of cochlear damage due to ototoxicity
  - highly frequency specific, relative to the audiogram
  - objective which contributes to reliability and feasibility even in very ill patients who cannot provide adequate behavioral responses

Clinical Concept

Limitations of High-Frequency Audiometry

- ☐ Lack of commercially available instrumentation
- ☐ Problems with stimulus calibration and standards
- ☐ Reduced reliability, and limited feasibility, of behavioral responses in very ill patients receiving potentially ototoxic drugs
- ☐ Cannot be performed in neonates and very young children

Did You Know?

Ototoxicity in Very Ill Children

- ☐ Hall et al. studied a series of 32 children ranging in age from 18 months to 17 years admitted to a burn intensive care unit.
- ☐ The children had acute, severe, thermal burns with a mean total body surface area (MTBSA) of 64%.
- ☐ Medical therapy included:
  - ✔ gentamicin
  - ✔ amikacin
  - ✔ vancomycin
  - ✔ amphotericin B
- ☐ Hearing therapy was evaluated with:
  - ✔ ABR
  - ✔ pure tone audiometry
  - ✔ speech audiometry
- ☐ 22% of the group showed serious decrease in hearing sensitivity during their ICU stay.
- ☐ Some children continued to show progression of sensory hearing loss months after hospital discharge and the last treatment with ototoxic drugs.

Source: Hall JW III, Herndon DN, Gary LB, Winkler JB. Auditory brainstem response in young burn-wound patients treated with ototoxic drugs. *International Journal of Pediatric Otorhinolaryngology 12:* 1986.

Key References

Ototoxicity (arranged topically and chronologically)

Early Studies

Schatz A, Bugie E, Waksman SA. Streptomycin, a substance exhibiting antibiotic activity against gram-positive and gram-negative bacteria. *Experimental Biology and Medicine* 55: 66–69, 1944.

Hawkins JE. Cochlear signs of streptomycin intoxication. *J Pharmacologic Therapy 100:* 38–41, 1950.

Stebbins WC, Miller JM et al. Ototoxic hearing loss and cochlear pathology in the monkey. *Ann of Otolaryngol, Rhinol, and Laryngol 78:* 1007–1019, 1969.

Schwartz GH, David DS et al. Ototoxicity induced by furosemide. *New Engl Med 282:* 1413–1414, 1970.

Fleishmann RW, Stadnick SW et al. Ototoxicity of cis-dichlorodiamineplatinum (II) in the guinea pig. *Toxicol and Appl Pharmacol 33:* 320–332,1975.

Fee WE. Aminoglycoside ototoxicity in the human. *Laryngoscope 90:* supplement 24, 1980.

High Frequency Audiometry

Jacobsen EJ, Downs MP, Fletcher JL. Clinical findings in high-frequency thresholds during known ototoxic drug usage. *J Auditory Res 9:* 379–385, 1969.

Fausti SA, Rappaport BZ. Detection of aminoglycoside ototoxicity by high frequency auditory evaluation: Selected case studies. *Am J Otolaryngol 5:* 177–182, 1984.

Fausti SA, Rappaport BZ (Eds). High frequency audiometry. *Seminars in Hearing 6:* 1985.

General References

Stringer SP, Meyerhoff WL, Wright CG. Ototoxicity. In: Paparella MM, Shumrick DA, Gluckman JL (eds). *Otolaryngology.* (3rd ed). Philadelphia: WB Saunders, p. 1653, 1991.

Rybak LP, Matz GJ. Effects of toxic agents. In: Cumming CW (ed). *Otolaryngology - Head and Neck Surgery (2nd ed), Vol 4.* St. Louis: Mosby Year Book, 1993, p. 2943.

Rybak LP (ed). Ototoxicity. *Otolaryngol Clin North Am 26*(5). Philadephia: WB Saunders, 1993.

References

AAO-ACO (American Academy of Otolaryngology and American Council of Otolaryngology). Guide for evaluation of hearing handicap. *JAMA 241*: 2055–2059, 1979.

Alho K, Sainio K, Sajaniemi N, Reinikainen K, Naatanen R. Event-related brain potential of human newborns to pitch change of an acoustic stimulus. *Electroencephalography and Clinical Neurophysiology 77*: 151–155, 1990.

Altschuler RA, Bobbin RP, Hoffman DW. (eds). *Neurobiolology of hearing: The cochlea*. New York: Raven Press, 1986.

Anderson H, Barr B, Wedenberg E. Intra-aural reflexes in retrocochlear lesions. In: Hamburg C, Wersall J (eds). *Nobel symposium 10: Disorders of the skull base region.* Stockholm: Almquist and Wiksell, 1969.

Arenberg IK, Ackley RS, Ferraro J. EcoG results in perilymph fistula: clinical and experimental studies. *Otolaryngology Head and Neck Surgery 99*: 435–443, 1988.

Arnold WJ. The spiral ganglion of the newborn baby. *The American Journal of Otology 3*: 266–269, 1982.

Austin DF. Diseases of the external ear. In: JJ Ballenger, JB Snow, Jr (eds). *Otorhinolaryngology: Head and Neck Surgery, 15*. Baltimore: Williams & Wilkins, 1996.

Barber HO, Stockwell CW. *Manual of electronystagmography*. (2nd ed). St. Louis: C.V. Mosby, 1990.

Beattie RC, Edgerton BJ, Svihovec DV. An investigation of Auditec of St. Louis recordings of Central Institute for the Deaf Spondees. *Journal of the American Audiology Society 1*: 97–101, 1975.

Bekesy G Von. A new audiometer. *Acta Oto-Laryngologica, 35:* 411–422, 1947.

Bekesy G Von. *Experiments in hearing*. New York: McGraw-Hill, 1960.

Berger KA. Speech discrimination task using multiple-choice key words in sentences. *J Auditory Res 3*: 247–262, 1969.

Berlin CI, Cullen JK, Jr, Ellis MS, Lousteau RJ, Yarbrough WM, Lyons GD Jr. Clinical application of recording human VIIIth nerve action potentials from the tympanic membrane. *Trans Amer Acad Ophthalmol Otolaryngol 87*: 401–410, 1974.

Bess FH, Josey AF, Humes LE. Performance intensity functions in cochlear and eighth nerve disorders. *Am J Otolaryngol 1*: 27–31, 1979.

Bess FH, Klee T, Culbertson JL. Identification, assessment, and management of children with unilateral sensorineural hearing loss. *Ear and Hearing 7*: 43–51, 1986.

Bess F, Lichtenstein M, Logan S. Audiology assessment of the elderly. In: Rintelmann W (ed). *Hearing assessment* (2nd ed). Austin, TX: Pro-Ed, 1991.

Bess FH, Tharpe AM. Unilateral hearing impairment in children. *Pediatrics 74*: 206–216, 1984.

Bjoraker DG, Modell JH. Planning and managing anesthesia. In: Polk HC, Gardner B, Stone HH. (eds), *Basic Surgery*. St. Louis: Quality Medical Publishing, pp. 28–60, 1993.

Blake R. Field B, Foster C, Platt, F, Wertz, P. Effect of FM auditory trainers on attending behaviors of learning-disabled children. *Language, Speech, and Hearing Services in Schools 22*: 111–114, 1991.

Bocca E, Calearo C, Cassinari V. A new method for testing hearing in temporal lobe tumors. *Acta Otolaryngologica 44*: 219–221, 1954.

Bonfils P, Uziel A, Pujol R. Evoked oto-acoustic emissions: A fundamental and clinical survey. *Acta Otolaryngologica 105*: 445–449, 1988

Boothroyd A. Developments in speech audiometry. *Sound 2*: 3–10, 1968.

Borg E. On the neuronal organization of the acoustic reflex: A physiological and anatomical study. *Brain Res 49*: 101–123, 1973.

Bosatra A, Russolo M, Poli P. Oscilloscopic analysis of the stapedius muscle reflex in brain stem lesions. *Arch Otolaryngol 102*: 284–285, 1976.

Brewer C, Resnick D. Speech discrimination tests. *Seminars in Hearing 4*: 1983.

Brookler, K and Rubin, W. (1991) Objective Confirmation of Symptoms. In: *Dizziness: Etiologic approach to management*. New York: Thieme Medical Publishers, Inc., 1991.

Brown AM et al. Acoustic distortion products can be used to monitor the effects of chronic gentamicin treatment. *Hearing Research 42*: 1989.

Burch-Sims PG, Hall JW III. Auditory mismatch negativity response in adults and normal versus brain injured infants. [Abstract]. *Audiology Today 6*: 1994.

Carhart R, Porter LS. Audiometric configurations and prediction of threshold for spondees. *J Speech Hear Res 14*: 486–495, 1971.

Carhart R. Observations on the relations between thresholds for pure tones and for speech. *J Speech Hear Disord 36*: 476–483, 1971.

Carhart R. Monitored live voice as a test of auditory acuity. *J Acoust Soc Amer 17*: 339–349, 1946.

Carhart R. Clinical determination of abnormal auditory adaptation. *Arch Otolaryngol 65:* 32–39, 1957.

Carhart R, Jerger J. Preferred method of clinical determination of pure-tone thresholds. *J Speech Hearing Disorders 24*: 330–345, 1959.

Chermak GD, Musiek FM. Managing central auditory processing disorders in children and youth. *Am J Audio 1*: 61–65, 1992.

Cipolle RJ, Canafax DM. Principles of pharmacotherapy. In: Paparella MM, Shumrick DA, Gluckman JL, Meyerhoff WL. (eds). *Otolaryngology* (volume 1, 3rd ed), Philadelphia: Saunders, pp. 599–604, 1991.

Clark JG. Uses and abuses of hearing loss classification. *Asha 23*: 493–500, 1981.

Coats A. On electrocochleographic electrode design. *J Acoust Soc Am 56*: 708–711, 1974.

Coats A. ENG examination technique. *Ear and Hearing. 7*: 143–150, 1986.

Colletti V. Stapedial reflex abnormalities in multiple sclerosis. *Audiology 14*: 63–71, 1975.

Colletti V. Tympanometry from 200 to 2000 Hz probe tone. *Audiology 15*: 106–119, 1976.

Committee on Hearing and Equilibrium. *Otolaryngology Head and Neck Surg 113*: 181–185, 1995.

Conn MJ, Dancer J, Ventry IM. A spondee list for determining speech reception threshold without prior familiarization. *J Speech Hear Disord 40*: 388–396, 1975.

Crain MR, Dolan KD. Internal auditory canal enlargement in Paget's disease apearing as bilateral acoustic neuromas. *Ann Otol Rhinol Laryngol 99*: 833–834, 1990.

Creten W, Van de Heyning P, Van Camp K. Immittance audiometry. *Scandinavian Audiol 14*: 115–121, 1985.

Csepe V. On the origin and development of the mismatch negativity. *Ear and Hearing 16*: 90–103, 1995.

Cyr DG. Vestibular system assessment. In: W Rintelmann (ed). *Hearing assessment* (2nd ed). Austin: Pro-Ed, pp. 739–803, 1991.

Cyr DG et al. Clinical application of computerized dynamic posturography. *ENTechnology*: Sept., pp. 36–47, 1988.

Cyr DG, Brookhouser PE, Harker LA, Gossman MA. Modified Semont procedure for patients with unilateral BPPV. Presented to the Middle Section Meeting of the Triological Society, January 22, 1994, Rochester, Minnesota.

Dallos P, Geisler CD, Matthews JW, Ruggero MA, Steele CR (eds). *The mechanics and biophysics of hearing*. New York: Springer-Verlag, 1990.

Davis H. Enhancement of evoked cortical potentials in humans related to a task requiring a decision. *Science 145*: 182–183, 1964.

Davis H. An active process in cochlear mechanics. *Hearing Research 9*: 79–90, 1983.

Davis H, Davis PA, Loomis AL, Harvey EN, Hobart G. Electrical reactions of the human brain to auditory stimulation during sleep. *J Neurophysiol 2*: 129–135, 1939.

Davis H, Deatherage BH, Eldredge DH, Smith CA. Summating potentials of the cochlea. *Amer J Physiol 195*: 251–261, 1958.

Davis PA. Effects of acoustic stimuli on the waking human brain. *J Neurophysiology 2*: 494–499,1939.

DeJonge R. Normal tympanometric gradient: A comparison of three methods. *Audiology 25*: 299–308, 1986.

DeLacure MD, Lee KJ. Pharmacology and therapeutics. In: Lee, K.J. (ed). *Essential Otolaryngology* (5th ed). New York: Elsevier Science Publishing, pp. 955–970.

DiSorga RM, Weir K. Medications and side effects related to hearing, auditory function, vestibular function, and central nervous system function. *Audiology Today 5*: 32–35, 1993.

Dix M, Hallpike C, Hood J. Observations upon the loudness recruitment phenomenon with especial reference to the differential diagnosis of disorders of the internal ear and the VIIIth nerve. *J Laryngol and Otology 62*: 671–686, 1948.

Downs M. Twentieth century pediatric audiology: Prologue to the 21st. *Seminars in Hearing 11*: 408-411, 1990.

Dubno JR, Dirks DD, Morgan DE. Effects of age and mild hearing loss on speech recognition in noise. *J Acoust Soc Amer 76*: 87–96, 1984.

Durrant JD. Extratympanic electrode support via vented earmold. *Ear and Hearing 11*: 468–469, 1990.

Egan JP. Articulation testing methods. *Laryngoscope 58*: 955–991, 1948.

Eimas PD, Siqueland PD, Juscyzk PW, Vigorito J. Speech perception in infants. *Science 171*: 303-306, 1971.

Epley JM. The Canalith Repositioning Procedure: For treatment of benign paroxysmal positional vertigo. *Otolaryngol Head Neck Surg 107*: 399–404, 1992.

Erber NP. Use of the auditory numbers test to evaluate speech perception abilities of hearing-impaired children. *J Speech Hear Disord 45*: 527–532, 1980.

Esslen E. Electrodiagnosis of facial palsy. In: A Miehlke. *Surgery of the Facial Nerve* (2nd ed). Urban and Schwarzenberg, 1973.

Fairbanks, DNF. Microbiology, infections, and antibiotic therapy. In: Bailey BJ (ed). *Head and neck Surgery—Otolaryngology*. Philadelphia: J.B. Lippincott, pp. 52–62, 1993.

Fairbanks G. Test of phonemic differentiation: The rhyme test. *J Acoust Soc Amer 30*: 596–600, 1958.

Fausti SA, Gray PS, Frey RH, Mitchell CR. Rise time and center-frequency effects on auditory brainstem responses to high-frequency tone bursts. *J Am Acad Audiol 2*: 24–31, 1991.

Fausti SA, Mitchell CR, Frey RH, Henry JA, O'Connor JL. Multiple-stimulus method for rapid collection of auditory brainstem responses using high-frequency (> or = 8k Hz) tone bursts. *J Am Acad Audiol 5*: 119–126, 1994.

Fausti SA, Rappaport BZ. Detection of aminoglycoside ototoxicity by high frequency auditory evaluation: Selected case studies. *Am J Otolaryngol 5*: 177–182, 1984.

Fausti SA, Rappaport BZ (eds). High frequency audiometry. *Seminars in Hearing 6*: 1985.

Fausti SA, Rappaport BZ, Frey RH, Henry JA, Phillips, DS, Mitchell CR, Olson DJ. Reliability of evoked responses to high-frequency (8–14 KHz) tone bursts. *J Am Acad Audiol 2*: 105–114, 1991.

Fee WE. Aminoglycoside ototoxicity in the human. *Laryngoscope 90*: (Suppl 24): 1980.

Feeney MP, Franks JR. Test-retest reliability of a distinctive feature difference test for hearing aid evaluation. *Ear and Hearing 3*: 59–65, 1982.

Feldman A. Impedance measurements at the eardrum as an aid to diagnosis. *J Speech Hear Res 6*: 315–327, 1963.

Ferraro J, Murphy G, Ruth R. A comparative study of primary electrodes used in extratympanic electrocochleography. *Seminars in Hearing 7*: 279–287, 1986.

Ferraro J, Best LG, Arenberg IK. The use of electrocochleography in the diagnosis, assessment, and management of endolymphatic hydrops. *Otol Clinics North Amer 16*: 69–82, 1983.

Fifer R, Jerger J, Berlin C, Tobey E, Campbell J. Development of a dichotic sentence identification test for hearing impaired adults. *Ear and Hearing 4*: 300–305, 1983.

Fineberg R, O'Leary DP, Davis LL. Use of active head movements for computerized vestibular testing. *Arch Otolaryngol Head Neck Surg 113*: 1063–1065, 1987.

Finitzo-Hieber, T, Gerling IJ, Matkin ND, Chaerow-Skalka E. A sound effects recognition test for the pediatric evaluation. *Ear and Hearing 1*: 271–276, 1980.

Fisch U. Facial paralysis in fractures of the petrous bone. *Laryngoscope 84*: 1974.

Fisch U. Maximal nerve excitability testing versus electroneuronography. *Arch Otolaryngol 106: 52*, 1980.

Fischer DS. Cancer chemotherapy. In: Lee KJ (ed). *Essential Otolaryngology* (5th ed). New York: Elsevier Science Publishing, pp. 255–372, 1991.

Fleishmann RW, Stadnick SW et al. Ototoxicity of cis-dichlorodiamineplatinum (II) in the guinea pig. *Toxicol Appl Pharmacol 33*: 320–332,1975.

Fletcher H. A method of calculating hearing loss for speech from an audiogram. *Acta Otolaryngol* (Suppl 90), 26–37, 1950.

Fletcher H. *Speech and hearing*. Princeton, NJ: Von Nostrand Reinhold, 1929.

Flexer C, Savage H. Using an ALD in speech-language assessment and training. *The Hearing Journal 45*: 26–35, 1992.

Fowler EP. The diagnosis of diseases of the neural mechanism by the aid of sounds well above threshold. *Trans Amer Otol Soc, 70*: 27–219.

French NR, Steinberg JC. Factors governing the intelligibility of speech sounds. *J Acoust Soc Amer 19*: 90–119, 1947.

Frijns JH, van Wijngaarden A, Peeters S. A multi-channel simultaneous data acquisition and waveform generation system designed for medical applications. *J Med Engineer & Technol 18*: 54–60,1994.

Fry DB. Word and sentence tests for use in speech audiometry. *Lancet 2:* 197–199, 1961.

Fry DB, Kerridge PMT. Tests for the hearing of speech by deaf people. *Lancet 1*: 106–109, 1939.

Gaeth J. A scale for testing speech discrimination. Final Report No. RD-2277-S, Society of Rehabilitation Services, Department of Health, Education and Welfare, 1970.

Galambos R, Makeig S, Talmachoff PJ. A 40-Hz auditory potential recorded from the human scalp. *Proc National Acad Science U.S.A 78*: 2643–2647, 1981.

Gardner H. Application of high-frequency consonant discrimination word list in hearing-aid evaluation. *J Speech Hear Disord 36*: 354–355, 1971.

Gascon G, Johnson R, Burd L. Central auditory processing and attention deficit disorder. *J Child Neurol 1*: 27–33, 1986.

Geisler CD, Frishkopf LS, Rosenblith WA. Extracranial responses to acoustic clicks in man. *Science 128*: 1210–1211, 1958.

Gibson WRP, Moffat DA, Ramsden RT. Clinical electrocochleography in diagnosis and management of Ménière's disease. *Audiology 16*: 389–401, 1977.

Gillet P. *Auditory processes*. Novato CA: Academic Therapy Publications, 1993.

Gilroy J. *Basic neurology*: New York, Pergamon, 1990.

Goin DW, Staller SJ, Asher DL, Mischkle RE. Summating potential in Meniere's disease. *Laryngoscope 92*: 1383–1389, 1982.

Gold T. Historical background to the proposal, 40 years ago, of an active model for cochlear frequency analysis. In: JP Wilson, DT Kemp (eds). *Cochlear mechanisms*. New York: Plenum, 1989.

Gold T. Hearing II. The physical basis of the action of the cochlea. *Proc Royal Soc Biology*: 492–498, 1948.

Goldstein R, Rodman LB. Early components of averaged evoked responses to rapidly repeated auditory stimuli. *J Speech Hear Res 10*: 697–705, 1967.

Goodman A. References zero levels for pure-tone audiometer. *Asha 7:* 262–263, 1955.

Gorlin RJ, Cohen MM, Levin LS. *Syndromes of the head and neck*. New York: Oxford University Press, 1990.

Gossman MA, Cyr D, White V, Brookhouser PE. Treating patients with BPPV: Non-medical/surgical approaches. Presented at American Academy of Audiology, April 29, 1994, Richmond, Virginia.

Gradenigo G, Allen SE. On the clinical signs of affections of the auditory nerve (German). *Arch Otorhinolaryngol 22*: 213–215, 1893.

Gray L. Development of a frequency dimension in chicken (Gallus gallus). *J Comp Psychol 105*: 85–88, 1991.

Gray L, Rubel EW. Development of absolute thresholds in chickens. *J Acoust Soc Amer 77*: 1162–1172, 1985.

Green DM. *An introduction to hearing*. Hillsdale, NJ: Lawrence Erlbaum Associates, 1976.

Grenman R, Lang H, Panelius M, Salmivally A, Laine H, Rintamaki J. Stapedius reflex and brainstem auditory evoked responses in multiple sclerosis patients. *Scand Audiol 13*: 109–113, 1984.

Griffiths J. Rhyming minimal contrasts: A simplified diagnostic articulation test. *J Acoust Soc Amer 42:* 236–241, 1967.

Haberman RS, Kramer MB. False-positive MRI and CT findings of an acoustic neuroma. *Am J Otol 10:* 301–303, 1989.

Hall JW III. Predicting hearing level from the acoustic reflex: A comparison of three methods. *Arch Otolaryngol 104*: 602–605, 1978.

Hall JW III. (Ed). Immittance audiometry. *Seminars in Hearing 8:* 1988.

Hall DE. *Musical acoustics: An introduction*. Belmont CA: Wadsworth Publishing Co., 1980.

Hall JW III. Acoustic reflex amplitude. II. Effect of age related auditory dysfunction. *Audiology 21*: 386–399, 1982.

Hall JW III. The acoustic reflex in central auditory dysfunction. In Pinheiro ML, Musiek FE (eds). *Assessment of central auditory dysfunction: Foundations and clinical correlates*. Baltimore: Williams & Wilkins, pp. 103–130, 1985.

Hall JW III. (ed). Contemporary tympanometry. *Seminars in Hearing 8*: 1988.

Hall JW III. Effects of age and sex on static compliance. *Arch Otolaryngol 105*: 601–605,1979.

Hall JW III. *Handbook of auditory evoked responses*. Needham, MA: Allyn & Bacon, 1992.

Hall JW III, Baer JE, Prentice C, Wilson D, Byrn A. Central auditory processing disorder: A case report. *Seminars in Hearing 14:* 254–264, 1993.

Hall JW III, Chandler D. Tympanometry in clinical audiology. In: Katz J (ed). *Handbook of clinical audiology* (4th ed). Baltimore: Williams & Wilkins, pp. 283–299, 1994.

Hall JW III, Prentice CH, Baer JE, Wilson DS, Smiley G, Cole R. Auditory findings in unusual syndromes: Review and case reports. *J Am Acad Audiol 5:* 1995.

Hall JW III, Weaver T. Impedance audiometry in a young population: effects of age, sex, and minor tympanogram abnormality. *J Otolaryngol 8*: 210–222, 1979.

Hamid AM. Determining side of vestibular dysfunction with rotatory chair testing. *Otolaryngol Head Neck Surg 105*: 40–43, 1991.

Hammill TA, Hussung RA, Sammeth CA. Rapid threshold estimation using the "chained-stimuli" technique for auditory brain stem response threshold. *Ear and Hearing 12:* 229–234, 1991.

Harris FP, Probst R. Transiently evoked otoacoustic emissions in patients with Meniere's Disease. *Acta Otolaryngologica 112*: 36–44, 1992.

Harris JP, Ruckenstein MJ. Sudden sensorineural hearing loss, perilymph fistula, and autoimmune inner ear disease. In: Ballenger JJ, Snow JB Jr (eds). *Otorhinolaryngology: Head and neck surgery* (15 ed). Baltimore: Williams & Wilkins, 1996.

Haskins H. A phonetically balanced test of speech discrimination for children. Unpublished master's thesis. Northwestern University, 1949.

Hausler R, Levine RA. Brain stem auditory potentials are related to interaural time discrimination in patients with multiple sclerosis. *Brain Res. 191*, 589–594, 1980.

Hawkins JE. Cochlear signs of streptomycin intoxication. *J Pharmacologic Therapy 100*: 38–41, 1950.

Hawkins DB. Comparisons of speech recognition in noise by mildly-to-moderately hearing-impaired children using hearing aids and FM systems. *J Speech Hear Disord 49*: 409–418, 1984.

Hess, K. (1979). Stapedius reflex in multiple sclerosis. *J Neurol Neurosurg Psychiat 42:* 331–337

Hirsch BE. Computed sinusoidal harmonic acceleration. *Ear and Hearing 7:* 198–203, 1986.

Hirsh I. *The measurement of hearing*. New York: McGraw-Hill Book Company, 1952.

Hirsh I, Davis H, Silverman S, Reynolds E, Eldert E, Benson R. Development of materials for speech audiometry. *J Speech Hear Disord 17:* 321–337, 1952.

Hodges A, Ruth R. Factors influencing the acoustic reflex. *Seminars in Hearing 8:* 339–357, 1987.

Hoke M, Pantev C, Ansa L, Lutkenhoner B, Herrmann E. A timesaving BERA technique for frequency-specific assessment of auditory threshoshold through tone-pulse series stimulation (TOPSTIM) with simultaneous gliding high-pass noise masking (GHINOMA). *Acta Oto-Laryngologica,* (Suppl 482): 45–56, 1991.

Holmquist J. Eustachian tube function assessed with tympanometry. *Acta Otolaryngologica 68*: 501–508, 1969.

Holte L, Margolis RH, Cavanaugh RM Jr. Developmental changes in multifrequency tympanograms. *Audiology 30:* 1–24, 1991.

Horner K, Cazals Y. Rapidly fluctuating thresholds at the onset of experimentally-induced hydrops in the guinea pig. *Hearing Research 26:* 319–325, 1987.

Horner K, Cazals Y. Distortion products in early stage experimental hydrops in the guinea pig. *Hearing Research 43:* 71–80, 1989.

Holtz MA, Harris FP, Probst R. Otoacoustic emissions: an approach for monitoring aminoglycoside-induced ototoxicity. *Laryngoscope 104:* 1994.

Hosford-Dunn HL, Runge CA, , Montgomery PA. A shortened rank-ordered word recognition list. *The Hearing Journal 36:* 15–19, 1983

Houck, J.R. Immunology and allergy. In: Lee KJ (ed). *Essential Otolaryngology* (5th ed). New York: Elsevier Science Publishing, pp. 273–296, 1991.

House A, Williams C, Hecker M, Kryter K. Articulation testing methods: Consonantal differentiation with closed-response set. *J Acoust Soc Amer 37:* 158–168, 1965.

House JW, Brackmann DE. Facial nerve grading system. *Otolaryngol Head Neck Surg 93:* 146–147, 1985.

Hughson W, Thompson EA. Correlation of hearing acuity for speech with discrete frequency audiograms. *Arch Otolaryngol 36:* 526–540, 1942.

Hughson W, Westlake H. Manual for program outline for rehabilitation of aural casualties both military and civilian. *Trans Am Acad Ophthalmol Otolaryngol* (Suppl 48): 1–15, 1944.

Jacobsen EJ, Downs MP, Fletcher JL. Clinical findings in high-frequency thresholds during known ototoxic drug usage. *J Auditory Research 9*: 379–385, 1969.

Jacobson GP, Privitera M, Neils JR, Grayson AS, Yeh H-S. The effects of anterior temporal lobectomy (ATL) on the middle-latency auditory evoked potential (MLAEP). *Electroencephalography and Clinical Neurophysiology 75:* 230–241, 1990.

Jacobson GP, Newman CW. The development of the dizziness handicap inventory. *Arch Otolaryngol Head Neck Surg 116:* 424–427, 1990.

Jacobson GP, Newman CW, Kartush J (eds). *Handbook of balance function testing.* St. Louis: Mosby/Yearbook, 1993.

Jacobson GP, Newman CW. Rotational testing. *Seminars in Hearing 12*: 199–224, 1991.

Jacobson JT (ed). Hereditary syndromes. *J Amer Acad Audiol 6*(1): 1–110, 1995.

Jeck L, Ruth R, Schoeny Z. High frequency sensitization of the acoustic reflex. *Ear and Hearing 4:* 98–101, 1983.

Jerger J. Bekesy audiometry in the analysis of auditory disorders. *J Speech Hearing Res 3:* 275–287, 1960.

Jerger J. Clinical experience with impedance audiometry. *Arch Otolaryngol 92:* 311–324, 1970.

Jerger JF. Research priorities in auditory science—The audiologist's view. *Ann Otol Rhinol Laryngol 89*(Suppl 74): 134–135, 1980.

Jerger J. Introduction to section IV: Impedance audiometry. In Alford BR, Jerger S (eds). *Clinical audiology: The Jerger perspective.* San Diego: Singular Publishing Group, 1993.

Jerger J, Anthony L, Jerger S, Mauldin L. Studies in impedance audiometry. III. Middle ear disorders. *Arch Otolaryngol 99:* 165–171, 1974.

Jerger J, Burney P, Mauldin L, Crump B. Predicting hearing loss from the acoustic reflex. *Arch Otolaryngol 99:* 11–22, 1974.

Jerger J, Harford E, Clemis J, Alford B. The acoustic reflex in eighth nerve disorders. *Arch Otolaryngol 99:* 409–413, 1974.

Jerger JF, Hayes D. The cross-check principle in pediatric audiometry. *Arch Otolaryngol 102:* 614–620, 1976.

Jerger J, Hayes D. Diagnostic speech audiometry. *Arch Otolaryngol 103:* 216–222, 1977.

Jerger J, Hayes D. Latency of the acoustic reflex in eighth-nerve tumor. *Arch Otolaryngol 109:* 1–5, 1983.

Jerger J, Jerger S. Clinical validity of central auditory tests. *Scand Audiol 4:* 147–163, 1975.

Jerger S, Jerger J. Diagnostic value of crossed vs. uncrossed acoustic reflexes. *Arch Otolaryngol 103:* 445–453, 1977.

Jerger J, Jerger S. Measurement of hearing in adults. In: Paparella MM, Shumrick DA (eds). *Otolaryngology* (2nd ed). Philadelphia: WB Saunders, Co., 1980.

Jerger S, Jerger J. Pediatric speech intelligibility test: Performance-intensity characteristics. *Ear and Hearing 3:* 325–333, 1982.

Jerger J, Jerger S. Acoustic reflex decay: 10-second or 5-second criterion? *Ear and Hearing 4:* 70–71, 1983.

Jerger S, Jerger J, Abrams S. Speech audiometry in a young child. *Ear and Hearing 4:* 56–66, 1983.

Jerger J, Johnson K, Jerger S. Effect of response criterion on measures of speech understanding in the elderly. *Ear and Hearing 9:* 49–56, 1988.

Jerger S, Jerger J, Lewis S. Pediatric speech intelligibility test. II. Effect of receptive language age and chronologic age. *International J Pediat Otorhinolaryngol 3:* 101–118, 1981.

Jerger J, Johnson K, Jerger S, Coker N, Pirozzolo F, Gray L. Central auditory processing disorder: A case study. *J Amer Acad Audiol 2:* 36–54.

Jerger J, Jerger S, Mauldin L. Studies in impedance audiometry. I. Normal and sensorineural ears. *Arch Otolaryngol 96:* 513–523, 1972.

Jerger S, Johnson K, Loiselle L. Pediatric central auditory dysfunction: Comparison of children with confirmed lesions versus suspected processing disorders. *Am J Otol 9* (Suppl): 63–71, 1988.

Jerger J, Lassman S, Harford E. On the detection of extremely small changes in sound intensity. *Arch Otolaryngol 69:* 200–211, 1959.

Jerger S, Lewis S, Hawkins J, Jerger J. Pediatric speech intelligibility test. I. Generation of test materials. *International J Pediat Otorhinolaryngol 2:* 217–230, 1980.

Jerger S, Martin R, Jerger J. Specific auditory perceptual dysfunction in a learning disabled child. *Ear and Hearing 8:* 78–86, 1987.

Jerger J, Northern JL (eds). *Clinical impedance audiometry.* Acton, MA: American Electromedics Corporation, 1980.

Jerger J, Oliver TA, Chmiel RA, Rivera VM. Patterns of auditory abnormality in multiple sclerosis. *Audiology 25:* 193–209, 1986.

Jerger J, Shedd J, Harford E. On the detection of extremely small changes in sound intensity. *Arch Otolaryngol 69:* 200–211, 1959.

Jirsa RE. The clinical utility of the P_3 AERP in children with auditory processing disorders. *J Speech Hearing Res 35:* 903–912, 1992.

Jirsa, R.E., Clontz, K.B. Long latency auditory event-related potentials from children with auditory processing disorders. *Ear and Hearing 11:* 222–232, 1990.

Joint Committee on Infant Hearing. 1994 Position Statement. *Audiology Today 6:* 6–9, 1994.

Jones KL. *Smith's recognizable patterns of human malformation* (4th ed). Philadelphia: WB Saunders, 1988.

Kalikow D, Stevens K, Elliott L. Development of a test of speech intelligibility in noise using sentence materials with controlled word predictability. *J Acoust Soc Amer 61:* 1337–1351, 1977.

Kamhi AG, Beasley DA. Central auditory processing disorder: Is it a meaningful construct or a twentieth century unicorn? *J Child Com Disord 9:* 5–13, 1985.

Kandel ER, Schwartz JH, Jessell TM (eds). *Principles of neural science* (3rd ed). Norwalk, CT: Appleton Lange, 1991.

Kartush J, Bouchard K. *Neuromonitoring in otology and head and neck surgery.* New York: Raven Press, 1992.

Katz DR, Elliott LL. Development of a new children's speech discrimination test. Paper presented at the convention of the American Speech-Language-Hearing Association, November 18–21, 1978, Chicago.

Katz JD, Lee KJ. Anesthesia for head and neck surgery. In: Lee, KJ (ed). *Essential otolaryngology* (5th ed). New York: Elsevier Science Publishing, pp. 875–900, 1991.

Kavanagh KT, Babin RW. Definitions and types of nystagmus and calculations. *Ear and Hearing 7:* 157–166, 1986.

Keating LW. Error frequency in CID W-22 lists. Unpublished data. Rochester, MN: Mayo Clinic, 1974 (cited in Olsen WO, Matkin ND. Speech audiometry. In: Rintelmann WF (ed). *Hearing Assessment* (2nd ed). Austin: Pro-Ed, p. 85, 1991.

Keith RW, (ed). Central auditory dysfunction. New York: Grune & Stratton, 1977.

Keith RW. Interpretation of the staggered spondee word (SSW) test. *Ear and Hearing 4:* 287–292, 1983.

Keith RW. A screening test for auditory processing disorders. The Psychological Corporation, Harcourt Brace Jovanovich, 1986.

Keith RW, Novak KK. Relationships between tests of central auditory function and receptive language. *Seminars in Hearing 5:* 243–250, 1984.

Keith RW, Rudy J, Donahue PA, Katbamna B. Comparison of SCAN results with other auditory and language measures in a clinical population. *Ear and Hearing 10:* 382–386, 1989.

Kemp DT. Stimulated acoustic emissions from within the human auditory system. *J Acoust Soc Amer 64:* 1386–1391, 1978.

Kileny P, Kemink JL. Artifacts and errors in the electronystagmographic (ENG) evaluation of the vestibular system. *Ear and Hearing 7:* 151–156, 1986.

Kileny PR, Paccioretti D, Wilson AF. Effects of cortical lesions in middle-latency auditory evoked responses (MLR). *Electroencephalography and Clinical Neurophysiology 66:* 108–120, 1987.

Kim Y, Aoyagi M, Koike Y. Measurement of cochlear basilar membrane traveling wave velocity by derived ABR. *Acta Otolaryngologica* (Suppl 511): 71–76, 1994.

Kofler F, Oberascher G, Pommer B. Brain-stem involvement in multiple sclerosis: a comparison between brain-stem auditory evoked potentials and the acoustic stapedius reflex. *J Neurol 231:* 145–147, 1984.

Konigsmark BW, Gorlin RJ. *Genetic and metabolic deafness*. Philadelphia: WB Saunders, 1976.

Kramer SJ. Frequency-specific auditory brainstem responses to bone-conducted stimuli. *Audiology 31:* 61–71, 1992.

Kraus N. Mismatch negativity in the assessment of central auditory function. *Am J Audiol 3:* 139–151, 1994.

Kraus N (ed). Special issue: Mismatch negativity as an index of central auditory function. *Ear and Hearing 16:* 1995

Kraus N, McGee TJ. Mismatch negativity in the assessment of central auditory function. *Am J Audiol 3:* 39–51, 1994.

Kraus N, Micco A, Koch D, McGee T, Carrell T, Sharma A. Wiet R, Weingarten C. The mismatch negativity cortical evoked potential evoked by speech stimuli. *Ear and Hearing 13:* 158–164, 1992.

Kraus N, Ozdamar O, Hier D, Stein L. Auditory middle latency responses (MLRs) in patients with cortical lesions. *Electroencephalography and Clinical Neurophysiology 54:* 275–297, 1982.

Krmpotic-Nemanic J, Kostovic I, Bogdanovic N, Fucic A, Judas M. Cytoarchitectonic parameters of developmental capacity of the human associative auditory cortex during postnatal life. *Acta Otolaryngologica (Stockh) 105:* 463–466, 1988.

Lambert PR. Nonlocalizing vestibular findings on electronystagmography. *Ear and Hearing 7:* 182–185, 1986.

Laukli E, Mair IWS. Ipsilateral and contralateral acoustic reflex thresholds. *Audiology 19:* 469–479, 1980

Lavigne-Rebillard, Pujol R. Auditory hair cells in human fetuses: Synaptogenesis and ciliogenesis. *J Electron Microscopy Technique 15:* 115–122, 1990.

Lee YS, Lueders H, Dinner DS, Lesser RP, Hahn J, Klemm G. Recording of auditory evoked potentials in man using chronic subdural electrodes. *Brain 107:* 115–131, 1984.

Legatt AD, Pedley TA, Emerson RG, Stein BM, Abramson M. Normal brain-stem auditory evoked potentials with abnormal latency-intensity studies in patients with acoustic neuromas. *Arch Neurol 45:* 1326–1330, 1988.

Lehiste I, Peterson G. Linguistic considerations in the study of speech intelligibility. *J Acoust Soc Amer 31:* 280–286, 1959.

Lempert J, Wever EG, Lawrence M. The cochleogram and its clinical application. *Arch Otolaryngol 51:* 307–311, 1959.

Lenoir M, Puel J-L, Pujol R. Stereocilia and tectorial development in the rat cochlea: A SEM study. *Anatomic Embryol 175:* 477–487, 1987.

Liden G. Speech audiometry, an experimental and clinical study with Swedish language material. *Acta Otolaryngologica* (Suppl 114): 1954.

Liden G, Nilsson G, Anderson H. Narrow band masking with white noise. *Acta Oto-Laryngologica 50:* 116–124, 1959.

Lightfoot GR. ABR screening for acoustic neuromata: The role of rate-induced latency shift measurements. *Brit J Audiol 26:* 217–227, 1992.

Lilly D. Multiple frequency, multiple component tympanometry: New approaches to an old diagnostic problem. *Ear and Hearing 5:* 300–308, 1984.

Lina-Granade G, Collet L, Morgon A. Auditory-evoked brainstem responses elicited by maximum-length sequences in normal and sensorineural ears. *Audiology 33:* 218–236, 1994.

Lindamood P. Auditory discrimination in depth program for phonologic awareness deficits. *Annals of Dyslexia:* 1991.

Ling D. Auditory coding and reading—an analysis of training procedures for hearing-impaired children. In: Ross M, Giolas TG (eds). *Auditory management of hearing-impaired children*. Baltimore: University Park Press, pp. 181–218, 1978.

Loftus B, Wazen JJ. A false-positive gadolinium-enhanced MRI: Acoustic neuroma versus cochleovestibular neuritis. *Otolaryngol Head Neck Surg 103:* 299, 1990.

Long GR, Tubis A. Modification of spontaneous and evoked otoacoustic emissions and associated psychoacoustic microstructure by aspirin consumption. *JASA 84:* 1988.

Luscher E, Zwislocki J. A simple method for indirect monaural determination of the recruitment phenomenon (difference limen in intensity in different types of deafness). *Acta Oto-laryngologica* (Stockh) 78 (Suppl): 156–168, 1949.

Lynn S, Pool A, Rose D, Brey R, Suman V. A randomized trial of the canalith repositioning procedure. *Otolaryngol Head Neck Surg*

Mabry RL. Principles of pharmacology and medical therapy. In: Bailey BJ (ed). *Head and Neck Surgery—Otolaryngology*. Philadelphia: J.B. Lippincott, pp. 44–51, 1993.

Margolis RH, Heller J. Screening tympanometry: Criteria for medical referral. *Audiology 26:* 197–208, 1987.

Margolis RH, Van Camp KJ, Wilson RH, Creten WL. Multifrequency tympanometry in normal ears. *Audiology 24:* 44–53, 1985.

Marsh RR. Signal to noise constraints on maximum length sequence auditory brain stem responses. *Ear and Hearing 13:* 396–400, 1991.

Marsh RR. Concurrent right and left ear auditory brain stem response recording. *Ear and Hearing 14: 169–174, 1993.*

Martin GK, Ohlms LA, Franklin DJ, Harris FP, Lonsbury-Martin BL. Distortion product emissions in humans III. Influence of sensorineural hearing loss. *Ann Otol Rhinol Laryngol 99*: 30–42, 1990.

Matz GJ, Ryback LP. Ototoxic drugs. In: Bailey BJ (ed). *Head and neck surgery—Otolaryngology*. Philadelphia: JB Lippincott, 1793–1801, 1993.

Maurer K, Schafer E, Hopf HC, Leitner H. The location by early auditory evoked potentials (EAEP) of acoustic nerve and brainstem demyelination in multiple sclerosis (MS). *J Neurol 223:* 43–58, 1980.

May M et al. The prognostic accuracy of the maximal stimulation test compared with that of the nerve excitability test in Bell's Palsy. *Laryngoscope 81:* 931–938, 1971.

McConnell F, Ward PH (eds). *Deafness in childhood.* Nashville, TN: Vanderbilt University Press, 1967.

McFadden D, Plattsmier HS. Aspirin abolishes spontaneous otoacoustic emissions. *JASA 76:* 1984

McGee ML. Electronystagmography in peripheral lesions. *Ear and Hearing 7:* 167–175, 1986.

McPherson D, Pang-Ching G. Development of a distinctive feature discrimination test. *J Auditory Res 19: 235–246, 1979.*

Melnick W. Instrument calibration. In: Rintelmann W (ed). *Hearing assessment* (2nd ed). Austin, TX: Pro-Ed, 1991.

Metz O. The acoustic impedance measured on normal and pathologic ears. *Acta Otolaryngologica 63* (Suppl): 1946.

Meyerhoff WL, Yellin MW. Summating potential/action potential ratio in perilymph fistula. *Otolaryngol Head Neck Surg 102:* 678–682, 1990.

Michael PL, Bienvenue GR. Real-ear threshold level comparisons between the Telephonics TDH-39 earphone with a metal outer shell and the TDH-39, TDH-49, and TDH-50 earphones with plastic outer shells. *J Acoust Soc Amer 61:* 1640–1642, 1977.

Michael PL, Bienvenue GR. Calibration data for the Telex 1470-A audiometric earphones. *J Acoust Soc Amer 67:* 1812–1815, 1980.

Moore EJ, Semela JJ, Rakerd B, Robb RC, Ananthanarayan AK. The I' potential of the brain-stem auditory-evoked potential. *Scand Audiol 21:* 153–156, 1992.

Morrongiello BA, Gotowiec A. Recent advances in the behavioral study of infant audition: The development of sound localization skills. *J Speech Lang Pathol Audiol 14:* 51–63, 1990.

Musiek FM. (ed). Selected topics in central auditory dysfunction. *Seminars in Hearing 5:* 1984.

Musiek FM. Hearing beyond the eighth nerve. *Amer J Otol 7:* 1986.

Musiek FM, Baran JA, Pinheiro ML. P300 results in patients with lesions of the auditory areas of the cerebrum. *J Amer Acad Audiology 3:* 5–15, 1992.

Musiek FM, Geurkink N, Keitel S. Test battery assessment of auditory perceptual dysfunction in children. *Laryngoscope 92:* 251–257, 1982.

Musiek FM, Gollegly KM, Baran JA. Myelination of the corpus callosum and auditory processing problems in children: Theoretical and clinical correlates. *Seminars in Hearing 5:* 231–241, 1984.

Musiek FM, Gollegly KM, Kibbe KS, Verkest-Lenz SB. Proposed screening test for central auditory disorders: Follow-up on the dichotic digits test. *Amer J Otol 12:* 109–113, 1991.

Musiek FM, Gollegly KM, Lamb LE, Lamb P. Selected issues in screening for central auditory processing dysfunction. *Seminars in Hearing 11:* 372–384, 1990.

Myklebust HR. *Auditory disorders in children: A manual for differential diagnosis.* New York: Grune & Stratton, 1954.

Naatanen R. Selective attention and evoked potentials in humans: A critical review. *Biological Review 2:* 237–307, 1975.

Naatanen R. The mismatch negativity: A powerful tool for cognitive neuroscience. *Ear and Hearing 16:* 6–18, 1995.

Naatanen R, Gaillard AWK, Mantysalo S. Early selective-attention effect on evoked potential reinterpreted. *Acta Psychologica 42:* 313–329, 1979.

Nashner LM. *Rationale and methodology for use of dynamic posturography: Patients with vestibular disorders.* Dizziness and Balance Disorders Conference in Denver, CO, 1988.

NIH Consensus Statement. (Volume 11, Number 1, March 1–3, 1993). "Early Identification of Hearing Impairment in Infants and Young Children."

Noffsinger D, Wilson RH, Musiek FE. Department of Veterans Affairs compact disc recording for auditory perceptual assessment: Background and introduction. *J Amer Acad Audiology 5:* 231–235, 1994.

Northern JL, Downs WP. *Hearing in children* (4th ed). Baltimore: Williams & Wilkins, 1991.

Northern JL, Hayes D. Universal hearing screening for infant hearing impairment: Necessary, beneficial, and justifiable. *Audiology Today 6:* 1994.

O'Leary DP, Davis LL. High-frequency autorotational testing of the vestibulo-ocular reflex. *Neurologic Clinics 8:* 297–312, 1990.

Ohlms LA, Lonsbury-Martin BL, Martin GK. The clinical application of acoustic distortion products. *Otolaryngol Head and Neck Surg 103:* 52–59, 1990.

Olsen W, Matkin ND. Speech audiometry. In: Rintelmann WF (ed). *Hearing assessment* (2nd ed). Austin, TX: Pro-Ed, 1991.

Olsen W, Noffsinger D, Kurdziel S. Acoustic reflex and reflex decay. *Arch Otolaryngol 101:* 622–625, 1975.

Olsen WO, Van Tassell DJ, Speaks CE. Preparation of isophonemic word list and sentence test materials. Paper presented at the Annual Convention of the American Speech-Language-Hearing Association, Toronto, Ontario, Canada, November 1982.

Olsen WO, Van Tassell DJ, Speaks CE. Further evaluation of isophonemic word list and sentence test materials. Paper presented at the Annual Convention of the American Speech-Language-Hearing Association, Cincinnati, Ohio, November 1983.

Owens E, Schubert E. Development of the California consonant test. *J Speech Hear Res 20:* 463–474, 1977.

Oyler RF, Oyler, AL, Matkin ND. Unilateral hearing loss: demographics and educational impact. *Language, Speech & Hearing in Schools 19:* 201–210, 1988.

Peck JE. Development of hearing. Part III. Postnatal development. *J Am Acad Audiol 6:* 113–123, 1995.

Pederson O, Studebaker G. A new minimal-contrasts closed-response-set speech test. *J Auditory Res 12:* 187–195, 1972.

Peterson HA, Marquardt TP. *Appraisal and diagnosis of speech and language disorders* (3rd ed). Englewood Cliffs, NJ: Prentice-Hall, 1994.

Physicians Desk Reference. Montvale, NJ: Medical Economics Data Production Co., 1994.

Piaget J, Inhelder B. *The psychology of the child.* New York: Basic Books, 1969.

Picton TW, Champagne SC, Kellett AJ. Human auditory evoked potentials recorded using maximum length sequences. *Electroencephalography and Clinical Neurophysiology 84:* 90–100, 1992.

Pinheiro ML, Musiek FM, (eds). *Assessment of central auditory dysfunction.* Baltimore: Williams & Wilkens, 1984.

Popelka G. Acoustic immittance measures: Terminology and instrumentation. *Ear and Hearing 5: 262–267, 1984.*

Portmann M, Aran JM. Electro-cochleography. *Laryngoscope 81:* 899–910, 1971.

Prather EM, Hendrick EL, Kerin CA. Articulation development in children aged two to four years. *J Speech Hearing Disorders 40:* 179–191, 1975.

Pratt H, Martin WH, Schwegler JW, Rosenwasser RH, Rosenberg SI, Flamm ES. Temporal correspondence of intracranial, cochlear and scalp-recorded human auditory nerve action potentials. *Electroencephalography and Clinical Neurophysiology 84:* 447–455, 1992.

Probst R, Lonsbury-Martin BL, Martin GK. A review of otoacoustic emissions. *J Acoust Soc Amer 89:* 2027–2067, 1991.

Probst R and Hauser R. Distortion product otoacoustic emissions in normal and hearing impaired ears. *Am J Otolaryngol 11:* 236–243, 1990.

Pujol R, Lavigne-Rebillard, M. Development of neurosensory structures in the human cochlea. *Acta Otolaryngologica (Stockh) 112:* 259–264, 1992.

Raffin M, Thornton AR. Confidence levels for differences between speech discrimination scores: A research note. *J Speech Hear Res 23:* 5–18, 1980.

Reger S. Loudness level contours and intensity discrimination of ears with raised auditory threshold. [Abstract]. *J Acoustical Soc Amer 7:* 73, 1937.

Resnick S, Dubno J, Hoffnung S, Levitt H. Phoneme errors on a nonsense syllable test. *J Acoust Soc Amer 58:* (Suppl) 114, 1975.

Riedel C, Wiley, T, Block M. Tympanometric measures of Eustachian tube function. *J Speech Hear Res 30:* 207–214, 1987.

Romand R (ed). *Development of auditory and vestibular systems II.* Amsterdam: Elsevier, 1991.

Rose DE, Schreurs KK, Miller LE. A ten-word speech discrimination screening test. *Audiology and Hearing Education* (winter): 15–16, 1979.

Rosenberg P. Abnormal auditory adaptation. *Arch Otolarngol 94:* 89, 1971.

Rosler G. Progression of hearing loss caused by occupational noise. *Scand Audiol 23:* 13–37, 1994.

Ross M, Lerman J. A picture identification test for hearing impaired children. *J Speech Hear Res 13:* 44–53, 1970.

Ruah CB, Schachern PA, Zelterman D, Paparella MM, Yoon TH. Age-related morphologic changes in the human tympanic membrane. *Arch Otolaryngol Head Neck Surg 117:* 627–634, 1991.

Rubel EW. Auditory system development. In: Gottlieb G, Krasnegor NA (eds). *Measurement of audition and vision in the first year of postnatal life: A methodological overview.* Norwood NJ: Ablex, pp. 53–90, 1985.

Rubin RJ, Bordley JE, Lieberman AT. Cochlear potentials in man. *Laryngoscope 71:* 1141–1164, 1961.

Runge CA, Hosford-Dunn, HL. Word recognition performance with modified CID W-22 word lists. *J Speech Hear Res 28:* 355–362, 1985

Rusk RD. *Introduction to college physics* (2nd ed). New York: Appleton-Century-Crofts, 1960.

Ruth RA, Dey-Sigman S, Mills JA. Neonatal ABR hearing screening. *The Hearing Journal* (November): pp. 39–40, 1985.

Ruth RA, Lambert PR. Comparison of tympanic membrane to promontory electrode recordings of electrocochleographic responses in patients with Meniere's disease. *Otolaryngol Head Neck Surg 100:* 546–552, 1989.

Rybak, L.P. Antibiotics. In: Paparella MM, Shumrick DA, Gluckman JL, Meyerhoff WL. (eds). *Otolaryngology*, (Vol 2, 3rd ed). Philadelphia: Saunders, 605–615, 1991.

Rybak LP (ed). Ototoxicity. *Otolaryngol Clini North Am 26*(5). Philadephia: WB Saunders, 1993.

Rybak LP, Matz GJ. Effects of toxic agents. In Cumming CW (ed). *Otolaryngology—head and neck surgery* (Vol 4, 2nd ed). St. Louis: Mosby Year Book, p. 2943, 1993.

Sanders JW. In Katz J (ed). *Handbook of clinical audiology.* Baltimore: Williams & Wilkens, 1972.

Sanes DH, Constantine-Paton M. Altered activity patterns during development reduce neural tuning. *Science 221:* 1184–1185, 1983.

Saunders GH. Determinants of objective and subjective auditory disability in patients with normal hearing. Doctoral thesis. Nottingham, England: University of Nottingham, 1989.

Saunders GH, Field DS, Haggard MP. A clinical test battery for Obscure Auditory Dysfunction (OAD): Development, selection and use of the tests. *Brit J Audiol 26:* 33–47, 1992.

Saunders GH, Haggard MP. The assessment of 'Obscure Auditory Dysfunction': Auditory and psychological factors. *Ear and Hearing 10:* 200–208, 1989.

Saunders GH, Haggard MP. The assessment of 'Obscure Auditory Dysfunction' (OAD). Case-control analysis of determining factors. *Ear and Hearing 13:* 241–254, 1992.

Saunders GH, Haggard MP. The influence of personality-related factors upon consultation for two different "marginal" organic pathologies with and without reports of auditory symptomatology. *Ear and Hearing 14:* 242–248, 1993.

Schatz A, Bugie E, Waksman SA. Streptomycin, a substance exhibiting antibiotic activity against gram-positive and gram-negative bacteria. *Experimental Biol Med 55:* 66–69, 1944.

Schuknecht HF. *Pathology of the ear* (2nd edition). Philadelphia: Lea & Febiger, 1993.

Schultz M, Schubert E. A multiple choice discrimination test (MCDT). *Laryngoscope 79:* 382–399, 1969.

Schwaber MK, Hall JW III. A simplified approach for transtympanic electrocochleography. *Amer J Otol 11:* 260–265, 1990.

Schwartz GH, David DS et al. Ototoxicity induced by furosemide. *New Engl J Med 282:* 1413–1414, 1970.

Semont A, Freyss G, Vitte E. Curing the BPPV with a Liberatory Maneuver. *Adv Oto-Rhino-Laryngol 42:* 290–293, 1988.

Sergeant L, Atkinson JE, Lacroix PG. The NSMRL tri-word test of intelligibility. *J Acoust Soc Amer 65:* 218–222, 1979.

Sesterhenn G, Breuninger H. The acoustic reflex at low sensation levels. *Audiology 15:* 523–533, 1976.

Shanks J. Tympanometry. *Ear and Hearing 5:* 268–280, 1984.

Shanks J. Aural acoustic immittance standards. *Seminars in Hearing 8:* 307–318, 1987.

Shanks J, Lilly D. An evaluation of tympanometric estimates of ear canal volume. *J Speech Hear Res 24:* 557–566, 1981.

Shephard NT, Telian SA. Balance disorders ("The dizzy patient"). In: Jacobson J, Northern J (eds). *Diagnostic audiology*. Boston: Little, Brown, 1990.

Siegel JH. Ear-canal standing waves and high-frequency sound calibration using otoacoustic emission probes. *J Acoust Soc Amer 95:* 289–2597, 1994.

Siegenthaler B, Haspiel G. Development of two standard measures of hearing for speech by children. Department of Health, Education and Welfare Project No. 2372, Contract OE5 10–003, 1966.

Silverman SR, Hirsh I. Problems related to the use of speech in clinical audiometry. *Ann Otol Rhinol Laryngol 64:* 1234–1244, 1955.

Sklare DA, Denenberg LJ. Auditory brain stem laboratory norms: When is the data base sufficient *Ear and Hearing 8:* 298–300, 1987.

Speaks C, Jerger J. Method for measurement of speech indentification. *J Speech Hear Res 8*: 185–194, 1965.

Stebbins WC, Miller JM et al. Ototoxic hearing loss and cochlear pathology in the monkey. *Ann Otolaryngol Rhinology, and Laryngol 78:* 1007–1019, 1969.

Steenerson RL, Van de Water SM, Sytsma WH, Fox EJ. Central vestibular findings on electronystagmography. *Ear and Hearing 7:* 176–181, 1986.

Stevens SS, Davis H. *Hearing: Its psychology and physiology.* New York: John Wiley & Sons, Inc, 1938.

Strasnick B, Glasscock ME, Haynes D, McMenomey SO, Minor LB. The natural history of untreated acoustic neuromas. *Laryngoscope 104:* 1115–1119, 1994.

Stringer SP, Meyerhoff WL, Wright CG. Ototoxicity. In: Paparella MM, Shumrick DA, Gluckman JL, Meyerhoff WL (eds). *Otolaryngology* (Vol 2, 3rd ed). Philadelphia: Saunders, 1653–1667, 1991.

Stypulkowski PH, Staller SJ. Clinical evaluation of a new ECoG recording electrode. *Ear and Hearing 8:* 304–310, 1987.

Tanaka Y, Susuki M, Inoue T. Evoked otoacoustic emissions in sensorineural hearing impairment: Its clinical implications. *Ear and Hearing 11:* 134–143, 1990.

Telian SA, Kileny PR, Niparko JK, Kemink JL, Graham MD. Normal auditory brainstem response in patients with acoustic neuroma. *Laryngoscope 99:* 10 – 14, 1989.

Templin MC. Certain language skills in children. Institute of Child Welfare Monograph Series, No. 26. Minneapolis: University of Minnesota, 1957.

Terkildsen K, Scott-Nielsen S. An electroacoustic impedance measuring bridge for clinical use. *Arch Otolaryngol 72:* 339–346, 1960.

Thompson GA. A modified SISI technique for selected cases with suspected acoustic neuroma. *J Speech Hear Disord, 28*: 299–302, 1963.

Thompson GA, Thompson M, McCall A. Strategies for increasing response behavior of 1- and 2-year-old children during visual reinforcement audiometry (VRA). *Ear and Hearing 13:* 236–240, 1992.

Thornton AR, Raffin MJM. Speech-discrimination scores modeled as a binomial variable. *J Speech Hear Res 21:* 507–518, 1978.

Thornton ARD, Slaven A. Auditory brainstem responses recorded at fast stimulation rates using maximum length sequences. *Brit J Audiol 27:* 205–210, 1993.

Tillman T, Carhart R. An expanded test for speech discrimination utilizing CNC monosyllabic words. Northwestern University Auditory Test No. 6. USAF School of Aerospace Medicine Technical Report, Brooks Air Force Base, Texas, 1966.

Tillman TW, Olsen WO. Speech audiometry. In Jerger J (ed). *Modern developments in audiology* (2nd ed). New York: Academic Press, 1973.

Trehub SE, Schneider BS (eds). *Auditory development in infancy.* New York: Plenum, 1985.

Tyler R. Measuring hearing loss in the future. *Brit J Audiol 2*(Suppl): 29–40, 1979.

Uziel A, Bonfils P. Assessment of endolymphatic cochlear hydrops by means of evoked acoustic emission. In: Nadol JB (ed). *Second International Symposium on Ménière's Disease*. Amsterdam: Kugler, pp. 379–383, 1989.

Van Camp KJ, Margolis RH, Wilson RH, Creten WL, Shanks JE. Principles of tympanometry. *ASHA Monographs No. 24:* 1986.

Van Camp K, Vanpeperstraete P, Creten W, Vanhuyse V. On irregular acoustic reflex patterns. *Scandinavian Audiol 4:* 227–232, 1975.

Van Camp K, Creten W, Van de Heyning P, Decraemer W, Vanpeperstraete P. A search for the most suitable immittance components and probe tone frequency in tympanometry. *Scand Audiol 12:* 27–34, 1983.

Van Campen LE, Sammeth CA, Hall JW III, Peek BF. Comparison of Etymotic insert and TDH supra-aural earphones in auditory brainstem response measurement. *J Amer Acad Audiol 3:* 315–323, 1992.

van Deelen GW, Ruding PRJW, Veldman JE, Huizing EH, Smoorenburg GF. Electrocochleographic study of experimentally induced endolymphatic hydrops. *Arch Otol Rhinol Laryngol 244:* 167–173, 1987.

von Roemling RW, Hrushesky WJM. Principles of chemotherapy and immunotherapy for head and neck cancer. In: Paparella MM, Shumrick DA, Gluckman JL, Meyerhoff WL (eds). *Otolaryngology* (Vol 2, 3rd ed). Philadelphia: Saunders, 1653–1669. 1991.

Weatherby L, Bennett, M. The neonatal acoustic reflex. *Audiology 9:* 103–10, 1980.

Werner LA, Gillenwater JM. Pure-tone sensitivity of 2- and 5-week-old infants. *Inf Behav Dev 13:* 355–375, 1990.

Wever E, Bray C. Auditory nerve impulses. *Science 71:* 215, 1930.

Wiley T, Goldstein R. Tympanometric and acoustic-reflex studies in neonates. *J Speech Hear Res 28: 265–272, 1985.*

Wiley TL, Stoppenbach DT, Feldhake LJ, Moss KA, Thordardottir ET. Audiologic practices: What is popular versus what is supported by evidence. *Amer J Audiol 4:* 26–34, 1994.

Wilson RH, Shanks J, Kaplan S. Tympanometric changes at 226 Hz and 678 Hz across 10 trials and for two directions of ear canal pressure change. *J Speech Hear Res 27:* 257–266, 1984.

Wilson DF, Hodgson RS, Gustafson MF, Hogue S, Mills L. The sensitivity of auditory brainstem response testing in small acoustic neuromas. *Laryngoscope 102:* 961–964, 1992.

Wilson RH, Antablin JK. A picture identification task as an estimate of word-recognition performance on nonverbal adults. *J Speech Hear Disord 45:* 223–238, 1980.

Woods PL, Clayworth CC, Knight RT, Simpson GV, Naeser MA. Generators of middle and long latency auditory evoked potentials: Implications from studies of patients with bitemporal lesions. *Electroencephalography and Clinical Neurophysiology 68:* pp. 132–148, 1987.

Yanagisawa E, Lee KJ. Noninfectious diseases of the ear. In: Lee KJ (ed). *Essential otolaryngology* (5th ed). New York: Elsevier Science Publishing, pp. 617–646, 1991.

Yanagisawa, E. (1991) Infections of the ear. In: Lee KJ (ed). *Essential otolaryngology* (5th ed). New York: Elsevier Science Publishing, 581–616.

Yost WA. *Fundamentals of hearing: An introduction* (3rd ed). San Diego: Academic Press, 1994.

Zwislocki J. An acoustic method for clinical examination of the ear. *J Speech Hear Res 6:* 303–314, 1963.

Index

A

B

E

F

I

J

K

L

M

N

O

P

Q

R

S

T

U

V

W

X

Z